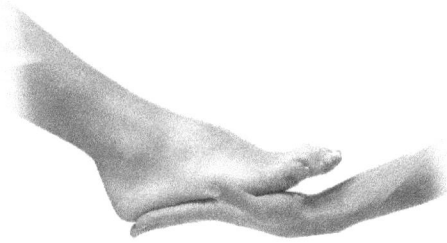

The
Diabetic Foot

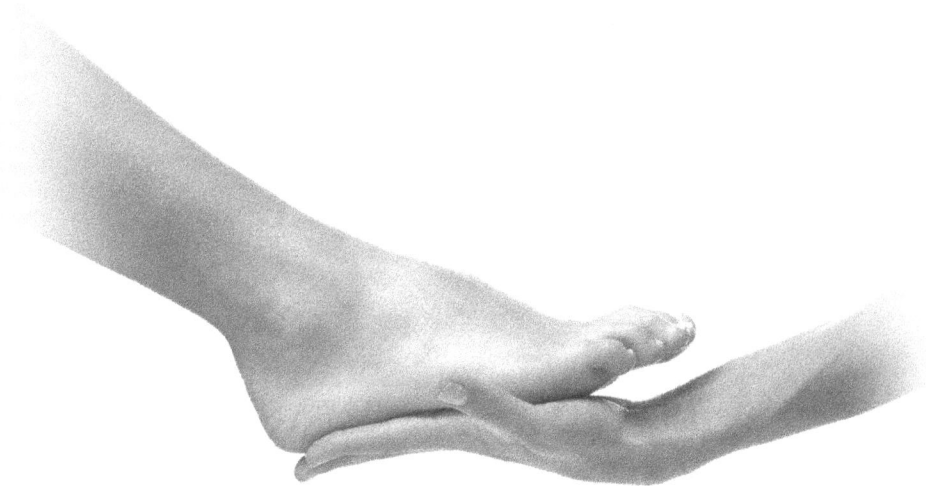

The
Diabetic Foot

Editor

Aziz Nather

National University of Singapore

World Scientific

NEW JERSEY · LONDON · SINGAPORE · BEIJING · SHANGHAI · HONG KONG · TAIPEI · CHENNAI

Published by

World Scientific Publishing Co. Pte. Ltd.

5 Toh Tuck Link, Singapore 596224

USA office: 27 Warren Street, Suite 401-402, Hackensack, NJ 07601

UK office: 57 Shelton Street, Covent Garden, London WC2H 9HE

British Library Cataloguing-in-Publication Data
A catalogue record for this book is available from the British Library.

THE DIABETIC FOOT

ISBN 978-981-4417-00-6

Typeset by Stallion Press
Email: enquiries@stallionpress.com

Printed in Singapore.

Dedication

This book is dedicated to the pioneers of the NUH Multi-Disciplinary Diabetic Foot Team who played an instrumental role to its success. The team was launched in May 2003. This book is also dedicated to Professor K Satku (former Head, Department of Orthopaedic Surgery: 2000–2004, current Director of Medical Services, Ministry of Health), who inspired me to take up this great venture.

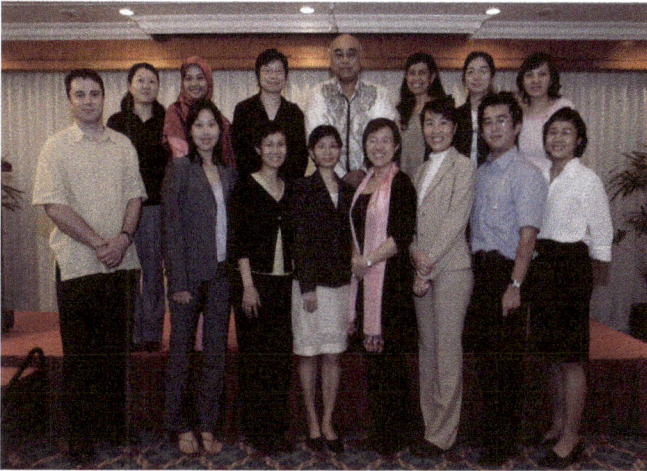

Pioneers of the NUH Multi-Disciplinary Team for Diabetic Foot Problems
(Photo taken on the 20th November 2004, at the First National and Regional Conference on Diabetic Foot Problems, Conference Dinner, Hilton Hotel).
From left to right:
Front row: Adam Jorgensen, Wendy Yue Lai Theng, Lim Pui Yee, Goh Mien Li, Lim Ling, Rose Low, Chris Lee, Elaine Tan
Back row: Wang Lihui, Fazlyn Johari, Chionh Siok Bee, Aziz Nather, Usha Menon, Chin Shu Yee, Torng Ai Hwa

I would also like to dedicate this book to my wife, Suraiya Rahman, my children, Sharnaz, Zameer and Azad and especially to my two grandchildren, Samira (7) and Aliya (5).

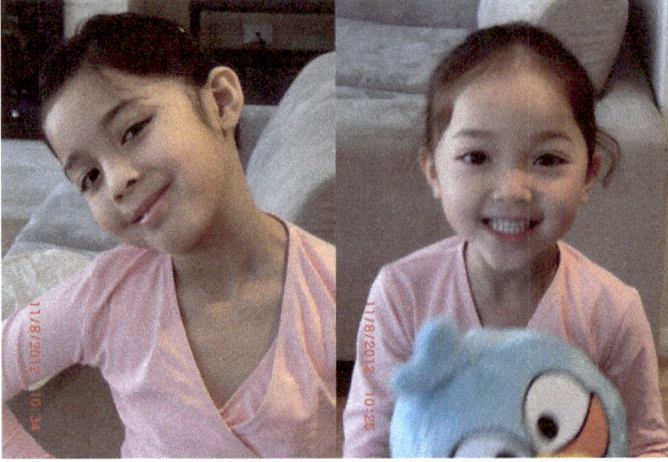

Contents

Preface

It has been nine years since Professor K Satku inspired me to develop a Diabetic Foot Team. The multi-disciplinary team, including an orthopaedic surgeon, an endocrinologist, an infection disease specialist, podiatrists and wound care nurses, was launched in May 2003. This was during the difficult period when SARS hit Singapore. We simultaneously launched a clinical pathway for diabetic foot problems. The experience we gained has been fulfilling.

A total of 12 publications on the subject has been published by the NUH Diabetic Foot Team, in addition to a book "Diabetic Foot Problems", A. Nather (ed) published by World Scientific in 2008. This book was launched during the 5th Asia Pacific Conference on Diabetic Limb Problems held in Singapore from 20th–22nd November 2008 (Organising Chairman: Dr Aziz Nather) with Professor K Satku, Director of Medical Services, Ministry of Health, as our Guest of Honour. This book became a best-seller and topped the list on World Scientific for the months of June and July, 2009.

"Diabetic Foot Problems" has been used as a textbook for our NUH Diabetic Foot Screening Courses run annually since March 2006 to train nurses to do foot screening for patients with diabetes. The 4th Regional Training Course for Diabetic Foot Screening Course was held in NUH from November 2010. This book has also become popular as a textbook for the National Diabetes Institute (NADI) Annual Foot Seminar/Workshops since May 2011 (3rd Annual Workshop).

The NUH Diabetic Foot Team not only catalysed the nation to set up the National Association for Diabetic Foot Problems but also galvanised the formation of the Asia Pacific Association for Diabetic Limb Problems (APADLP) in November 2004. Both associations were founded during the First National and Regional Conference on Diabetic Foot Problems held in Singapore from 20–21st November 2004 with Dr Balaji Sadasivan, Minister of State for Health as our Guest of Honour. APADLP has grown from year to year — 2nd Asia Pacific Conference for Diabetic Limb Problems (APCDLP) in Putrajaya, Malaysia in December 2005 (Organising Chairman: Dr R. Ramanathan), 3rd APCDLP in Ancor, Indonesia in November 2006 (Organising Chairman: Dr Mulyono Soedirman), 4th APCDLP in Hong Kong in November 2007 (Organising Chairman: Dr Josephine Ip Wing Yuk), 5th APCDLP in Singapore, 6th APCDLP in Beijing, China in 2009 (Organising Chairman: Dr Xu Zhangrong), 7th APCDLP in Kuantan, Malaysia in 2010 (Organising Chairman: Dr Ahmad Hafiz Zulkifly) and the 8th APCDLP in Bandung, Indonesia in December 2011 (Organising Chairman: Dr Bambang Tiksnadi).

This new book is written in a user friendly style to benefit not just doctors but also nurses, patients and care-givers. There is a section 'Guide to Operative Surgery' that is useful for surgeons and in particular, residents-in-training. It also has a section 'Wound Care' of interest to all health professionals, especially nurses and podiatrists. Finally, it has 'A Patient's Guide' section which will be of benefit to all patients and caregivers. Topics in this section include: care of your diabetes, care of your foot, choosing your own footwear, doing your own dressing and rehabilitating your below knee amputation. The appendix records our history of the NUH Multi-Disciplinary Diabetic Foot Team and the Asia Pacific Association on Diabetic Limb Problems.

This year, the 9th APCDLP will be held in Hong Kong in November 2012 with Dr Samson Chan as the Organising Chairman. I am glad to announce that the 10th Anniversary — 10th APCDLP will be held in Singapore, the country that gave birth to this association, in October 2013 (Organising Chairman: Dr Aziz Nather).

I would like to thank in particular my four co-authors who helped me write several chapters of this book, namely Ms April Voon Siew Lian, Ms Amaris Lim Shu Min, Ms Teo Zhen Ling and Ms Amy Pannapat Chanyarungrojn — the 8th NUH Diabetic Foot Research Team (2012).

This book will be officially launched during the Opening Ceremony of the 10th APCDLP!

Aziz Nather
Editor
Chairman, NUH Diabetic Foot Team
Corresponding Member, International Working Group
on the Diabetic Foot (IWGDF),
The Netherlands
Senior Consultant
Division of Foot and Ankle
Department of Orthopaedic Surgery
Yong Loo Lin School of Medicine
National University of Singapore

About the Editor

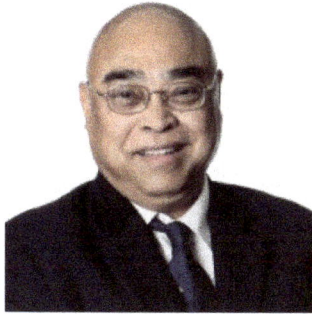

Associate Professor Aziz Nather

- Chairman of ASEAN Plus Expert Group Forum on Management of Diabetic Foot Wounds
- Launched Inaugural ASEAN Plus Expert Group Forum on Management of Diabetic Foot Wounds on 10 November 2012 in Hilton Hotel, Singapore in conjunction with First National Training Workshop on Management of Diabetic Foot Wounds for Nurses and Allied Health Professionals held in National University Health System, Singapore
- Founding President and current Honorary Secretary of Asia Pacific Association of Diabetic Limb Problems
- Organising Chairman of 10th Asia Pacific Conference on Diabetic Limb Problems to be held in National University Health System, Singapore on 10–12 November 2013
- Chairman of NUH Diabetic Foot Team since May 2003
- Senior Consultant, Division of Foot & Ankle, University Orthopaedics, Hand and Reconstructive Microsurgery Cluster, National University Health System, Singapore.

List of Contributors

EDITOR AND AUTHOR:
Aziz Nather
Chairman
NUH Diabetic Foot Team

Corresponding Member
International Working Group on the
    Diabetic Foot
The Netherlands

Senior Consultant
Division of Foot and Ankle
Department of Orthopaedic Surgery
Yong Loo Lin School of Medicine
National University of Singapore
NUHS Tower Block, Level 11
1E Kent Ridge Road
Singapore 119228
dosnathe@nus.edu.sg

8th NUH DIABETIC FOOT
RESEARCH TEAM:

Chanyarungrojn Amy Pannapat
amychanya@gmail.com

Lim Shu Min Amaris
amarislimshumin@gmail.com

Teo Zhen Ling
zhenling.teo@gmail.com

Voon Siew Lian April
april.voon@hotmail.com

Department of Orthopaedic Surgery
Yong Loo Lin School of Medicine
National University of Singapore
NUHS Tower Block, Level 11
1E Kent Ridge Road
Singapore 119228

OTHER CONTRIBUTORS:
Cardosa Mary Suma
Consultant Anaesthesiologist
Hospital Selayang
Selayang-Kepong Highway
68100 Gombak

Selangor, Malaysia
mary.cardosa@gmail.com

Chan Wei Ying Joanna
House Officer
Department of Orthopaedic Surgery
Yong Loo Lin School of Medicine
National University of Singapore
NUHS Tower Block, Level 11
1E Kent Ridge Road
Singapore 119228

Chen Wei Xian Ruth
Resident
Department of Orthopaedic Surgery
Yong Loo Lin School of Medicine
National University of Singapore
NUHS Tower Block, Level 11
1E Kent Ridge Road
Singapore 119228

Chin Yu Xuan
Department of Orthopaedic Surgery
Yong Loo Lin School of Medicine
National University of Singapore
NUHS Tower Block, Level 11
1E Kent Ridge Road
Singapore 119228
yuxuanchin@gmail.com

Hey Hwee Weng Dennis
Registrar
Department of Orthopaedic Surgery
Yong Loo Lin School of Medicine
National University of Singapore

NUHS Tower Block, Level 11
1E Kent Ridge Road
Singapore 119228
hwee_weng_hey@nuhs.edu.sg

Ho Pei Jackie
Consultant
Department of Cardiac, Thoracic
 and Vascular Surgery
National University Heart Centre
5 Lower Kent Ridge Road
Singapore 119074
jackie_ho@nuhs.edu.sg

Ho Sharlene
Department of Orthopaedic Surgery
Yong Loo Lin School of Medicine
National University of Singapore
NUHS Tower Block, Level 11
1E Kent Ridge Road
Singapore 119228
september_sharlene@yahoo.co.uk

Hong Choon Chiet Andrew
Medical Officer
Department of Orthopaedic Surgery
Yong Loo Lin School of Medicine
National University of Singapore
NUHS Tower Block, Level 11
1E Kent Ridge Road
Singapore 119228

Lai Yuen Fun Alexis
Podiatrist
Rehabilitation Centre

National University Hospital
5 Lower Kent Ridge Road
Singapore 119074
alexis_lai@nuhs.edu.sg

Lee Choon Wei Chris
NUH Tissue Bank
Department of Orthopaedic Surgery
National University Hospital
5 Lower Kent Ridge Road
Singapore 119074
leechoonwei@hotmail.com

Leung Ping Chung
Chairman
Management Committee
Institute of Chinese Medicine
The Chinese University
   of Hong Kong
Tai Po Road, Hong Kong
pingcleung@cuhk.edu.hk

Lim Kean Seng Andrew
Associate Consultant
Department of Orthopaedic Surgery
Yong Loo Lin School of Medicine
National University of Singapore
NUHS Tower Block, Level 11
1E Kent Ridge Road
Singapore 119228
Andrew_KS_LIM@nuhs.edu.sg

Nair Harikrishna K Ragavan
President
Malaysia Society of Wound Care
   Professionals

Hospital Kuala Lumpur
50586 Jalan Pahang
Wilayah Persekutuan
Kuala Lumpur, Malaysia
hulk25@hotmail.com

Quah Yan Ling
Department of Orthopaedic Surgery
Yong Loo Lin School of Medicine
National University of Singapore
NUHS Tower Block, Level 11
1E Kent Ridge Road
Singapore 119228
yanling1@hotmail.com

Singh Gurpal
Consultant
Department of Orthopaedic Surgery
Yong Loo Lin School of Medicine
National University of Singapore
NUHS Tower Block, Level 11
1E Kent Ridge Road
Singapore 119228
gurpal25@singnet.com.sg

Steenkamp Johan
Podiatrist
Rehabilitation Centre
National University Hospital
5 Lower Kent Ridge Road
Singapore 119074
johan_steenkamp@nuhs.edu.sg

Sussman Geoff
Director Wound Research
Wound Foundation of Australia

Monash University
geoff.sussman@vcp.monash.edu.au

Toh Lynn Li
Podiatrist
Rehabilitation Centre
National University Hospital
5 Lower Kent Ridge Road
Singapore 119074
lynn_li_toh@nuhs.edu.sg

Tsao Tiffany
Principal Podiatrist
Rehabilitation Centre
National University Hospital
5 Lower Kent Ridge Road
Singapore 119074
tiffany_tsao@nuh.com.sg

Wong Keng Lin Francis
Resident
Department of Orthopaedic Surgery
Yong Loo Lin School of Medicine
National University of Singapore
NUHS Tower Block, Level 11
1E Kent Ridge Road
Singapore 119228

Zameer Aziz
Medical Officer
Department of Cardiovascular
    Thoracic Surgery
Singapore General Hospital
Outram Road, Outram Park
Singapore 169608
zam.aziz@gmail.com

Section 1

Overview of Diabetes

1

Diabetes and Its Complications: A Global Problem

Aziz Nather, April Voon Siew Lian and Joanna Chan Wei Ying

Department of Orthopaedic Surgery
Yong Loo Lin School of Medicine
National University of Singapore

Diabetes

Diabetes currently affects 366 million people worldwide or 8.3% of the world's adult population (Fig. 1). This figure is expected to increase to 9.9% by 2030 (Fig. 2, Table 1), owing to environmental factors such as sedentary lifestyles and changing dietary patterns.[1] Now the fourth leading cause of death in most developed countries, diabetes has been considered the "global epidemic of the 21st century".

Singapore has one of the highest prevalence of diabetes in the developed world. 11.3% of residents aged between 18 and 69 years old had diabetes in 2010[2] (Table 2). It is one of the top ten causes of death locally[3] (Table 3).

Complications

Raised blood glucose levels associated with diabetes may damage the heart and blood vessels (cardiovascular disease and peripheral vascular disease), kidneys (nephropathy), eyes (retinopathy) and nerves (neuropathy). Peripheral vascular disease and neuropathy can lead to serious foot problems in diabetic patients.

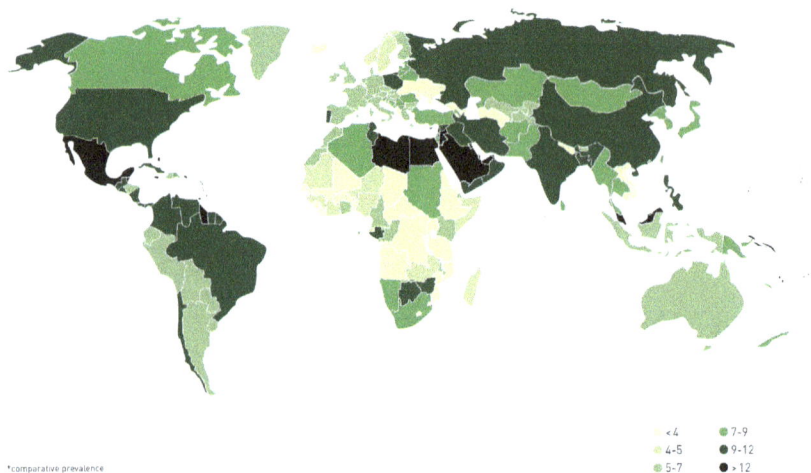

Figure 1. Prevalence (%) of diabetes (20–79 years) in 2011

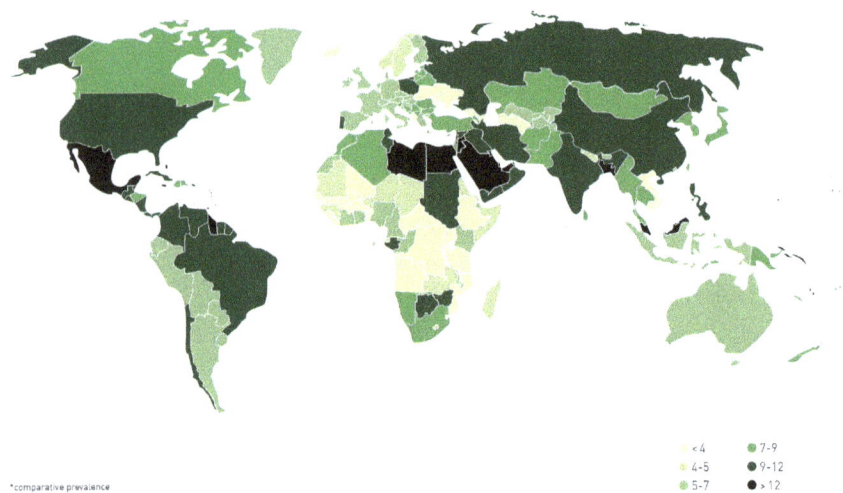

Figure 2. Prevalence (%) of diabetes (20–79 years) in 2030

Source: http://www.idf.org/diabetesatlas/5e/diabetes.

Such complications of diabetes can reduce the quality of life of the patient and his family. They may also cause severe disability or death. Every year, approximately 3.8 million adults die from diabetes-related causes.[4]

Table 1. Global prevalence of diabetes (2011 and 2030)

	2011	2030
Total world population (billions)	7.0	8.3
Adult population (20–79 years, billions)	4.4	5.6
Number of people with diabetes (millions)	366	552
Global prevalence of diabetes (%)	8.3	9.9

Table 2. Disease burden in Singapore

Prevalence among adults aged 18 to 69 years (%)	1998	2004	2010
Hypertension	27.3	24.9	23.5
Diabetes	9.0	8.2	11.3
High total cholesterol	25.4	18.7	17.4
Obesity	6.0	6.9	10.8
Daily smoking	15.2	12.6	14.3

Table 3. Principal causes of death in Singapore

% of total deaths	2008	2009	2010
Cancer	29.3	29.3	28.5
Ischaemic heart disease	20.1	19.2	18.7
Pneumonia	13.9	15.3	15.7
Cerebrovascular disease (including stroke)	8.3	8.0	8.4
Accidents, poisoning and violence	5.8	5.7	5.5
Other heart diseases	4.0	4.4	4.8
Chronic obstructive lung disease	2.5	2.4	2.5
Urinary tract infection	2.1	2.5	2.5
Nephritis, nephrotic syndrome and nephrosis	2.1	2.3	2.2
Diabetes mellitus	2.7	1.7	1.0

Ulceration

Foot ulcers are very common among diabetic patients, affecting about 15% of all diabetic patients in developed countries. They are a major cause of amputations. Approximately 85% of all amputations begin with an ulcer.[5]

Amputation

A diabetic patient is up to 40% more likely to receive a lower limb amputation.[5] Currently, it is estimated that every 20 seconds a lower leg is lost due to diabetes globally.[4] In Singapore, 700 lower limb amputations are performed annually due to diabetes.[6]

Lower limb amputations often cause mortality in diabetic patients: 70% of them die within five years after an amputation.[5]

Social Impact

Patients with amputation are often unable to work. They have limited mobility and lead a less active social life. Patients with chronic foot ulcers face similar problems. Many are permanently disabled. There is a high incidence of depression. Their quality of life is significantly reduced as a result.[5]

Economic Impact

Diabetic foot complications are a significant economic burden for both the patient and society. This is due to the cost of long-term treatment of ulcers, hospitalisation and surgery, rehabilitation and the increased need for home care and social services.

3–4% of all diabetics have a foot problem and use 12–15% of the healthcare resources. The average cost for primary healing in the USA ranges between US$7,000 and US$10,000. The cost of an amputation due to diabetes is estimated to be between US$30,000 and US$60,000. The estimated cost of the diabetic foot in the USA is some US$6 billion a year if one includes the cost to the individual and the loss in quality of life.[7]

Conclusion

Foot complications are one of the most serious and costly complications of diabetes. A good national programme is required for the management of diabetic foot problems. One must employ a two-pronged strategy. The most important strategy is prevention with the use of education programmes for diabetes as well as programs for care of the foot and footwear. This must be directed nation-wide to the whole community. In addition, where we have failed to prevent the complication, such complications must be handled by a multi-disciplinary team in hospitals running a diabetic foot clinic and diabetic foot ward rounds.

In National University Hospital (NUH) in Singapore, the NUH Diabetic Foot Team was able to reduce the below knee amputation rate from 31.15% in 2002 (pre-diabetic foot team formation) to 11.01% in 2007 (post team formation). Efforts are now directed to make sure that all patients diagnosed with diabetes must receive annual foot screening in order to reduce the development of foot complications.[8]

References

1. The Global Burden, Diabetes Atlas, International Diabetes Federation (2011).
2. Disease Burden, Singapore Health Facts, Ministry of Health Singapore (2012).
3. Principal Causes of Death, Singapore Health Facts, Ministry of Health Singapore (2012).
4. Diabetes: The Epidemic of the 21st Century, International Working Group on the Diabetic Foot (2011).
5. International Diabetes Federation and International Working Group on the Diabetic Foot, *Diabetes and Foot Care: Time to Act* (International Diabetes Federation, 2005).
6. 2001 Annual Report, Ministry of Health Singapore.
7. 2005 World Diabetes Day on Diabetic Foot Care, International Working Group on the Diabetic Foot (2005).
8. A. Nather, S. B. Chionh, K. L. Wong, X. B. Chan, L. Shen, P. A. Tambyah, A. Jorgensen and A. Nambiar, Value of team approach combined with clinical pathway for diabetic foot problems: a clinical evaluation, *Diabet. Foot Ankle* 1:5731-5 (2010).

2

What is Diabetes?

Sharlene Ho, Quah Yan Ling and Aziz Nather

Department of Orthopaedic Surgery
Yong Loo Lin School of Medicine
National University of Singapore

Definition

Diabetes mellitus is a chronic disease, which occurs when the pancreas does not produce enough insulin, or when the body cannot effectively use the insulin it produces. This leads to an increased concentration of glucose in the blood (hyperglycaemia) (World Health Organisation).

Understanding blood glucose and insulin

After a meal, a portion of food a person eats is digested in the intestine (Fig. 1) into glucose, which is then absorbed into the bloodstream. Some of it will be taken up by cells to produce energy to meet the metabolic demands of the body. The rest is stored in the form of glycogen for future use.

For normal functioning of the body, blood glucose is tightly regulated within the range of 3.5–8.0 mmol/L (63–144 mg/dL), despite the varying demands of food, fasting and exercise. This is achieved by the action of insulin, which is a hormone produced by the pancreas. In the fasting state, the main action of insulin is to regulate glucose release from glycogen stores. After a meal, it facilitates glucose uptake into the cells, thereby maintaining blood glucose within an optimal range.

When blood glucose level rises after a meal, the pancreas will respond by increasing its production and secretion of insulin to bring down the blood glucose level. On the other hand, when blood glucose level drops in between meals, insulin production and secretion will decrease.

However, in diabetes, either the pancreas produces little or no insulin (Type 1 diabetes) or the cells do not respond normally to the insulin (Type 2 diabetes), resulting in hyperglycaemia. This chronic hyperglycaemia causes damage to various organs especially kidney, eye, nerves, heart and blood vessels.

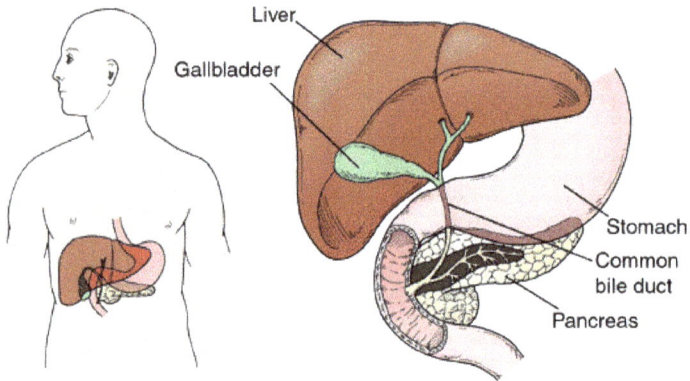

Figure 1. Insulin from the pancreas in relation to digestion of food in the intestine. Adapted from http://www.clivir.com/lessons/show/what-are-the-symptoms-of-diabetes.html

Types of Diabetes Mellitus

There are 2 main types of diabetes mellitus, Type 1 and Type 2. In addition, there are other specific types of diabetes such as gestational diabetes and maturity onset diabetes of the young.

Type 1 Diabetes

Epidemiology

Type 1 diabetes occurs mostly in children and adolescents. It can, however, also occur at any age, even in the 8th and 9th decades of life. In addition, type 1 diabetes is associated with other autoimmune disorders such as Graves' disease, Hashimoto's thyroiditis and Addison's disease.

Pathogenesis

Type 1 diabetes is due to destruction of cells in the pancreas that produce insulin (known as β cells). It usually leads to absolute insulin deficiency. This

β cell destruction is either attributable to an autoimmune process or due to an unknown cause.

Type 2 Diabetes

Epidemiology

Type 2 diabetes is the most common form of diabetes. Its frequency varies in different racial or ethnic subgroups. It often has a strong familial and genetic predisposition.

Pathogenesis

Type 2 diabetes ranges from predominantly insulin resistant with relative insulin deficiency to predominantly insulin secretory defect with insulin resistance. Insulin resistance refers to a condition in which the body's cells cannot properly use insulin. This results in decreased uptake of blood glucose into the cells. Initially, blood glucose remains normal because the pancreas is able to compensate by producing more insulin. However as the disease progresses, the pancreas becomes fatigued and is unable to produce sufficient insulin. This results in relative insulin deficiency and hyperglycaemia. This is how diabetes develops.

In type 2 diabetes, there is interaction between genetic and environmental factors. Specific genes that predispose to diabetes are still under research. So far it is certain that diabetes is a polygenic (involves many genes) and multifactorial disease. Environmental factors such as diet and exercise further modulate the presentation of diabetes.

Risk Factor For Developing Type 2 Diabetes

Overweight/obesity (body mass index $>25.0 \, \text{kg/m}^2$)
Hypertension ($>140/90 \, \text{mmHg}$)
A first degree relative with diabetes mellitus
Previous gestational diabetes mellitus
Coronary heart disease
Polycystic ovary disease

(*Continued*)

(Continued)

Dyslipidaemia (HDL cholesterol <1.0 mmol/l, and/or triglyceride level
>2.30 mmol/l)
Previously identified impaired fasting glycaemia (IFG) or impaired
glucose tolerance (IGT)

Singapore Ministry of Health Clinical Practice Guidelines 3/2006

First degree relative = a spouse, parent, sibling, or child.
Gestational diabetes mellitus = a condition in which women without previously diagnosed
diabetes exhibit high blood glucose levels during pregnancy.
Polycystic ovary disease = a condition commonly characterised by obesity, menstrual
abnormalities, infertility, male pattern hair growth, insulin resistance, and enlarged ovaries.
Dyslipidaemia = an abnormal amount of lipids (e.g. cholesterol and/or fat) in the blood.
High Density Lipoprotein (HDL) = a combination of lipids and protein which carries
cholesterol to the liver where it is removed from the body.
Triglyceride = the form in which the majority of fat exists in the body.

Clinical presentation of diabetes

Patients with all types of diabetes may present with the classical symptoms of:

1. Polyuria (passing large amount of urine)
When blood glucose level exceeds the amount that the kidneys can handle,
glucose leaks into the urine. Since glucose is an osmotically active substance,
it holds on to water and reduces reabsorption of water in the kidneys, thereby
increasing urine output. This is known as osmotic diuresis.

2. Polydipsia (increased thirst)
There is increased thirst due to the resulting loss of fluid and electrolytes.

3. Polyphagia (increased hunger)
As there is decrease uptake of glucose into the cells, cells become 'starved' and
send signals to the brain to increase appetite.

4. Loss of weight
Insulin deficiency also causes break down of fats and muscles. This, together
with fluid depletion, results in weight loss.

In type 1 diabetes, the presentation tends to be acute, with a shorter
duration of symptoms. In addition, if left untreated, patients may present
with symptoms of diabetic ketoacidosis (DKA) such as ketoacidosis, ketonuria

and hyperventilation. Ketoacidosis occurs when the liver breaks down fats and proteins into ketone bodies. These can be used by the brain cells as a substitute for glucose as there is impaired glucose uptake. This excess ketone bodies can significantly acidify the blood (ketoacidosis), resulting in hyperventilation to remove the excess acid in the form of carbon dioxide from the body. The excess ketone bodies are also removed in the urine (ketonuria).

In type 2 diabetes, the presentation tends to be subacute, with a longer duration of symptoms. Polyuria, polydipsia, polyphagia and loss of weight are typically present. Some patients may also present with chronic complications of diabetes (see Chapter 3). However, with a more effective screening programme in place, more and more people with hyperglycaemia are picked up at the asymptomatic stage.

Diagnosis of diabetes

In patients with typical symptoms, diabetes can be diagnosed if any one of the following is present:

1. Casual plasma glucose >11.1 mmol/l
2. Fasting plasma glucose >7.0 mmol/l
3. Oral glucose tolerance test >11.1 mmol/l

In individuals without symptoms, 2 positive tests on 2 separate days are needed for diagnosis.

Important notes to diagnosis:

a. Casual is defined as any time of the day, without regard to the interval since the last meal.
b. Fasting is defined as no calorie intake for at least 8 hours.
c. In oral glucose tolerance test, 75 g of glucose is ingested and plasma glucose is measured before and 2 hours later.
d. Capillary blood glucose/hypocount is not one of the diagnostic criteria.
e. Glycated haemoglobin (HbA1c) has been accepted as a diagnostic test for diabetes according to the latest WHO recommendation (2011) and American Diabetes Association guidelines. HbA1c of 6.5% is the cut off point for diagnosing diabetes.

IFG and IGT (Table 1) are pre-diabetic stages, indicating higher risk for future development of diabetes.

Figures 2 and 3 are flow charts for the diagnosis of diabetes, IFG and IGT.

Table 1.   Intermediate categories of glucose tolerance

	Fasting plasma glucose (mmol/l)	2-hour plasma glucose (mmol/l)
Impaired Fasting Glycaemia (IFG)	6.1–6.9	<7.8
Impaired Glucose Tolerance (IGT)	<7.0	7.8–11.0

Singapore Ministry of Health Clinical Practice Guidelines 3/2006

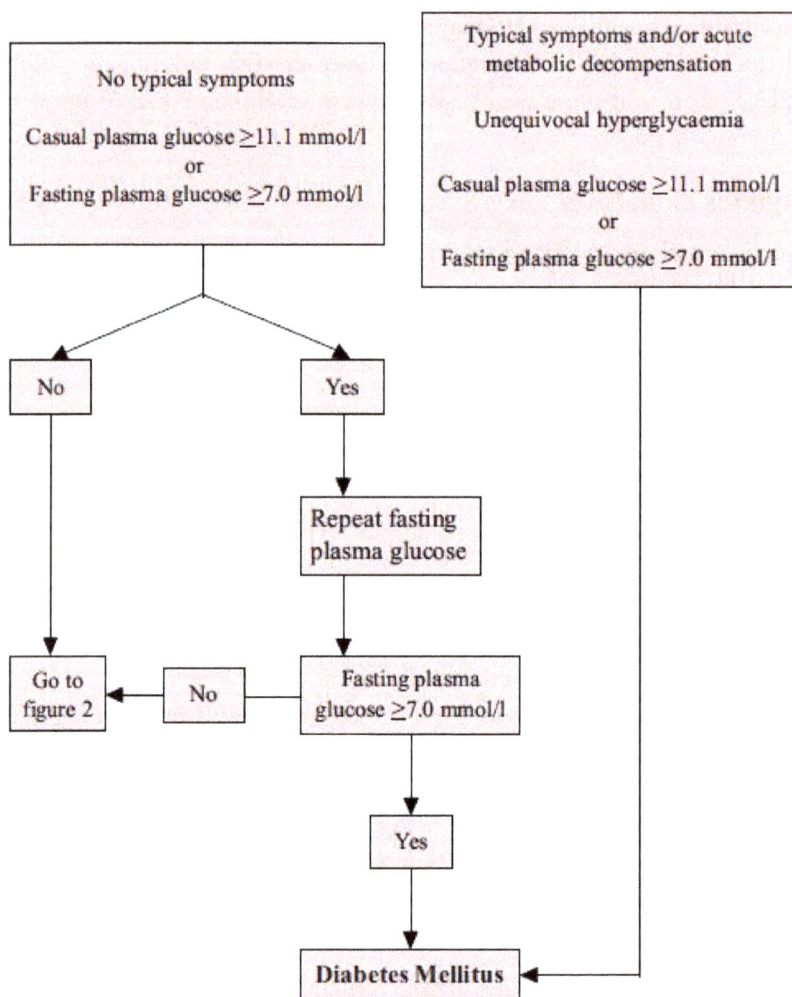

Figure 2.   Flow chart for diagnosis of diabetes
Singapore Ministry of Health Clinical Practice Guidelines 3/2006

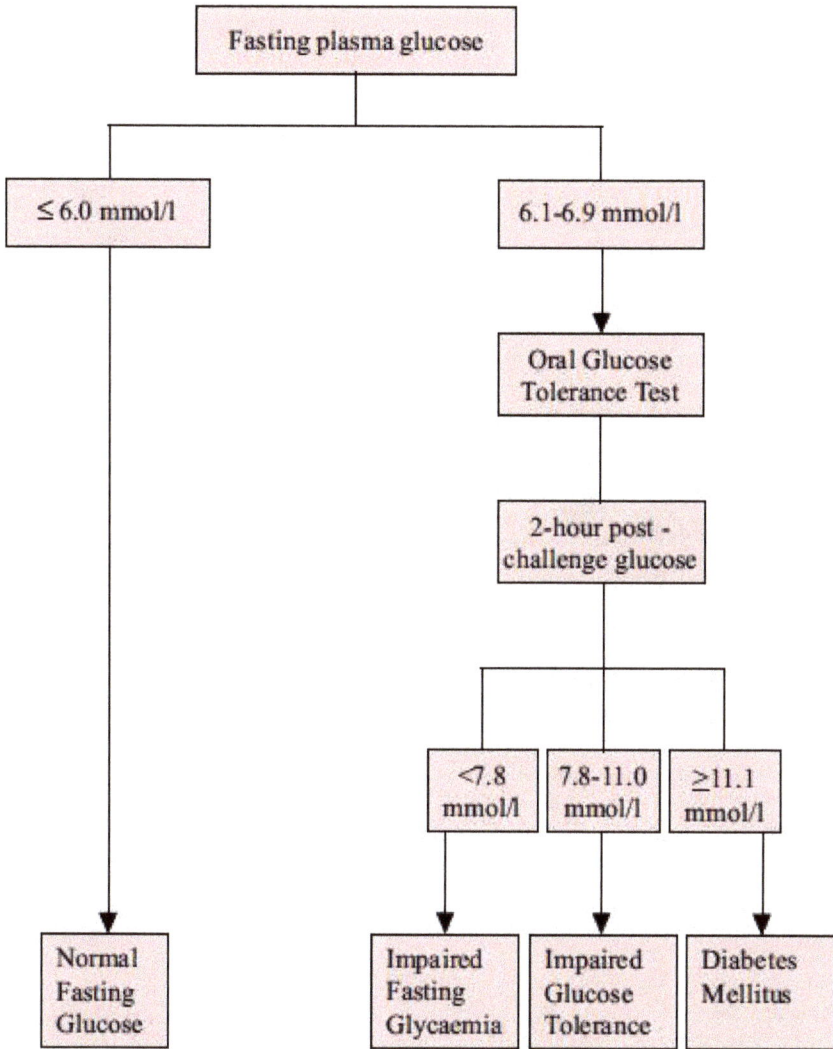

Figure 3. Flowchart for individuals suspected to have diabetes but whose fasting plasma glucose <7.0 mmol/l
Singapore Ministry of Health Clinical Practice Guidelines 3/2006

3

Complications of Diabetes Mellitus

Quah Yan Ling, Sharlene Ho, Ruth Chen Wei Xian and Aziz Nather

Department of Orthopaedic Surgery
Yong Loo Lin School of Medicine
National University of Singapore

Diabetes is a life-long condition that requires careful control. Without proper management, many complications can arise. Almost every organ in the body may be affected, resulting in disability or even death.

Patients with diabetes can suffer from acute and/or chronic complications.

Acute complications	Chronic complications
1. Diabetic ketoacidosis (DKA)	**Macrovascular complications (damage to large blood vessels)**
	1. Coronary heart disease
2. Hyperglycaemic hyperosmolar state (HHS)	2. Cerebrovascular disease
	3. Peripheral vascular disease
	Microvascular complications (damage to small blood vessels)
3. Hypoglycaemia	1. Kidney: diabetic nephropathy
	2. Eye: diabetic retinopathy and other eye problems
	3. Nerve problems: diabetic neuropathy
	Other complications
	1. Foot problems: diabetic foot
	2. Frequent, recurrent and persistent infections

Acute Complications

1. Diabetic ketoacidosis (DKA)

DKA is a life threatening condition that usually occurs in patients with type 1 diabetes. It is often seen in the following circumstances:

  i. previously undiagnosed diabetes
 ii. when insulin therapy is not adhered to or when the dose is inadequate
iii. intercurrent illness

In DKA, there is reduced glucose uptake into the cells due to insufficient insulin, leading to a state of 'cellular starvation'. As a result, the body breaks down fats and proteins into ketone bodies to be used as substrates for energy instead. This process is known as ketogenesis. When large amounts of ketone bodies accumulate, it significantly acidifies the blood, causing ketoacidosis, which is toxic to the body.

Look out for the following symptoms:

Early presentations:

- Polyuria
- Polydipsia
- Weight loss
- Nausea and vomiting
- Nonspecific abdominal pain
- Fatigue and weakness
- Breathlessness

Late presentations:

- Confusion
- Disorientation
- Diabetic coma

2. Hyperglycaemic hyperosmolar state (HHS)

Like DKA, HHS is also a life threatening condition. However, it tends to affect patients with type 2 diabetes. It is characterised by severe hyperglycaemia without ketoacidosis.

In HHS, hyperglycaemia induces osmotic diuresis and patients present with polyuria or excessive urination. This leads to volume depletion and dehydration, which are further worsened by inadequate fluid intake to replace the fluid lost. As a result, blood osmolarity increases, hence the name hyperglycaemic hyperosmolar state. Ketoacidosis is absent because unlike in DKA, some insulin is still produced by the pancreas which prevents production of excessive ketone bodies.

The most common precipitating cause of HHS is an underlying infection. Other causes include non-compliance, undiagnosed diabetes, medications and co-existing disease.

Look out for the following symptoms:

Early presentations:

- Polyuria
- Polydipsia
- Weight loss
- Weakness
- Visual disturbances
- Leg cramps
- No nausea and vomiting, abdominal pain and breathlessness (unlike DKA)

Late presentations:

- Neurological symptoms such as drowsiness, delirium, seizures and weakness on one side of the body
- Diabetic coma

3. Hypoglycaemia

Hypoglycaemia is defined as blood glucose <3.0 mmol/L. In patient with diabetes, hypoglycaemia usually occurs as a complication due to treatment. This can occur when:

i. meals are skipped, delayed or insufficient
ii. physical activity is increased
iii. too much insulin has been administered

Look out for the following symptoms:

Early presentations:

- Hunger
- Shakiness
- Anxiety
- Sweating
- Dizziness
- Sleepiness
- Mental confusion
- Weakness
- Headache
- Irritability
- Increased heart rate
- Cold skin
- Double vision

In severe cases:

- Seizures
- Coma
- Death

Treatment of hypoglycaemia involves rapid delivery of easily absorbed sugar such as 3 teaspoons of sugar, 4 teaspoons of honey, 5 teaspoons of milo or half a can of soft drink.

Chronic Complications

Macrovascular complications

Macrovascular complications arise from damage to large blood vessels in the body. High blood glucose levels cause deposition of fatty materials (plaques) on the inner surface of blood vessel walls. This leads to narrowing and hardening of blood vessels, which reduces blood flow and increases the risk of clogging. This process is known as atherosclerosis.

Type 2 diabetes is recognised as a major risk factor for atherosclerotic disease. In Singapore, almost 60% of people with diabetes die due to

(a) **Normal artery**

Artery wall

Normal blood flow

Artery cross-section

Abnormal blood flow

Plaque

(b) **Narrowing of artery**

Narrowed artery

Plaque

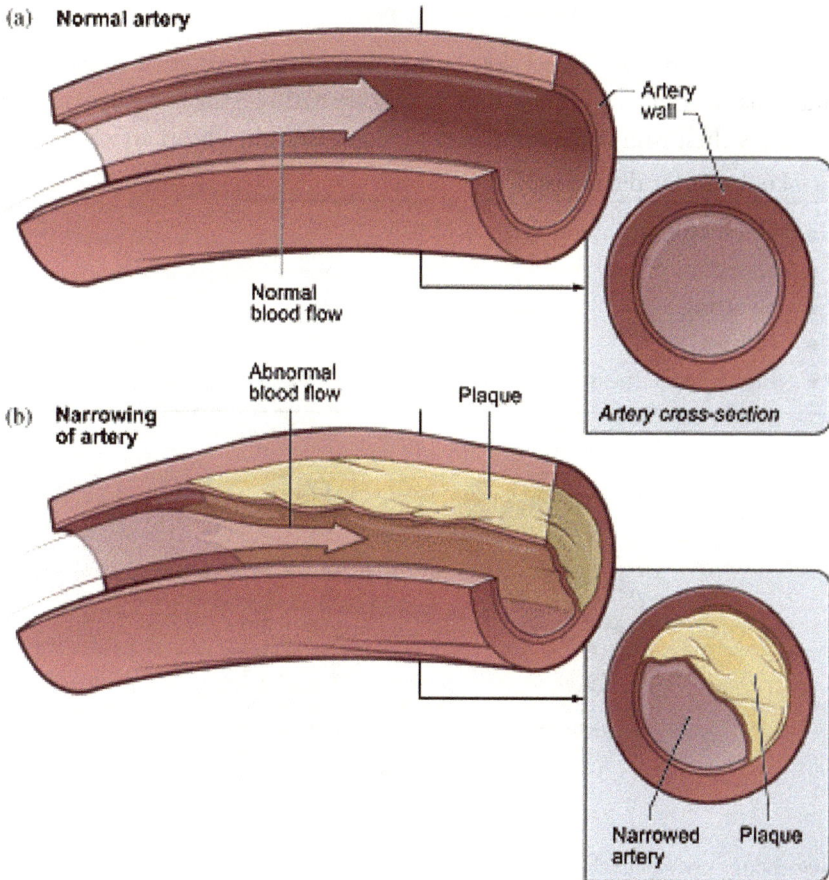

Source: http://www.nhlbi.nih.gov

cardiovascular disease (MOH CPG guidelines). In addition to diabetes, many have other conditions that increase their likelihood of developing heart disease and stroke. These include hyperlipidemia, hypertension, obesity, smoking and a family history of heart disease.

What types of blood vessel disease occur in people with diabetes?

Atherosclerosis can lead to coronary artery disease (blockage of blood flow to the heart), cerebrovascular disease (blockage of blood flow to the brain) and peripheral arterial disease (blockage of blood flow to the legs).

1. Coronary artery disease

Coronary arteries are blood vessels that supply the heart with oxygen and nutrients it needs for normal functioning. Partial blockage of these arteries produces chest pain while complete blockage results in a heart attack.

Look out for the following symptoms:

- Chest pain or discomfort
- Shortness of breath
- Sweating
- Nausea
- Light-headedness

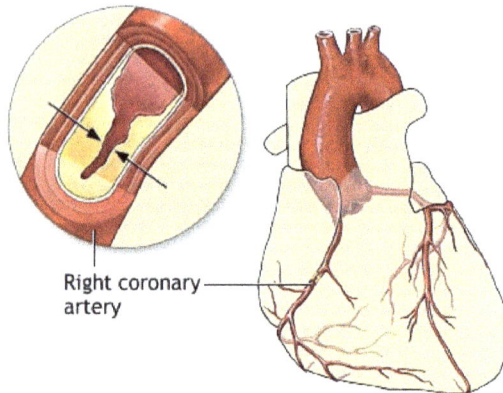

Right coronary artery

Source: http://www.nlm.nih.gov

2. Cerebrovascular disease

Limited blood flow to the brain can result in strokes or Transient Ischaemic Attacks (TIA). A stroke occurs when a blood vessel in the brain or neck is blocked or burst, leading to sudden cut-off of blood supply to the brain. Brain cells become deprived of oxygen and die. TIA occurs when there is a temporary blockage of a blood vessel to the brain. This causes a brief, sudden change in brain function such as numbness or weakness on one side of the body. These symptoms resolve quickly and permanent damage is unlikely.

Look out for following symptoms:

- Sudden weakness or numbness on one side of the body
- Sudden confusion

(*Continued*)

(Continued)

- Sudden difficulty in talking or understanding
- Sudden dizziness, loss of balance, or trouble walking
- Sudden visual disturbances such as double vision
- Sudden severe headache

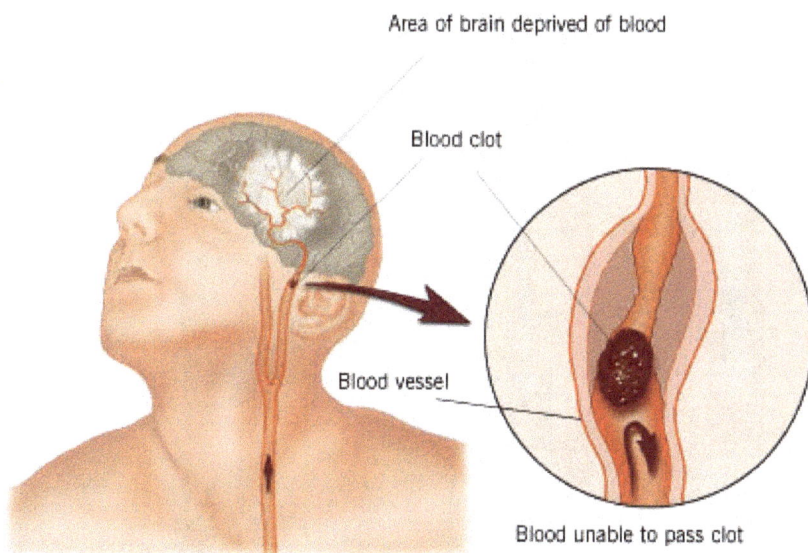

Source: http://behavioralphys.wikispaces.com

3. Peripheral arterial disease (PAD)

PAD occurs due to poor blood circulation in the legs and feet. Many people with PAD do not have symptoms. Others, however, may develop pain in the calves when walking, which improves by resting.

Poor circulation in the legs and feet also increases the risk of amputation.

Look out for the following signs and symptoms:

- Weak or tired legs
- Difficulty walking or balancing
- Cold and numb feet or toes
- Slow-healing sores and ulcers
- Foot pain at rest

(Continued)

(Continued)

- Black skin on feet or toes (indicates gangrene)
- Loss of hair, shiny skin, nail changes and hyperpigmented skin (patches of dark skin)

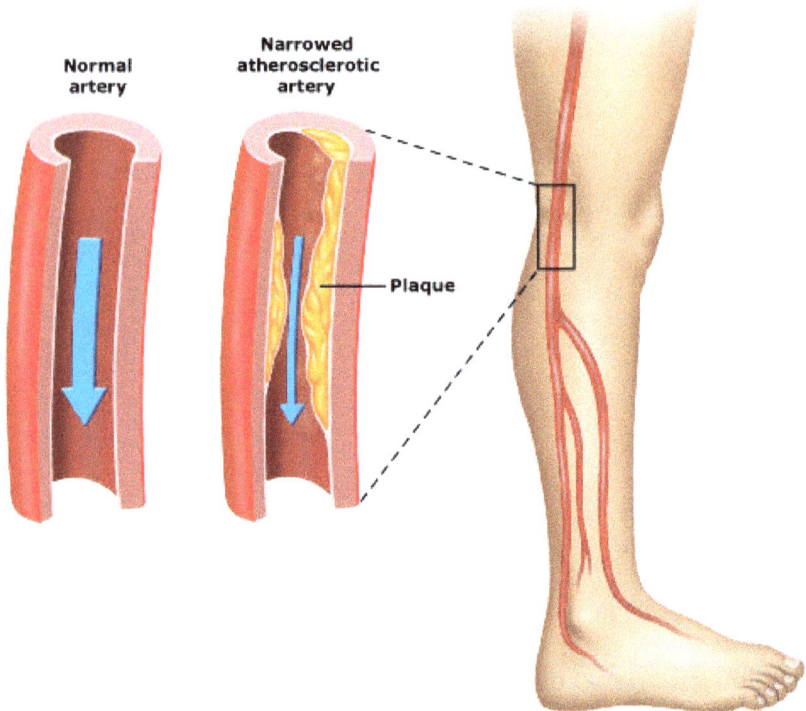

Source: http://drmiri.com

Microvascular complications

Microvascular complications arise from damage to small blood vessels of the body, in particular the kidneys, eyes and nerves.

1. Kidney: diabetic nephropathy

Nephropathy refers to damage of the kidneys. In Singapore, diabetes is the most common cause of end stage renal disease (ESRD). It accounted for nearly half (47.2%) of ESRD in 2000.

How does diabetes cause nephropathy?

Blood is brought to the kidneys to be filtered by millions of tiny blood vessels known as glomerular capillaries. Glomerular capillaries contain even tinier holes in them which act as filters. Waste products that are filtered become part of the urine. On the other hand, useful substances such as proteins and red blood cells remain in the blood as they are too big to pass through the filters. In diabetes, this filter system becomes damaged over time.

Over several years, small amounts of protein (albumin) start to leak into the urine. This first stage of kidney disease is called microalbuminuria (defined as low levels of urine albumin from 30 to 299 mg/day or 20 to 199 μg/min). At this stage, treatments are available to prevent it from getting worse.

However, without specific interventions, 80% of these people will progress to a later stage of the disease over another period of 10 to 15 years. This is known as macroalbuminuria in which the urine albumin level reaches >300 mg/l. The kidneys' filtering function also starts to drop, leading to retention of various waste products in the body. At this stage, treatments are less effective, and ESRD usually follows. People with ESRD will require kidney transplants or dialysis to have their blood filtered by a machine. On average, it takes a total of more than 15 to 25 years before kidney failure set in.

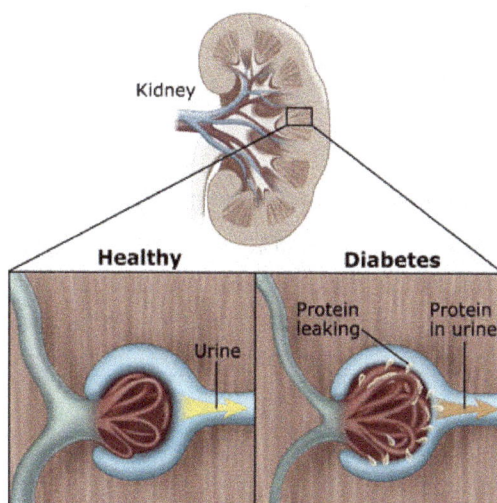

Source: http://www.deo.ucsf.edu

What are the symptoms?

Diabetic nephropathy takes many years to develop because there is a large reserve of renal tissue.

When glomerular capillaries start to fail, the kidneys work harder. There are usually no symptoms until almost all function is gone. Only then do symptoms manifest.

Look out for the following symptoms:

- Swelling around the eyes, abdomen, legs, ankles and feet
- Urination problems e.g. unable to pass urine, or passing urine more frequently, pain or burning sensation when urinating, foamy, bloody or dark urine
- Fatigue
- Insomnia
- Breathlessness
- Loss of appetite
- Metallic taste in the mouth
- Nausea or vomiting
- Weakness
- Dizziness
- High blood pressure
- Itching or rashes
- Pain, mostly in legs, back and around the kidney area

2. Eye: diabetic retinopathy and other eye problems

Retinopathy or damage to the retina is a common complication of diabetes. Without proper treatment, it can worsen and cause blurring of vision and even blindness. In 2006, an estimated 2.5 million people worldwide are blind from diabetic retinopathy. In Singapore, retinal conditions including diabetic retinopathy is the main cause of blindness in adults.

Anatomy of the eye:

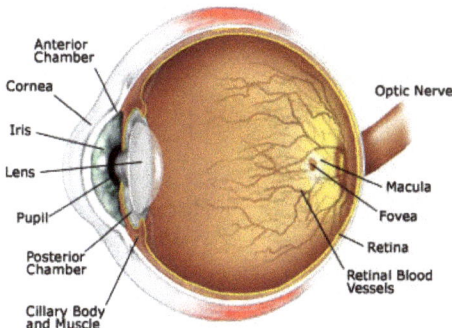

Anterior Chamber

Cornea

Iris

Lens

Pupil

Posterior Chamber

Ciliary Body and Muscle

Optic Nerve

Macula

Fovea

Retina

Retinal Blood Vessels

Retina: the lining at the back of the eye. Its function is to detect light coming into the eye
Vitreous: a jelly-like fluid that fills the back of the eye
Lens: transparent biconcave structure behind the iris that focuses light onto the retina
Iris: contractile, circular diaphragm forming the coloured portion of the eye and containing a circular opening, the pupil, in its center
Optic nerve: the nerve that carries images from the eye to the brain
Macula: central portion of the retina, rich in cones, which are specialized nerve endings that detect colour

Source: http://www.healthtree.com

How does diabetes cause retinopathy?

In diabetic retinopathy, chronically elevated blood glucose levels weaken and damage the small blood vessels in the retina, resulting in the following problems:

- Small localized, sac-like dilatation of blood vessels (Microaneurysms)
- Minor fluid leakage from damaged blood vessels
- Minor bleeding from damaged blood vessels (Hemorrhages)
- Swelling of the macula
- Some blood vessels may become clogged, impairing blood flow and oxygen to the retina

As the disease progresses:

- Low oxygen condition stimulates formation of new blood vessels. However, these new vessels are abnormal, delicate and prone to bleeding. In severe cases, they may bleed into the vitreous humour and affect vision.
- Scar tissues can form from the ruptured blood vessels and pull the retina away from the back of the eye, causing retinal detachment. This may cause floating spots, flashing lights or severe vision loss.

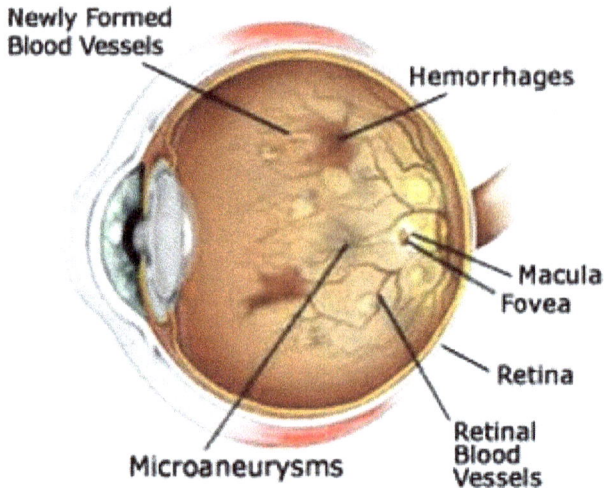

Source: http://www.elements4health.com

Other diabetic eye problems that can occur are:

- Cataracts
  Patients with diabetes have higher risk of developing cataract compared to the general population. In cataracts, there is increased opacity or clouding of the lens, thereby affecting vision.
- Glaucoma
  In patients with diabetes, new blood vessels may grow on the iris and interfere with the normal drainage of fluid out of the eye, causing build up of pressure in the eye, known as glaucoma. This pressure can damage the optic nerve and lead to blindness.

Look out for the following symptoms:

- blurry or double vision
- rings, flashing lights or blank spots
- dark or floating spots
- pain or pressure in one or both eyes
- difficulty seeing things in the corner of the eyes

Normal vision

Blurry vision

3. Nerve problems: diabetic neuropathy

Neuropathy refers to nerve damage. It is one of the earliest complications of diabetes.

Function of nerves

The primary function of nerves is communication. Nerves connect the brain and spinal cord to the rest of the body. Together, the brain and spinal cord form the central nervous system (CNS), which helps to integrate information and coordinate activities in our body.

All nerve fibres outside the CNS form the peripheral nervous system (PNS). PNS consists of:

- **sensory nerves** that transmit signals from sensory organs to the brain, thus enabling us to perceive the environment around us.
- **motor nerves** that transmit signals from the brain to the muscles, thereby controlling muscle contraction and movement.
- **autonomic nerves** that transmit signals from the brain to internal organs, which function largely below the level of consciousness (automatic/involuntary). They regulate activities such as digestion, urination, sexual response, heart rate and perspiration.

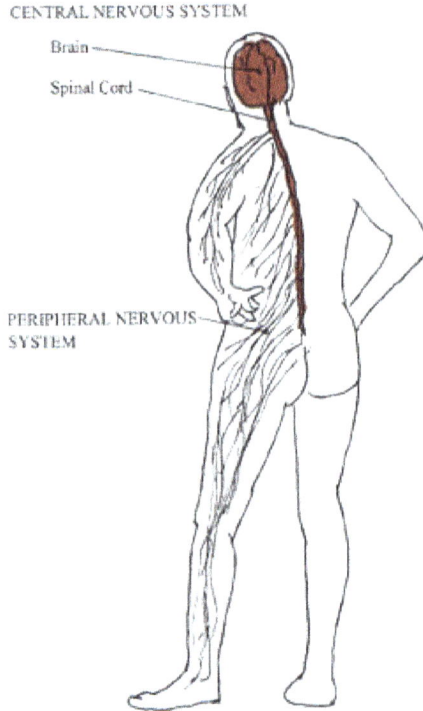

CENTRAL NERVOUS SYSTEM

Brain

Spinal Cord

PERIPHERAL NERVOUS SYSTEM

Source: http://library.thinkquest.org

How does diabetes cause neuropathy?

Chronic hyperglycaemia can cause direct damage to the nerves. Excess blood glucose can also injure the walls of tiny blood vessels that supply the nerves, resulting in nerve ischemia and damage.

In diabetic neuropathy, the PNS is mainly affected. Patients may present with symptoms involving the sensory, motor and autonomic nerves.

Look out for the following symptoms:

- Numbness, tingling, or pain in the toes, feet, hands and fingers, usually described as 'gloves and stoking' sensory disturbance
- Muscle wasting in feet or hands
- Weakness
- Nausea, vomiting, indigestion or bloatedness

(*Continued*)

(Continued)

- Constipation or diarrhea
- Urination problems
- Sexual problems such as erectile dysfunction in men or vaginal dryness in women
- Giddiness due to a drop in blood pressure after standing or sitting up

Other Complications

1. Infections

People with diabetes are more susceptible to infections such as pneumonias, tuberculosis, pyelonephritis and diabetic ulcers due to poor immunity. In addition, wounds take a longer time to heal due to poor blood supply.

Look out for the following signs and symptoms:

- Fever
- Viral signs and symptoms including headache, cough, fatigue, chills, body aches
- Nausea, vomiting or diarrhoea
- Urinary symptoms such as cloudy or foul smelling urine, increased frequency or burning sensation on passing urine
- Swelling, redness, tenderness, rash
- Foul smelling and /or discharging skin wound
- Sore mouth, white patches in the mouth
- Acute onset of confusion

2. Diabetic foot

About 700 lower extremities amputations are performed each year in Singapore for patients with diabetic foot problems. Major amputation due to diabetes is also a worldwide problem, with estimates as high as 1 amputation every 20 seconds. Patients with diabetes are more prone to developing frequent and serious foot problems due to their increased risk of peripheral vascular disease, neuropathy and infections. Diabetic foot problems include cellulitis, abscess, wet or dry gangrene, ulcer, osteomyelitis, septic arthritis, necrotising fasciitis and Charcot Joint Disease.

4

Management of Diabetes Mellitus

Aziz Nather, Sharlene Ho and Quah Yan Ling

Department of Orthopaedic Surgery
Yong Loo Lin School of Medicine
National University of Singapore

Management of diabetes can be divided into treatment and prevention, as shown in Fig. 1.

Treatment

Lifestyle

1. *Diet*

A well balanced diet is important for everyone, including patients with diabetes. This can be achieved by following the food pyramid recommendations (Fig. 2).

Of all nutrients, carbohydrates have the most effect on blood glucose level as carbohydrates are digested to form glucose. Carbohydrates can be divided into two main types — simple and complex. Simple carbohydrates include table sugar, honey and sugars found in fruits and milk. Complex carbohydrates include rice, wholemeal bread, noodles, oats, and vegetables such as corn, yam, peas and beans. Patients with diabetes are advised to eat more complex carbohydrates and less simple carbohydrates. This is

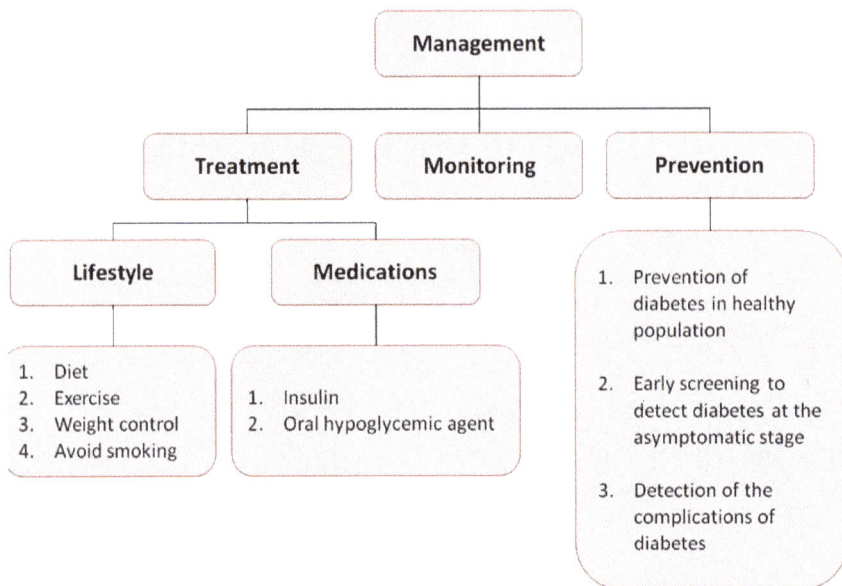

Figure 1. Flow diagram for management of diabetes

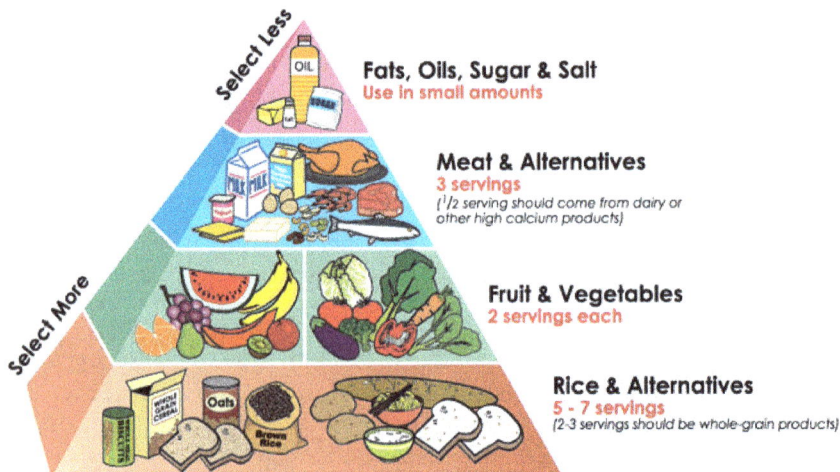

Figure 2. Food pyramid

Source: http://www.hpb.gov.sg

because complex carbohydrates are more slowly digested and absorbed into the bloodstream, thereby preventing a sudden rise in blood sugar levels after a meal. Eating small frequent meals can also prevent fluctuations in blood sugar levels.

In addition, patients with diabetes have to be more conscious of the amount of fats, oil, sugar and salt they take in their diet as they have higher risk of developing heart disease and stroke.

2. Exercise

Patients with diabetes are encouraged to maintain a healthy lifestyle by exercising regularly.

The guidelines for exercise are as follows:

- Frequency: 3–5 days per week (daily if low intensity).
- Intensity: 60–85% of maximum heart rate (till patient feels warm or sweats and breathes deeply).
- Time: 20–60 minutes each time, fairly continuously.
- Type: aerobic exercises like walking, jogging, swimming, cycling, ball and racket games.

Singapore Ministry of Health Clinical Practice Guidelines 3/2006

However, there are certain precautions patients with diabetes should take note of. These include usage of proper footwear, reduction of medications prior to exercise and prompt recognition of hypoglycaemic symptoms during exercise.

3. Weight control

Maintaining a healthy weight is beneficial for the control of blood glucose levels. In fact, weight loss has been shown to reduce insulin resistance. Weight loss can be achieved by eating less and exercising more.

4. Avoid smoking

As nicotine in cigarettes promotes both macrovascular and microvascular disease in patients with diabetes, they should avoid smoking.

Medications

In type 1 diabetes, the pancreas fails to produce insulin, hence synthetic insulin has to be given as replacement. In type 2 diabetes, oral hypoglycaemic agents are given initially when lifestyle modifications fail to keep the blood glucose levels under control. However, as diabetes progresses, it reaches a stage where the pancreas is unable to produce sufficient insulin, thus requiring synthetic insulin.

1. Insulin

There are many types of synthetic insulin available in the market (Table 1), which differ in onset, peak and duration of action. Different patients require different types of insulin and regimes to match their daily requirements. To achieve effective diabetes control, it is important to understand how these different types of insulin work. There are 4 main types of insulin — rapid acting, short acting, intermediate acting and long acting (Table 2).

There are many different insulin regimes prescribed by doctors. These regimes mimic the normal insulin requirement of the body in the fasting state and after a meal. Our body requires insulin throughout the day and night. In normal people, the pancreas produces a basal or background level of insulin. This helps to control blood sugar level as our body still needs energy even when we are not eating. After a meal, blood sugar rises. In response, more insulin is produced and this is referred to as a 'bolus'.

Table 1. Types of insulin

Types of insulin		Onset	Peak	Duration
Rapid acting	1) Insulin lispro (Humalog)	5–15 mins	1–2 hours	3–5 hours
	2) Insulin aspart (NovoRapid)	10–20 mins	1–3 hours	3–5 hours
Short acting	1) (Humulin R) 2) (Actrapid)	30–60 mins	2–4 hours	6–8 hours
Intermediate acting	1) NPH (Humulin N or Insulatard) 2) Lente (Humulin L or Monotard)	1–4 hours	8–12 hours	12–20 hours
Long acting	1) (Humulin U)	3–5 hours	10–16 hours	18–24 hours
	2) (Ultratard)	3–5 hours	10–16 hours	18–24 hours
	3) Insulin glargine (Lantus)	1–4 hours	Peakless	24 hours
	4) Insulin detemir (Lemevir)	1–4 hours	Peakless	18–24 hours

Source: Singapore Ministry of Health Clinical Practice Guidelines 3/2006[1]

To provide basal or background insulin, intermediate or long acting preparations are used. These are typically given at night to help control blood sugar level while sleeping. They may also be given during the day if extra cover is needed.

To control the rapid rise of blood sugar level after a meal, short or rapid acting preparations are given before meals — breakfast, lunch and dinner.

Insulin cannot be taken by mouth. It is usually given as an injection, using syringe and needle or pen injectors, into the layer of fat under the skin at the following sites: abdomen, outer sides of thighs, buttocks, back of upper arms (Fig. 3).[2]

Avoid injecting at the same spot each time as this may lead to a loss or accumulation of fatty tissues, causing a lump or dent in the skin.

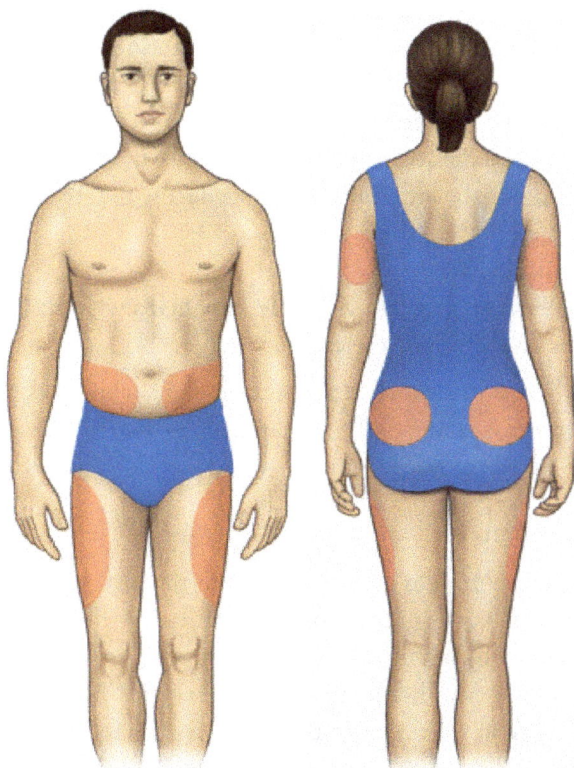

Figure 3. Sites of insulin injection

Source: www.uptodate.com

2. Oral hypoglycaemic agents

For type 2 diabetes, patients are usually given oral tablets to help control their blood glucose level. These are known as oral hypoglycaemic agents. They include:

- Insulin secretagogues
  Insulin secretagogues work by stimulating the release of insulin from the pancreas. There are 2 types of insulin secretagogues: (1) sulphonylureas (e.g. tolbutamide, glibenclamide, glipizide, glimepiride); (2)nonsulphonylureas (e.g. nateglinide, repaglinide). One of the major side effects is increased risk of hypoglycaemia.
- Biguanides
  Biguanides (e.g. metformin) result in a net decrease of blood glucose level. They work by reducing glucose production from the liver, delaying glucose absorption from the intestines and increasing the usage of glucose by cells in the body. Biguanides should be used with caution in people with kidney and liver impairment.
- Alphaglucosidase inhibitors
  Alphaglucosidase inhibitors (e.g. acarbose) slow the digestion and absorption of glucose in the intestines, thereby reducing the rise in blood glucose level after a meal.
- Thiazolidinediones
  Thiazolidinediones (e.g. rosiglitazone, pioglitazone) makes tissues more sensitive to insulin so glucose can be absorbed.

Of these oral hypoglycaemic agents, the most commonly used are sulphonylureas and metformin. The table below summarises their mechanism of action, advantages and possible side effects.

Blood glucose monitoring

Blood glucose monitoring is an integral part in the management of diabetes. It promotes better blood glucose control. Methods include self monitoring and regular follow up with the doctor. Self monitoring can be easily done by patients themselves at home using a glucometer. This allows patients to participate actively in their own care. During regular follow ups, blood tests are done to measure the glycated haemoglobin level known as HbA1c. This is useful in assessing the blood glucose control over the past 3 months. Table 3 summarizes the targets of blood glucose control in Singapore.

Table 2. Types of oral hypoglycaemic agents

Oral hypoglycaemic agents	Mechanism of action	Advantages	Possible side effects	Of note
Sulphonylurea Tolbutamide Glipizide Gliclazide Glibenclamide	Stimulate the release of insulin from the pancreas	Well established	Likely to cause low blood glucose (hypoglycaemia)	Always carry a source of carbohydrate with you in case of hypoglycaemic episodes
			Weight gain	Inform your doctor if your blood glucose levels are consistently low
Biguanide Metformin	Reduce glucose production from the liver	Well established	Gastrointestinal symptoms e.g. nausea, diarrhea, abdominal cramps, bloating	Take with food to minimize gastrointestinal symptoms
	Delay glucose absorption from the intestines	Weight loss (additional benefit for obese patients)	Metallic taste	Inform your doctor if you are going for scanning procedure involving the use of contrast/dye (e.g. CT scan, angiogram) as it needs to be stopped
	Increase the usage of glucose by cells in the body	Not likely to cause low blood glucose	Lactic acidosis-serious but rare complication, more likely to occur in patients with heart problems, and abnormal kidney and liver function	

Table 3.   Targets of blood glucose control

Test	(Ideal non-diabetic levels)	Assessment of glucose control		
		Optimal (target goal for majority of patients)	Suboptimal (adequate goal for some patients)‡	Unacceptable (action needed in all patients)
HbA$_{1c}$* (%)	4.5–6.4	6.5–7.0	7.1–8.0	>8.0
Pre-meal glucose† (mmol/l)	4.0–6.0	6.1–8.0	8.1–10.0	>10.0
2-hour post-meal† glucose (mmol/l)	5.0–7.0	7.1–10.0	10.1–13.0	>13.0

Notes:

*Normal reference range obtained from NUH and SGH laboratories using Biorad Variant 11[R]

Other laboratories should establish their own non-diabetic reference intervals

†Values pertaining to capillary blood sample

‡Adequate goal in elderly patients and individuals with advanced diabetic complications or other co-morbidities

Singapore Ministry of Health Clinical Practice Guidelines 3/2006

Prevention of Diabetes

1. *Prevention of diabetes in healthy population*

Lifestyle modifications such as eating a balanced diet, doing regular exercise, maintaining a healthy weight and avoiding smoking (as described above) can help prevent diabetes.

2. *Early screening to detect diabetes at the asymptomatic stage*

Table 4 shows individuals who are at risk of developing diabetes. Type 2 diabetes is largely underdiagnosed as it is usually asymptomatic at the early stages. Early detection and treatment can prevent complications of diabetes. As it is not cost effective to screen everyone, the following criteria are useful to identify individuals at higher risk of developing diabetes.

Table 4. Criteria for testing for diabetes in asymptomatic, undiagnosed individuals

Testing for diabetes should be considered:

1. Individuals at age 45 years and above, particularly in those with a BMI ≥ 25 kg/m^{2*}; if normal, it should be repeated at 3-year intervals.
2. Individuals at a younger age or be carried out more frequently in individuals who are overweight (BMI ≥ 25 kg/m^{2*}) and have additional risk factors:

- have a first-degree relative with diabetes
- are physically inactive
- are members of a high-risk ethnic population (e.g. African-American, Hispanic American, Native American, Asian American, Pacific Islander)
- have delivered a baby weighing >9 lb (>4.08 kg) or have been diagnosed with gestation diabetes mellitus
- are hypertensive ($\geq 140/90$ mmHg)
- have an HDL cholesterol level ≤ 35 mg/dl (0.90 mmol/l) and/or a triglyceride level ≥ 250 mg/dl (2.82 mmol/l)
- have Polycystic Ovary Syndrome
- on previous testing, had Impaired Glucose Tolerance (IGT) or Impaired Fasting Glycaemia (IFG)
- have a history of vascular disease

*May not be correct for all ethnic groups
Source: Report of the Expert Committee on the Diagnosis and Classification of Diabetes Mellitus. Diabetes Care 2003; 26 (Suppl 1): S5-20

Table 5.   Risk reduction per 1% decrease in HbA1c

Study	Eye	Kidney	Nerve	Heart
DCCT	27%–38%	22%–28%	29%–35%	40%
UKPDS	19%	26%	18%	14%

3. *Detection of the complications of diabetes*

Diabetic patients are recommended to go for eyes, kidneys, heart and foot screening annually to enable early detection of the complications of diabetes.

4. *Prevention of complications of diabetes mellitus*

Reduction of HbA1c levels is the key to preventing complications of diabetes, as shown by the United Kingdom Prospective Diabetes Study (UKPDS)[3] for Types 2 Diabetes, and the Diabetes Control and Complications Trial (DCCT)[4] for Type 1 Diabetes (Table 5).

References

1. Singapore Ministry of Health Clinical Practice Guidelines 3/2006.
2. David K. McCulloch, MD, Insulin therapy in type 2 diabetes mellitus, www.uptodate. com, Dec 12, 2011.
3. UK Prospective Diabetes Study Group (UKPDS 33), Intensive blood-glucose control with sulphonylureas or insulin compared with conventional treatment and risk of complications in patients with type 2 diabetes, *Lancet* **352**:837–53 (1998).
4. The Diabetes Control and Complications Trial Research Group, The effect of intensive treatment of diabetes on the development and progression of long-term complications in insulin-dependent diabetes mellitus, *N. Engl. J. Med.* **329**:977–86 (1993).

Section 2

Basic Science of Diabetic Foot

5

Anatomy of the Foot

Aziz Nather, Amaris Lim Shu Min and Zameer Aziz

Department of Orthopaedic Surgery
Yong Loo Lin School of Medicine
National University of Singapore

Introduction

The structure of the foot is superficially similar to that of the hand. However, detailed comparison shows that the two are markedly different anatomically, biomechanically and functionally. It is therefore not surprising that hand surgery departments all over the world deal only with hand surgery and not foot surgery. Instead, surgery of the foot comes under the domain of the ankle and foot division. It is, however, interesting to note that Hong Kong is unique in this particular aspect, as hand and foot problems are handled by a single, combined division of hand and foot surgery.

Surface Anatomy

Medial Side and Sole of the Foot (Fig. 1)

— *Medial Malleolus* — the medial surface of the lower extremity of the tibia
— *Medial longitudinal arch of the foot*
— *Metatarso-phalangeal joint of the big toe* — the joint found between the base of the 1st proximal phalanx and the head of the 1st metatarsal bone
— *Ball of the foot* — padded portion of sole of foot underneath the heads of the metatarsal bones, from the 1st to 5th metatarsals

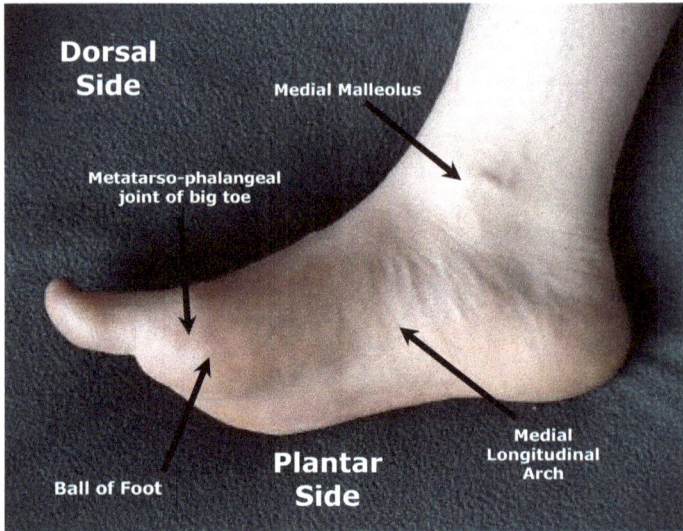

Figure 1. Medial side and sole of foot

Lateral Side and Dorsum of Foot (Fig. 2)

— *Lateral Malleolus* — the lower extremity of the fibula
— *Styloid process of the fifth metatarsal bone*
— *Interphalangeal Joints* — the joints between the phalanges of the toes
— *Metatarso-phalangeal joints of toes*
— *Tendo Achilles*

Portions of the Foot

The foot can be divided into 3 portions (Fig. 3):

— *Forefoot*: metatarsal bones and phalanges
— *Midfoot*: tarsal bones in front of the ankle joint
— *Hindfoot*: tarsal bones below and behind the ankle joint

Bones of the Foot

Forefoot (Fig. 4)

The forefoot consists of five rays of the foot – each consisting of a metatarsal bone together with its phalanx attached distally.

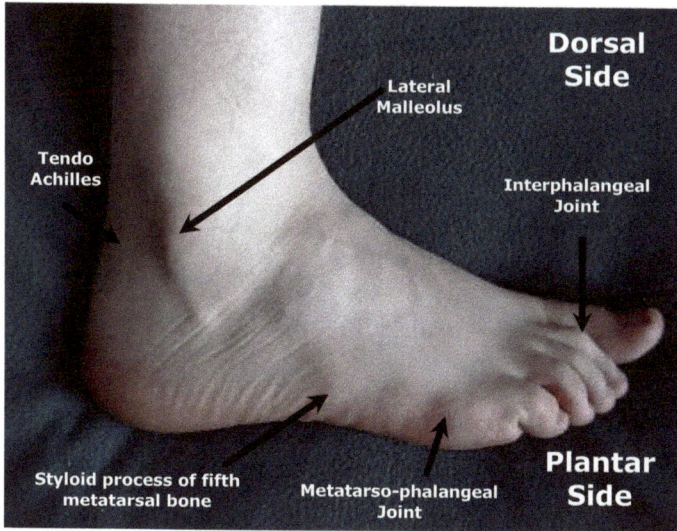

Figure 2. Lateral side and dorsum of foot

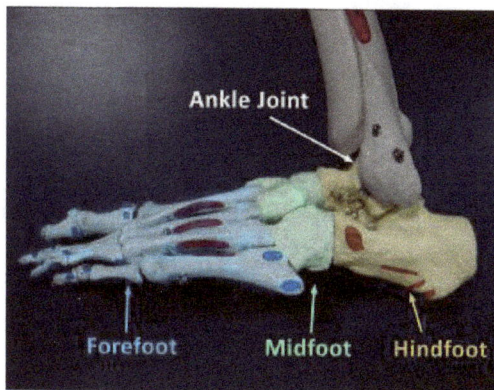

Figure 3. Portions of foot

Metatarsals:

These are a set of five long bones between the tarsal bones and the phalanges. The five bones are numbered (1st to 5th) starting from the medial side.

Phalanges:

These are the bones in the toes. The big toe (hallux), also known as the "Great Toe", contains 2 phalanges — the distal and proximal phalanx. Together with

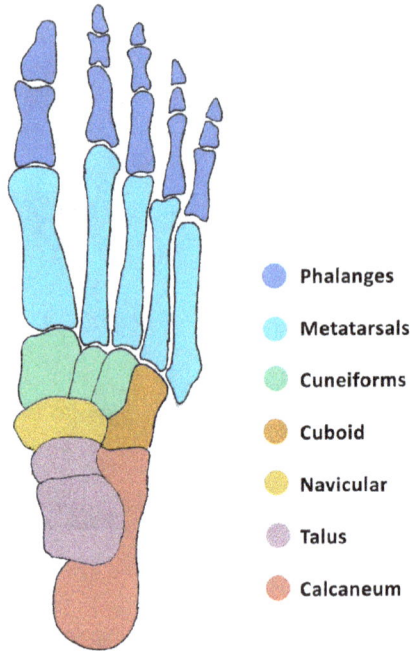

Figure 4. Bones of the foot

the first metatarsal head, the big toe plays a key role in weight-bearing and in propulsion of the foot.

The other toes each contain 3 phalanges — the proximal, middle and distal phalanges.

A "Ray Amputation" is an amputation that goes through the metatarsal bone — either the neck, the shaft or the base of the metatarsal. In contrast, a "Toe Disarticulation" refers to a disarticulation through the metatarso-phalangeal joint.

Midfoot (Fig. 4)

The tarsus consists of seven bones, making up the posterior half of the foot. The distal row contains four bones: the medial cuneiform, intermediate cuneiform, lateral cuneiform and the cuboid. These bones lie side by side and form the transverse arch of the foot, which is convex dorsally. On the medial side of the foot, the navicular bone is interposed between the talus and the three cuneiforms to form the medial longitudinal arch of the foot.

Hindfoot (Fig. 4)

The proximal row of the tarsus consists of the talus and the calcaneum, with the talus lying above the calcaneum. The calcaneum projects posteriorly to form the calcaneal tuberosity, the point where the tendo achilles is inserted.

Arches of the Foot

The arches of the foot are made up of the tarsal and metatarsal bones, and are strengthened by ligaments and tendons to support the weight of the body.

The longitudinal arch consists of the medial arch and the lateral arch. The medial longitudinal arch is formed by the medial three metatarsals (1st to 3rd), the three cuneiforms, the navicular, the talus and the calcaneus. The lateral longitudinal arch, on the other hand, is formed by the 4th and 5th metatarsals, the cuboid and the calcaneus.

The arches are maintained by the plantar aponeurosis (Fig. 5), which runs from the calcaneum posteriorly to the metatarsals anteriorly — much like a bowstring.

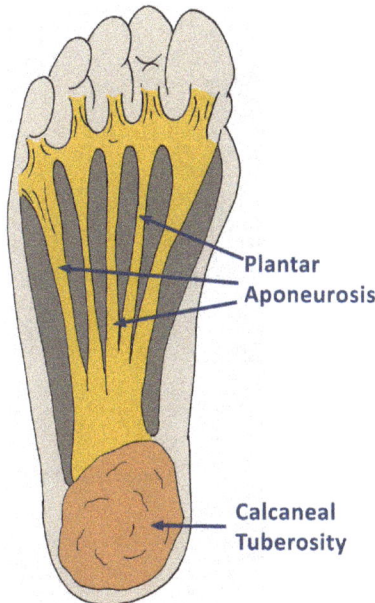

Plantar Aponeurosis

Calcaneal Tuberosity

Figure 5. Plantar aponeurosis of foot

Joints of the Foot

Lisfranc Joint (Fig. 6)

The tarsal bones of the distal row — the 3 cuneiforms and the cuboid — articulate with the five metatarsal bones to form the tarso-metatarsal joints. These are plane joints — also known together as the "Lisfranc Joint". Amputation of the foot through this plane is known as a "Lisfranc's Amputation".

Chopart's Joint (Fig. 6)

The talo-navicular joint consists of the articulation between the head of the talus posteriorly and the navicular bone anteriorly. This likes beside the calcaneo-cuboid joint between the calcaneus posteriorly and the cuboid anteriorly. The talo-navicular joint and the calcaneo-cuboid joint together form the "Chopart's Joint". Amputation through this joint is known as a "Chopart Amputation".

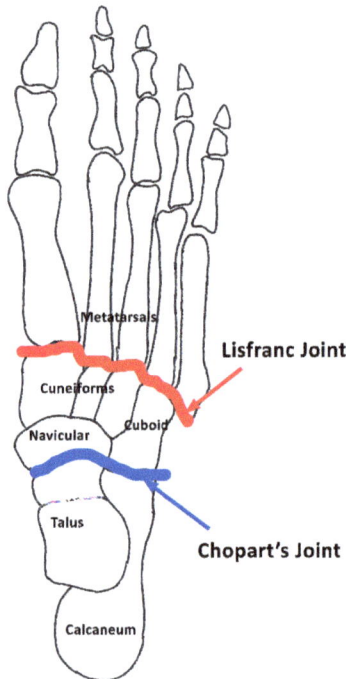

Figure 6.　Joints of the foot

Ankle Joint

The talus articulates with the articular surface of the tibia to form the ankle joint.

Muscles of the Leg

Muscles of the leg are divided into three groups: anterior, lateral and posterior. These muscles have tendinous insertions to the foot.

Anterior Muscles (Fig. 7)

The anterior muscles include the tibialis anterior, the extensor digitorum longus, the extensor hallucis longus, and the peroneus tertius. The first three work together to dorsiflex and invert the foot. The extensor hallucis longus

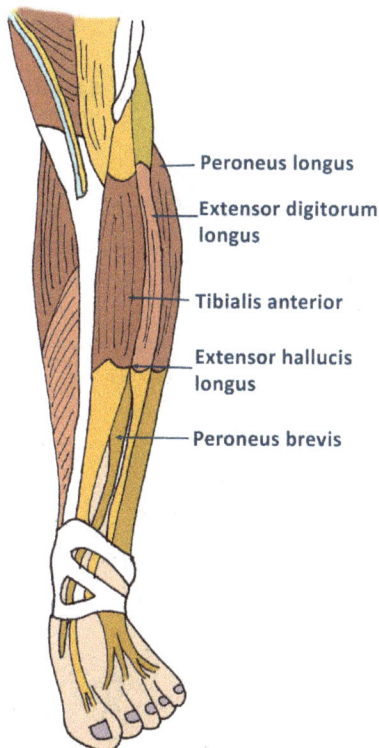

Figure 7. Anterior and lateral muscles of leg

additionally extends the big toe. These muscles are innervated by the deep peroneal nerve. The tibialis anterior is tendinous in the lower one-third of the leg and inserts into the medial cuneiform and base of first metatarsal.

Lateral Muscles (Fig. 7)

The lateral muscles consist of the peroneus longus and brevis, which evert and plantar flex the foot. They are innervated by the superficial peroneal nerve.

Posterior Muscles

The posterior muscles can be subdivided into two groups- superficial and deep. The superficial group consists of the gastrocnemius, soleus and plantaris (Fig. 8). These muscles are the main plantar flexors and are innervated by

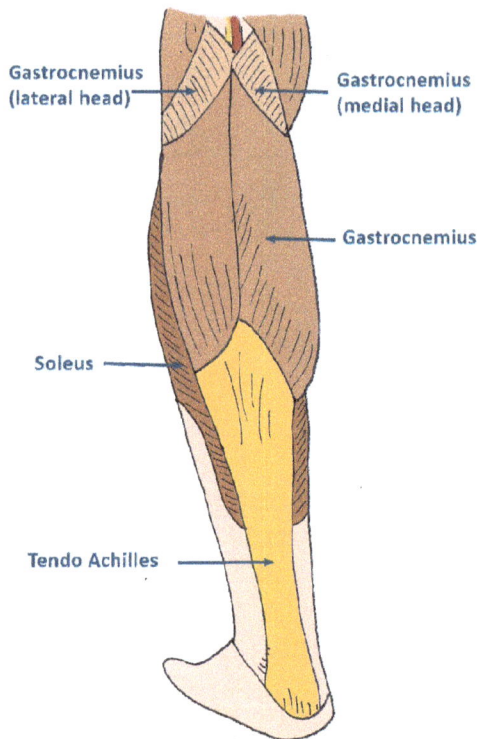

Figure 8.   Posterior muscles of leg (superficial)

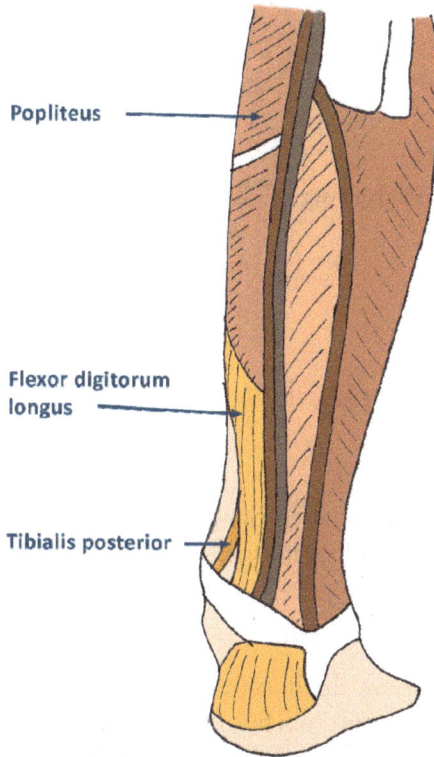

Figure 9. Posterior muscles of leg (deep)

branches of the tibial nerve. The gastrocnemius and the soleus converge distally to form the Tendo Achilles or Tendo Calcaneus, the strongest tendon in the body. The Tendo Achilles inserts into the posterior border of the calcaneum.

The deep group consists of the popliteus, flexor digitorum longus and tibialis posterior (Fig. 9). They are supplied by the branches of the tibial nerve. The flexor digitorum longus functions to flex the 2nd to 5th toes. The tibialis posterior passes behind the medial malleolus and inserts into the tuberosity of the navicular bone. It inverts and plantar-flexes the foot.

Muscles of the Foot

In addition to muscles that arise in the leg and terminate in the foot, the foot has intrinsic foot muscles — muscles that arise and terminate in the foot.

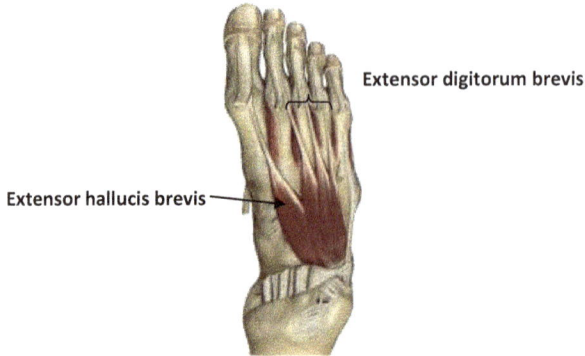

Figure 10. Dorsal foot muscles

The muscles in the foot are divided into two groups — the dorsal group and the plantar group. All foot muscles contribute to movement of toes.

Dorsal Foot Muscles (Fig. 10)

There are two muscles in the dorsum of the foot — the Extensor hallucis brevis and the Extensor digitorum brevis. They assist the long extensor muscles (Extensor digitorum longus) in extending the toes. The Extensor hallucis brevis helps to extend the big toe while the Extensor digitorum brevis extends the 2nd, 3rd and 4th toes.

Plantar Foot Muscles

The plantar muscles are arranged in 4 layers, as follows:

First Layer (Fig. 11)

Name of muscle	Function of muscle
Abductor hallucis (AbH)	Abduct big toe
Flexor digitorum brevis (FDB)	Flex lateral four toes
Abductor digiti minimi (ADM)	Abduct little toe

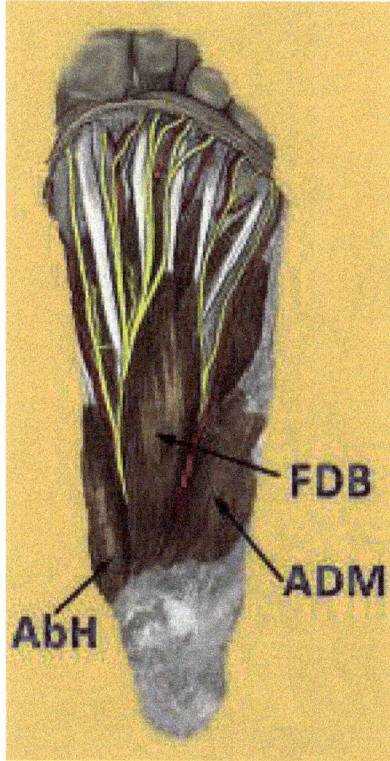

Figure 11.   First layer of muscles in the foot
Adapted from http://academic.amc.edu

Second Layer (Fig. 12)

Name of muscle	Function of muscle
Quadratus plantae (accessory flexor) (QP)	Assists flexor digitorum longus in flexing lateral 4 toes
Lumbricals (L)	Extend toes at interphalangeal joints

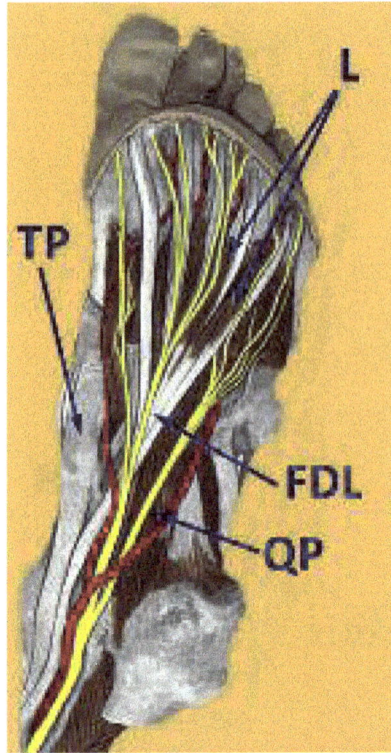

Figure 12.   Second layer of muscles in the foot

Adapted from http://academic.amc.edu

Third Layer (Fig. 13)

Name of muscle	Function of muscle
Flexor hallucis brevis (FHB)	Flex metatarso-phalangeal joint of the big toe
Adductor hallucis (Add)	Adduct big toe
Flexor digiti minimi brevis (FDMB)	Flex metatarso-phalangeal joint of 5th toe

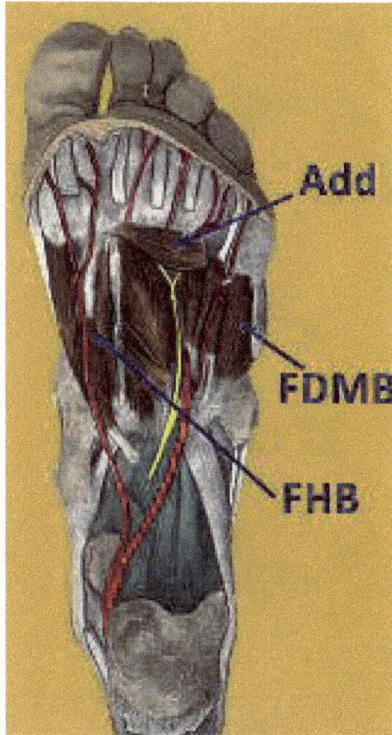

Figure 13. Third layer of muscles in the foot

Adapted from http://academic.amc.edu

Fourth Layer (Fig. 14)

Name of muscle	Function of muscle
Dorsal interossei (DI)	Flex metatarso-phalangeal joints and extend interphalangeal joints
Plantar interossei (PI)	Flex metatarso-phalangeal joints and extend interphalangeal joints

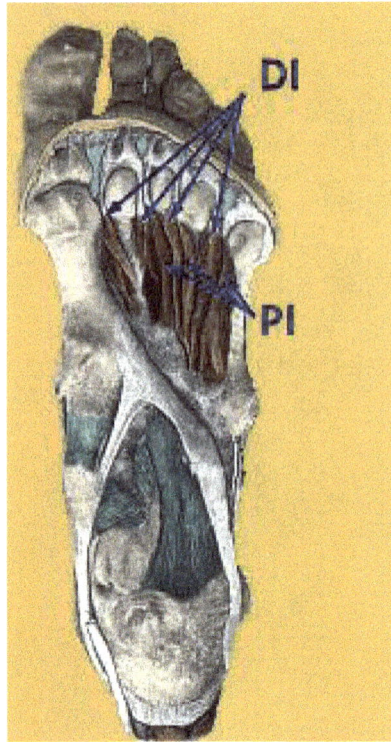

Figure 14.   Fourth layer of muscles in the foot

Adapted from http://academic.amc.edu

Blood Vessels of the Foot

Anterior Tibial Artery (Fig. 15)

The anterior tibial artery continues down the front of the leg behind the extensor retinaculum to the front of the ankle, where it becomes the dorsalis pedis artery. It carries blood from the popliteal artery to the anterior part of the leg and the dorsum of the foot.

Posterior Tibial Artery (Fig. 15)

The posterior tibial artery continues down the back of the leg and passes behind the medial malleolus deep to the flexor retinaculum. It divides into the medial

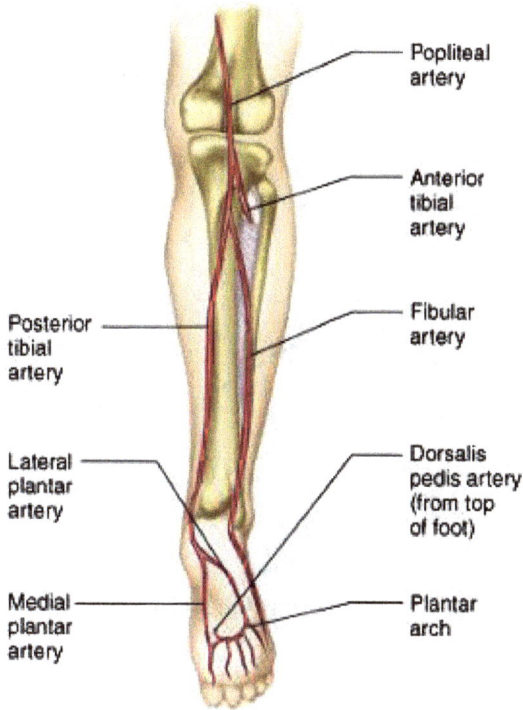

Figure 15. Arteries of the leg and foot

Copyright ©2001 Benhamin Cummings, an imprint of Addison Wesley Longman, Inc.

and lateral plantar arteries. The posterior tibial artery supplies blood from the popliteal artery to the posterior aspect of the leg and the plantar side of the foot.

Fibular Artery (Peroneal Artery) (Fig. 15)

The fibular artery is a large branch of the posterior tibial artery that arises just below the knee. It lies medial to the fibula, providing it with a nutrient artery. The fibular artery also supplies blood to the lateral part of the leg.

Plantar Arch (Fig. 16)

The plantar arch is an arterial arch in the sole of the foot. It is formed by the anastamosis between the lateral plantar artery and the deep plantar branch of

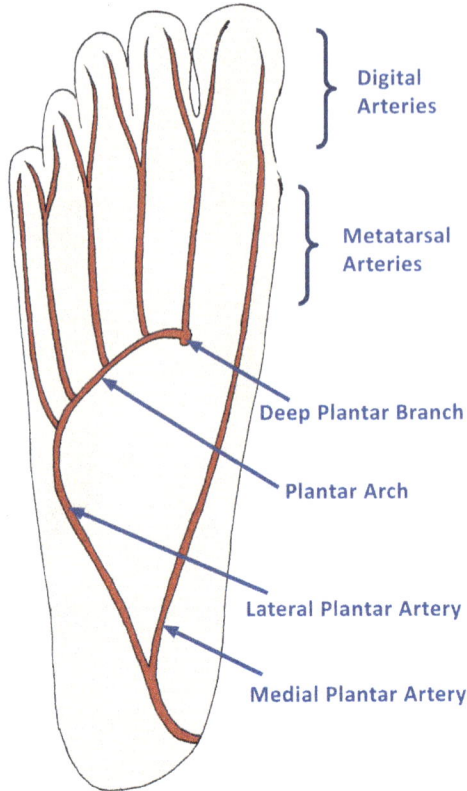

Figure 16.   Arteries in the foot

the dorsalis pedis artery. The plantar arch supplies the sole of the foot and extends medially from the 5th to the 1st metatarsal. The arch gives rise to the metatarsal arteries, which each branch into two digital arteries, supplying the toes of the foot.

Saphenous Veins (Fig. 17)

The great saphenous vein passes in front of the medial malleolus and continues up the medial side of the leg. It functions to drain the medial end of the dorsal venous arch, and empties into the femoral vein. The small saphenous vein originates from the lateral end of the dorsal venous arch, running behind the

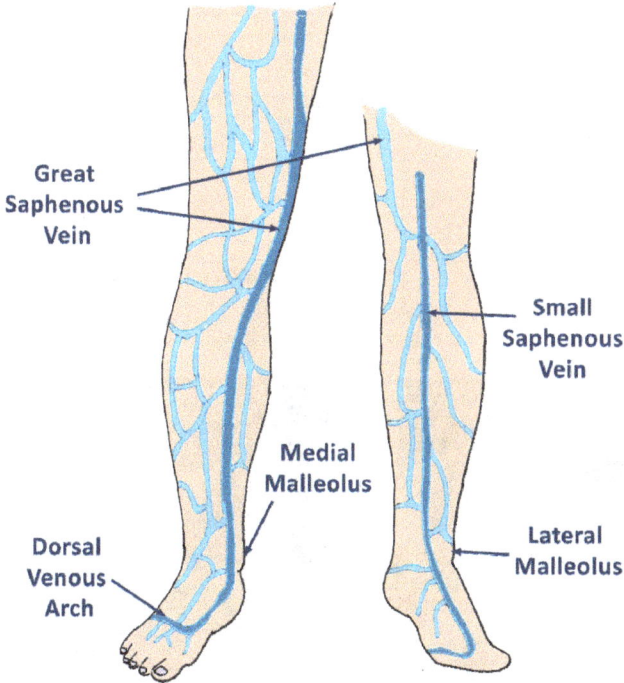

Figure 17. Saphenous veins

lateral malleolus. It continues up the posterior side of the leg, before joining with the popliteal vein behind the knee.

Angiosomes of the Foot

Introduction

In 1987, Ian Taylor and John Palmer introduced the angiosome concept. An angiosome is a three-dimensional anatomic unit of tissue (consisting of skin, subcutaneous tissue, fascia, muscle and bone) fed by a source artery.[1] 40 angiosomes were identified in the body. In 2006, Attinger and colleagues identified 6 angiosomes of the ankle and foot.[2]

Angiosomes of the Foot

The 6 angiosomes of the foot originate from three main arteries — the posterior tibial artery, the anterior tibial artery and the peroneal artery.

Posterior Tibial Artery

The posterior tibial artery supplies 3 angiosomes in the medial ankle and the plantar foot (Fig. 18). It has three main branches that each supply different portions of the plantar foot:

Medial Calcaneal Artery (MC):   Heel
Medial Plantar Artery (MP):   Instep
Lateral Plantar Artery (LP):   Lateral plantar surface and plantar forefoot

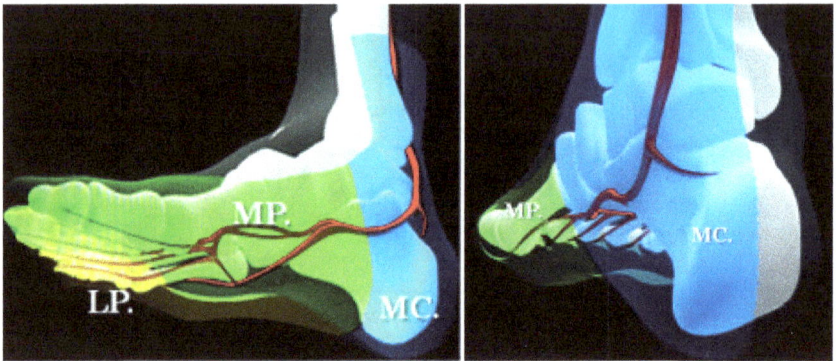

Figure 18.   Branches of the posterior tibial artery[2]

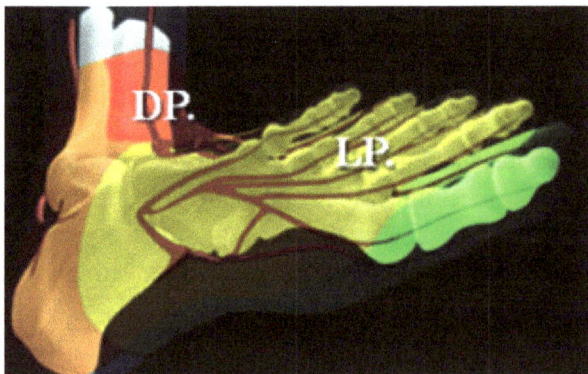

Figure 19.   Lateral plantar artery[2]

Anterior Tibial Artery and Dorsalis Pedis

The anterior tibial artery originates from the popliteal artery, and supplies the anterior ankle. Its angiosome encompasses the area overlying the anterior compartment of the foot. The anterior tibial artery forms the dorsalis pedis artery (DP) (Fig. 20), supplying the dorsum of the foot.

Peroneal Artery

The peroneal artery has 2 main branches that supply the anterolateral part of the foot as well as the lateral rear foot:

Lateral Calcaneal Branch (LC):   Plantar heel
Anterior Perforating Branch: Anterior ankle

Applications of Angiosomes

The angiosome principle is useful in making safe incisions in normal and vascularly compromised patients. It provides the basis for designing incisions and tissue exposure that preserve blood flow for surgical wounds to heal. There should be adequate blood flow to either side of the incision to optimize healing.

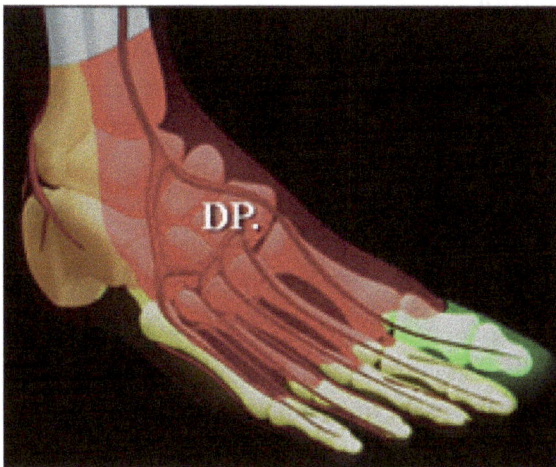

Figure 20.   Dorsalis pedis artery[2]

Incisions should therefore be made along the border between 2 adjacent angiosomes to allow maximum blood flow to each side of the incision.[3]

The angiosome principle is also useful in planning flap reconstruction of the foot and ankle. It is vital to ensure that underlying arterial flow toward the base of the flap is antegrade, and not retrograde, so that blood flow to the flap is not cut off. Understanding the angiosome principle can also help surgeons decide which artery to use for a particular flap.[3]

In a diabetic foot, the angiosome principle is important in healing foot ulcers. By understanding the principle of angiosomes and the vascular anatomy of the foot, wound healing and foot salvage will be easier to predict.[4] The angiosome principle is important for planning optimal revascularization of ischaemic wounds. Revascularization of the major artery directly supplying the ischaemic and ulcerated angiosome is more likely to successfully heal ischaemic lower extremity wounds than revascularizing other major arteries. Attinger *et al.* examined the results of direct versus indirect consecutive revascularization of 52 limbs. The study found that the amputation rate in the group with indirectly bypassed wounds was four times that of the group with directly revascularized wounds. They therefore supported the suggestion that direct revascularization of the affected angiosome leads to higher limb salvage rates.[3]

Nerves of the Foot

The tibial nerve divides into two main nerves that supply the sole of the foot: medial and lateral plantar nerves. These two nerves arise beneath the flexor retinaculum and run forward within the sole of the foot.

Medial Plantar Nerve (Fig. 18)

The medial plantar nerve lies between the abductor hallucis and the flexor digitorum brevis.

Muscular Branches: Supply the Abductor hallucis, Flexor digitorum brevis, Flexor hallucis brevis and the first Lumbrical.

Sensory Branches of the Great Toe: Supplies medial side of hallux.

Three common digital nerves: Each split into 2 digital nerves to supply 1st to 4th toes.

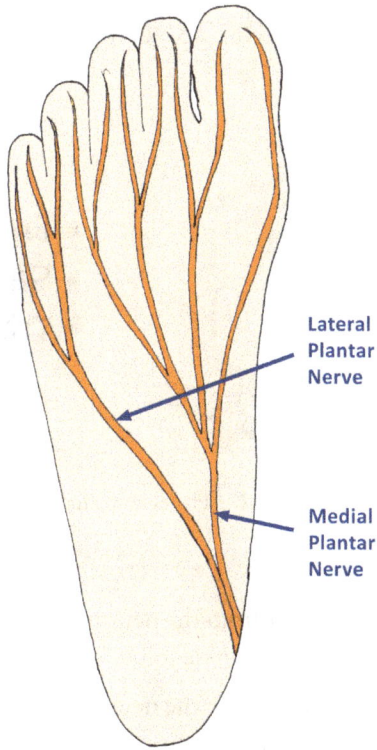

Figure 21. Plantar nerves

Lateral Plantar Nerve (Fig. 21)

The lateral plantar nerve reaches the base of the fifth metatarsal bone.

Muscular Branches: Supply the Quadratus plantae, abductor digiti minimi, interossei, 2nd, 3rd, 4th Lumbricals, and the Adductor hallucis.

Sensory Branches: Supply the 5th toe and the lateral half of the 4th.

Planes in the Foot

(a) Frontal plane
(b) Sagittal plane
(c) Transverse plane (Fig. 22)

Planes In Foot

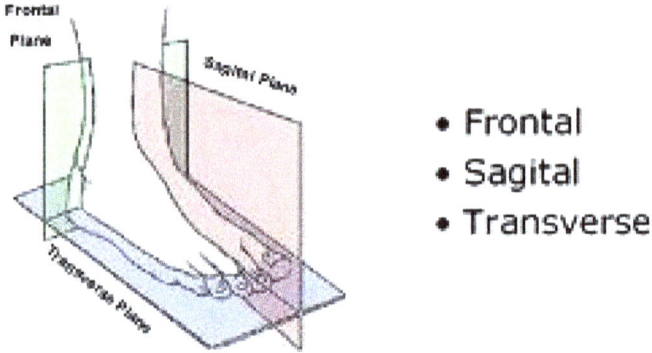

Figure 22.   Planes in the foot

Motions of Ankle and Foot

Dorsiflex: Extension of the foot from the neutral position in the sagittal plane of the foot. Motion occurs in the ankle joint.

Plantar-flex: Flexion of the foot from the neutral position in the sagittal plane of the foot. Motion occurs in the ankle joint.

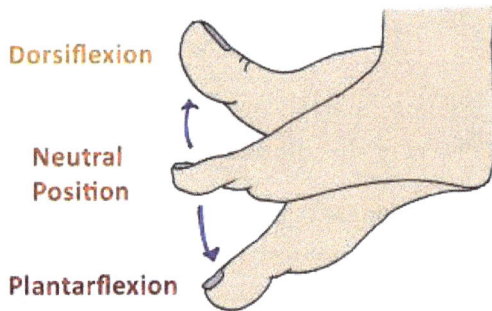

Figure 23.   Dorsiflexion/plantarflexion at ankle joint

Eversion: Lateral rotation of the foot in the frontal plane. Motion occurs in the subtalar joint.

Inversion: Medial rotation of the foot in the frontal plane. Motion occurs in the subtalar joint.

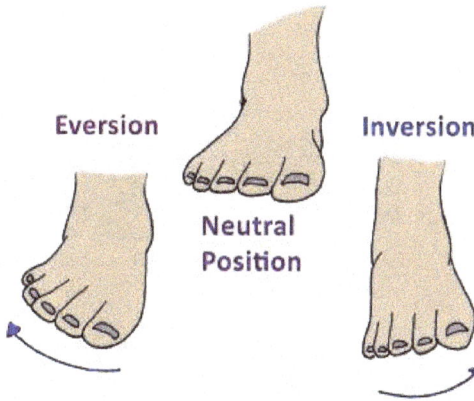

Figure 24. Eversion/inversion at sub-talar joint

Abduction: Lateral deviation of the foot in the transverse plane. Movement occurs in the tarso-metatarsal joint.

Adduction: Medial deviation of the foot in the transverse plane. Movement occurs in the tarso-metatarsal joint.

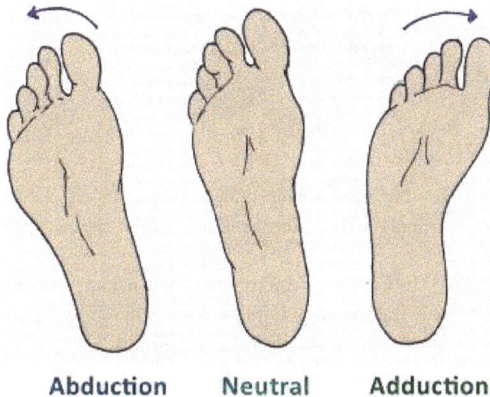

Figure 25. Abduction/adduction at tarsometatarsal joint

Pronation of the foot — A triplane movement consisting of abduction, dorsiflexion and eversion of the foot.

Triplane movement:

- Abduction
- Dorsiflexion
- Eversion

Pronation

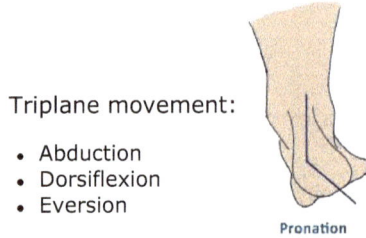

Figure 26. Protonation of foot

Supination of the foot — A triplane movement consisting of adduction, plantarflexion and inversion of the foot.

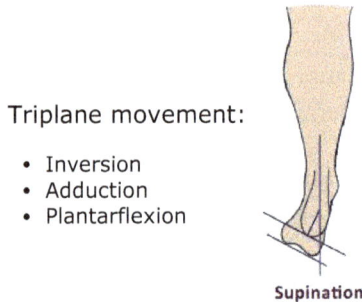

Triplane movement:

- Inversion
- Adduction
- Plantarflexion

Supination

Figure 27. Supination of foot

References

1. O. Iida, M. Uematsu and H. Terashi, The Angiosome Concept: A look at how this concept is being used to treat patients with critical limb ischaemia, *Endovascular Today*, Sept 2010: pp. 96–100.
2. V. Alexandrescu and G. Hubermont, Primary infragenicular angioplasty for diabetic neuro-ischemic foot ulcers following the angiosome distribution: a new paradigm for the vascular interventionist? *Diabetes Metab. Syndr. Obes.* 4:327–36 (2011).
3. C. E. Attinger, K. K. Evans and E. Bulan, Angiosomes of the foot and ankle and clinical implications for limb salvage: reconstruction, incisions, and revascularization, *Plast. Reconstr. Surg.* 117(7 suppl):261S–93S (2006).
4. L. Tudhope, Diabetic foot ulcers — the importance of angiosomes in healing foot ulcers, *Wound Healing Southern Africa* 1(2):13–14 (2008).

6

Biomechanics of the Foot

Aziz Nather, Amaris Lim Shu Min and Johan Steenkamp

Department of Orthopaedic Surgery
Yong Loo Lin School of Medicine
National University of Singapore

Introduction

Biomechanics is the application of mechanical principles of physics to living structures. It deals with internal and external forces acting on the human body. More specifically, biomechanics of the foot specifically focus on the interaction of the foot and lower extremity during ambulation. It studies how movements and forces in the foot affect each other.

In treating diabetic foot problems, it is important to first understand the normal biomechanics of the foot and lower extremity. This is then compared to the abnormal forces acting on the foot in patients with diabetic pathology.

Biomechanics of the Normal Foot

There are 26 bones within the foot, working together to support the body weight of an individual and perform daily activities such as walking, jogging, running and jumping.

Joints Involved in Biomechanics (Fig. 1)

The ankle joint and subtalar joint play important roles in the movements of the foot.

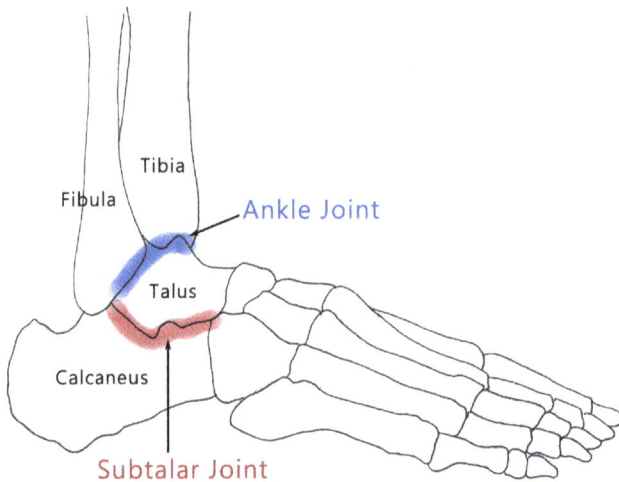

Figure 1. Ankle joint and subtalar joint

The ankle joint allows dorsiflexion (foot to move upwards) and plantarflexion (foot to move downwards). Extensor muscles in the anterior compartment of the leg produce dorsiflexion, while muscles in the posterior compartment produce plantarflexion. This is essential for bipedal ambulation.

The subtalar joint allows for pronation (rotation of foot inwards and downwards) and supination (rotation of foot outwards and upwards) of the foot to occur. This allows the foot to carry out its principal function of shock absorption during heel strike.

Arches of the Foot (Fig. 2)

The medial arch of the foot consists of the medial 3 metatarsals anteriorly and the calcaneum posteriorly. The lateral arch is flatter and comprises the lateral 2 metatarsals anteriorly and the calcaneum posteriorly. The arches are maintained by the plantar aponeurosis, attached to the metatarsals anteriorly and the calcaneum posteriorly. This causes the foot to arch like a bowstring.

Gait Cycle

A gait cycle starts when one foot strikes the ground. It ends when the same foot strikes the ground again. It consists of 2 phases — the stance phase and the swing phase. The stance phase is the period during which the foot is in contact

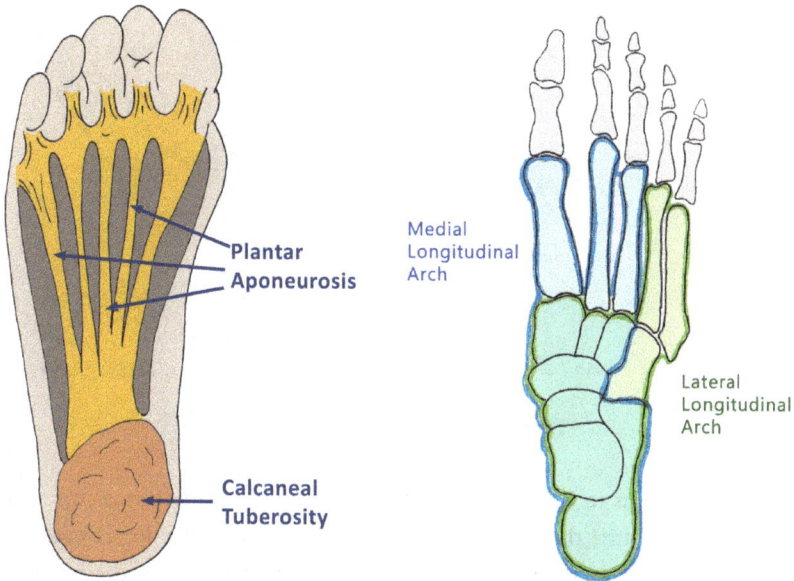

Figure 2. Arches of foot

with the ground. The swing phase starts when the foot is lifted in the air — it is the phase where the foot is not in contact with the ground. In normal gait, stance phase is about 60% and swing phase takes up the remaining 40%.

Stance Phase

The stance phase consists of 3 sub-phases: the contact phase, the midstance phase and the propulsion phase (Fig. 3).

Contact Phase

The contact phase begins with the heel strike, when the heel makes contact with the ground. This phase is completed as the remainder of the foot makes contact with the ground. During this phase, the foot pronates at the subtalar joint, the ankle joint is in a neutral position and the leg is internally rotating.

Midstance Phase

The midstance phase begins when the entire foot makes contact with the ground. The body weight is transferred fully onto the foot as the opposite foot

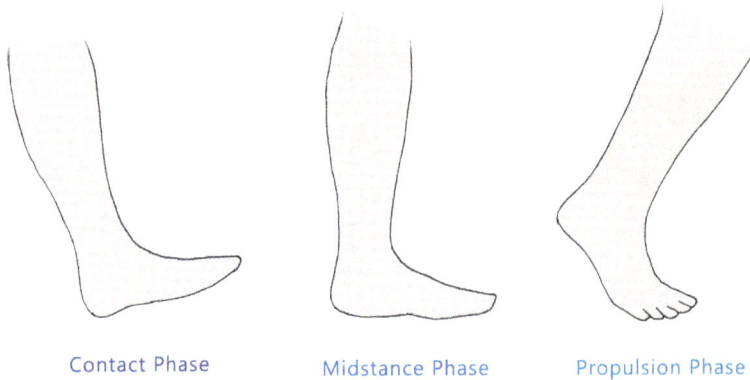

Contact Phase   Midstance Phase   Propulsion Phase

Figure 3.   Stance phase of gait cycle

toes-off and begins its swing phase. During this phase, the foot is supinating at the subtalar joint, the ankle joint is dorsi-flexed and the leg is externally rotating. The foot acts as a lever to propel the body forward during the propulsion phase.

Propulsion Phase

The propulsion phase follows. It constitutes the final 35% of the stance phase. It begins with the heel-off of the supporting foot. It ends with the toe-off of the supporting foot, and with the heel strike of the opposite foot. During the propulsion subphase, the foot is supinated at the subtalar joint, and the ankle joint is plantar-flexed. Body weight is shifted to the opposite foot as it contacts the ground. The foot is subjected to the greatest shear and vertical forces. As the forefoot is the part of the foot in contact with the ground, this relatively small area is subjected to the greatest pressure.

Swing Phase

The swing phase begins immediately after toe-off of the supporting foot, and ends with the heel strike of the same foot. It consists of the acceleration phase and the deceleration phase.

The acceleration phase occurs as the moving limb gains speed after leaving the ground. During deceleration phase, the limb slows down and returns to the ground. When the heel contacts the ground, the swing phase ends and a new gait cycle begins.

Tasks of the Gait Cycle

Three tasks are accomplished through the course of a gait cycle — weight acceptance, single limb support, and limb advancement (Fig. 4).

Weight Acceptance

Weight acceptance occurs during the stance phase of the gait cycle, over the period of initial contact and loading response. It involves the transfer of body weight onto a limb that has just completed swing phase, and is aligned unstably.

    Initial contact refers to the instant the foot contacts the ground, while *loading response* is the period following initial contact, before the opposite limb leaves the ground. (Fig. 5)

Single Limb Support

During single limb support, one limb supports the entire body weight and provides stability. It occurs during the stance phase of the gait cycle, and includes the phases of midstance, terminal stance, and pre-swing.

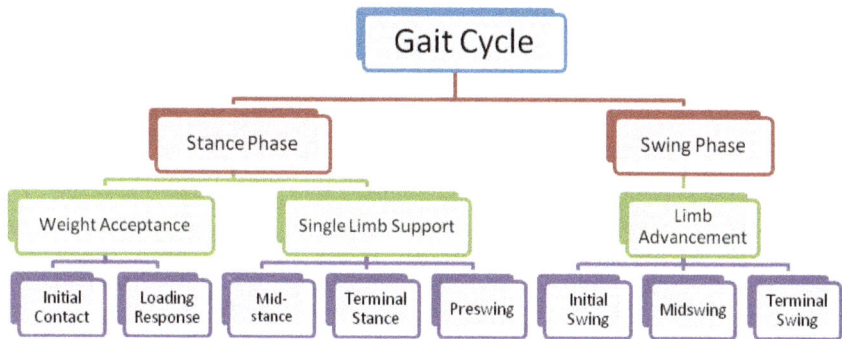

Figure 4. Tasks of gait cycle

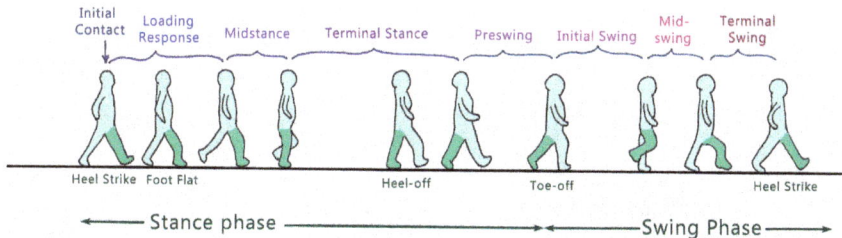

Figure 5. Gait cycle

Midstance occurs as the opposite limb is lifted, until both ankles are aligned in the frontal plane. *Terminal stance* is the period following ankle alignment in the frontal plane, until the opposite limb touches the ground. *Pre-swing* occurs when both feet are on the ground — it immediately follows initial contact of the opposite limb, before the limb in stance phase enters swing phase. (Fig. 5)

Limb Advancement

During limb advancement, the limb swings through three positions as it moves to the front of the body. It occurs over the swing phase, during initial swing, mid-swing and terminal swing. (Fig. 5)

Transmission of Forces in the Foot

During everyday activity, the plantar surface of the foot is subjected to forces from the ground acting upon it. This is known as ***ground reaction force***. (Fig. 6)

When standing, this force is equal to the individual's body weight, which is equally distributed. 50% of the body weight is absorbed by the foot. Higher pressures are experienced at the heel and forefoot.

Forces experienced by the foot during ambulation are higher than those experienced during standing. During the stance phase, the entire body weight

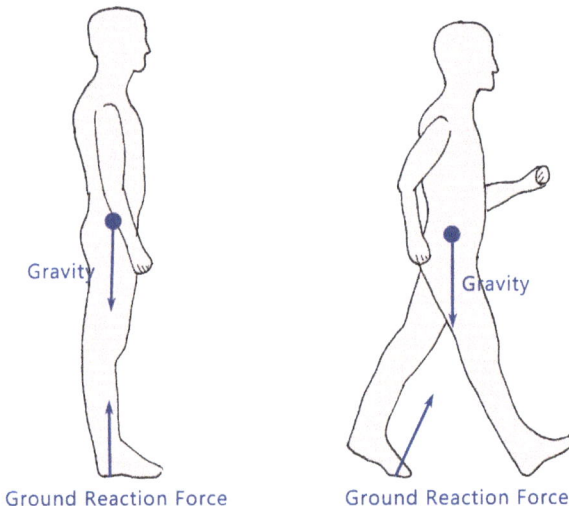

Figure 6.   Ground reaction force

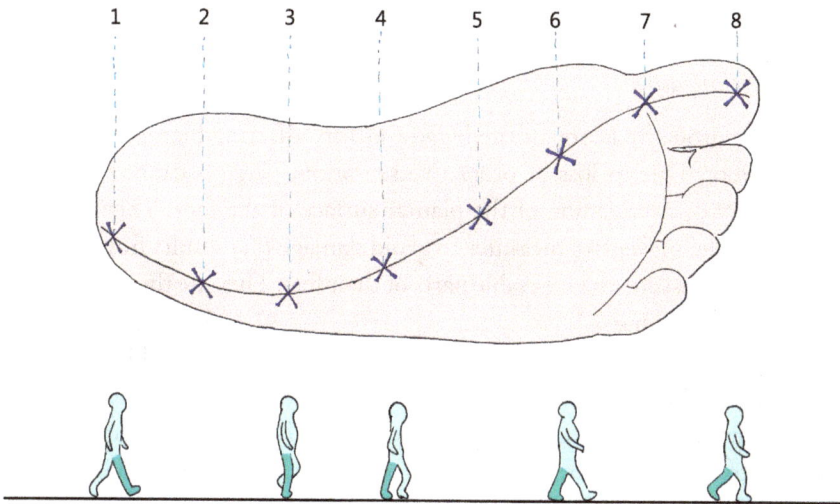

Figure 7. Transmission of forces through foot

is borne by a single foot. With transition from one phase of the gait cycle to another, different parts of the foot are subjected to greater forces at different times during the gait cycle.

In the above diagram (Fig. 7), transmission of forces through the foot to the ground is plotted at each point in the stance phase of the gait cycle.

During contact phase (1–3), heel strike occurs at the postero-lateral aspect of the heel. Most of the weight is borne by the outer edge of the heel. As the foot pronates (rotates downward and inward) due to internal rotation of the subtalar joint, weight is shifted to the medial edge of the foot. The arches of the foot flatten to distribute the force of heel strike. The ball of the foot makes contact with the ground.

During midstance phase (4–5), weight shifts from the posterior of the foot to the forefoot.

During propulsion phase (6–8), the foot acts as a lever, with the posterior part of the foot exerting force, and the ball of the foot acting as the fulcrum.

The foot is not just subjected to vertical forces. It also experiences shear forces maximum during the contact and propulsion phases. However, these forces are lower in magnitude compared to the vertically-directed ones.

Biomechanics of Pathological Diabetic Foot

Sensory Neuropathy

Sensory neuropathy is one of the biggest factors affecting biomechanics in a diabetic foot. Due to loss of protective sensation, patients cannot feel pain from injury or overloading of the plantar surface of the foot. They are thus unable to take preventive measures to avoid damage that results from overuse or excessive pressure on vulnerable parts of their feet. They are therefore prone to developing wounds.

High pressures occlude microvasculature in normal feet while standing and walking. With intact sensation, normal people are able to realize that certain parts of their foot are becoming ischaemic. They can then change their position to relieve pressure at those areas, restoring blood supply to ischaemic tissues. A diabetic patient with neuropathy would be unaware that areas of his foot are becoming ischaemic. He will not make changes to his position in order to restore blood flow to the ischaemic areas.

Autonomic Neuropathy

Autonomic neuropathy results in abnormally dry skin. This dry skin is more vulnerable to stress and strains. It can therefore develop cracks or fissures – a portal of entry for infection.

Motor Neuropathy

Motor neuropathy causes structural changes to the foot. Muscle wasting of the intrinsic muscles in the foot may cause hammertoes, claw toes, lesser joint dislocations, hallux valgus deformity and even collapse of the medial arch in the midfoot. These structural changes subject the foot to increased plantar pressure. Inappropriate footwear to accommodate these deformities is a major cause of ulceration.

Pathogenesis of the Diabetic Foot

Glycosylation

In patients with diabetes, glycosylation of collagen in the joint tissues occurs. This causes decreased elasticity and flexibility of the tissues. This results in stiffness of various joints in the foot such as the metatarso-phalangeal, subtalar and ankle joints. This results in altered biomechanics in the feet. Stiffness of the joints decreases the ability of the foot to adapt to undulating terrain, thus predisposing the foot to injuries.

Reduced mobility at the ankle and at the first metatarso-phalangeal joints can interfere with normal rollover of the foot during the Gait cycle. This results in higher plantar pressures, especially under the hallux during the toeing-off phase of propulsion, and higher risk of ulceration.

Charcot Joint Disease

The development of Charcot foot causes skeletal deformities. Normal biomechanics are altered. Awkward prominences are prone to increased forces and hence ulceration. Ulceration is also due to the loss of protective sensation in a Charcot foot.

Plantar Tissues

The plantar soft tissues in normal feet help to absorb shock and protect the foot from damage. In patients with diabetic neuropathy, fibrotic changes occur in the plantar fat pad. The plantar soft tissues also become stiffer and thinner in elderly patients with diabetes.[1,2] The plantar soft tissue is less able to absorb shock and deal with the strong forces exerted on the foot during contact and propulsion phases of the Gait cycle. Decreased plantar tissue thickness also causes increased plantar pressure. This increases the risk of ulceration.

Callosity

Uneven pressures exerted on the foot may result in a build up of calluses. In patients with diabetes, fatty infiltration of intrinsic muscles of the feet results in atrophy of the foot muscles.[3] This results in development of claw toes or hammertoes. The metatarsal heads are subjected to increased plantar pressure. Calluses may develop. Deformities in the foot due to Charcot Joint Disease are also predisposed to the formation of calluses.

Murray et al 1996 showed that the presence of plantar callus predisposed to foot ulceration. Callus formation may lead to high plantar foot pressures. The callus itself may also act an extrinsic source of stress. The development of callosities thus predisposes the affected areas to injury and ulceration.[4]

Partial amputations from neglected diabetic feet can also result in increased pressures in the remaining metatarsals further predisposing to ulceration.[5]

Techniques for Measurement of Pressure

Measurement techniques include *platform* types and *in-sole* types. Such pressure measurement techniques are extremely useful in identifying areas of high pressure, and hence high risk areas of the foot. Steps can then be taken to unload these areas, thus preventing injury from repetitive over-loading.

Platform Measurement Technique

The platform type measures foot-floor pressure and identifies areas of the foot subjected to high pressures (Fig. 8). However, the disadvantage of this method is its inability to measure pressure once corrective orthotic devices have been applied.

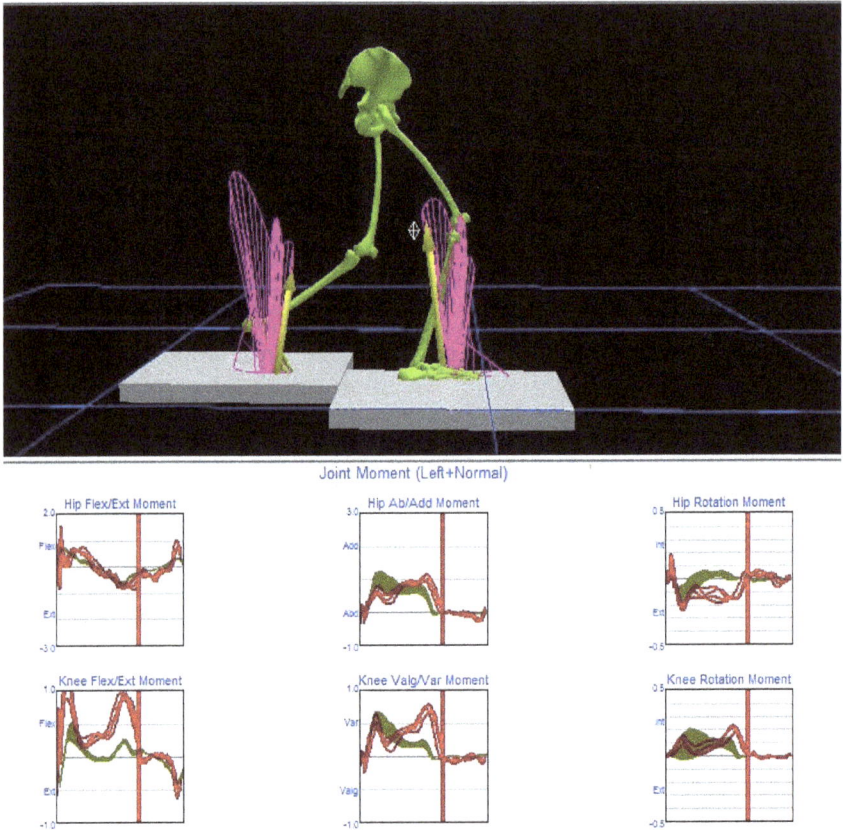

Figure 8. Platform pressure measurement technique

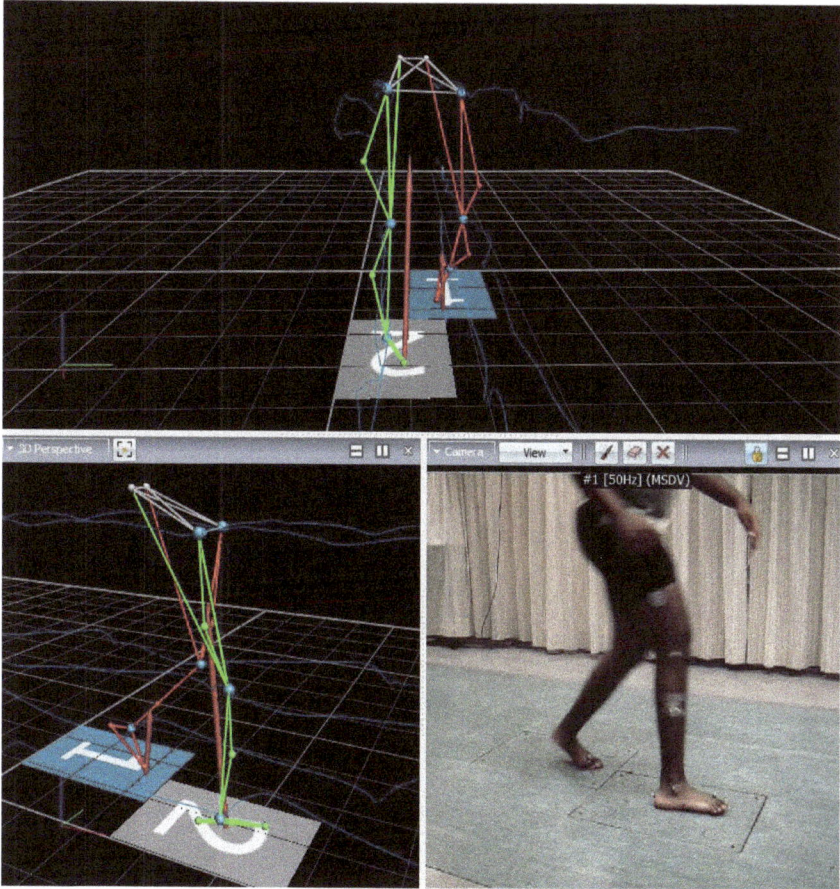

Figure 9.   NUH gait lab

The Department of Orthopaedic Surgery, NUH has a gait laboratory with a 3-camera Vicon System equipped with a Kistler Force Plate (Fig. 9). It is useful for measurement of forces transmitted to the foot during the Gait cycle. However, it is not useful for measuring effectiveness of custom-mode insoles or custom-made shoes for treatment of diabetic ulcers and deformities.

Insole Measurement Technique

The in-sole type is more practical and useful. It not only analyzes the pressures the foot is subjected to during various parts of the Gait cycle. It also allows for measurements to be made with the use of footwear. Measurements can then be

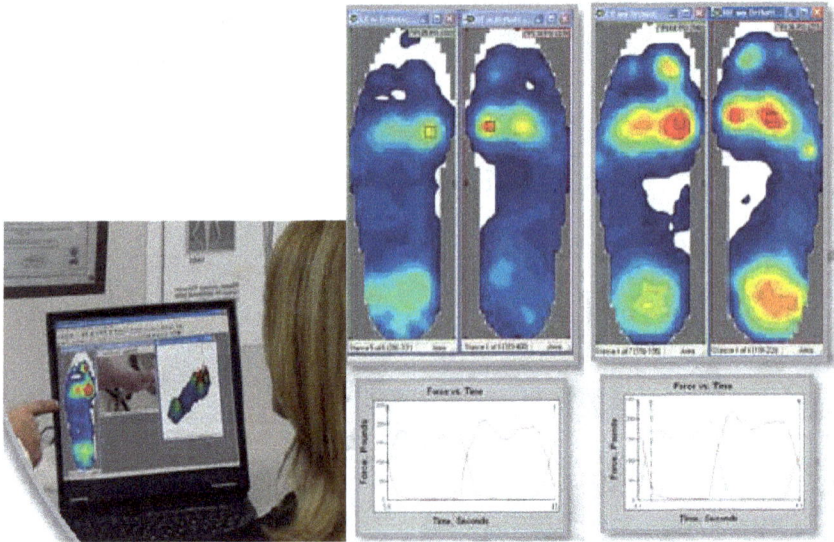

Figure 10.   F-Scan analysis

repeated after corrective orthotic devices have been applied. It can objectively measure the effectiveness of these devices.

F-scan Analysis (Fig. 10)

F-scan analysis makes use of paper-thin sensors placed inside footwear to capture dynamic in-shoe pressure distribution. Measurements can also be made after the application of orthotic devices such as insoles. F-scan analysis allows the force to be quantified, and determines the distribution and timing of contact pressure. In this way, orthotic footwear performance can be improved.

Conclusion

The key to management of the diabetic foot lies in the ability to identify the "foot-at-risk". This is only possible with a thorough knowledge of the biomechanics of the normal foot and that of the diabetic foot.

The development of diabetic foot problems is multi-factorial. Prevention of the formation of ulcers is of utmost importance. Attention to altered biomechanics can prevent the development of callosities and ulcers.

References

1. Y. P. Zheng, Y. K. Choi, K. Wong, S. Chan and A. F. Mak, Biomechanical assessment of plantar foot tissue in diabetic patients using an ultrasound indentation system, *Ultrasound Med. Biol.* 26:451–6 (2000).
2. A. Gefen, M. Megido-Ravid, M. Azariah, Y. Itzchak and M. Arcan, Integration of plantar soft tissue stiffness measurements in routine MRI of the diabetic foot, *Clin. Biomech.* (Bristol, Avon) 16:921–5 (2001).
3. H. Andersen, M. Gjerstad and J. Jakobsen, Atrophy of foot muscles. A measure of diabetic neuropathy, *Diabetes Care* 27:2382–5 (2004).
4. H. J. Murray, M. J. Young, S. Hollis and A. J. Boulton, The association between callus formation, high pressures and neuropathy in diabetic foot ulceration, *Diabet. Med.* 13:979–82 (1996).
5. C. H. M. van Schie, A review of the biomechanics of the diabetic foot, *Int. J. Low. Extrem. Wounds* 4:160–70 (2005).

7

Pathogenesis

Aziz Nather and Amaris Lim Shu Min

Department of Orthopaedic Surgery
Yong Loo Lin School of Medicine
National University of Singapore

Introduction

To manage a Diabetic Foot Problem effectively, one must first understand its pathogenesis — the "Diabetic Foot Triad"[1] (Fig. 1). 3 risk factors — Neuropathy, Vasculopathy and Immunopathy — contribute to varying degrees in different patients.

In some patients, one component dominates (e.g. dry gangrene due to ischaemia), whilst a combination of two risk factors may be responsible in others (e.g. wet gangrene due to ischaemia and infection). All 3 factors — neuropathy, ischaemia and infection — may contribute, resulting in Diabetic Foot Problems such as abscess and gangrene (Fig. 2).

Neuropathy

Neuropathy usually spells the start of a diabetic foot problem. Abbot *et al.* (2002)[2] showed that 90% of patients with diabetes with foot ulcers have peripheral neuropathy. Neuropathy includes motor, sensory and autonomic neuropathy.

Motor Neuropathy

Motor neuropathy presents as weakness of the foot muscles. Other clinical manifestations include clawing of the toes and wasting of intrinsic muscles.

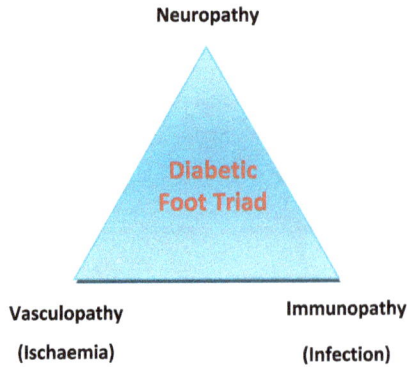

Figure 1.   The diabetic foot triad

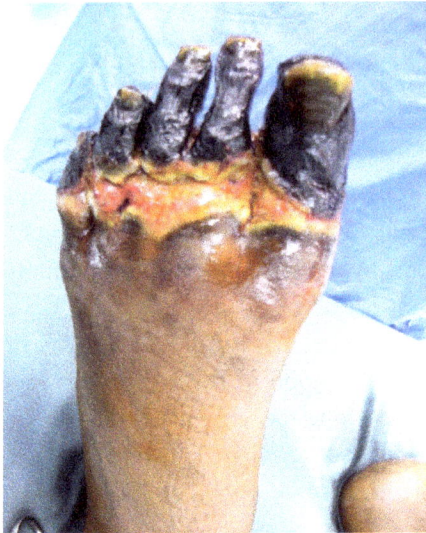

Figure 2.   Patient with diabetes showing forefoot gangrene and infection in a foot with sensory neuropathy

Sensory Neuropathy

The incidence of sensory neuropathy in Diabetic Foot Problem is 42.1% in our local study.[3] Sensory neuropathy may present as a "glove and stocking" sensory disturbance in the feet, where the sensation of wearing an invisible "stocking" is felt. The sensory disturbance consists of hyperaesthesia (abnormal increase in sensitivity, hypoaesthesia (reduced sensitivity), anaesthesia (completely lacking sensitivity to touch) or paresthesia (pins and needles sensation).

Autonomic Neuropathy

Autonomic neuropathy manifests itself as dryness of the skin.

Vasculopathy

Peripheral Vascular Disease

PVD refers to the obstruction of large vessels (eg. aorta, femoral arteries) and medium-sized blood vessels (e.g. popliteal, dorsalis pedis, and posterior tibial). In PVD, atherosclerosis (the hardening of artery walls) occurs, leading to ischemia (Fig. 3). The patient may present with vascular claudication, or more commonly rest pain.

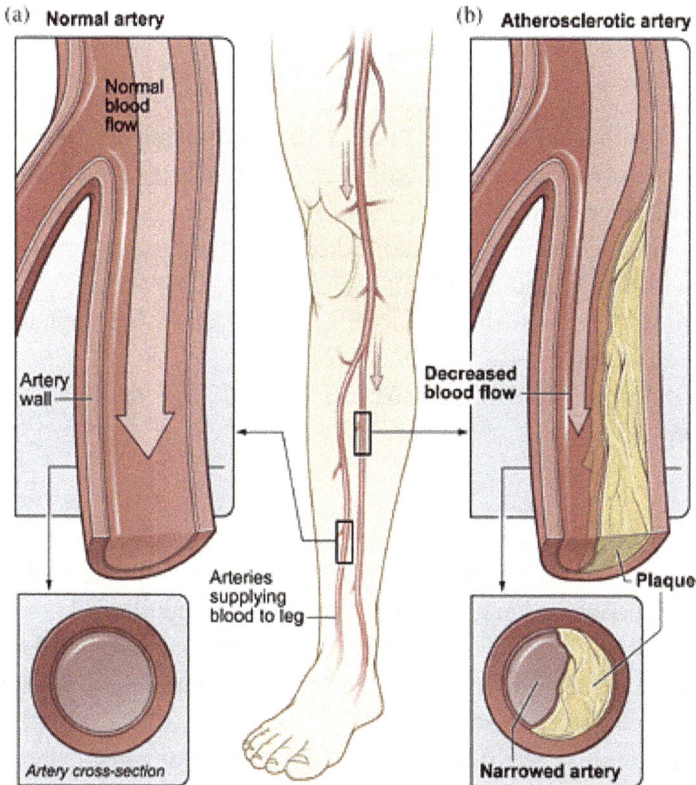

Figure 3.   Atheroschlerosis

Source: National Heart Lung and Blood Institute, USA, http://www.nhlbi.nih.gov/health/health-topics/topics/pad/

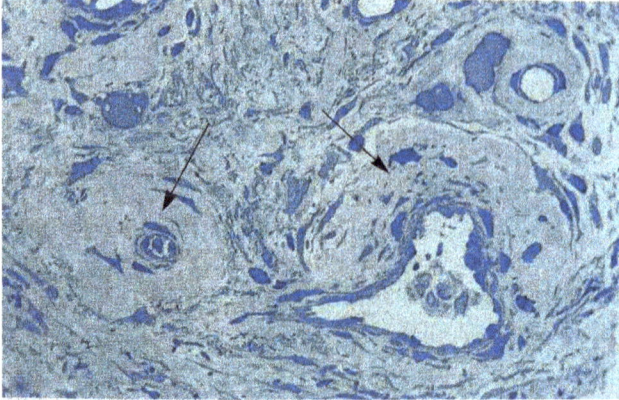

Figure 4. Showing thickening of basement membrane of endothelium

Microangiopathy

Microangiopathy may also occur. It is a disease affecting smaller blood vessels such as arterioles, venules and capillaries. Vessel walls thicken and weaken until they leak protein and blood, and obstruct the flow of blood in the body (Fig. 4). Terminal arterioles become blocked due to thickening of the basement membrane of the endothelium.

14% of diabetics with foot ulcers have Peripheral Vascular Disease — Abbot *et al.* (2002).[2] Nather *et al.* (2007)[3] in a study of 202 patients with DFP found that 54.2% of patients had an Ankle Brachial Index of <0.8 (indicating ischaemia).

Immunopathy

Patients with diabetes are inherently susceptible to infection due to defects in leukocyte function, although the exact mechanism is unknown. These defects lead to abnormalities in phagocytosis, neutrophil dysfunction (inability to kill and digest microorganisms engulfed by phagocytosis) and deficient chemotaxis (cell movement) and adherence of white blood cells.

The pathogens responsible for diabetic foot infections are predominantly gram positive cocci:

- Staphylococcus *aureus* (Fig. 5a)
- Group B Streptococcus *pyogenes*

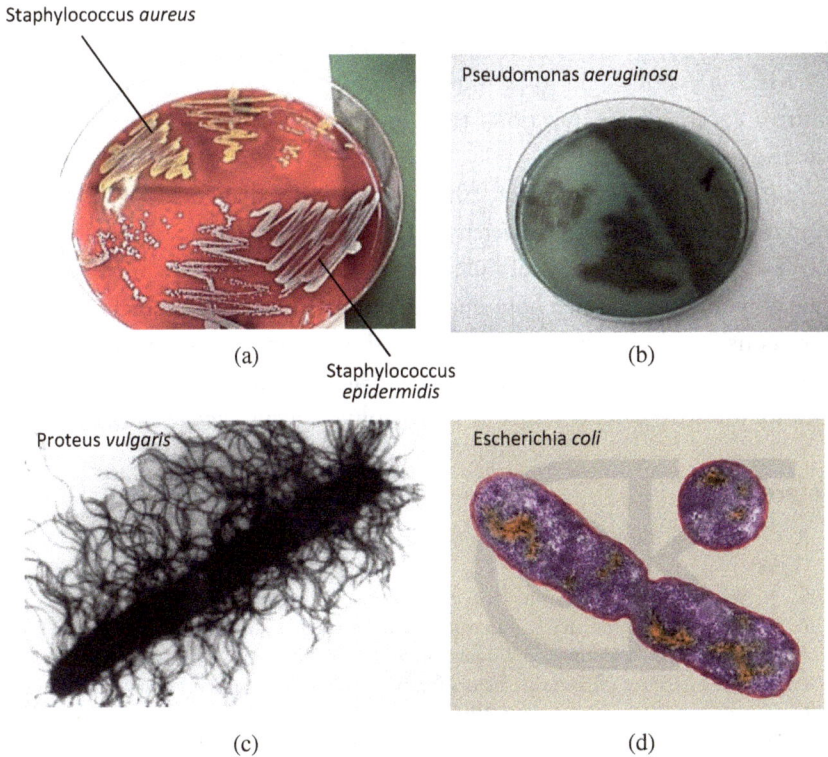

Figure 5. (a) Staphylococcus *aureus* and Staphylococcus *epidermidis* (b) Pseudomonas *aeruginosa* (c) Proteus *vulgaris* (d) Escherichia *coli*

- Group A Streptococcus *agalactiae*
- Methicillin Resistant Staphylococcus *aureus* (MRSA) — usually in patients who have been previously hospitalised

Patients are also susceptible to infections by gram-negative rods:

- Pseudomonas *aeruginosa* (Fig. 5b)
- Proteus *vulgaris* (Fig. 5c)
- Escherichia *coli* (Fig. 5d)

Anaerobes are present in 40% of diabetic foot infections:

- Bacteroides *fragilis*
- Peptostreptococcus are also present in some cases

The most common microorganisms in diabetic foot infections are Staphylococcus *aureus* (gram-positive) and Pseudomonas *aeruginosa* (gram-negative).

Mild infections tend to be monomicrobial and are mainly due to gram-positive cocci. Severe infections tend to be polymicrobial.[4] Gram-positive bacteria still dominate.

In a prospective study of 100 patients with diabetic foot infections treated at the National University Hospital of Singapore, Zameer *et al.* (2011)[5] found that 48% of infections were monomicrobial while 52% were polymicrobial. When both monomicrobial and polymicrobial infections were considered together as one entity, the commonest pathogens in this cohort were Staphylococcus *aureus* (39.7%), Bacteroides *fragilis* (30.3%), Pseudomonas *aeruginosa* (26.0%) and Staphylococcus *agalactiae* (21.0%).

References

1. R. G. Frykberg, Diabetic foot ulcers: current concepts, *J. Foot Ankle Surg* **37**(5):440–46 (1998).
2. C. A. Abbott, A. L. Carrington, H. Ashe, S. Bath, L. C. Every, J. Griffiths, A. W. Hann, A. Hussein, N. Jackson, K. E. Johnson, C. H. Ryder, R. Torkington, E. R. Van Ross, A. M. Whalley, P. Widdows, S. Williamson and A. J. Boulton, North-West diabetes foot care study. Incidence of, and risk factors for, new diabetic foot ulceration in a community-based patient cohort, *Diabet. Med.* **19**(5):377–84 (2002).
3. A. Nather, S. B. Chionh, Y. H. Chan, J. L. L. Chew, C. B. Lin, S. H. Neo and E. Y. Sim, Epidemiology of diabetic foot problems and predictive factors for limb loss, *J. Diabetes Complications* **22**:77–82.
4. R. G. Frykberg, An evidence-based approach to diabetic foot infections, *Am. J. Surg.* **186**(5A):44S–54S (2003).
5. Z. Aziz, W. K. Lin, A. Nather and Y. H. Chan, Predictive factors for lower extremity amputations in diabetic foot infections, *Diabet. Foot Ankle* **2**:7463 (2011).

8

Basic Science of Wound Healing

Teo Zhen Ling, Aziz Nather and Hey Hwee Weng Dennis

Department of Orthopaedic Surgery
Yong Loo Lin School of Medicine
National University of Singapore

Introduction

The treatment of the diabetic foot is mainly the treatment of wounds. To make wounds heal, one must understand the art and science of wound healing.

There are 3 phases in wound healing: Inflammation, Proliferation and Maturation. Clinically, there is considerable overlap between each of these phases. Wound healing is a dynamic process. It can progress forward and backward depending on the intrinsic and extrinsic factors present.

The inflammatory phase starts at the time of injury and usually lasts for 2–4 days. Proliferation begins around day 3. Maturation begins about 3 weeks after injury and may continue for six months to one year. (Table 1 and Fig. 1).[1,2]

Inflammatory Phase

The inflammatory phase is the cleansing and migratory phase. It serves to remove bacteria and limit the extent of tissue damage.

Table 1. Phases of wound healing

Phases of wound healing	Onset	Main cells involved
Inflammation	Day 1–7	• Platelets • Neutrophils • Macrophages
Proliferation	Day 3–21	• Fibroblasts • Myofibroblasts • Epidermal cells • Vascular endothelial cells
Maturation	Day 21 to 1 year	• Fibroblasts

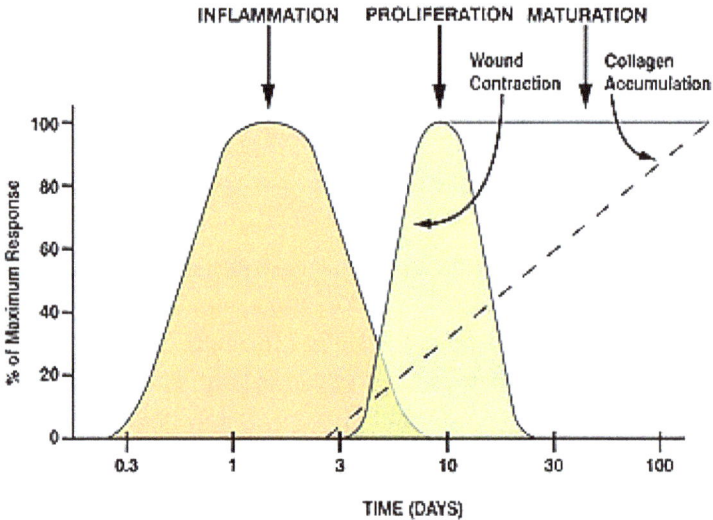

Figure 1. Phases of wound healing
(*Source: http://www.clinimed.co.uk*)

Blood vessels in the wound bed first contract to form a fibrin clot to achieve haemostasis. Once bleeding is stopped, the blood vessels then dilate to allow macrophages, neutrophils, growth factors, enzymes and nutrients to enter the wound.

Platelets are activated and degranulation occurs. The activated platelets release cytokines (Fig. 2 and Table 2), including transforming growth factor

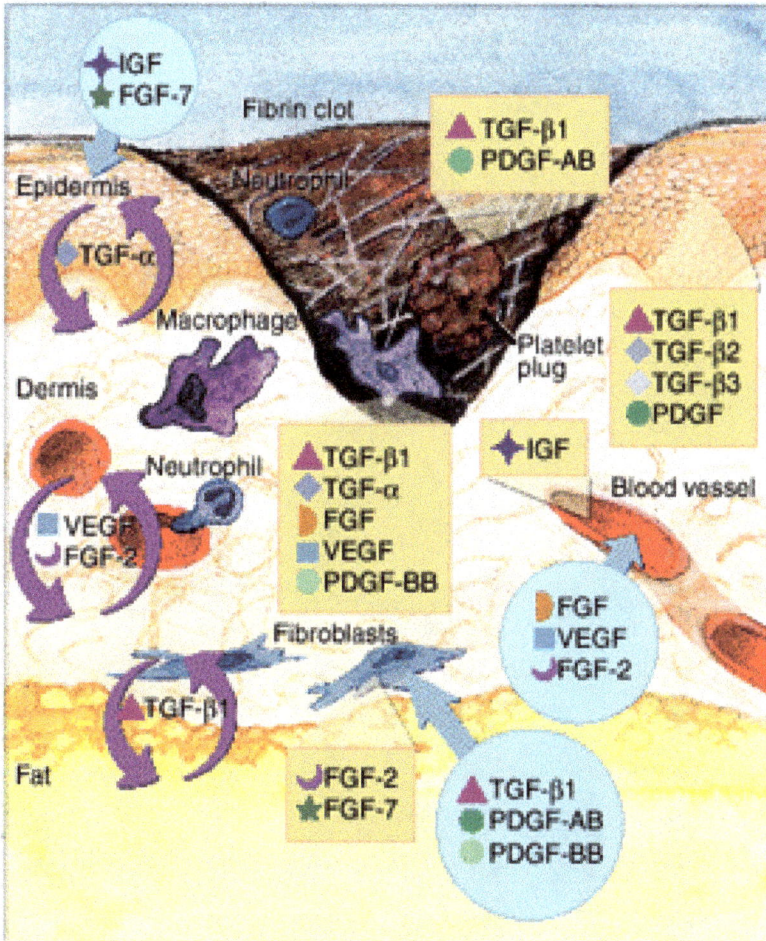

Figure 2. Factors released by various cells during inflammatory and proliferative phases
(*Source*: *Sharon Wahl. http://www.scienceboard.net*)

beta (TGF-β), platelet-derived growth factor (PDGF) and vascular endothelial growth factor (VEGF). Cytokines trigger the recruitment of inflammatory cells to the wound. The 2 main cells are neutrophils and macrophages.

Neutrophils begin the cleansing process. First, they engulf and digest contaminants and foreign debris in the wound. They then kill bacteria by producing free radicals. Neutrophils also secrete proteases to break down damaged tissue. Upon completion of these tasks, they undergo apoptosis.

Table 2. Source of various cytokines present during wound healing

				Cell Source –
Cytokines	Platelets	Mast Cells	PMN	Monocytes/Macrophages
TGF-βs	•	•	•	•
PDGF	•	•		•
EGF	•			•
TGF-α	•			•
VEGF	•	•	•	•
IGF-I	•			•
FGFs	•	•		•
Angiopoietin	•			•
FGF-7/KGF				
Endothelin		•		•
TNF-α		•	•	•
IL-1β	•	•	•	•
IL-6		•		•
IL-4		•	•	
IL-8		•	•	•
IL-10		•		•
SLPI	• *		• r	• r
MCP-1	• *	•	•	•
MIP-1α		•	•	•
MIP-2		•	•	•
IL-18		•	•	•
IFN-α/β		•		•

r = rodent, * = trace

(*Source*: Sharon Wahl. http://www.scienceboard.net)

Macrophages (Fig. 3) also help to clean the wound. Platelets release growth factors (PDGF) to attract monocytes to the wound. These monocytes subsequently mature into macrophages. Macrophages ingest bacteria, debris and dead neutrophils via phagocytosis. Macrophages then release growth factors and cytokines to stimulate and attract other cell types involved in the next phase.

Due to the host response mounted, any devitalized, necrotic and sloughy tissue is autolysed.

The dilation of blood vessels forms exudate in the wound, causing the tissue to swell (oedema). It also causes other signs of inflammation — erythema, maceration, warmth, pain and possible loss of function.

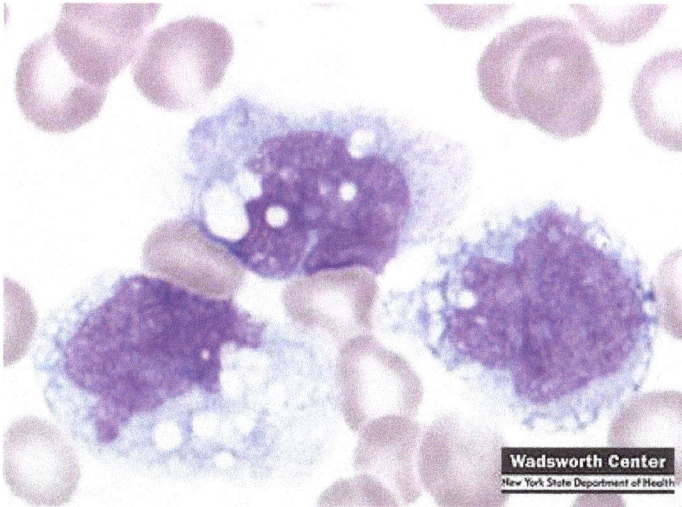

Figure 3.　Microscopic view of monocytes in the process of maturing into macrophages (*Source*: *http://www.wadsworth.org/chemheme/heme/microscope/monoblast.htm*)

Proliferative Phase

The proliferative phase is the phase of mesenchymal cell recruitment, proliferation and matrix synthesis.

Angiogenesis is initiated by factors (PDGF, VEGF, TGF-β, TGF-α, fibroblast growth factor (FGF)) released by platelets and further proliferated by similar factors released by mainly macrophages. This allows for the formation of new granulation tissue (Fig. 4) with collagen, extracellular matrix and blood vessels.

Fibroblasts are crucial in this phase. They migrate to the wound and proliferate under the influence of cytokines: FGF, insulin-like growth factor 1 (IGF1) and PDGF. Fibroblasts produce collagen that provides strength and structure to the granulation tissue formed.

Myofibroblasts located at the periphery of the wound carry out wound contraction by drawing the wound edges together via contractile features. Wound contraction (Fig. 5) occurs at an average rate of 0.6-0.7 mm per day,[3] varying in accordance to the shape of the wound and the laxity of the surrounding skin.

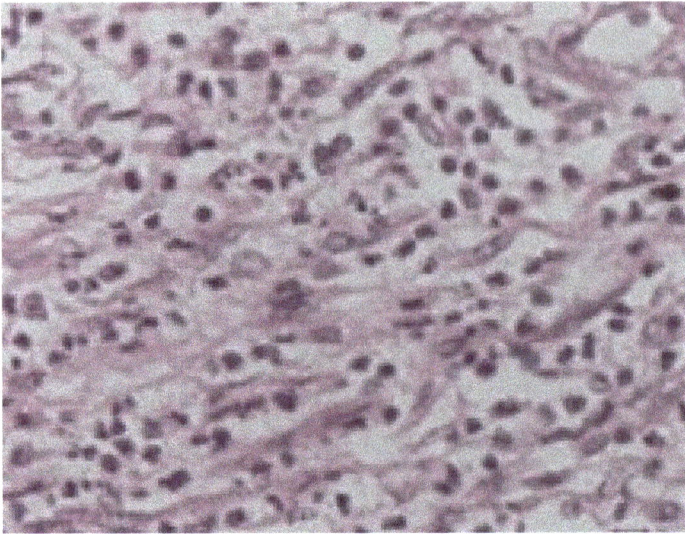

Figure 4. Microscopic view of a granulation tissue
(*Source*: *Robbins Pathologic Basis of Disease. http://pathology.class.kmu.edu.tw/ch01/Slide3.htm*)

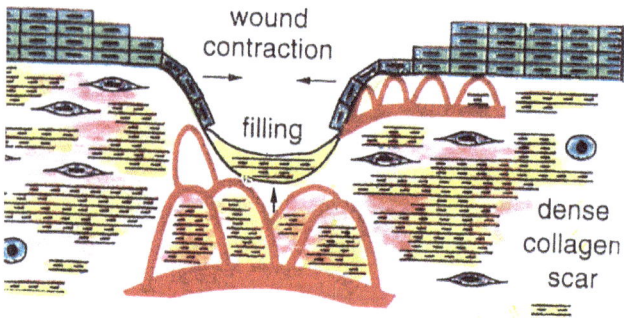

Figure 5. Wound contraction
(*Source*: *http://www.burnsurgery.org*)

Epithelialisation then occurs to resurface the wound. Epidermal cells grow over the top of the granulation tissue, preventing fluid loss and bacterial invasion of the wound.

Maturation Phase

Maturation is the final phase of wound healing. It involves wound remodelling.

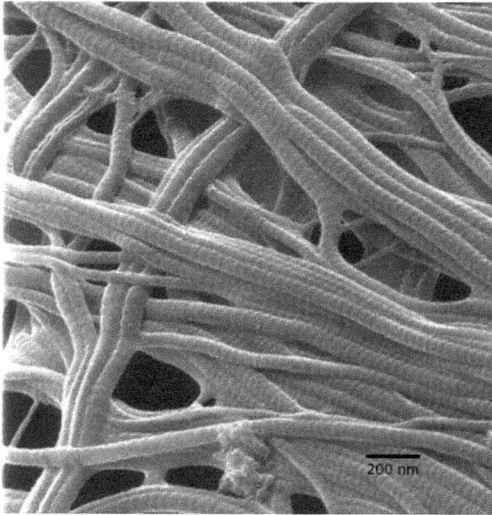

Figure 6. Electron micrograph of collagen fibres
(*Source*: *http://www.zeiss.co.kr*)

Scar tissue formation begins. The initial haphazard collection of collagen (Fig. 6) is degraded and replaced by a resynthesised collagen matrix, parallel to skin stress lines. Wound remodelling can continue for up to 1 year. The wound strength never returns to that of uninjured skin, reaching a maximum of only 80% strength.[4]

References

1. http://www.clinimed.co.uk/Wound-Care/Education/Wound-Essentials/Phases-of-Wound-Healing.aspx.
2. A. Gabriel, J. Mussman, L. Z. Rosenberg and J. Torre, Wound Healing and Growth Factors. *Medscape Reference*: article 1298196 (2011).
3. W. Naylor, D. Laverty and J. Mallett, *The Royal Marsden Hospital Handbook of Wound Management in Cancer Care* (Blackwell Science, London, 2001), pp. 12.
4. T. Dinh, H. Pham and A. Veves, Emerging treatments in diabetic wound care, *Wounds* 14:2–10 (2002).

Section 3

Classification

.

9

Classification Systems

April Voon Siew Lian and Aziz Nather

Department of Orthopaedic Surgery
Yong Loo Lin School of Medicine
National University of Singapore

Introduction

A good classification system takes into account the major risk factors involved in causing a diabetic foot problem — namely vasculopathy, neuropathy and immunopathy. Such a classification system serves to provide good guidelines for the management of these problems.

Most classification systems classify ulcers. These include the Wagner-Meggitt Wound Classification and the University of Texas Wound Classification. The King's College Classification, designed in 2000, takes into account other clinical features of the diabetic foot, such as cellulitis and gangrene.

Classification Systems

Several classification systems have been used for diabetic foot problems, including King's College Classification,[1] Wagner-Meggitt Classification,[2,3] University of Texas Classification[4] and PEDIS Classification.[5] The author prefers to use the King's College Classification as it is simple to use, its stages reflect different types of clinical presentations and it indicates the relevant type of management needed.

Table 1. King's college classification

Stage	Description
Stage 1	Normal foot
Stage 2	High risk foot
Stage 3	Ulcerated foot
Stage 4	Cellulitic foot
Stage 5	Necrotic foot
Stage 6	Major amputation

King's College Classification

The King's College Classification (Table 1) is a simple staging system. It is based on the types of clinical presentation of the diabetic foot — ulcer, cellulitis, gangrene and amputation.

The advantage of this system is that it is simple to use and is useful for planning the appropriate treatment for each stage.

Its disadvantage is that it has not been well-validated.

Stage 1: Normal Foot

There is no risk factor in the normal foot (Fig. 1). There is no neuropathy. Both foot pulses are palpable. There is no deformity, callosity or swelling.

Stage 2: High-Risk Foot

One or more risk factors for ulceration are present — namely sensory neuropathy or ischaemia (Fig. 2). In the latter, one or both distal pulses are not palpable. There may be deformity, callosity, previous ulceration or previous amputation in the foot.

Stage 3: Ulcerated Foot

This stage (Fig. 3) presents with skin breakdown or an ulcer. Ulceration usually occurs on the plantar surface in the neuropathic foot and on the dorsum of the foot in infection.

Stage 4: Cellulitic Foot

There is cellulitis with infection of the skin and subcutaneous tissue (Fig. 4).

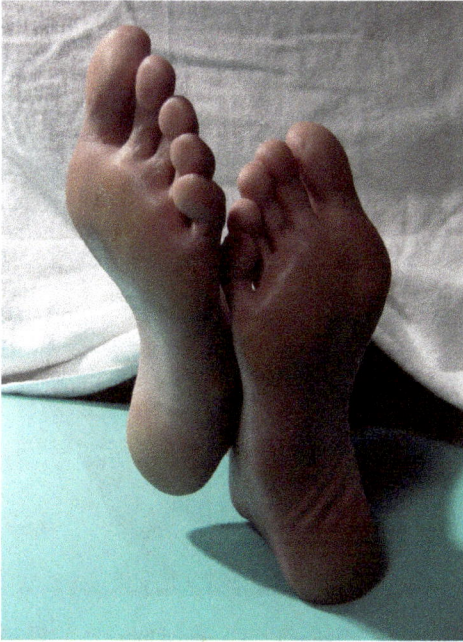

Figure 1. Normal foot

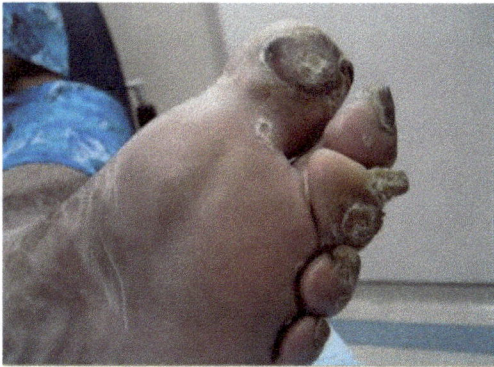

Figure 2. High-risk foot

Stage 5: Necrotic Foot

This is characterised by the presence of necrosis or gangrene (Fig. 5). Common sites of involvement are toes (one or more) and heel of the foot. They present as dry gangrene (no superimposed infection) or as wet gangrene (with superimposed infection).

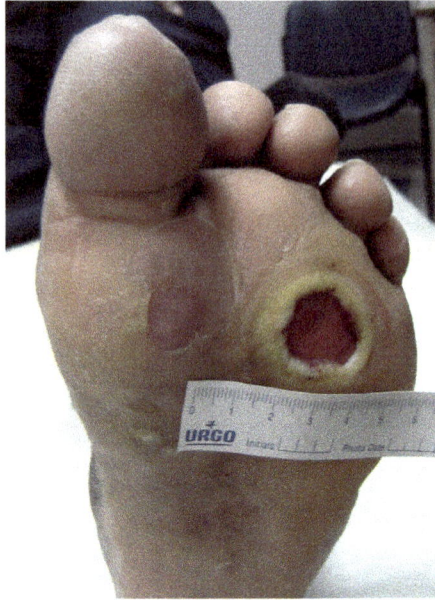

Figure 3. Ulcerated foot

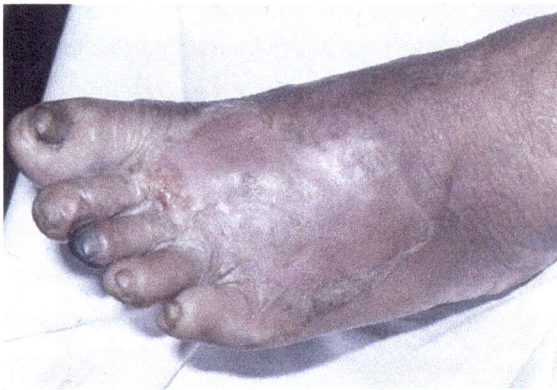

Figure 4. Cellulitic foot

Stage 6: Major Amputation

Major amputation (Fig. 6) is defined as one taking place above the ankle joint — namely below knee, through knee and above knee amputation. Causes of below knee amputation include agonising pain in the foot, overwhelming infection in the foot and extreme necrosis or gangrene involving the foot.

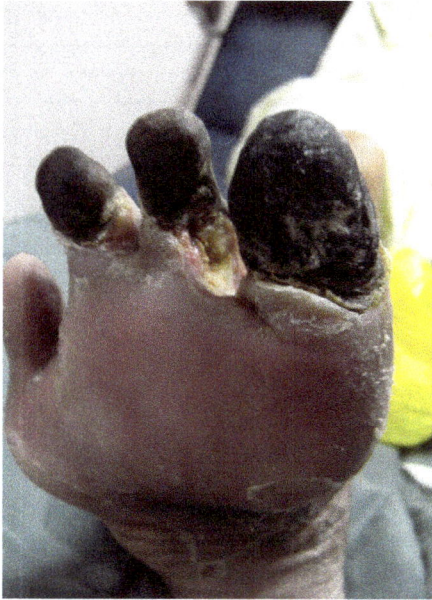

Figure 5.   Necrotic foot

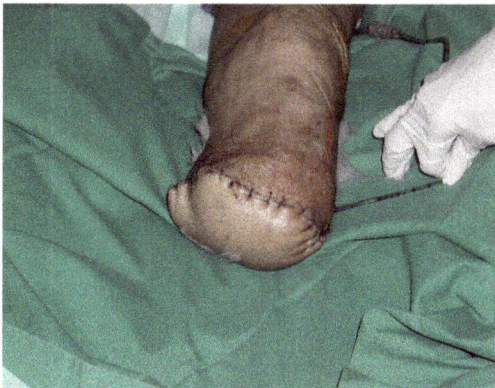

Figure 6.   Major amputation

Wagner-Meggitt Wound Classification

This classification (Table 2 and Fig. 7) was first described by Meggitt in 1976 and popularised by Wagner in 1981. It is a six-grade system that classifies ulcers according to the depth and extent of wound.

Table 2. Wagner-Meggitt wound classification

Grade	Description of ulcer
Grade 0	Pre- or post-ulcerative lesion completely epithelialised
Grade 1	Partial/ full-thickness ulcer confined to the dermis, not extending to the subcutis
Grade 2	Ulcer of the skin extending through the subcutis with exposed tendon or bone No abscess formation or osteomyelitis
Grade 3	Deep ulcer with abscess formation or osteomyelitis
Grade 4	Localised gangrene of the toes or partial foot gangrene
Grade 5	Whole foot gangrene

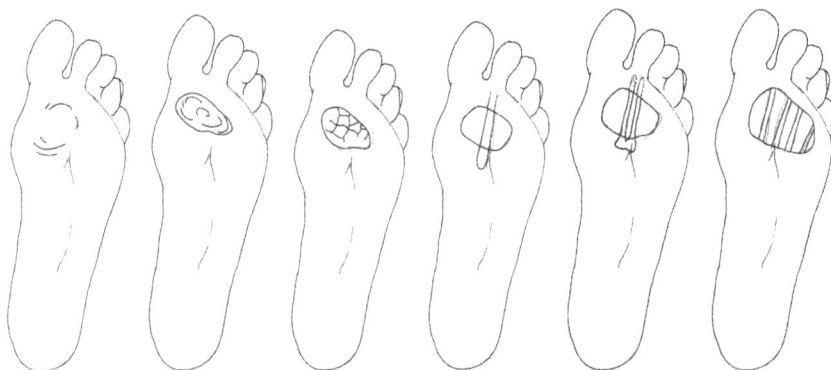

Figure 7. Wagner-Meggitt wound classification

Advantages of the Wagner-Meggitt Wound Classification include its simplicity in usage. It also provides a guide for practitioners to plan treatment.[6]

Disadvantages include the fact that infection is only taken into account in Grade 3 and ischaemia in Grades 4 and 5.[7] There is also controversy on the validation of this classification system.[8,9]

University of Texas Wound Classification

The University of Texas (UT) Wound Classification (Table 3) evaluates the wound for depth, infection, and ischaemia. Wounds are first graded as 0, 1, 2, or 3 according to the depth of the wound. It is further categorised into four stages (A to D) according to the presence of infection and ischaemia.

Table 3.   University of Texas wound classification

	Grade			
Stage	0	1	2	3
A	Pre- or post-ulcerative lesion completely epithelialised	Superficial wound not involving tendon, capsule or bone	Wound penetrating to tendon or capsule	Wound penetrating to bone or joint
B	With infection	With infection	With infection	With infection
C	With ischaemia	With ischaemia	With ischaemia	With ischaemia
D	With infection and ischaemia	With infection and ischaemia	With infection and ischaemia	With infection and ischaemia

The UT system has been well validated. Armstrong *et al.*[10] found that patients whose wounds probed to bone were more than 11 times more likely to receive a mid-foot or higher level amputation. Patients with both infection and ischaemia were approximately 90 times more likely to receive a mid-foot or higher level amputation.

The disadvantage of this system is that it is difficult to use in clinical practice because of the complexity of the grading system employed. It is perhaps better suited for research purposes. Another disadvantage is that it does not take into account the presence or absence of neuropathy. It also does not take into account the location and size of the ulcer involved.

PEDIS Classification

The PEDIS Classification (Table 4) was developed by the International Working Group of the Diabetic Foot (IWGDF) in 2003 for clinical research purposes. It includes five categories: Perfusion, Extent/size, Depth/tissue loss, Infection and Sensation. Within each category, wounds are graded based on severity using objective techniques described in The International Consensus on the Diabetic Foot.

Developed for research purposes, the system is highly complicated to use. The PEDIS system relies on up-to-date investigations for classification, including ankle-brachial index (ABI), toe-brachial index (TBI) and transcutaneous oxygen pressure ($TcPO_2$).

Table 4. PEDIS classification

Perfusion

Grade 1	No symptoms of peripheral arterial disease (PAD)
Grade 2	Symptoms or signs of PAD, but not critical limb ischaemia (CLI)
Grade 3	Evidence of CLI

Extent/size   Wound size (in cm^2)

Depth/tissue loss

Grade 1	Superficial, full-thickness ulcer
Grade 2	Deep ulcer, penetrating to subcutaneous structures, involving fascia, muscle or tendon
Grade 3	Bone or joint exposed

Infection

Grade 1	No symptoms or signs of infection
Grade 2	Infection involving skin and subcutaneous tissue only
Grade 3	Erythema >2 cm Infection involving deeper structures eg. abscess, osteomyelitis, septic arthritis or fasciitis
Grade 4	Foot infection with signs of systemic response

Sensation

Grade 1	No loss of protective sensation
Grade 2	Loss of protective sensation

The Infectious Disease Society of America (IDSA) Guidelines have used the PEDIS system to recommend treatment according to the severity of infection.[11] For Infection, Grade 1 does not usually require antibiotics. Grades 2 and 3 with less severe infections can be continued with oral antibiotics. Grade 4 with severe infection and critical limb ischaemia usually require hospitalisation and intravenous antibiotics.

Conclusion

The classification system most popularly used for clinical practice is the Wagner-Meggitt Wound Classification. The King's College Classification is gaining popularity. The University of Texas Wound Classification and the PEDIS Classification are not commonly used in the clinical setting. They are more suited for research.

References

1. M. E. Edmonds and A. V. M. Foster, *Managing the Diabetic Foot* (Blackwell Science, 2000).
2. B. Meggitt, Surgical management of the diabetic foot, *Br. J. Hosp. Med.* **16**:227–32 (1976).

3. F. W. Wagner, The dysvascular foot: a system for diagnosis and treatment, *Foot Ankle* 2(2):64–122 (1981).
4. L. A. Lavery, D. G. Armstrong and L. B. Harkless, Classification of diabetic foot wounds: the University of Texas San Antonio diabetic wound classification system, *Ostomy Wound Manage.* 43(2):44–53 (1997).
5. N. C. Schaper, Diabetic foot ulcer classification system for research purposes: a progress report on criteria for including patients in research studies, *Diabetes Metab. Res. Rev.* 20(Suppl I):S90–5 (2004).
6. N. Katsilambros, E. Dounis, K. Makrilakis, N. Tentolouris and P. Tsapogas, *Atlas of the Diabetic Foot*, 2nd Edition (Wiley-Blackwell, 2010).
7. D. G. Armstrong and E. J. G. Peters, Classification of wounds of the diabetic foot, *Curr. Diab. Rep.* 1(3):233–8 (2001).
8. J. H. Calhoun, J. Cantrell, J. Cobos, J. Lacy, R. R. Valdez, J. Hokanson and J. T. Mader, Treatment of diabetic foot infections: Wagner classification, therapy, and outcome, *Foot Ankle* 9(3):101–6 (1988).
9. S. O. Oyibo, E. B. Jude, I. Tarawneh, H. C. Nguyen, L. B. Harkless and A. J. Boulton, A comparison of two diabetic foot ulcer classification systems: the Wagner and the University of Texas wound classification systems, *Diabetes Care* 24(1):84–8 (2001).
10. D. G. Armstrong, L. A. Lavery and L. B. Harkless, Validation of a diabetic wound classification system. The contribution of depth, infection, and ischaemia to risk of amputation (see comments), *Diabetes Care* 21(5):855–9 (1998).
11. B. A. Lipsky, A. R. Berendt, H. G. Deery, J. M. Embil, W. S. Joseph, A. W. Karchmer, J. L. LeFrock, D. P. Lew, J. T. Mader, C. Norden and J. S. Tan, IDSA guidelines: diagnosis and treatment of diabetic foot infections, *Clin. Infect. Dis.* 39:885–910 (2004).

10

Foot At Risk

Aziz Nather and April Voon Siew Lian

Department of Orthopaedic Surgery
Yong Loo Lin School of Medicine
National University of Singapore

Introduction

The 'Foot At Risk' is defined as the foot with the potential to ulcerate. This is because a high percentage of diabetic foot ulcers lead to lower limb amputations.

- Foot ulceration is a common complication of all diabetics (12–25%)[1]
- 84% of non-traumatic limb amputations in diabetics are preceded by foot ulcers[2]

Foot ulcers involve a break in the skin's protective covering that extends into or through the dermis and may involve the underlying structural tissues.

Identification of Foot At Risk

There are 4 key features for risk of ulceration:

- Loss of protective sensation (peripheral neuropathy)
- One or both distal pulses not palpable (peripheral arterial disease)
- Presence of foot deformity or callosity
- Inability to reach foot or visual impairment

Peripheral neuropathy has been shown to be the most common risk factor and was present in 78% of foot ulceration cases.[3] This long-term complication of diabetes occurs in up to 58% of all diabetic patients.[4] The presence of peripheral neuropathy is evaluated under 'Part III Assessment: Neurological Assessment' in the foot screening protocol outlined in the next section.

Lower-limb ischaemia, a severe form of peripheral arterial disease, is a significant risk factor present in 35% of foot ulceration cases.[3] Peripheral arterial disease occurs in 10.4% of diabetic patients in Singapore.[5] Smoking, hypertension and hyperlipidemia commonly increases the risk of peripheral arterial disease in diabetics.[4] The presence of peripheral arterial disease is evaluated under 'Part IV Assessment: Vascular Assessment' in the foot screening protocol.

Foot deformities in diabetic patients lead to focal areas of high pressure. Foot ulcers can develop when foot deformities are coupled with lack of sensation.[4] The presence of foot deformities is evaluated under 'Part II Assessment: Clinical Evaluation' in the foot screening protocol.

IWGDF Risk Stratification Tool

The International Working Group on the Diabetic Foot (IWGDF) developed a risk stratification tool (Fig. 1) to predict the risk of foot ulceration in diabetic

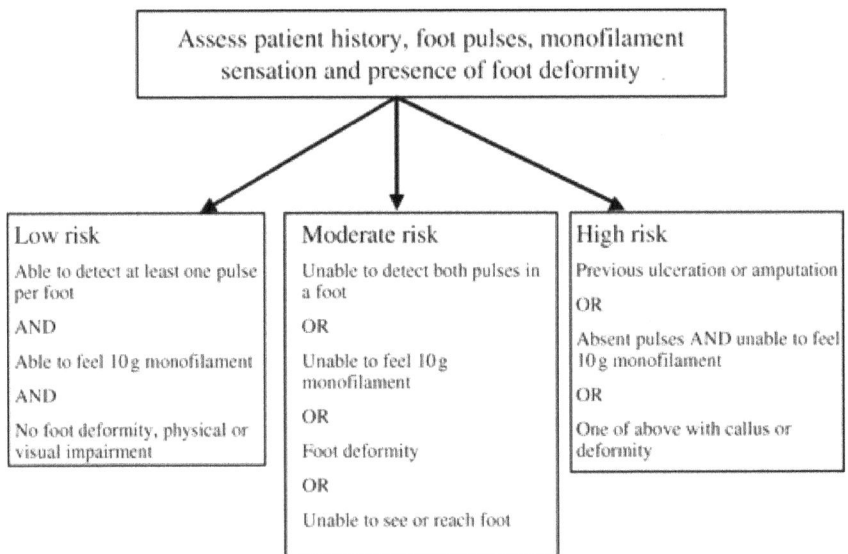

Figure 1. Foot risk stratification scheme

Source: Leese *et al.*, 2007. http://care.diabetesjournals.org/content/30/8/2064.long

patients. Patients are classified into three categories (low, moderate and high risk) based on 4 clinical criteria:

- Patient history
- Foot pulses
- 10 points Semmes Weinstein 5.07 monofilament test
- Foot deformity

Low Risk

At least one pulse is palpable. Patient is able to feel the 10g monofilament. No foot deformity is present. Patients with low risk have a 99.6% chance that they will not develop foot ulcers.[6]

Moderate Risk

No pulse is palpable. Patient is unable to feel the 10g monofilament. He may be unable to see or reach his foot. Patients with moderate risk are 6 times more likely to suffer from foot ulceration than patients with low risk.[6]

High Risk

Patient has a history of previous ulceration or previous amputation. No pulse is palpable. Patient is unable to feel the 10g monofilament. Callosity or deformity may be present (Fig. 2). Patients with high risk are 83 times more likely to suffer from foot ulceration than patients with low risk.[6]

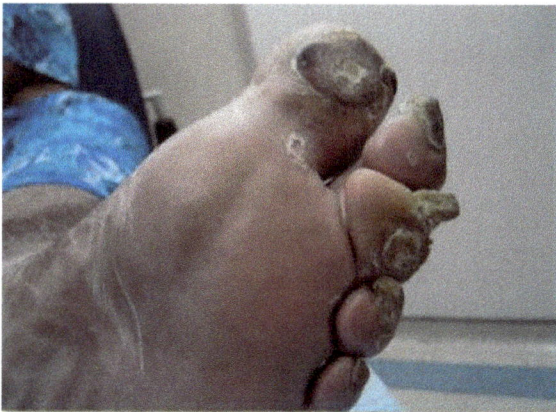

Figure 2. High risk foot showing callosities and trophic nails

Conclusion

All patients with diabetes must undergo to annual foot examination. In this way, we can detect the 'foot at risk' early and seek early intervention to avoid the development of diabetic foot complications. This in turn will reduce the major amputation rate.

References

1. N. Singh, D. G. Armstrong and B. A. Lipsky, Preventing foot ulcers in patients with diabetes, *JAMA* **293**(2):217–28 (2005).
2. H. Brem, P. Sheehan, H. J. Rosenberg, J. S. Schneider and A. J. Boulton, Evidence-based protocol for diabetic foot ulcers, *Plast. Reconstr. Surg.* **117**(7 Suppl):193S–209S (2006).
3. G. E. Reiber, L. Vileikyte, E. J. Boyko, M. del Aguila, D. G. Smith, L. A. Lavery and A. J. Boulton, Causal pathways for incident lower-extremity ulcers in patients with diabetes from two settings, *Diabetes Care* **22**(1):157–62 (1999).
4. D. G. Armstrong and L. A. Lavery, Diabetic foot ulcers: prevention, diagnosis and classification, *Am. Fam. Physician* **57**(6):1325–32, 1337–8 (1998).
5. S. Tavintharan, N. Cheung, S. C. Lim, W. Tay, A. Shankar, E. S. Tai and T. Y. Wong, Prevalence and risk factors for peripheral artery disease in an Asian population with diabetes mellitus, *Diab. Vasc. Dis. Res.* **6**(2):80–6 (2009).
6. G. P. Leese, F. Reid, V. Green, R. Mcalpine, S. Cunningham, A. M. Emslie-Smith, A. D. Morris, B. Mcmurray and A. C. Connacher, Stratification of foot ulcer risk in patients with diabetes: a population-based study, *Int. J. Clin. Pract.* **60**(5):541–5 (2006).

Section 4

Clinical Presentation

11

Types of Clinical Presentation

Aziz Nather and Amaris Lim Shu Min

Department of Orthopaedic Surgery
Yong Loo Lin School of Medicine
National University of Singapore

Introduction

Diabetic foot problems may be due to infection, ischaemia or trauma. Clinical presentations include cellulitis, abscess, dry or wet gangrene, ulcer, osteomyelitis, septic arthritis, Charcot Joint Disease and necrotising fasciitis.

Soft Tissue Infection

Cellulitis (Fig. 1)

Cellulitis is the inflammation of connective tissue including the skin dermal and subcutaneous layers. It occurs when bacteria enters a wound, for example a cut, a burn or a blister. The microorganism most commonly present is Streptococcus *pyogenes*. The skin is red, painful, warm and tender.

Abscess (Fig. 2)

An abscess is an accumulation of pus. Pus formation is a protective mechanism to prevent the spread of bacteria. The infected tissue is separated from the healthy tissue. The white blood cells, dead cells and bacteria

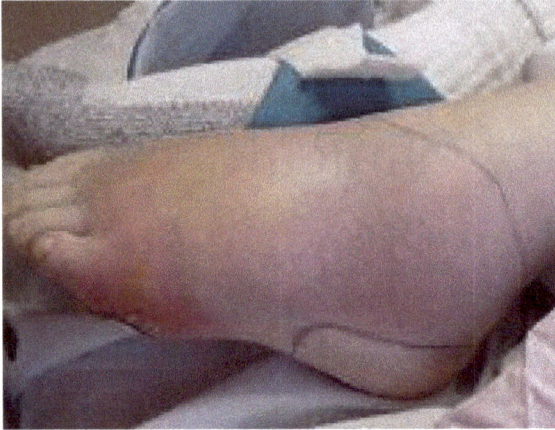

Figure 1.   Cellulitis of the foot

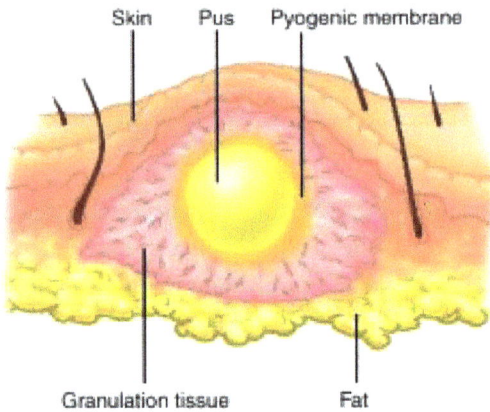

Figure 2.   Abscess

Source: Dorland's Medical Dictionary for Health Consumers, http://medical-dictionary. thefreedictionary.com/abscess

form a collection of pus — the abscess. This presents as a swelling in the foot.

Superficial Abscess (Fig. 3)

A superficial abscess is a pus swelling on the skin or just under the skin. It is known as a blister or a boil. It is painful, swollen, red, warm and tender.

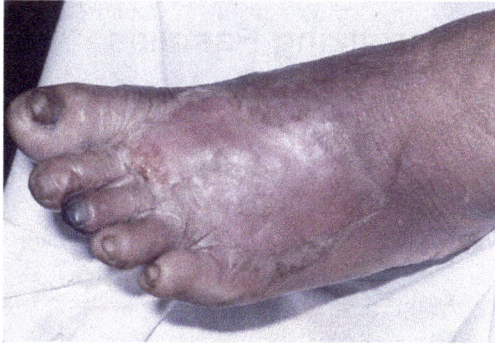

Figure 3.   Superficial abscess dorsum of foot

Muscle Abscess: Pyomyositis (Deep Abscess)

Pyomyositis is the formation of an abscess within a muscle. It is deep-seated. A swelling may be felt. There is often no inflammation of the overlying skin. It is often diagnosed because of deep tenderness and raised white blood cell (WBC) count, C-reactive protein (CRP) and erythrocyte sedimentation rate (ESR) on investigation.

Necrotising Fasciitis

Necrotising Fasciitis (NF) is one of the most dangerous conditions that can develop in a limb. It is commonly known as flesh-eating disease. Diabetes is the most common co-morbidity. Other co-morbidities include cancer, alcoholism and Human Immunodeficiency Virus infection. NF can be classified into 2 types, depending on the cause of infection:

- Type 1: Polymicrobial infection with both aerobic and anaerobic bacteria.
- Type 2: Monomicrobial infection. Most cases are due to Group A Streptococcus.

NF is a progressive inflammatory infection which spreads rapidly in the deep fascia. There is secondary necrosis of the subcutaneous tissues (Fig. 4). The presence of palpable crepitation due to the collection of air in the subcutaneous tissue is a classical clinical feature. Radiologically, gas shadows are seen in the subcutaneous plane due to the presence of gas-forming organisms.

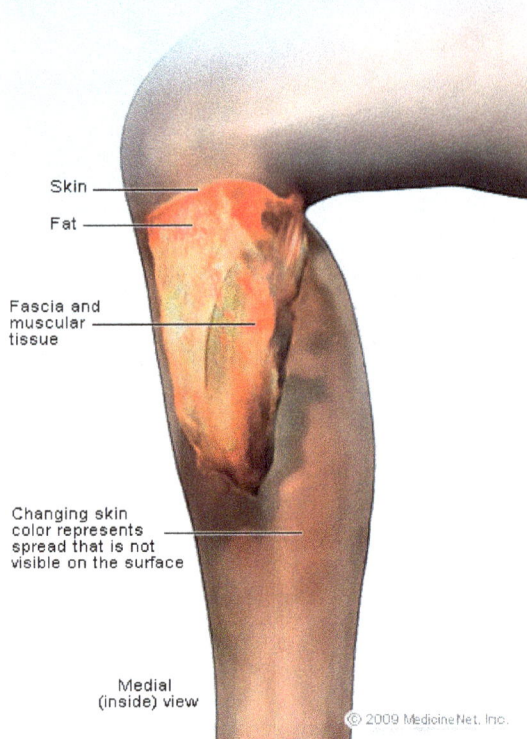

Figure 4.   Illustration of necrotising fasciitis
Source: MedicineNet Inc, www.medicinenet.com

The patient looks toxic and is febrile. Early symptoms include severe pain in the foot. Haemorrhagic blisters are clinical signs that often appear late on the second or third day (Fig. 5). The patient may develop hypotension due to septicaemic shock. The WBC and CRP count is often markedly raised, with WBC $>15 \times 10^9$/L and CRP > 100 mg/L.

It is important to make the diagnosis early. After fluid resuscitation and institution of antibiotics, the key to treatment is aggressive surgical debridement. In late presentations of NF, amputation of the limb may be necessary to remove the exceptionally high bacterial load and overwhelming toxicity. The mortality rate in NF can be as high as 20–40%.

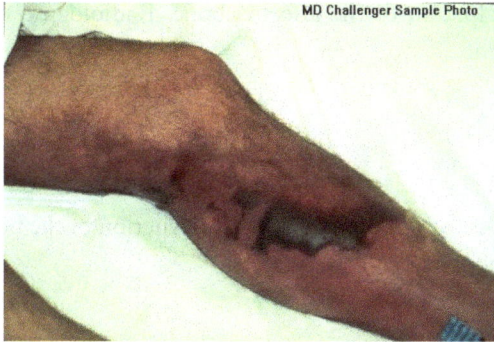

Figure 5. Necrotising fasciitis of the leg and thigh showing haemorrhagic blisters of the skin

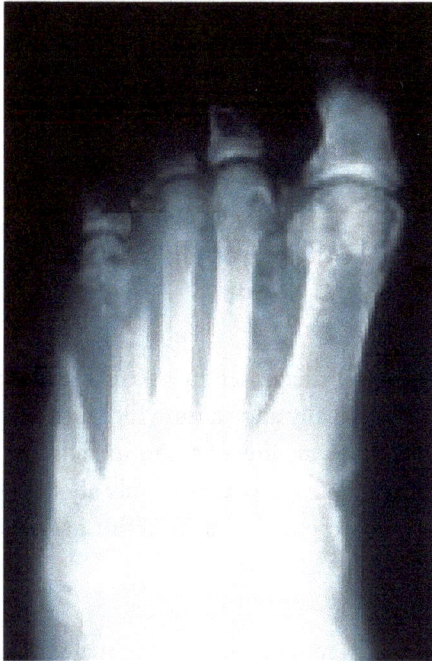

Figure 6. Showing pathological fracture of the fourth metatarsal due to osteomyelitis

Bone Infection

Osteomyelitis (Fig. 6)

Osteomyelitis is infection of the bone. The bones commonly involved are the calcaneum, metatarsals, and proximal phalanges. It is manifested by deep tenderness on palpation of the affected bone. Radiological changes include erosion of the bone.

Joint Infection

Septic Arthritis

Septic arthritis is infection of a joint with destruction of the bones adjacent to the joint. Common joints involved are:

- Metatarsophalangeal Joint
- Proximal Interphalangeal Joint

Clinically, movement of the affected joint causes severe pain. The range of motion of the joint is severely restricted. Radiologically, one sees destruction of both bones adjacent to the joint.

Ischaemia

Gangrene

Gangrene is death of a tissue part (necrosis), due to lack of blood supply to the tissue. Gangrene can be either dry gangrene or wet gangrene.

Dry gangrene (Fig. 7)

In dry gangrene, the aim of management is to keep the tissue dry or uninfected by applying spirit dressings daily and waiting for "auto-amputation" to occur. With auto-amputation, the gangrenous stump falls off, leaving a healed underlying wound. This, however, occurs in only about 5–10% of cases. Dry gangrene often becomes infected eventually, resulting in wet gangrene.

Wet gangrene (Figs. 8 and 9)

Wet gangrene often spreads more rapidly, as the stagnant blood promotes the growth of bacteria. Toxic by-products secreted by the bacteria may spread to the blood and cause septicaemia. Wet gangrene requires a surgical amputation, leaving a surgical wound.

Site of gangrene

Common sites of gangrene are the toe(s) and the heel.

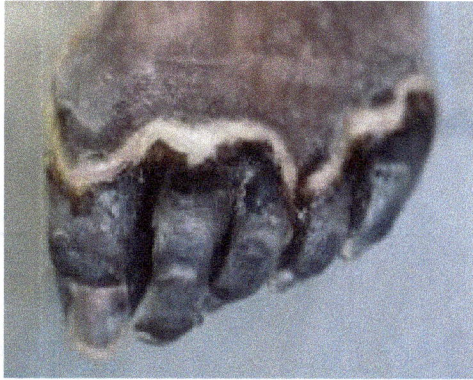

Figure 7. Dry gangrene of all 5 toes

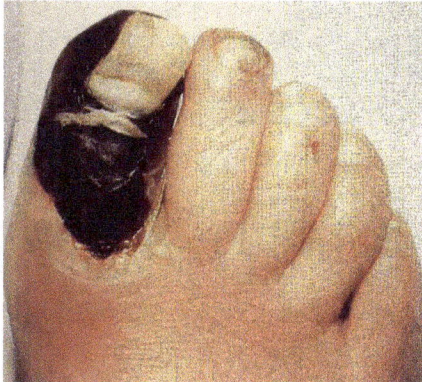

Figure 8. Wet gangrene of big toe

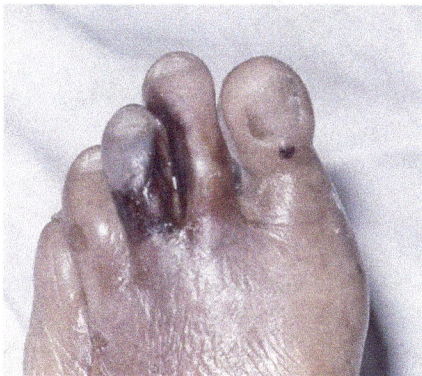

Figure 9. Wet gangrene of 2nd and 3rd toes

Trauma

Charcot Joint Disease (Figs. 10 and 11)

Charcot Joint Disease (CJD) or neuropathic joint is a progressive musculoskeletal condition. It refers to the progressive degeneration of a joint, starting

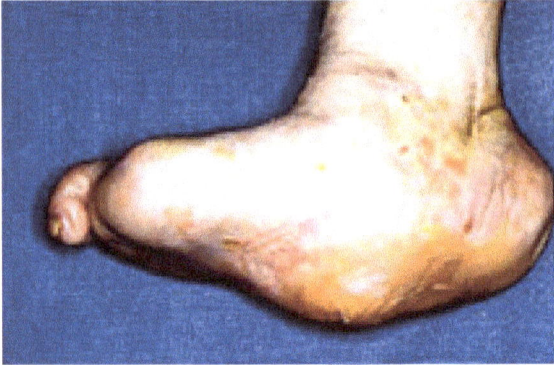

Figure 10. Rocker bottom foot deformity in patient with Charcot Joint Disease

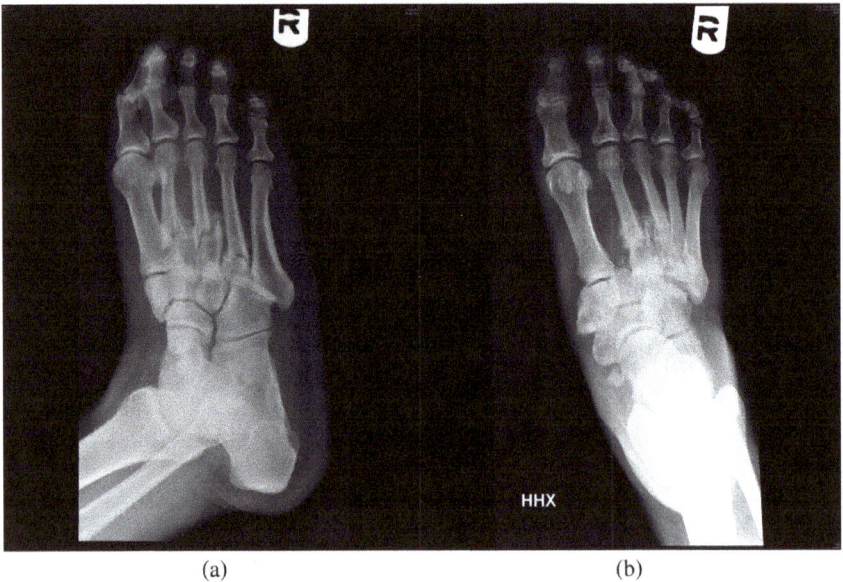

(a)   (b)

Figure 11. (a) Showing fracture of 2nd and 3rd metatarsals. (b) Showing tarso-metatarsal dislocation of 2nd to 5th metatarsals in a patient with Charcot Joint Disease

with bone destruction, bone resorption, and eventually deformity. In severe cases, rocker bottom foot deformity occurs.

CJD usually results from a loss of sensation in the lower limb. It can occur in one or more of the following regions:

- Forefoot
- Midfoot
- Hindfoot

Ulcers

Infective Ulcers (Fig. 12)

Infective ulcers are usually found on the dorsum of the foot, in the 1st web space, and over the heel.

Neuropathic Ulcers (Fig. 13)

These usually occur in the sole of the foot.

Ischaemic Ulcers

Ischaemic ulcers result when there is a lack of blood flow to the feet. Patients suffering from atherosclerosis have a higher chance of developing ischaemic ulcers. In the foot, the signs of chronic ischaemia are shininess of the skin, loss of hair, increased skin pigmentation and trophic nail changes.

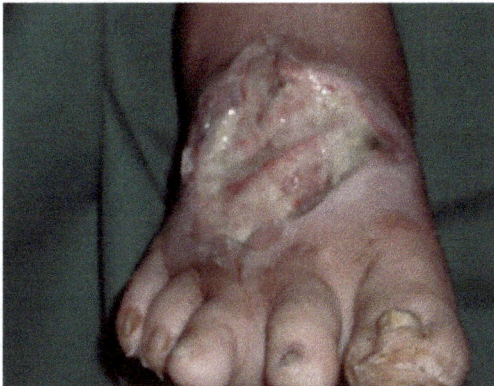

Figure 12. Infective ulcer on dorsum of foot

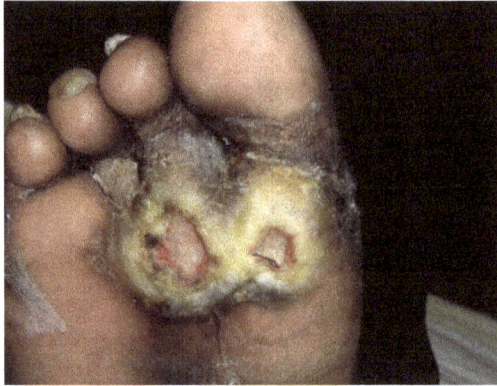

Figure 13. Neuropathic ulcer on sole of foot

Traumatic Ulcers

Traumatic ulcers can occur from the friction of wearing ill-fitting or poorly-designed footwear. For example:

Site of ulcer	Type of shoes/sandals
1st web space:	Japanese slippers/flip flops
Dorsum of foot:	Slippers with dorsal straps
Heel:	Slippers with ankle straps

Ulcers can also arise from self-inflicted trauma, when patients cut their own nails or callosities using non-sterile equipment they have at home. Traumatic ulcers may also result from ingrown toe-nails and infected callosities and ulcers. They often become infected.

Decubitus Ulcers

Decubitus ulcers form when too much pressure is constantly placed on the skin. They can be found over the heel and over the lateral aspect of the base of the 5th metatarsal. Decubitus ulcers often become infected.

12

Clinical Examination of a Diabetic Foot Problem

Aziz Nather and Amy Pannapat Chanyarungrojn

Department of Orthopaedic Surgery
Yong Loo Lin School of Medicine
National University of Singapore

Introduction

In examining a diabetic foot problem (DFP), the usual method of using "look, feel, move and Radiographs" — Apley's system of examination for orthopaedics[1] (for examination of a hip joint, a knee joint or a spine) may not be appropriate. The system of examination recommended is:

- General examination of the patient
- Local examination of the limb
- Examination for vasculopathy
- Examination for sensory neuropathy
- Examination for immunopathy

History Taking

It is important to take a comprehensive medical history.

What is the patient's profile?

Patients are usually in the 5th and 6th decades of life.[2] Males and females are equally affected.[2]

What is the patient's socioeconomic status?

There is a significantly higher incidence of DFPs in Malays and Indians as compared to the other ethnic groups in Singapore. The incidence in Chinese was found to be significantly lower.[3] DFPs mainly occur in the lower socioeconomic group. The highest level of education in DFP patients is usually up to secondary school level only. They tend to have a low average monthly household income of less than SGD2000.[3]

Where is the pain?

It is important to localise the site of the pain:

- Toe(s)
- Dorsum of the foot
- Sole of the foot
- Heel

Is there vascular claudication?

Vascular claudication is pain in the calf that comes on after walking a specific distance (claudication distance). This is due to inadequate blood flow to the limb. The pain disappears when he stops walking. Vascular claudication, although a common symptom of the ischaemic limb, is not common in patients with DFPs.

Is there rest pain?

Rest pain is common in patients with DFPs. It refers to continuous pain in the distal part of the limb – toes or forefoot. The pain is present at rest, throughout the day and night. This continuous, severe and aching pain often stops him from walking and sleeping. The patient usually hangs the leg over the side of the bed, as putting the leg below the level of the heart allows the blood to gravitate into the limb and may offer some relief of pain. He prefers to sleep in a sitting position rather than lying down in bed. Sometimes, the rest pain is so severe that the patient begs for an amputation.

Is there swelling?

In cellulitis, the generalised swelling in the foot is associated with redness, warmth and pain (Fig. 1). A localized swelling is usually due to an abscess or infection of the underlying bone (osteomyelitis).

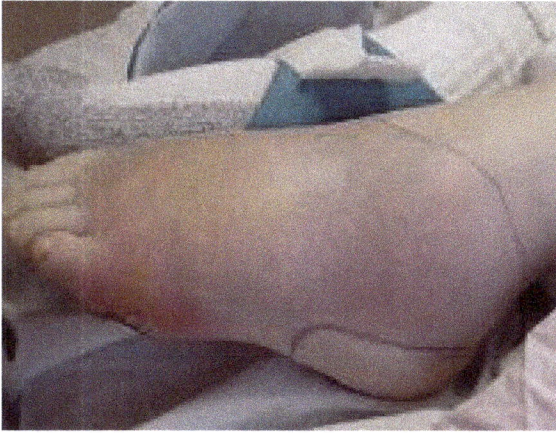

Figure 1. Cellulitis

Swelling of a joint with pain on movement of the joint is usually due to septic arthritis of the joint. This commonly involves the metatarsophalangeal joints or the proximal interphalangeal joints of the foot.

Fever, chills and rigors may be present. Often, no systemic response is seen in the elderly and in patients with diabetes, as these patients are usually immunocompromised.

Is there deformity?

Clawing of toes may be present due to motor neuropathy.

A large swollen foot with deformity is due to Charcot Joint Disease (CJD). CJD can also be bilateral (Fig. 2). Deformity can lead to a loss of the arch of the foot, and in advanced cases, a rocker bottom foot deformity develops (Fig. 3).

Is there an ulcer?

An ulcer is a common presentation.

Site of ulcer

Localise the site of the ulcer:

- Dorsum of foot (Fig. 4)
- Sole of foot (Fig. 5)

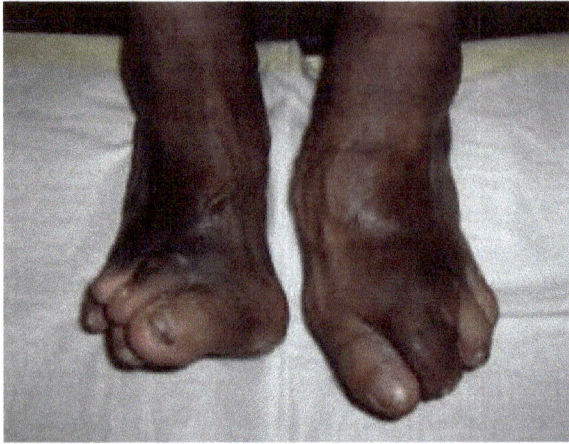

Figure 2.   Bilateral deformed feet due to CJD showing clawing of toes and hallux valgus deformity

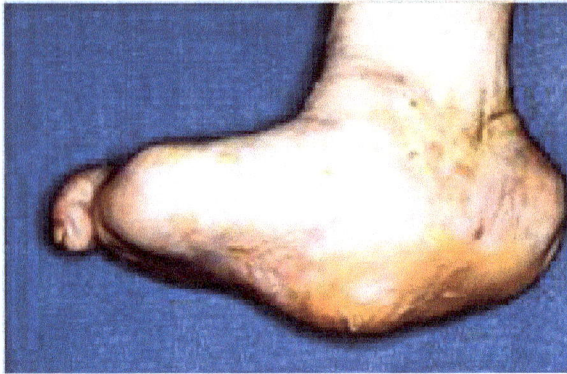

Figure 3.   Rocker bottom deformity in patient with CJD

- Base of 5th metatarsal
- Lateral malleolus
- Heel

Contents of ulcer

Is there discharge from the ulcer?

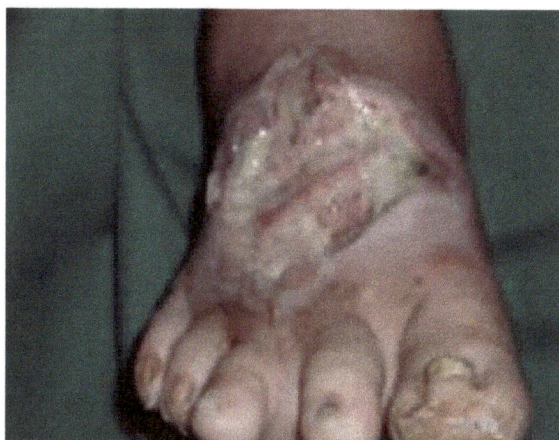

Figure 4.   Ulcer of dorsum of foot showing infection and slough

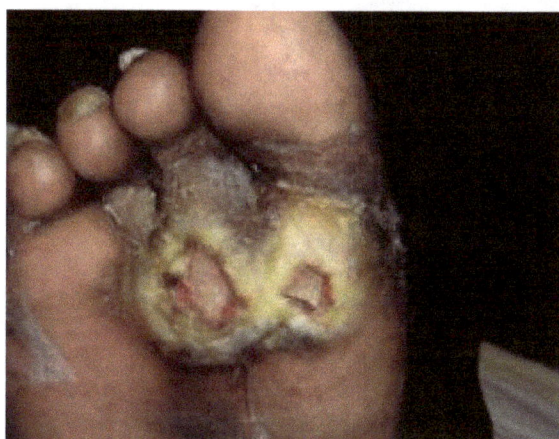

Figure 5.   Ulcer on sole of foot (neuropathic ulcer)

When discharge is present, note the colour and smell of the discharge.

Staphylococcus *aureus*:	Thick, brown, little odour
Pseudomonas *aeruginosa*:	Greenish, rotten fruit smell or "metallic" smell
Bacteroides *fragilis* (Anaerobe):	"Faecal" smell

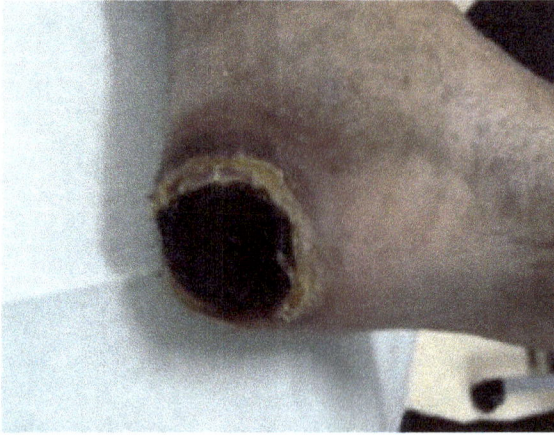

Figure 6. Dry gangrene of heel

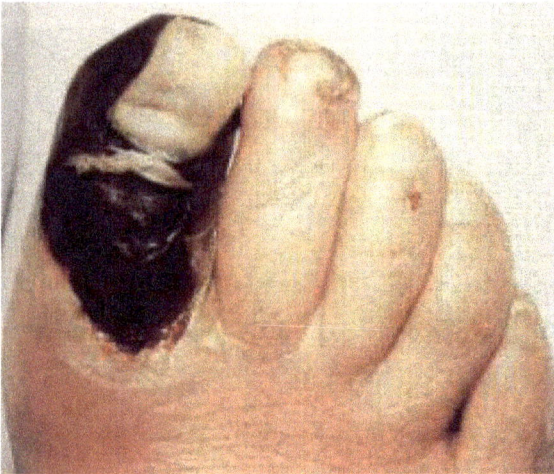

Figure 7. Wet gangrene of big toe

Is there gangrene?

Is the gangrene dry (with no superimposed infection) (Fig. 6) or wet (with super-imposed infection) (Fig. 7)?

Is there pain?
In gangrene, pain is usually felt at the junction of dead and living tissues (pain receptors function in living tissue only).

Is there numbness?

Does the patient experience "pins and needles" sensation in the foot?

Is there decreased sensation in the foot?

What is the extent of sensory disturbance felt?

The different extents of sensory disturbance are:

- Involving toes only
- Up to mid-foot
- Up to ankle
- Up to mid-shin
- Up to knees

A patient usually experiences "glove and stocking" sensory disturbance symmetrically in both limbs. A DFP presents with sensory disturbance with a bilateral "stocking" distribution. Of these, about 10% present with hand problems. The latter may experience sensory disturbance with "glove" distribution.

What is the degree of sensory disturbance felt?

A patient experiences "pins and needles" (paraesthesia), increased sensitivity to pain (hyperaesthesia) in mild cases, decreased sensitivity to pain (hypoaesthesia) or complete loss of feeling (anaesthesia) in severe cases.

What is the duration of sensory disturbance felt?

Note how long the patient has suffered from diabetes. The presence of sensory disturbance is related to the duration of diabetes.[4] The longer the duration, the higher is the incidence of sensory disturbance.

Has the patient sustained recent trauma?

Trauma is usually sustained at home (e.g. when the patient kicks the side of the bed or slips and falls in the bathroom). Often, the trauma goes unrecognized because the patient has sensory neuropathy and does not feel the pain.

Patients with DFPs tend to walk barefoot. It is not uncommon to see nails and foreign objects embedded in the foot on radiographs, without the patient knowing how they got there.

Has the patient sustained self-inflicted trauma?

This includes the cutting of a callosity or digging of a toe nail using non-sterile equipment at home. This is often the start of the foot problem.

Does the patient self-medicate?

Many patients like to self-medicate. Malays tend to apply coffee powder on their ulcers, the Indians apply turmeric and the Chinese apply herbs from Traditional Chinese Medicine to heal their wounds. Such applications can cause infections.

What is the type of footwear worn?

Does the patient wear shoes?

Note the type of footwear worn by the patient. Nather, Kathryn and Zameer 2005[5] found that about 70% of diabetics do not wear shoes outside the house. They only wear slippers.

What is the type of slippers worn?

- Japanese slippers with a strap across the first web space commonly cause ulceration of the first web space.
- Slippers with dorsal straps and ankle straps lead to ulceration over the ankle and dorsum of foot.

What is the type of diabetes mellitus present?

Most patients have Type 2 Diabetes (non-insulin dependent diabetes).[2–5]

What is the type of diabetic medication used?

Record the diabetic medications used.

- Is the patient on diabetic diet only?
- Is the patient on oral hypoglycaemic agents only?
- Is the patient on oral drugs supplemented with insulin injections?

Does the patient monitor control of his diabetes?

Is the patient using a urine dipstick?

Does the patient monitor capillary blood glucose levels?
How often does the patient monitor his glucose levels?

Does the patient know his HbA1C level?

When was the last HbA1C test performed?
HbA1C level reflects the control of diabetes over the last 3 months. In patients
with no diabetes, HbA1C is 3.5–5.5%. In patients with diabetes, HbA1C of
less than 7% is good.

What are the symptoms of poorly-controlled diabetes?
The symptoms are polyuria (excessive production and passing of urine),
polydipsia (excessive thirst) and polyphagia (excessive desire to eat).

What are the complications of diabetes present?

The complications are:

- Cataracts — Impairment of vision
- Diabetic Retinopathy — Damage to retina
- Diabetic Nephropathy — Sallow appearance
- Diabetic Neuropathy — "Glove and stocking" sensory disturbance in feet
- Diabetic Vasculopathy — Vascular claudication or rest pain

What are the co-morbidities present?

The co-morbidites are:

- Hypertension
- Ischaemic Heart Disease
- Chronic Renal Failure
- Cerebrovascular Accident (CVA)

Diabetes + Renal Failure

A patient with diabetes is immunocompromised. Renal failure also leads to
immunocompromise. The combination of diabetes and renal failure gives a
poor prognosis, as the patient is "double-immunocompromised".

In patients undergoing renal dialysis, post-operative bleeding is a common
complication leading to haematoma formation. The patient's wound healing

rate is also compromised. In a patient who has undergone below knee amputation (BKA), the chance of wound healing is only about 50–60%. The patient must be warned about the need for a further operation such as a revision BKA or an above knee amputation (AKA), before the surgeon performs the primary BKA.

Diabetes + Hypertension

On its own, diabetes and hypertension each predisposes the patient to atherosclerosis (hardening of arteries). The combination of diabetes and hypertension causes an increased risk to atherosclerosis or peripheral vascular disease. These patients thus have a greater risk of requiring a BKA.

Diabetes + CVA

The combination of stroke with diabetes is also bad, as severely physically disabled patients have an increased risk to pressure ulceration and bedsores.

What are the risk factors of diabetes?

The risk factors are:

- Hypertension
- Smoking
- Hyperlipidaemia

What is the functional status of the patient?

Is he a walker?
Is the patient a community walker or is he housebound?
Is he wheelchair-bound?
Is he bed-ridden?

What is the patient's occupation?

Jobs that put workers at high risk of BKA include taxi drivers, housewives, cooks, manual labourers, and factory workers wearing safety boots (the latter frequently causes callosity and ulceration).

A housewife who cooks is at risk of BKA from hazards in the kitchen. She is exposed to dangers of boiling water, frying oils and other accidents in the kitchen.

A taxi driver who needs to continually exert pressure on the foot by stepping on the accelerator, brake or clutch may need to change his job to avoid a BKA.

A factory worker experiences ulceration from wearing safety boots. He may also require a change of job to avoid a BKA.

Family History

Is there a family history of diabetes?

One or both parents and one or more siblings could have diabetes.

What is the lifespan of parents with diabetes?

Look into the lifespan of any parent with diabetes. If the parent died at the age of 88, the chances of the patient living to 70 years old or more is good.

*Does the patient have a care-giver?*a

Identify the care-giver — spouse, daughter, daughter-in-law, etc, who can help in managing the diabetes or diabetic foot problem (e.g. in performing daily dressings of the wound).

Clinical Examination

Only after completing a detailed medical history can one proceed to examine the patient. This must be done carefully and meticulously in a systematic manner.

Firstly, the examiner must conform to a proper dress code to avoid the risk of spreading infection from this patient to others. It is easy for the doctor to be contaminated by the ulcer or discharging abscess.

The examiner must not wear:

- Long-sleeved shirt (short sleeves only)
- Long tie (bow tie allowed)
- Watch or bracelets (no watch or bracelet on either arm)

He must wash his hands with Hibiscrub or with alcohol hand rub before approaching the patient.

General Examination

A general examination of the patient must be performed, before one proceeds to examine the foot. One must not rush to examine the foot, even in a short case for an MBBS examination. The student must first perform a general examination before proceeding to a local foot examination.

    General inspection must include:

- Is the patient toxic, ill, anxious or well?
- Is he febrile?
- Is he alert or drowsy? (This is caused by hypoglycaemia or ketoacidosis.)
- Is there acidotic breathing? (This is due to ketoacidosis — hyperventilation present with smell of ketones in his breath.)
- Is there a sallow appearance? (This is due to renal impairment.)
- Is there pallor? (Depress the eyelid and look for conjunctival pallor.)
- Is there dehydration? (Ask the patient to stick out his tongue to look for a parched tongue.)
- Examine the eyes for cataracts. (If cataracts are present, fundoscopy cannot be performed; if no cataracts are present, perform fundoscopy to look for diabetic retinopathy.)
- Examine the sclera for jaundice.

Vital Signs

- Assess the Blood Pressure
  - Look for postural hypotension (a fall in blood pressure) when changing from a supine to an erect posture
  - Take the pressure on both sides
- Examine the Pulse Rate
  - Look for tachycardia (abnormally fast pulse rate at rest)
- Examine the Respiratory Rate
  - Look for tachypnoea (rapid breathing)

Palpation of All Pulses

Examine all pulses starting with:

- Neck:
  - Carotids (feel for thrill, auscultate for bruit)

- Upper limb:
  — Axillary
  — Brachial
  — Radial
  — Ulnar
- Abdominal aorta
- Lower limb:
  — Femoral
  — Popliteal
  — Dorsalis pedis
  — Posterior tibial

Record the palpation of each pulse as:

- ++ (normal)
- + (weak)
- − (not palpable)

Cardiovascular Examination:

- Locate the apex beat (normally found on the left 5th intercostal space, midclavicular line)
- Look for cardiomegaly (abnormal enlargement of the heart)
- Listen to heart sounds for murmurs

Chest Examination:

- Look for bronchopneumonia (chest infection)
- Look for pleural effusion (fluid accumulation in the pleural cavity)
- Look for chronic obstructive lung disease (COLD) (obstruction of airflow that interferes with normal breathing)

Abdominal Examination:

- Examine for hepatosplenomegaly (enlargement of the liver and spleen)

Local Examination

After the general examination, proceed to perform a local examination.

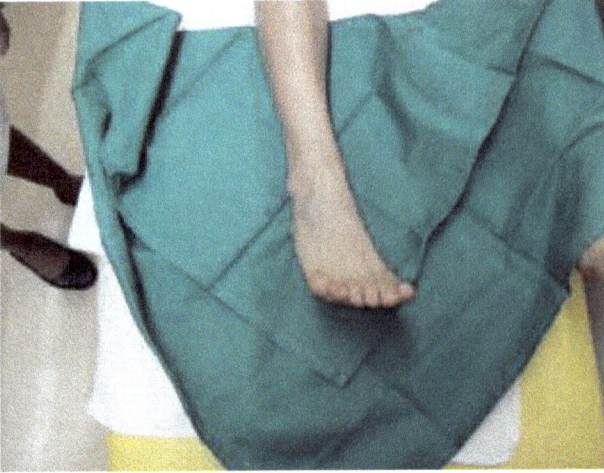

Figure 8a.   Foot placed on sterile dressing towel for examination

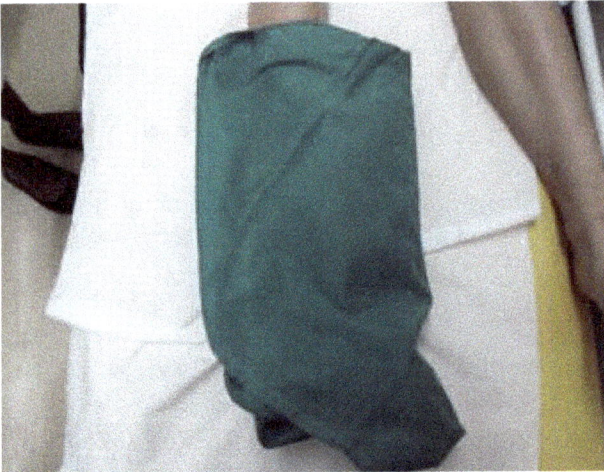

Figure 8b.   Foot wrapped in dressing towel on completion of the examination

Before starting, wear gloves and bring a sterile green towel to the bedside. Remove the dressing and place the exposed limb on a sterile green towel (Fig. 8a), to prevent the limb from contaminating the bed. After completing the examination, the foot is wrapped in the green towel (Fig. 8b) before the new dressing is applied. The soiled dressings are placed in a plastic bag beside the limb on the bed.

After completing the examination, wrap the foot in the green towel. Remove the gloves and discard them into the plastic bag. The bag is then thrown into a biohazard container Wash hands with Hibiscrub. Only then does the examiner record his findings.

For local examination, perform local inspection first. After performing local inspection, instead of doing "look, feel, move and Radiographs" as one does systematically for examination of a hip joint, a knee joint or a spine, proceed to examine the following:

- Assessment for Vasculopathy
- Assessment for Sensory Neuropathy
- Assessment for Immunopathy

Local Inspection

Look for signs of:

- Chronic Ischaemia

    — Trophic nail changes
    — Shininess of skin
    — Loss of hair
    — Increased pigmentation of the skin

- Motor Neuropathy

    — Clawing of toes (Fig. 9)
    — Wasting of intrinsic muscles

- Autonomic Neuropathy

    — Dryness of skin

- Deformity

    — Increased size in one foot (due to Charcot Joint Disease)
    — Rocker bottom foot (Fig. 3)
    — Hallux valgus (bunion)

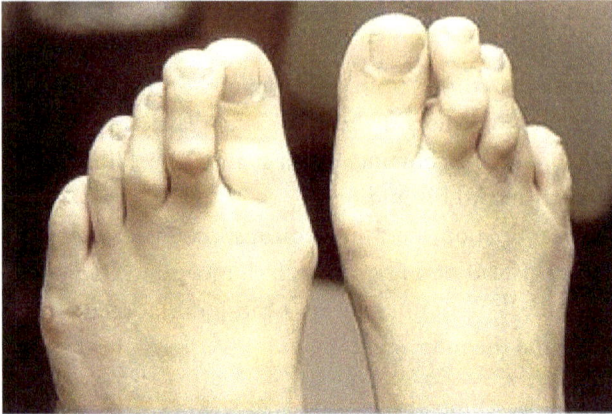

Figure 9.   Clawing of toes

Source: The Parkgate Chiropody Practice, 2012. http://www.parkgatechiropody.co.uk/conditions.html [2012]

Inspect the following:

1. Dorsum of foot: For cellulitis, blister, abscess, and ulceration
2. Sole of foot: For callosity, cellulitis, blister and abscess
3. Web spaces in between toes: For ulceration and fungal infection
4. Toes: For wet or dry gangrene, number of toes involved
5. Toe-nails: For dystrophic changes, paronychia
6. Heel: For ulcer, abscess and wet or dry gangrene

Describe the ulcer (Fig. 10) accurately and systematically:

- **Site**
    — Dorsum foot and ankle (infective)
- **Size**
    — 7 cm × 4 cm
- **Edge**
    — Clean cut, not inverted or everted
    — Parts of edge ischaemic
- **Floor**
    — Presence of slough and tendon

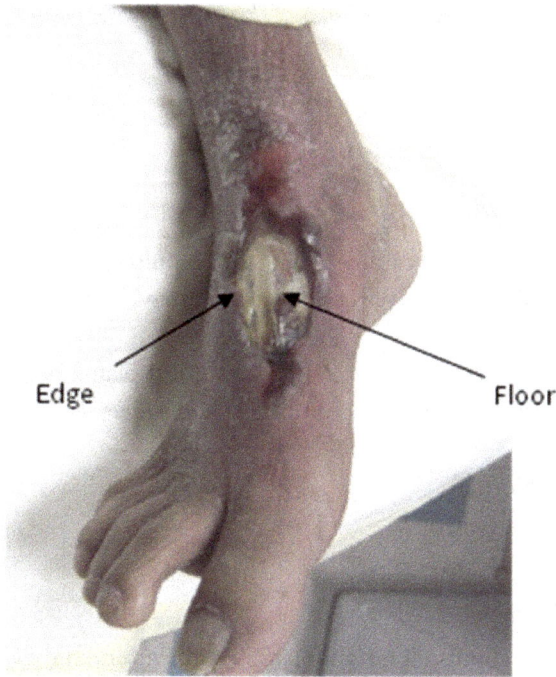

Figure 10. Ulcer on dorsum of foot with ischaemic edges and with slough and tendon in floor

The floor is what is visible in the ulcer. The base (beneath the floor) is not visible but palpable. (Eg. In a carpeted room, the "floor" is the carpet and the concrete beneath the carpet is the "base".)

- **Presence of Pain**
  - Painful ulcer: Infective, Ischaemia
  - Non-painful ulcer: Neuropathic

Examination for Vasculopathy

Examine all patients with DFPs carefully for vasculopathy.

Colour of skin

Pink colour: Normal
Pale: Ischaemia

Temperature of skin (feel temperature of skin with back of palm)

Warm: Normal
Cold: Ischaemia

Pulp capillary refill

It is better to perform the capillary refill on the pulp of the toe instead of the toe-nail. Toe nails may be dystrophic and are often coloured in patients with diabetes.

Press the tip of the pulp for 2 seconds until it blanches and observe the time taken for the blanched area to turn back to pink.

<2 seconds: Normal
>2 seconds: Ischaemia

Palpation of pulses

Palpate the femoral pulse. The landmark is in the groin, midway between the pubic tubercle and the anterior superior iliac spine (the mid-inguinal point). This is the easiest pulse to feel.

Palpate the popliteal pulse. This is the more difficult pulse to feel as it is deep seated. The knee should be flexed to about 90°. Both thumbs should be placed on either side of the tibial tuberosity and the other fingers on the popliteal fossa. Using the other fingers, gently press to relax the hamstrings and press against the tibia to feel the pulse.

Palpate the dorsalis pedis artery (Fig. 11a). Locate the mid-point of the anterior ankle line, passing along the front of the ankle between the medial malleolus and the lateral malleolus (Point A, Fig. 11b). Often, the anterior tibial pulse is palpable at this point.

Draw a line between this point (Point A, Fig. 11b) to the first interdigital cleft. The doraslis pedis pulse can usually be felt one-third down this line from the anterior ankle line (Point B, Fig. 11b).

Palpate the posterior tibial artery (Fig. 12a). This is also difficult to feel as it is slightly deep seated. Practice is needed to perfect this examination. Place the hip in external rotation, the knee in flexion and the foot in dorsiflexion.

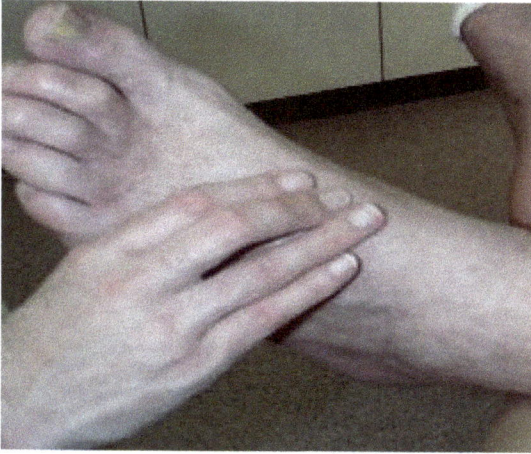

Figure 11a. Palpation of dorsalis pedis artery

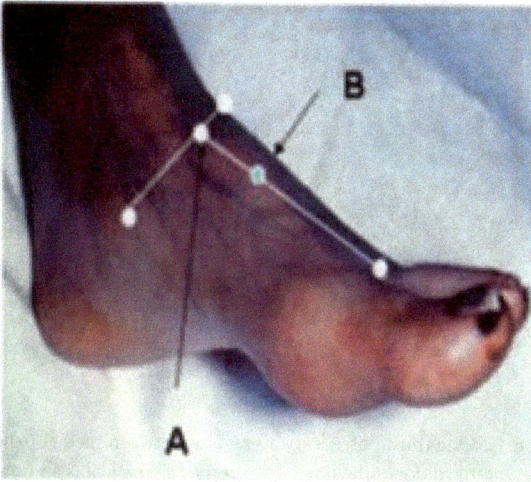

Figure 11b. Point A: Midpoint of line between malleoli. Point B: One third down the line from A to first interdigital cleft

The landmarks for this pulse are:

- One-third along the line between the tip of the medial malleolus and the Tendo Achilles (Point C, Fig. 12b), or
- One-third along the line between the tip of the medial malleolus and the point of the heel (calcaneum) (Point D, Fig. 12b).

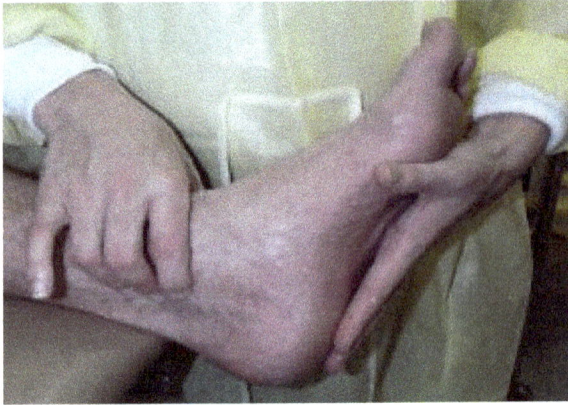

Figure 12a. Palpation for posterior tibial artery

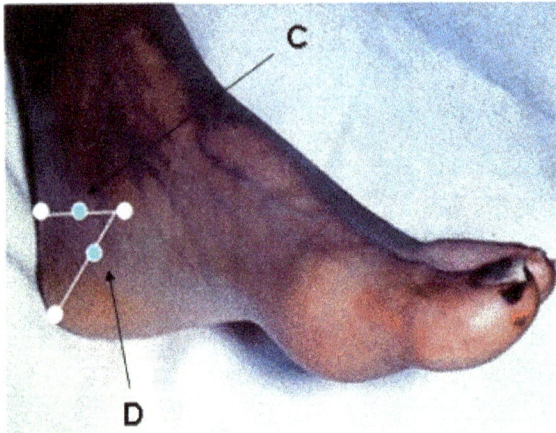

Figure 12b. Point C: One third posteriorly along line between medial malleolus and Tendo Achilles. Point D: One-third down the line between medial malleolus and point of heel

Record all the pulses using the stick diagram (Fig. 13).

The presence of palpable pulses is important to decide whether a ray amputation or other distal amputation (e.g. transmetatarsal, Syme) can be performed with good wound healing.

- 2 pulses palpable — Very good chance of success (70–80%)
- 1 pulse palpable — Fairly good chance of success (50–60%)

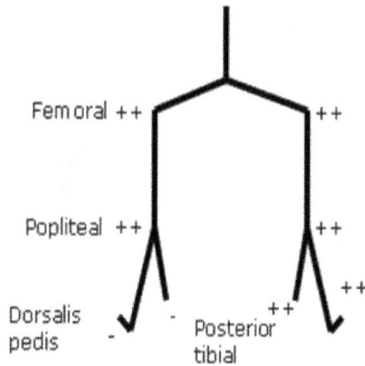

Figure 13. Stick diagram showing absent pulses in right foot

- No pulse palpable   — No chance of success
                        — Refer to vascular surgeon
                        — Distal amputation should not be performed. BKA should be performed if revascularisation fails

Buerger's Test

A **Buerger's Test** should be done when one or both pulses are clinically not palpable. There are 2 components to this test.

First Component

With the patient supine, raise the lower limb and look for pallor of the sole and toes (Fig. 14). Record the vascular angle at which the feet turn pale.

Normal: 90°   Pink
Ischaemia: 15–30°   Pallor

A Buerger's angle of less than 20° indicates severe ischaemia.

Second Component

Sit the patient up and hang the legs down the side of the couch.

Normal: Leg remains healthy pink.
Ischaemia: Leg slowly turns from white to pink due to reactive hyperaemia. Time taken (capillary refill time) is noted.
             A capillary refill time of 15 to 30 seconds or more indicates severe ischaemia.

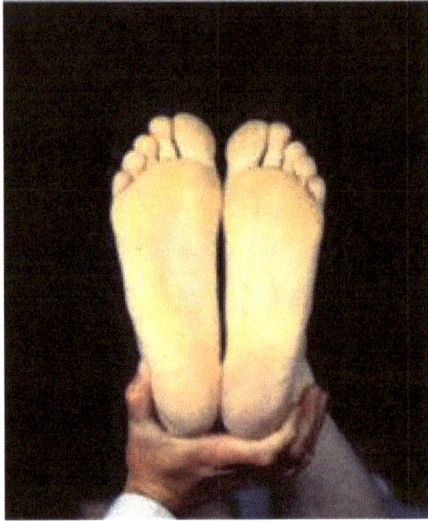

Figure 14. Both feet turning pale at an angle of 30°

Examination for Sensory Neuropathy

All patients with DFPs must be carefully evaluated for sensory neuropathy. The assessments for sensory neuropathy are:

- Semmes Weinstein 5.07 Gauge Monofilament Test (SWMT)
- Pin Prick Test
- Vibration Sense Test
- Position Sense Test
- Deep Tendon Reflex Test

Semmes Weinstein 5.07 Gauge Monofilament Test (SWMT)

The monofilament test makes use of a 5.07 Gauge Nylon Monofilament to test for touch sensation (Table 1). A positive monofilament test is more accurate than pinprick, vibration sense and position sense combined to detect sensory neuropathy.[6]

Method:

- Apply sufficient force — 10 g (Fig. 15a) until the filament bends with the patient's eyes closed.

Table 1. End organs for sensory neuropathy tests

Stimulus modality	Test conducted	End organ type
Touch	Semmes Weinstein 5.07 Gauge Monofilament Test (SWMT)	• Meissner corpuscle end-organs • Pacinian corpuscle end-organs
Pain	Pin prick test (using neurotip)	• Free nerve ending nociceptors
Vibration	Vibration sense test using tuning fork	• Meissner corpuscle end-organs • Pacinian corpuscle end-organs
Position Sense	Joint proprioception test	• Muscle spindle receptors • Joint capsule mechanoreceptors • Cutaneous tactile receptors

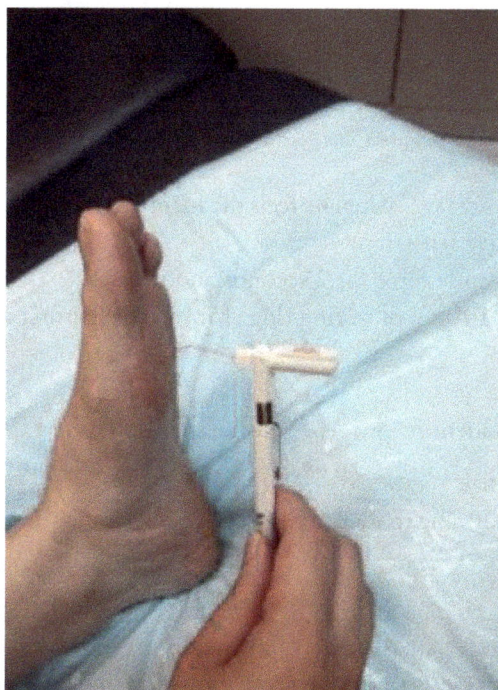

Figure 15a. Ten grams of force applied until filament bends

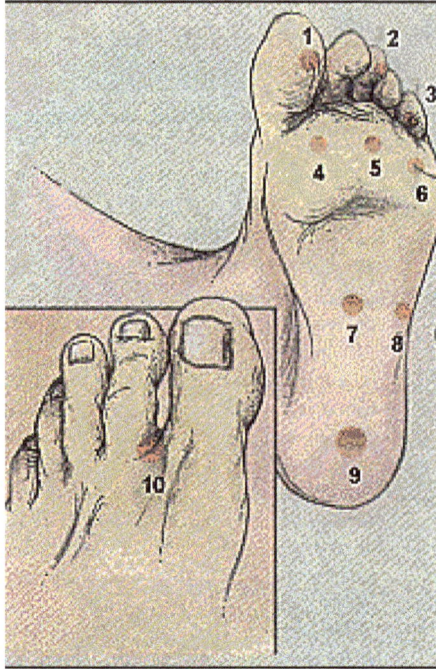

Figure 15b.　Ten sites for SWM testing

- Ask patient to say "yes" when he feels the filament. Inability to feel indicates loss of protective sensation.
- Apply only a gentle force for 2 seconds and release.
- Complete the 10 sites of testing (Fig. 15b) in a consistent manner.

Normal response

Patient is able to identify $\frac{8}{10}$, $\frac{9}{10}$, $\frac{10}{10}$ of the sites tested.

Abnormal response

The patient is only able to identify $\frac{7}{10}$, or less out of the sites tested.

Pin Prick Test

The Pin Prick Test makes use of a pin (neurotip) to test for pain sensation. It assesses the degree of numbness present — increased sensitivity to pain (hyperaesthesia), decreased sensitivity to pain (hypoaesthesia) or complete loss of feeling (anaesthesia).

In addition, it maps out the extent of the sensory disturbance present in each foot. The numbness present may involve the toes only or can be up to the forefoot, ankle, mid-shin or knee level. It is usually present bilaterally in a "glove and stocking" distribution.

Method:

- Use a neurotip disposable pin (Fig. 16a).
- Ask the patient to close their eyes and report whether they feel a sharp or dull pain (Fig. 16b).

Vibration sense

Vibratory sensation (pallesthesia) is tested by using a 128 Hz tuning fork and placing the vibrating instrument over a bone or bony prominence, such as the tips of toes, malleoli and tibial crest.

Method:

- Use a 128 hertz vibration fork.
- Apply the vibrating instrument over the bony prominence (Fig. 17).

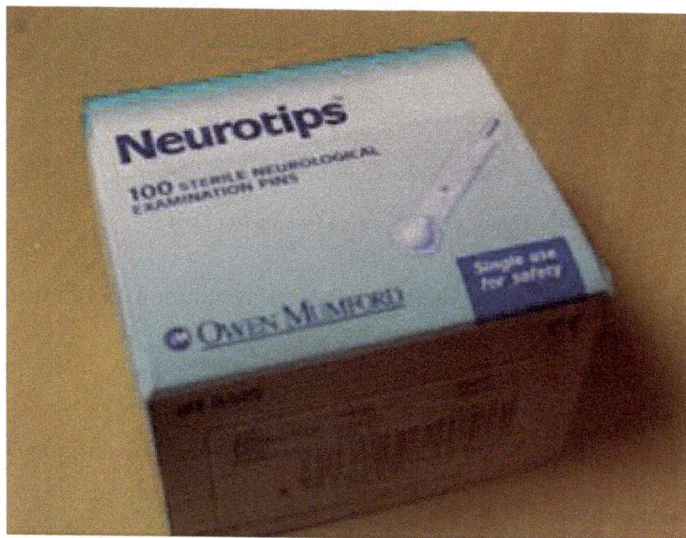

Figure 16a. Neurotips

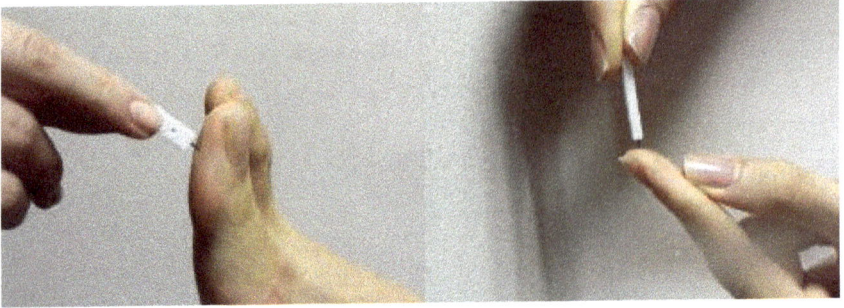

Figure 16b.   Pin prick test

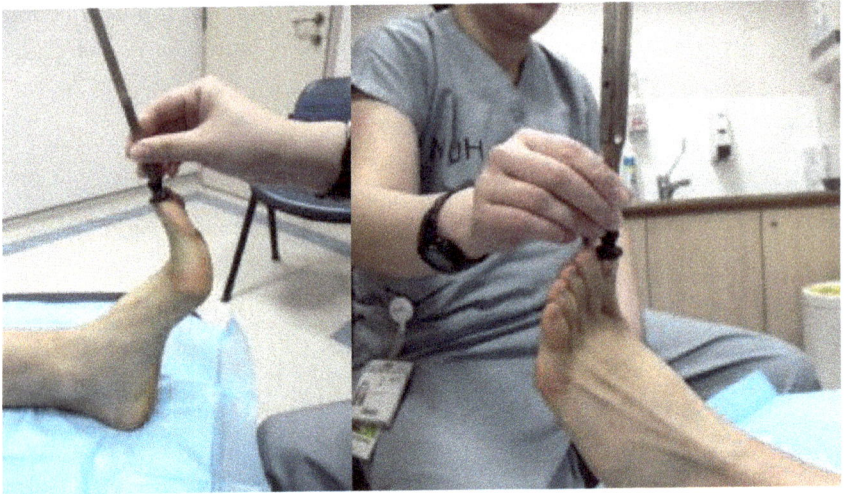

Figure 17.   Vibration (tuning fork) test

• Ask the patient to report whether they feel the vibration and then to report when it stops.

Normal response

The patient is able to report whether he receives a vibration stimulus or not.

Abnormal response

Patient is unable to identify or report when the vibration is felt and when it stops.

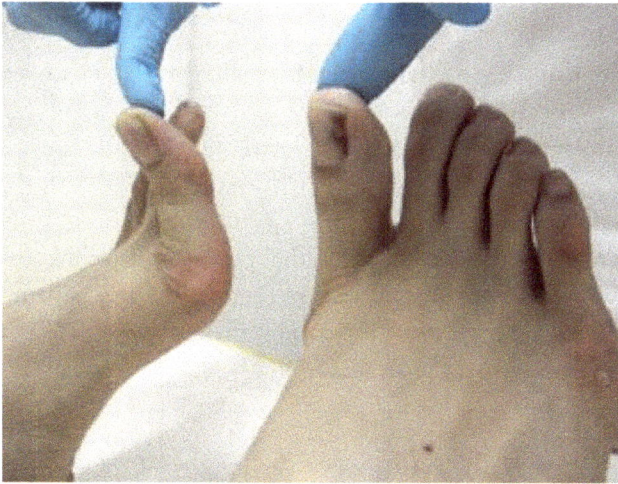

Figure 18a. Position sense test, hallux dorsiflexion (up)

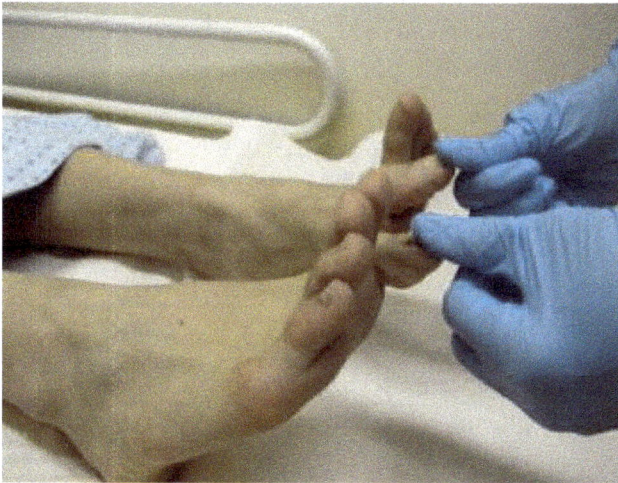

Figure 18b. Position sense test, hallux plantar flesion (down)

Position sense of toes

The test for position sense (joint proprioception) is done by holding the most distal joint of a digit (distal interphalangeal joint) by its sides and moving it slightly up (Fig. 18a) or down (Fig. 18b).

Method:

- Demonstrate the test with the patient watching so that he understands the procedures of the test.
- Then perform the test with his eyes closed.

Normal response

The patient can accurately identify the position of hallux (big toe) as manipulated by the examiner during the assessment. The patient should be able to detect and report the smallest of movement of the toe tested and report the direction of movement to the examiner — either as "up" or "down".

Abnormal response

The patient is unable to identify the position of the hallux (big toe).

Deep Tendon Reflexes Test (Ankle Jerk Reflex Test)

The ankle jerk can be affected in a patient with sensory neuropathy. The Tendo Achilles muscle is stretched and this leads to a reflex contraction of the muscle.

Method:

- Direct the patient into a sitting position on the examination table.
- Explain the examination technique to the patient.
- Ask patient to close their eyes.
- Gently stretch the Achilles tendon by passive dorsiflexion of the ankle. This should be done by gently delivering a strike to the Achilles tendon (Fig. 19).
- Record whether reflex is present (++), diminished (+) or absent (−).

It is the microvascular changes occuring with diabetes that lead to end organ damage of the peripheral nerves. End organs are encapsulated terminal nerve filaments of sensory nerves. The end organs involved in the various tests performed for sensory neuropathy are as shown in Table 1.

Examination for Immunopathy

In assessing immunopathy one must exclude:

- Deep abscess
- Osteomyelitis

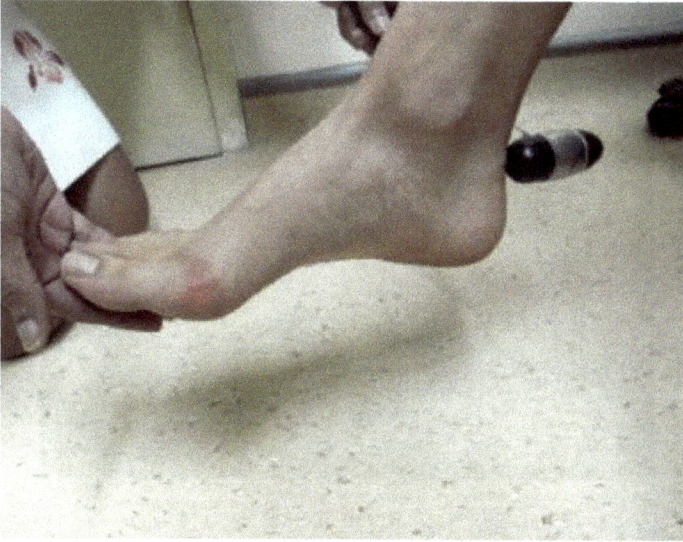

Figure 19. Ankle jerk reflex test

- Septic arthritis
- Necrotising fasciitis

Palpate for deep tenderness in the foot to exclude osteomyelitis of the underlying bones.

Move the interphalangeal joints and metatarsophalangeal joints gently to look for pain on movement of the joint. Severe pain is an indication of septic arthritis.

Start with the dorsum of the foot (Fig. 20). Move the interphalangeal joints and metatarsophalangeal joints of the 1st ray to look for septic arthritis of the interphalangeal and metatarsophalangeal joints. Then, perform deep palpation of the bones from the distal phalanx and proximal phalanx to the metatarsal and tarsal (ankle) bones to look for osteomyelitis of the underlying bones. Repeat this process with each ray — 2nd, 3rd, 4th and 5th. Gently squeeze the metatarsal bones from the 1st to the 5th rays to look for deep infection in between the rays.

Repeat the whole deep palpation of all rays in the sole of the foot (Fig. 21).

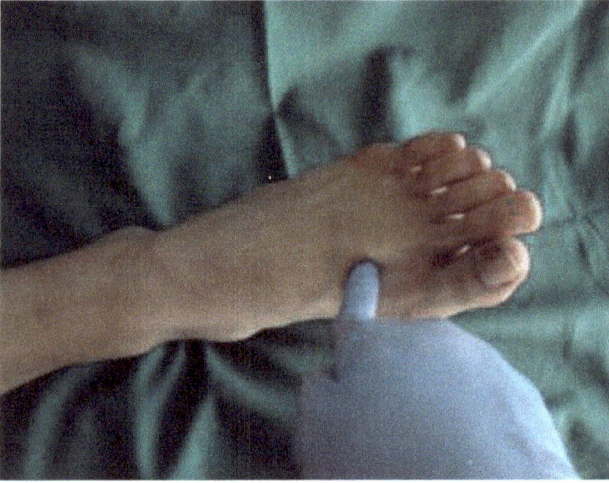

Figure 20.   Deep palpation ray by ray — dorsum

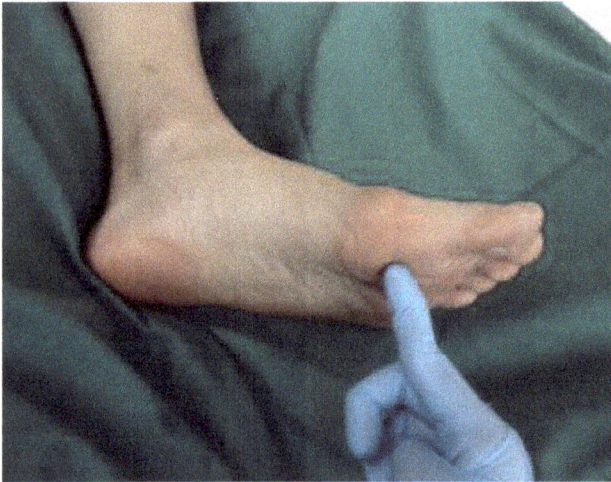

Figure 21.   Deep palpation ray by ray — sole

The most common joints involved in septic arthritis are the metatarsophlangeal joints and the proximal interphalangeal joints of the foot.

The most common bones involved in osteomyelitis are the metatarsal bones and the proximal phalanges.

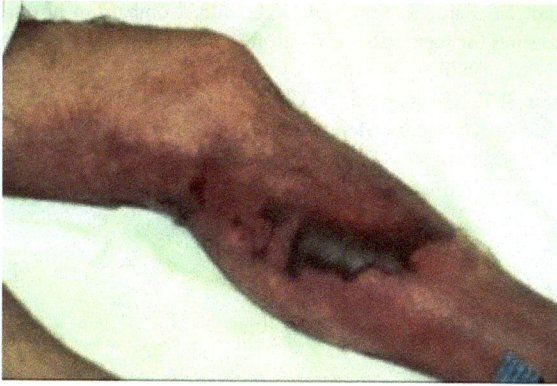

Figure 22. Necrotising fasciitis, showing haemorrhagic blister of the skin

In necrotising fasciitis (Fig. 22), the overlying skin often has cellulitis. In delayed cases, haemorrhagic blisters are commonly present. This is characteristic of necrotising fasciitis. There is severe tenderness and tension of the underlying deep fascia. This subcutaneous tenderness is also characteristic of this condition.

In a diabetic foot ulcer, a bone seen or palpated is usually infected (osteomyelitis). In a "Probe Test", if a sterile metal probe or the gloved finger reaches a bone, that bone is considered to have osteomyelitis (Caputo *et al.* 1994).[7]

References

1. L. Solomon, D. J. Warwick, S. Nayagam and A. G. Apley, *Apley's System of Orthopaedics and Fractures*, 8th Edition (Hodder Arnold, London, New York, New Dehli, 2001).
2. A. Nather, S. B. Chionh, Y. H. Chan, J. L. L. Chew, C. B. Lin, S. H. Neo and E. Y. Sim, Epidemiology of diabetic foot problems and predictive factors for limb loss, *J. Diabetes Complications* **22**:77–82 (2008).
3. A. Nather, S. B. Chionh, K. L. Wong, S. Q. O. Koh, Y. H. Chan, X. Y. Li and A. Nambiar, Socioeconomic profile of diabetic patients with and without foot problems, *Diabet. Foot Ankle* **1**:5523 (2010).
4. A. Nather, S. H. Neo, B. C. Siok, S. C. F. Liew, E. Y. Sim and J. L. L. Chew, Assessment of sensory neuropathy in diabetic patients without diabetic foot problems, *J. Diabetes Complications* **22**:126–31 (2008).
5. K. Stone, A Nather, Z. Aziz and A Erasmus, Footwear in patients with diabetic foot problems, 35th Annual General Meeting of Malaysia Orthopaedic Association, 12 May 2005, Miri, Sarawak, Malaysia.

6. J. M. Sosenko, M. Kato, R. Sato and D. E. Bild, Comparison of quantitative survey threshold measures for their associates with foot ulceration in diabetic patients, *Diabetes Care* **13**:1057–61 (1990).

7. G. M. Caputo, P. R. Cavanagh, J. S. Ulbrecht, G. W. Gibbons and A. W. Karchmer, Assessment and management of foot disease in patients with diabetes, *N. Engl. J. Med.* **331**(13):854–60 (1994).

13

Foot Screening

Aziz Nather and April Voon Siew Lian

Department of Orthopaedic Surgery
Yong Loo Lin School of Medicine
National University of Singapore

Introduction

As recommended by the Ministry of Health Clinical Practice Guidelines for Managing Diabetes Mellitus 2006,[1] all patients with diabetes are recommended to undergo annual foot screening to detect the 'foot at risk'[2] for referral to the podiatrist, the orthopaedic surgeon or the vascular surgeon as early as possible. With foot screening, we can reduce the rate of foot complications and thereby lower the extremity amputation rate.[3]

The National University Hospital (NUH) Diabetic Foot Team implemented a foot screening programme in 2006[4] with the following objectives:

1. To provide foot screening and foot care education to all diabetics
2. To detect diabetics with 'foot at risk' for early intervention to prevent development of diabetic foot complications
3. To provide prompt treatment to diabetics who have already developed foot complications
4. To reduce the number of major lower limb amputations

Foot Screening

To detect risk factors, one must perform foot screening. Foot screening has been shown to significantly lower major amputation rate.[5]

NUH provides a complete foot screening package that includes neurological assessment, vascular assessment, foot risk assessment and foot care education. The NUH protocol for foot screening is as follows:

Part I Assessment: History Taking

1. Demography
   Patient's basic personal information is requested for medical records purpose. The basic personal information includes:

   - Marital status
   - Education level
   - Care giver's detail
   - Relationship with the care giver

2. Medical history
   This includes:

   - Date of patient's diagnosis of diabetes
   - Current treatment for diabetes

   Patient's diabetes complications and other medical conditions will be reviewed. Patient will also be asked questions about lifestyle, such as smoking and drinking (Fig. 1).

3. History of foot condition
   Patient will be asked about lower limb symptoms, such as:

   - Presence of any "pins and needles" sensation
   - Pain or cramping of the calf while walking

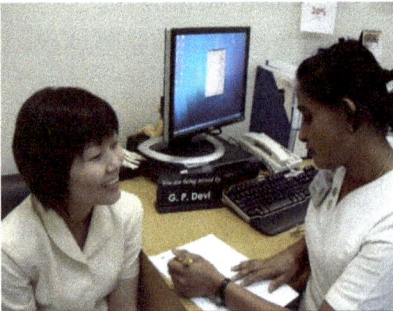

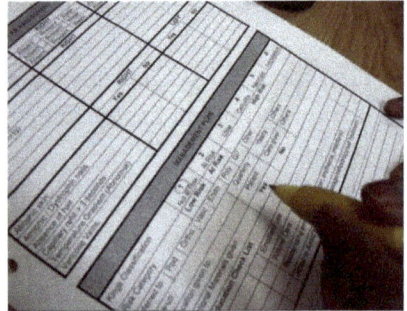

Figure 1.   Trained nurse taking down patient's history

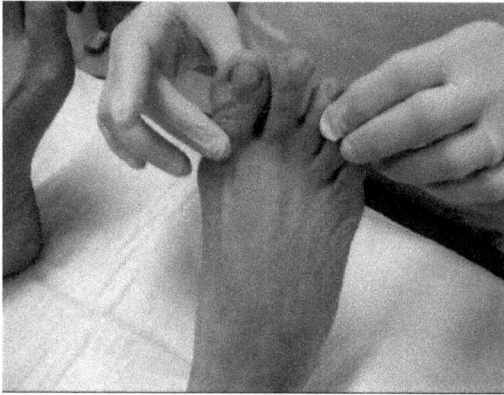

Figure 2.   General foot assessment

- previous wounds/amputations
- Footwear for home and outdoors
- Use of any insoles or prosthetic devices

Part II Assessment: Clinical Examination

1. General foot assessment (Fig. 2)
   Patient will be assessed for skin conditions, such as:

   - Maceration
   - Redness
   - Swelling
   - Dryness
   - Nail fungal infection
   - Corn and callus

2. Biomechanical assessment (Fig. 3)
   Patient will be assessed for any foot structure deformities. Three common foot deformities are:

   - Bunion
   - Lesser toe deformity
   - Charcot joint

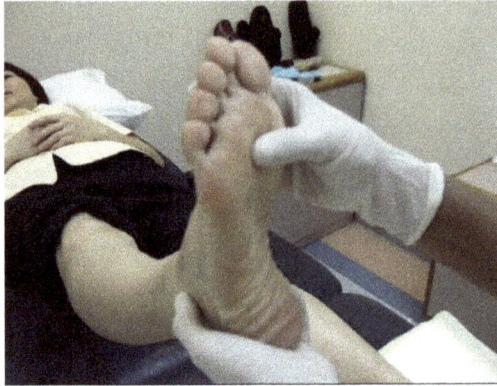

Figure 3. Biomechanical assessment

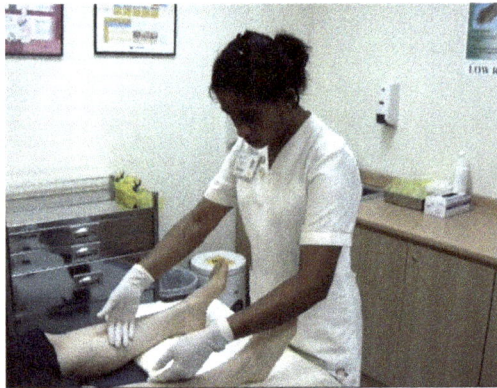

Figure 4. Muscle wasting test

Part III Assessment: Neurological Assessment

Five tests will be performed to assess the neurological condition in the patient's feet:

- Muscle wasting test (Fig. 4)
- Proprioception test (Fig. 5)
- Monofilament test (Fig. 6)
- Vibration perception test (Fig. 7)
- Knee and ankle reflex tests (Fig. 8)

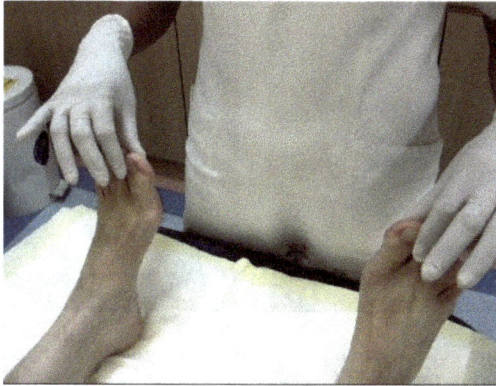

Figure 5. Proprioception test

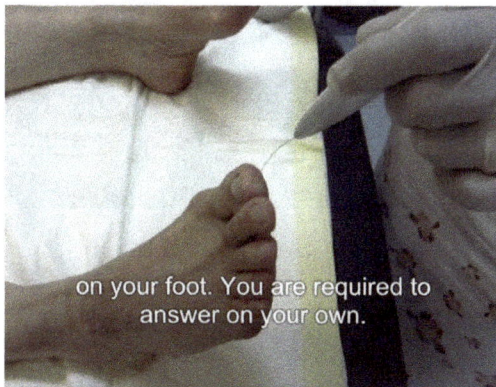

Figure 6. Ten points Semmes Weinstein 5.07 monofilament test (SWMT)

Part IV Assessment: Vascular Assessment

This aims to detect the 2 distal pulses using a probe (Fig. 9):

- Dorsalis pedis pulse
- Posterior tibial pulse

The ankle-brachial index (ABI) and toe-brachial index (TBI) will also be calculated.

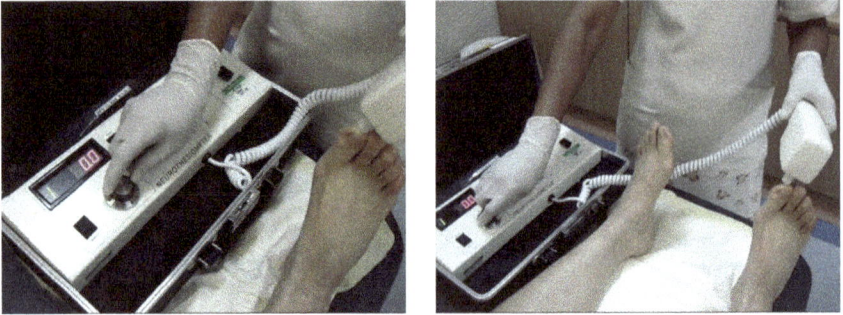

Figure 7.   Vibration perception test using neurothesiometer

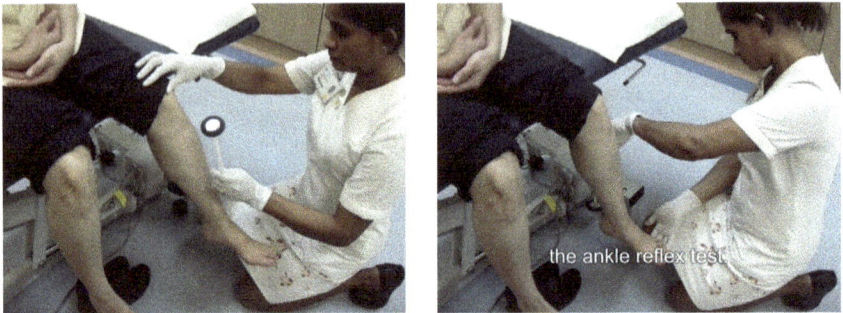

Figure 8.   Knee and ankle reflex tests

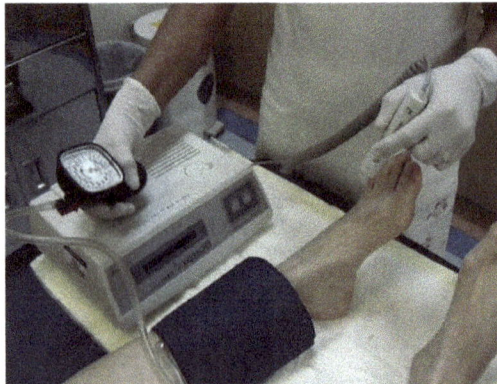

Figure 9.   Detecting distal pulses using Doppler ultrasound

Part V Assessment: Management Plan

After completing the foot screening, the examiner will explain any abnormality detected to the patient and suggest appropriate management for this. Patient's diabetic foot assessment results will also be classified according to both the King's College Classification (Table 1) and the International Working Group of the Diabetic Foot (IWGDF) risk stratification tool (Fig. 10).

If needed, medical referrals will be made to a podiatrist, orthopaedic surgeon, vascular surgeon or endocrinologist (Table 2). The patient may also

Table 1. King's College classification

Stage	Description
Stage 1	Normal foot
Stage 2	High risk foot
Stage 3	Ulcerated foot
Stage 4	Cellulitic foot
Stage 5	Necrotic foot
Stage 6	Major amputation

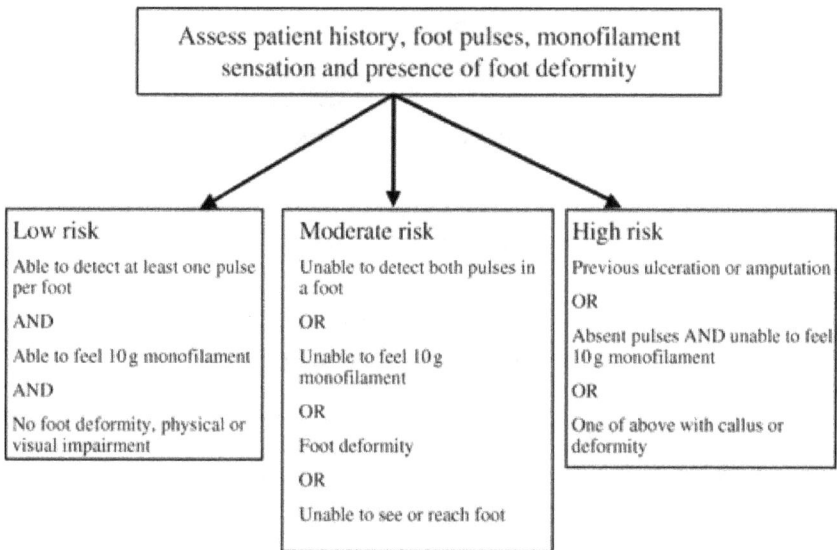

Assess patient history, foot pulses, monofilament sensation and presence of foot deformity

Low risk	Moderate risk	High risk
Able to detect at least one pulse per foot	Unable to detect both pulses in a foot	Previous ulceration or amputation
AND	OR	OR
Able to feel 10 g monofilament	Unable to feel 10 g monofilament	Absent pulses AND unable to feel 10 g monofilament
AND	OR	OR
No foot deformity, physical or visual impairment	Foot deformity	One of above with callus or deformity
	OR	
	Unable to see or reach foot	

Figure 10. Foot risk stratification scheme
Source: Leese *et al.* (2007). http://care.diabetesjournals.org/content/30/8/2064.long

Table 2. Recommended referrals

Indication	Referral recommended
Callosity	Podiatrist
Deformity	Orthopaedic surgeon
Ulcer or previous ulceration	Orthopaedic surgeon
Previous amputation	Orthopaedic surgeon
One pulse or no pulse	Vascular surgeon

be referred to a polyclinic or general practitioner. A follow-up appointment date for diabetic foot assessment will be given to the patient.

NUH Foot Screening Experience

Nather *et al.* (2010)[6] studied 2137 diabetics (3926 feet) screened from 2006 to 2008 using the NUH foot screening protocol. The foot screening was conducted by a trained staff nurse. All patients were classified according to King's College Classification.

Our results showed majority of patients were in the 5th (27.9%) and 6th (30.0%) decades of life. 2064 patients (96.6%) suffered from type 2 diabetes and 73 patients (3.4%) type 1 diabetes. Neuropathy was found in 1307 feet (33.3%) based on SWMT. Vasculopathy (ABI < 0.8) was found in 510 feet (13.0%). TBI < 0.7 was found in 546 feet (13.9%).

According to King's Classification, 1069 patients (50.0%) were Stage 1: Normal foot, 615 patients (28.8%) were Stage 2: Foot at risk, 212 patients (9.9%) were Stage 3: Ulcerated foot, 83 patients (3.9%) were Stage 4: Cellulitic foot, 11 patients (0.3%) were Stage 5: Necrotic foot and 147 patients (6.9%) classified as Stage 6: Major amputation.

Following foot screening, 83 patients (3.9%) were referred to specialists — 75 to podiatrists, 5 to vascular surgeons and 3 to orthopaedic surgeons.

NUH Foot Screening Courses

NUH Diabetic Foot Team started training nurses to be proficient in foot screening in March 2006. This venture was supported by a grant from the National Healthcare Group (NHG) to provide the 3 member hospitals with equipment required to run foot screening. The manpower for doing the foot screening came from the individual hospitals themselves. A special curriculum was designed including lectures and practical sessions to learn how to use monofilament test, neurothesiometer, and Doppler ultrasound for measuring ABI and TBI. This course ends with a theory and practical examination.

The 1st NUH Diabetic Foot Screening Course was launched in March 2006. This 2-week training course trained 9 staff nurses from 3 hospitals in Singapore — National University Hospital, Tan Tock Seng Hospital and Alexandra Hospital. In addition, 2 occupational therapists from Universiti Kebangsaan Malaysia (UKM) enrolled in this course. It was a great success.

Subsequently, an annual Regional Training Course for Diabetic Foot Screening was conducted by the NUH Diabetic Foot Team for Singapore and nurses from 3 regional countries, namely Malaysia, Indonesia and Hong Kong. The 5th Regional Training Course for Diabetic Foot Screening was held from 21–25 November 2011. There were a total of 14 participants — 6 from Singapore, 7 from Malaysia and 1 from Indonesia. As of December 2011, a total of 116 nurse clinicians had been trained by the NUH foot screening courses. This included 62 nurses in Singapore from polyclinics, as well as hospitals like the National University Hospital, Tan Tock Seng Hospital, Alexandra Hospital, Singapore General Hospital and Changi General Hospital. 31 nurse clinicians and 2 occupational therapists from Malaysia, 5 nurse clinicians and 2 orthopaedic surgeons from Indonesia, as well as 4 nurse clinicians from Hong Kong had also been trained.

Conclusion

Foot screening is an important part of the diabetic service that should be provided for all patients diagnosed with diabetes. All diabetics must be subjected to annual foot screening. Risk factors can be detected early for prompt attention by the relevant specialists — the podiatrist, orthopaedic surgeon or vascular surgeon. In this way, diabetic foot complications can be prevented thereby reducing the incidence of major amputations.

The NUH Diabetic Foot Team continues to play an important role in training nurses in Singapore to specialise in foot screening for patients with diabetes. It also provides training for healthcare professionals from regional countries, namely Malaysia, Indonesia and Hong Kong.

References

1. Ministry of Health, Singapore, Clinical Practice Guidelines for Managing Diabetes Mellitus (2006).
2. H. M. Rathur and A. J. Boulton, The neuropathic diabetic foot, *Nat. Clin. Pract. Endocrinol. Metab.* **3**(1):14–25 (2007).
3. R. Ogrin and A. Sands, Foot assessment in patients with diabetes, *Aust. Fam. Physician* **35**(6):419–21(2006).
4. A. Nather, J. C. C. Cheng, G. P. Devi, S. B. Chionh and A. Erasmus, Foot screening for diabetics. In: A. Nather (ed.), *Diabetic Foot Problems* (World Scientific Publishing, Singapore, 2008), pp. 169–77.
5. C. J. McCabe, R. C. Stevenson and A. M. Dolan, Evaluation of a diabetic foot screening and protection programme, *Diabet. Med.* **15**(1):80–4 (1998).
6. A. Nather, S. B. Chionh, P. L. M. Tay, Z. Aziz, J. W. H. Teng, K. Rajeswari, A. Erasmus and A. Nambiar, Foot screening for diabetics, *Ann. Acad. Med. Singapore* **39**:472–5 (2010).

14

Investigations

Aziz Nather and Amy Pannapat Chanyarungrojn

Department of Orthopaedic Surgery
Yong Loo Lin School of Medicine
National University of Singapore

Introduction

After clinical examination of the patient and making a diagnosis, investigations are performed. These include blood tests, culture and sensitivity tests and radiographs.

Blood Tests

Investigations include:

- Markers of infection
  - Full blood count

	Normal range	
o White Blood Cell (WBC)	3.40 – 9.60	$\times 10^9$/L
o Haemoglobin (Hb)	Male: 12.9 – 17.0	g/dL
	Female: 11.3 – 13.5	g/dL
o *Leukocytosis*	WBC > 10.00	$\times 10^9$/L

- Acute phase reactants

	Normal range	
o Erythrocyte sedimentation rate (ESR)	5 – 15	mm/hr
o C-reactive protein (CRP)	0 – 10	mg/L

- Urea and electrolytes

	Normal range	
o Urea	2.0 – 6.5	mmol/L
o Sodium (Na)	135 – 150	mmol/L
o Chloride (Cl)	98 – 107	mmol/L
o Potassium (K)	3.5 – 5.0	mmol/L
o Creatinine (Cr)	50 – 90	μmol/L

- HbA1C

	Normal range
o *Patients without diabetes*	3.5 – 5.5%
o *Patients with diabetes*	< 7.0%

- Capillary blood glucose test
  — Monitoring is performed 4 times daily and charted (tds +10 pm in diabetes chart) (Fig. 1)

	Normal range	
o Glucose	4.0 – 7.8	mmol/L

- Total proteins

	Normal range	
o Albumin	38 – 48	g/L

Culture and Sensitivity (c/s) Studies

- Blood for c/s
  — This procedure is done under sterile conditions

Hypocount Chart
(Blood glucose chart)

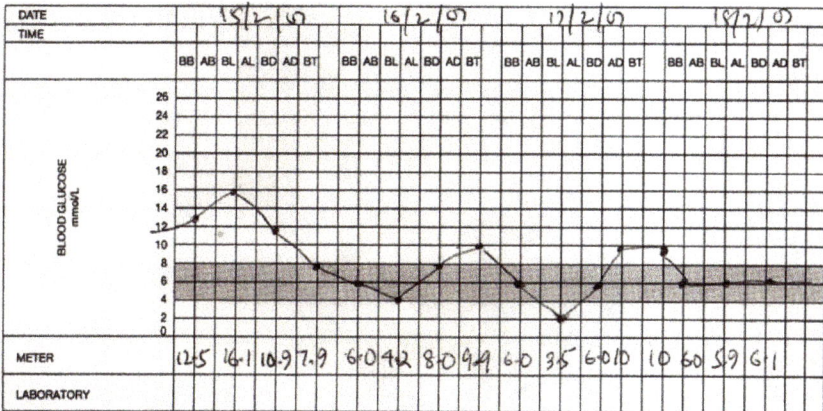

Figure 1. Hypocount chart in patient with DFP showing good control

— It is done in all cases — even in the absence of a spike of fever. This is because elderly and diabetic patients often have infection without systemic response

• Swab for c/s

— A swab is taken from the ulcer or pus discharging from a wound
— Culture is done for both aerobic and anaerobic organisms (Fig. 2), and the sensitivity of organism(s) present to various antibiotics are performed

Taking a wound swab

— A culture must be taken before antibiotics are started
— First, clean the ulcer and the surrounding skin with normal saline
— Press the wound at the edges to squeeze pus out from the centre portion
— Take the swab from the deepest portion of the ulcer, and not from the edges (Fig. 2) to avoid contamination by commensals harboured in the neighbouring skin
— Send the swab for c/s for aerobic and anaerobic organisms

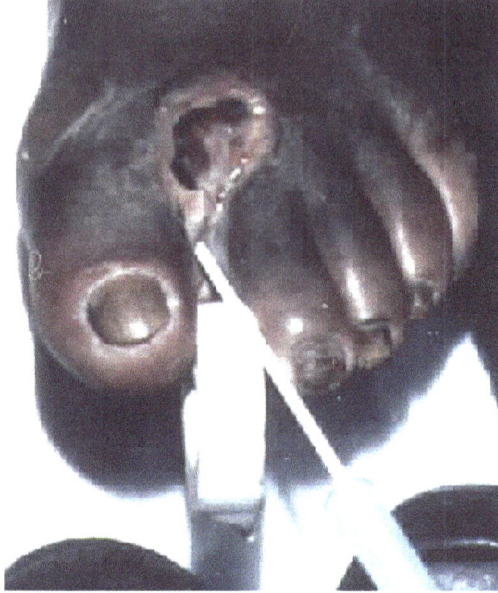

Figure 2.   Wrong way of taking swab for c/s. swab stick applied to the edge of the ulcer

- Taking a tissue specimen
  — Tissue specimen is more accurate than a swab
  — After cleaning with normal saline, a piece of tissue is cut from the floor of the ulcer and sent for culture

Radiological Tests

- Radiographs of the foot — anteroposterior (AP) and oblique views, or radiographs of the ankle (AP and lateral views) are taken (Figs. 3a to 3c)

  Look for the following features on radiographs:
  — Loss of soft tissue plane
  — Calcification of vessels — dorsalis pedis (DP) or posterior tibial (PT) artery (Fig. 3a)
  — Erosion of adjacent bones abutting a joint: septic arthritis (Fig. 3b)
  — Erosion of bone: Osteomyelitis (Fig. 3c)
  — Presence of gas implies an ominous or serious life-threatening infection

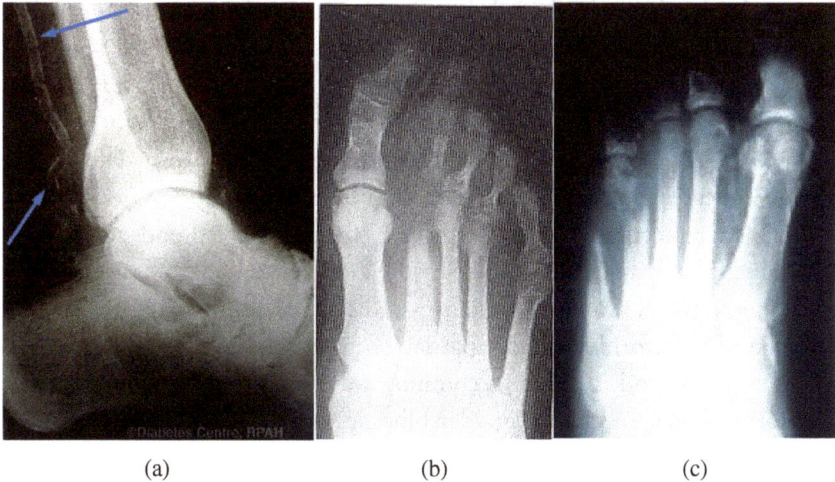

(a)   (b)   (c)

Figure 3. (a) Showing calcification of posterior tibial artery, (b) erosion of metatarsal head and base of proximal phalanx: septic arthritis of 2nd metatarsophalangeal joint, and (c) pathological fracture of the 4th metatarsal bone due to osteomyelitis and gas in between the 3rd and 4th rays: necrotising faciitis of the foot

— Necrotising faciitis (Fig. 3c)
— Dislocation of joint, bone destruction: Charcot Joint Disease (CJD)

Chest Radiographs and Electrocardiograms should also be performed.

Other Investigations

Ankle Brachial Index (ABI)

The ABI is a non-invasive evaluation of blood flow. The index is calculated by dividing the highest systolic pressure of two pedal arteries — DP and PT by the brachial systolic pressure in the arm ($\frac{Ankle\ Systolic\ Pressre}{Brachial\ Systolic\ Pressure}$). The ankle systolic pressure is measured using a cuff and a hand-held continuous wave Doppler ultrasound probe placed over the pedal vessels (Fig. 4).

The interpretation of ABI values are:

- 0.8 to 1.2   Normal
- < 0.8   Ischaemia
- < 0.5   Critical ischaemia

ABI results should not be the only investigation method used to make a clinical decision, as the results can be misleading. Medial wall calcification is present in many patients with long-term diabetes. This results in an artificially elevated systolic pressure and ABI value.

An ABI above 1.2 (eg. 2.0) does not indicate a good or normal flow. Such a value indicates presence of calcification in the vessel.

It is more accurate to look at the waveform generated and not just the ABI value. The waveforms obtained by the Doppler can be triphasic, biphasic or monophasic. A triphasic waveform indicates a healthy artery (Fig. 5a). A biphasic waveform indicates partial obstruction (Fig. 5b). This is still regarded as safe and is the most common waveform present. A monophasic waveform indicates occlusion (sudden blockage of a blood vessel) and increased

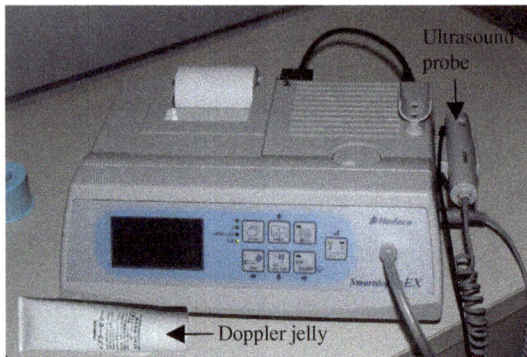

Figure 4.   ABI machine with ultrasonic probe and doppler jelly

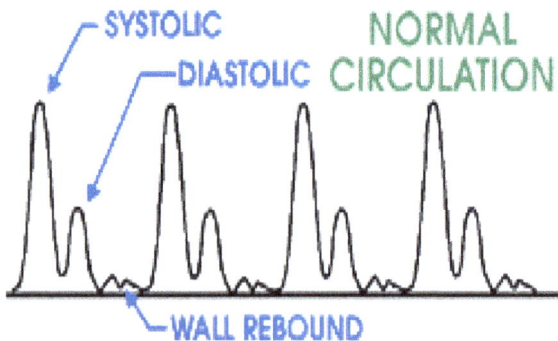

Figure 5a.   Triphasic

PARTIALLY OBSTRUCTED

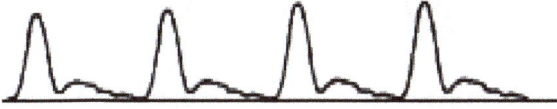

Figure 5b. Biphasic

INCREASED OBSTRUCTION

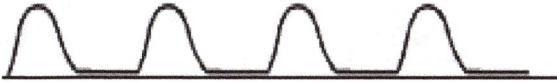

Figure 5c. Monophasic (loss of diastolic flow)

SEVERE OBSTRUCTION

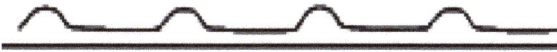

Figure 5d. Monophasic (waveform flattened then disappears)

obstruction of blood flow (Fig. 5c). The flatter the waveform, the smaller the volume of flow (Fig. 5d).

Method:

- With the patient supine, remove shoes and stockings. Wait for at least 10 minutes before taking blood pressure measurements
- Apply blood pressure cuff snugly on the upper arm (Fig. 6a)
- Inflate the cuff, gradually lower the pressure and record the systolic reading obtained from the Doppler probe

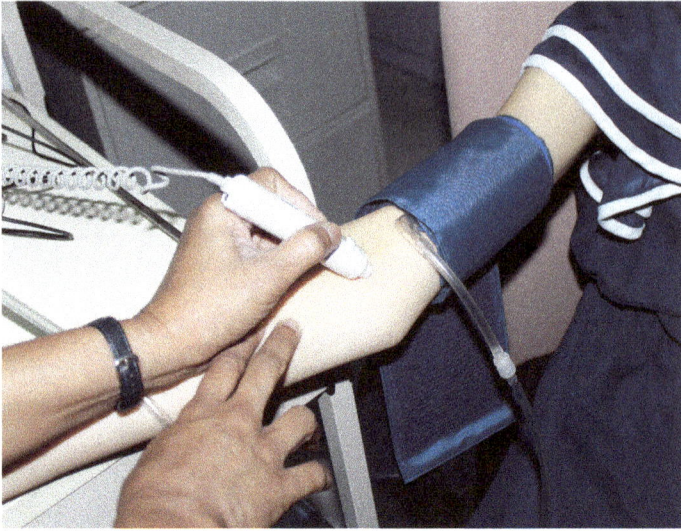

Figure 6a. Taking the systolic pressure of the brachial artery

- Apply the same cuff snugly on the ankle on the same side of the body
- Palpate the area behind the medial malleolus to find the PT pulse. Inflate the cuff, gradually lower the pressure and record the systolic reading (Fig. 6b)
- Palpate the dorsum of the same foot for the DP pulse. Inflate the cuff, gradually lower the pressure and record the systolic reading (Fig. 6c)
- Apply cuff on the opposite ankle and record the PT and DP pressures

The advantages of ABI include:

- Method is non-invasive
- It is quick and easy to perform
- It provides reliable and reproducible results
- It is inexpensive

The disadvantages of ABI are:

- Results can be falsely elevated in patients with calcified vessels
- It is operator dependent

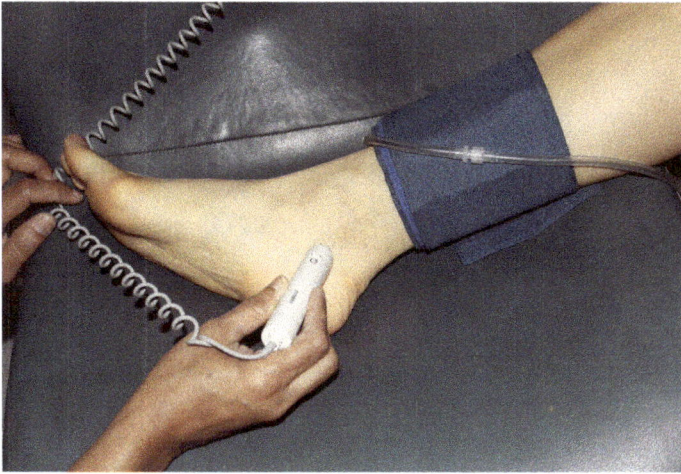

Figure 6b. Taking the systolic pressure of the posterior tibial artery

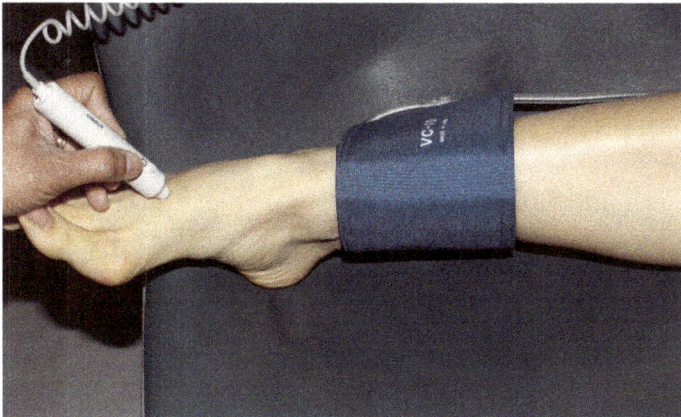

Figure 6c. Taking the systolic pressure of the dorsal pedis artery

Toe Brachial Index (TBI)

Unlike ABI which uses ultrasound, TBI is based on infra-red light using photoplethysmography. It measures digital blood flow.

The index is calculated by dividing the highest systolic pressure of the big toe by the brachial systolic pressure ($\frac{Toe\ Systolic\ Pressre}{Brachial\ Systolic\ Pressure}$). The toe systolic pressure is measured using a cuff and a small photoplethysmograph (PPG) probe placed over the tip of the big toe.

The TBI measures tissue perfusion at the toe level. In the toes, the small digital arteries are not affected by medial wall calcification, unlike pedal arteries. The TBI is a more accurate measure of tissue perfusion in the toes than the ABI.

The interpretation of TBI values are:

- ≥ 0.7   Normal
- 0.4 to 0.6   Ischaemia
- ≤ 0.3   Critical ischaemia

The toe pressure can be expected to be 60% to 80% of the ankle pressure and an absolute toe pressure of 30 mmHg or higher is required for normal wound healing.

Method:

- With the patient supine, remove shoes and stockings Wait for at least 10 minutes before measuring blood pressure
- Place the blood pressure cuff snugly on the upper arm
- Inflate the cuff, gradually lower the pressure and record the systolic reading
- Place the small toe cuff snugly around the base of the big toe (Fig. 7)
- Place the small PPG probe over the tip of the toe (Fig. 7)
- Inflate the cuff, gradually lower the pressure and record the systolic reading

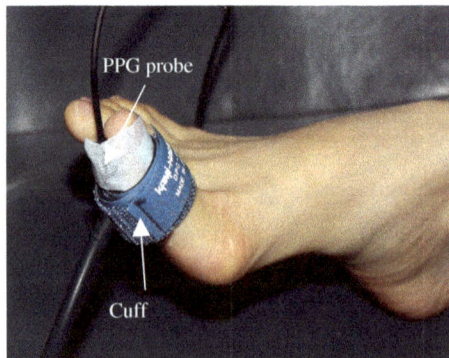

Figure 7.   Photoplethymography toe pressure measurement

- Place the toe cuff to the opposite big toe and record the toe pressure on the other side

The advantages of TBI are:

- The method is non-invasive
- It reflects tissue perfusion at toe level more accurately than ABI
- There is no calcification of the digital arteries

Biothesiometer (Vibration Perception Threshold)

The Biothesiometer (Fig. 8) measures a patient's vibration perception threshold (VPT). This is an index of sensory neuropathy.[1]

Method:

- Apply the probe on the big toe
- Turn the dial to increase the intensity of vibration until it can be felt
- Instruct the patient to report as soon as vibration is felt. The reading on the dial is recorded

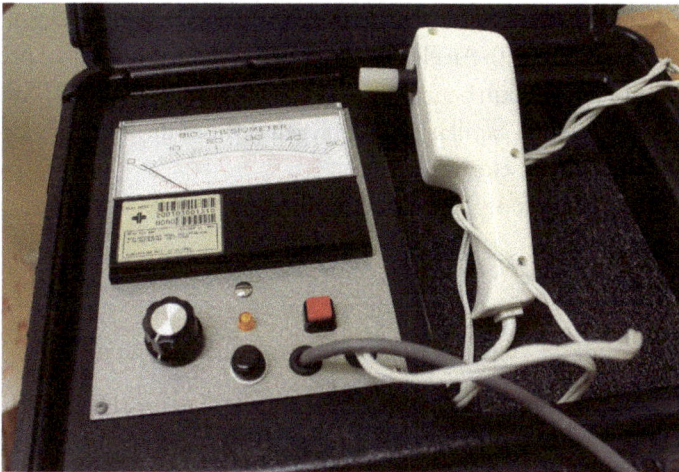

Figure 8. Biothesiometer

The interpretation for biothesiometer readings (in volts) are:

- 0 – 24 V   Normal range
- 25 – 50 V   Abnormal range

The advantages of using a biothesiometer are:

- It is non-invasive
- It is quick and easy to use — takes only a few minutes
- It is a portable and battery operated machine

The disadvantage of using a biothesiometer is its high costs as compared to other methods such as the Semmes Weinstein 5.07 Gauge Monofilament Test (SWMT) and the Neurotip Pin Prick Test. A biothesiometer costs about SGD4200.

Transcutaneous Oxygen (TcPO$_2$) Measurements

For wounds to heal, the microcirculation needs to provide important nutrients and oxygen to the tissue. Oxygen is vital for the formation of granulation tissue and provides resistance to fight infection.[2] Wound healing is dependent on tissue perfusion as this determines the amount oxygen delivered to the wound. Therefore, tissue oxygen levels are useful in determining healing potential in diabetic foot.

The TcPO$_2$ is the measurement of the partial pressure of oxygen on the surface of the skin (Fig. 9). An electrode is placed on the skin in close proximity to the wound site. The skin beneath the electrode is heated to 44°C. This causes vasodilation within the capillary bed. Oxygen diffuses through the skin and is measured by the Clark electrode.

The interpretation of TcPO$_2$ values (in mmHg) are:

> 50 mmHg   Normal

< 40 mmHg   Impaired wound healing

< 30 mmHg   Critical ischaemia (inadequate tissue perfusion)

TcPO$_2$ is a key component of Hyperbaric Oxygen Therapy (HBOT). It is used to determine if patients are suitable for HBOT. There is a direct correlation between the effectiveness of HBOT and the predicted healing potential by the TcPO$_2$.[3]

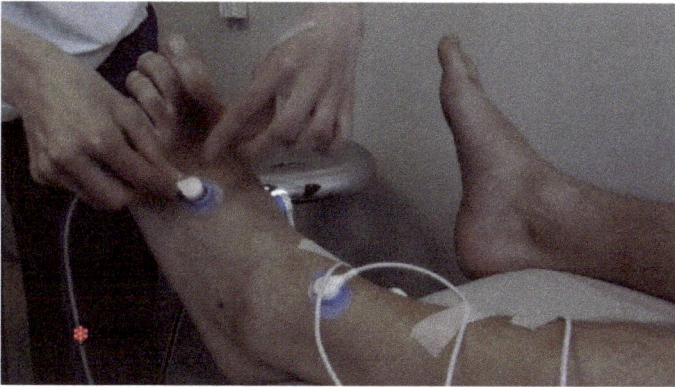

Figure 9. TcPO$_2$ measurements

For healing to take place, a TcPO$_2$ of more than 30mmHg is required. The advantages of TcPO$_2$ are:

- The method is non-invasive
- It is a more accurate measure of tissue perfusion than ABI/TBI

The disadvantages include:

- There is a need for the machine to be recalibrated daily
- It is inaccurate for patients presenting with shock, acidosis, hypoxia, hypothermia, oedema or anaemia

References

1. A. Kasalovà, Biothesiometry in the diagnosis of peripheral neuropathies, *Cas. Lek. Cesk.* **141**(7):223–5 (2002).
2. F. Gottrup, Oxygen in wound healing and infection, *World J. Surg.* **28**:312–5 (2004).
3. B. M. Smith, L. D. Desvigne, B. Slade, J. W. Dooley and D. C. Warren, Transcutaneous oxygen measurements predict healing of leg wounds with hyperbaric therapy, *Wound Repair Regen.* **4**(2):224–9 (1996).

15

Charcot Joint Disease

Aziz Nather and Amaris Lim Shu Min

Department of Orthopaedic Surgery
Yong Loo Lin School of Medicine
National University of Singapore

Introduction

Charcot Joint Disease (CJD) or neuropathic joint is a progressive musculoskeletal condition that is characterised by severe damage and disruption of the joints and surrounding bones. It is a spectrum of diseases ranging from mild changes identifiable only on radiological examination to gross deformities of the foot easily detectable on both clinical and radiological examination. Pathology of CJD starts from the loss of protective sensation which leads to gradual damage and disruption of the joints and surrounding bones. CJD can involve any joint. However, in the lower extremity, it occurs most commonly in the foot and ankle regions.

Historical Background

In 1868, Jean-Martin Charcot[1] (1825–1893), a French neurologist, gave the first detailed description of the neuropathic aspect of CJD. The disease was therefore named after him.

In 1936, William Riely Jordan[2] described the association between neuropathic arthropathy and diabetes mellitus. He attributed a typical painless Charcot joint of the ankle in an elderly woman with diabetes to be "a diabetic process of a neurologic trophic nature". From then on, diabetes has been considered to be the leading cause of neuropathic osteo-arthropathy or CJD.

Epidemiology and Aetiology

CJD may occur bilaterally (Fig. 1). It is associated with longstanding duration of diabetes and peripheral neuropathy. In the early stages, CJD is characterised by acute inflammation which eventually leads to bone and joint fracture, dislocation, instability and gross deformities.[3]

Any pathology that causes sensory or autonomic neuropathy can lead to CJD. CJD occurs as a complication of diabetes, syphilis, chronic alcoholism, leprosy, meningomyelocele, spinal cord injury, syringomyelia, renal dialysis, and congenital insensitivity to pain.

In the past, Charcot joints in the lower limb were most commonly the result of Tabes Dorsalis. However, this condition is very rare nowadays. Diabetic neuropathy is now considered to be the most common cause of CJD

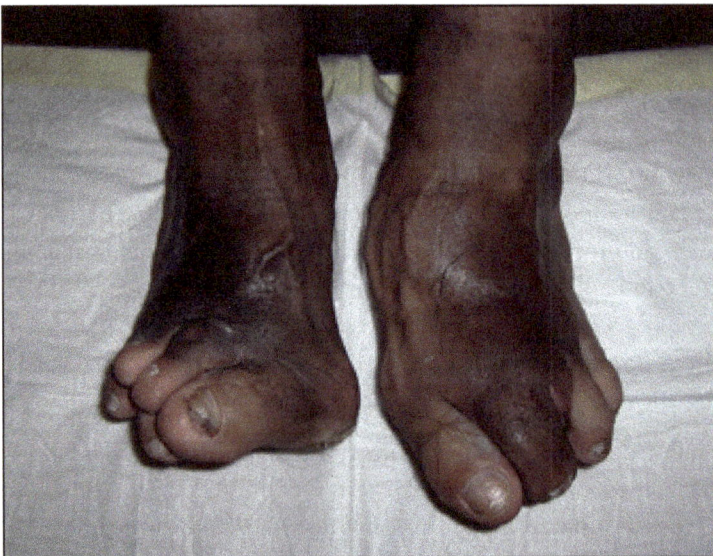

Figure 1. Severe deformity of the forefoot, medial convexity of the mid-foot, left ankle deformity and distended veins in a patient with bilateral CJD involving the feet

of the foot, while Charcot joints in the upper limb are classically caused by Syringomyelia.

Pathogenesis

Three major theories exist regarding the pathophysiology of CJD:

- Neurotraumatic Theory (German)
- Neurovascular Theory (French)
- Modern Theory

While peripheral neuropathy develops over decades, the progression of Charcot foot can occur in a matter of weeks or months initiated by a minor trauma, such as twisting the foot.

Neurotraumatic theory

Charcot believed that the development of enlarged joints was initiated by "spontaneous fracture". Johnson[4] in 1967 explained further that a stress fracture caused by microtrauma in an insensate foot could go undetected due to loss of peripheral sensation and proprioception. The patient continues to traumatize the bone and soft tissues, leading to hyperaemia. Inadequate protection of the fractured bone causes recovery and healing to be impaired.[5]

A vicious cycle arises due to continuous microtrauma and impairment of the repair responses. This occurs repeatedly, causing more and more damage to the bone, joints and the surrounding tissues, eventually resulting in Charcot joint destruction.[5]

Neurovascular theory

The neurovascular theory suggests that a dysregulated autonomic nervous system causes the extremities to receive increased blood flow. This in turn leads to a mismatch in bone destruction and synthesis, resulting in osteopenia (lower bone mineral density). The atrophic and osteopenic bone easily becomes traumatised. Bone and joint trauma may therefore occur easily with minimal activities like walking.[5]

Modern theory

The modern theory is a combination of the above-mentioned two theories.

History

The diagnosis of CJD is often based on clinical features. These include profound unilateral swelling, increased skin temperature (by 3–7°C), erythema, joint effusion and foot and ankle deformity in an insensate extremity. Such clinical signs, in the presence of an intact skin, are often pathognomonic of acute CJD. In addition, plain radiographs are valuable in confirming the presence of CJD.

Concomitant ulceration is common in patients with CJD. Ulceration complicates the diagnosis of CJD, as osteomyelitis is more likely to occur when ulceration is left untreated and affects deep tissues and bones. Radiologically, it may be a challenge to differentiate CJD in the foot from osteomyelitis.

As the disease progresses, the longitudinal and transverse arches of foot may collapse, resulting in a rocker bottom foot.

Clinical Phases of CJD

The clinical presentation of foot CJD can be divided into three phases:

- Acute CJD
- Bone Destruction/Deformity
- Stabilisation

Acute phase

The acute phase presents with unilateral swelling, erythema, increase in local skin temperature, bounding pulses, prominent veins and joint effusion. In CJD, prominent veins are caused by venous shunting.

Pain or discomfort may be minimal due to underlying neuropathy. Patients usually note a recent foot or ankle injury. There is swelling, but with minimal pain.

In the absence of ulceration, it may be difficult to differentiate CJD from cellulitis and deep vein thrombosis, since all three present with a red, warm

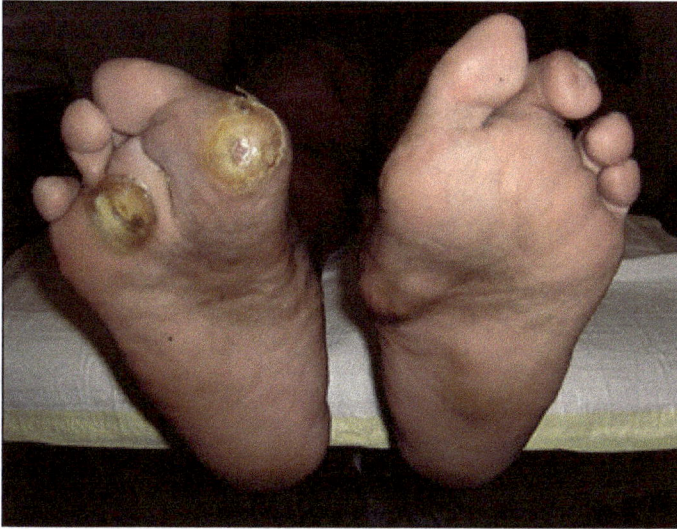

Figure 2. Clawing and overriding toes with medial convexity of the left mid-foot. Callosities are noted over the right first and forth metatarsal heads of the right foot

and swollen foot. In addition, plain radiographs may be normal in cellulitis and in the early stages of acute CJD.

Bone destruction/deformity phase

In this phase, the foot is swollen and warm. Collapse of the medial arch of the foot becomes more apparent. This progression of deformity results in a rocker-bottom foot (Fig. 2).

This correlates with radiological findings of bone fragmentation, new bone formation, subluxation and dislocation. These changes develop within weeks of the onset of this condition.

The involvement of tarso-metatarsal joints leads to broadening of the mid-foot, giving rise to a medial convexity. The involvement of the metatarso-phalangeal and inter-phalangeal joints together with imbalance of the muscles in the feet leads to toe deformities e.g. claw toes (Fig. 2). This deformity increases pressure at the tip of the toes. In the presence of neuropathy, these sites become ulcer prone.

In this phase, the involved bones and joints become unstable, requiring some form of immobilisation.

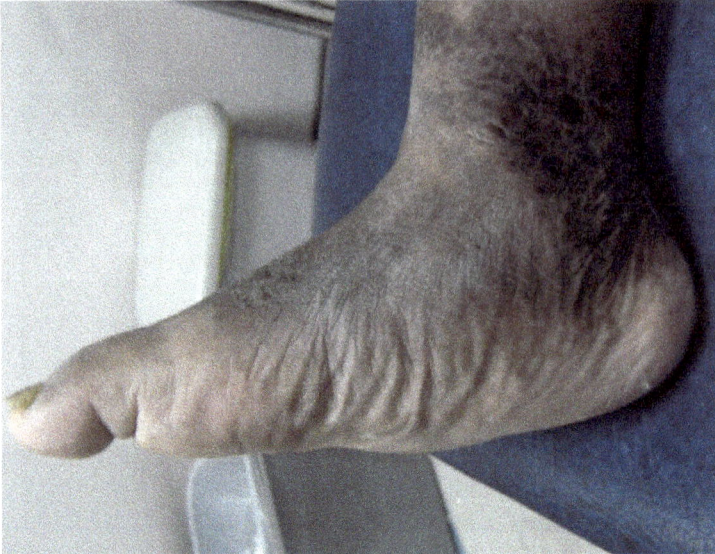

Figure 3. Patient with collapse of the medial arch of the foot in the Stabilization Phase. There is no cellulitis. The foot is not inflamed or swollen

Stabilization phase

In this phase, the foot is no longer red or swollen. The deformity may be marked, but the patients are asymptomatic. Bone integrity is strengthened and the involved joints develop into pseudoarthroses or become fused (Fig. 3).

Radiological Presentation

Radiographically, CJD can present in two different ways:

Atrophic

Atrophic patterns have characteristic dissolution of bone and joint surfaces, commonly seen in the more lateral metatarsal regions.

Hypertrophic

The hypertrophic pattern is more common and can present anywhere within the foot. The radiographic features of a Charcot joint can be described by

Yochum and Rowe using the *6 'D's of Hypertrophy*:[6]

- Increased Density (Subchondral sclerosis)
- Destruction
- Debris (Intra-articular loose bodies) production
- Dislocation
- Distention of joint
- Disorganization

Classification System Based on Radiographic Pathology

Eichenholtz Classification System[7]

The hypertrophic pattern of CJD is typically defined according to the Eichenholtz classification system. This classification system is the first and the most commonly used classification system for CJD. It is based on radiographic appearance as well as physiologic stages of the process.

The original Eichenholtz classification system consisted of 3 stages: the Developmental, Coalescent and Reconstructive stages. Stage 0, the At-Risk Stage, was later added to the classification system. The purpose of this classification system is to determine the patient's prognosis and to gauge the optimal timing for arthrodesis. Surgical intervention is most effective when performed during early stage 1 or late stage 3 disease.

Stage 0: At-Risk Stage

This stage is used to describe a patient with peripheral neuropathy who has sustained an acute sprain or fracture in the ankle or foot, but has not developed characteristic bone radiographic changes. This prodromal period might be considered a "**Charcot *in situ***" stage. Diagnosis of the condition during this period, in which no deformity has yet developed, could prevent further progression of the destructive inflammatory process.

Stage 1: Developmental (Acute) Stage

In the developmental phase of Charcot destruction, hyperaemia (increased blood flow to certain tissues) due to autonomic neuropathy weakens bones

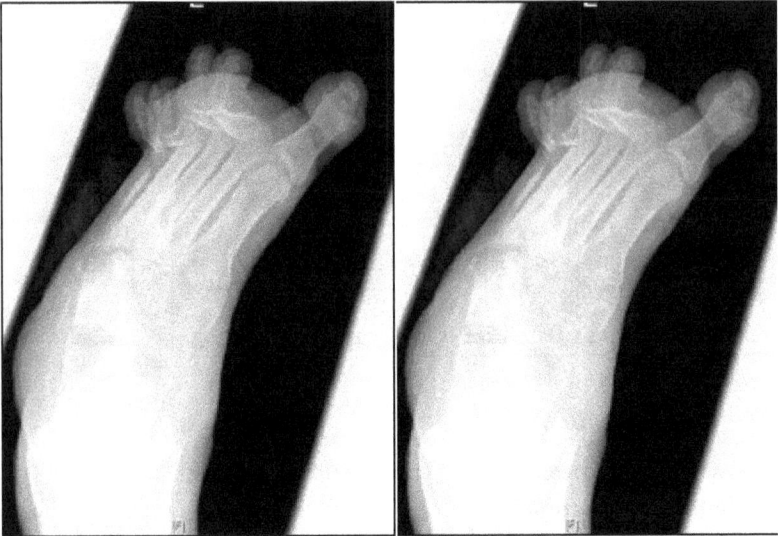

Figure 4.   Plain radiographs showing claw deformity of the toes, visible joint disruption and bony fragmentation involving the fore-foot and the mid-foot (Developmental Phase; Brodsky's Type 5, Saunders' and Mrdjencovich's Pattern 1)

and ligaments. This leads to diffuse swelling, joint laxity, subluxation, and frank dislocation. The patient presents with an acute inflammatory process. Bone fragmentation and joint disruption are visible in radiographs (Fig. 4), with osseous debris surrounding the affected joint.

Stage 2: Coalescent (Quiescent) Stage

In the Coalescent or Quiescent Phase, the osseous debris is resorbed and the larger fragments fuse together (Fig. 5). There is a decrease in warmth, redness, and swelling. Radiographs will show sclerotic bone surrounding the joint, resorption of intra-articular debris, callus formation and fusion of larger bony fragments. Patterns of trabeculation (formation of small and often microscopic tissue element) may also be seen across the fractured margins on radiographs.

Stage 3: Reconstructive Stage

The Remodelling Phase can last months to years. There is continued resolution of inflammation. Bone integrity is strengthened and joints are re-established either in the form of pseudoarthroses or actual fusions. Radiographs show the

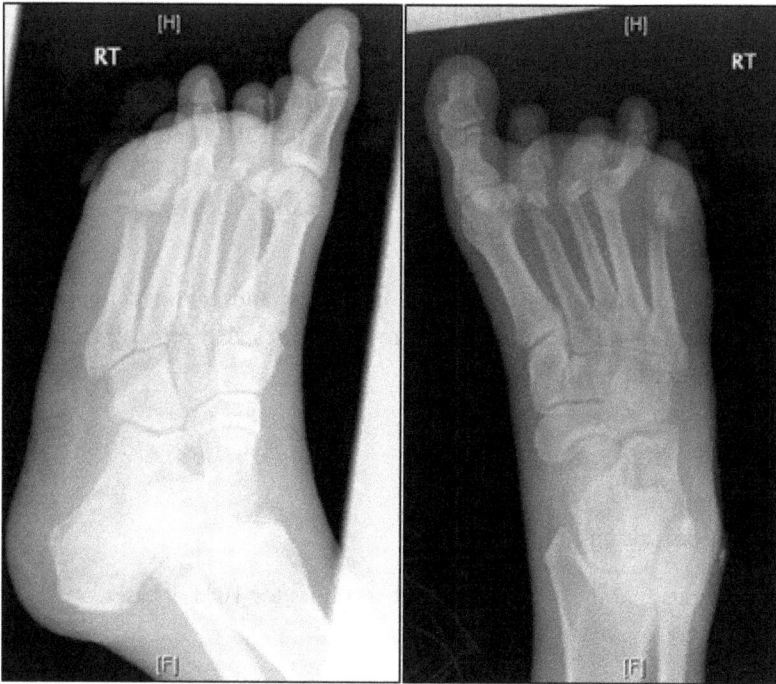

Figure 5. Plain radiographs showing deformities of the fore-foot. There is a visible joint disruption. The osseous debris has been resorbed (Coalescence Phase; Brodsky's Type 5, Saunders' and Mrdjencovich's Pattern 1)

remodeling of bone, bony ankylosis and hypertrophic proliferation. The foot is therefore once again stable, but deformed.

The progression of healing during the reconstruction phase is determined by the joints involved. Generally, patients with forefoot and midfoot involvement respond favourably, whereas hindfoot and ankle involvement is associated with a poorer prognosis. This is due to the severe destruction of ligamentous structures which offer a large proportion of support and joint integrity in the hindfoot and ankle.

Classification Systems Based on Anatomic Pathology

Brodsky's System of Classification[8]

Brodsky's System of classification is based on the four most common regions affected. It classifies different cases of Charcot's foot into 5 groups.

Type 1 — Tarsometatarsal (Lisfranc's) Joints (Fig. 6)

Approximately 60% of cases of Charcot's foot occur in this region. Residual deformity in this area manifests as a collapse of the longitudinal arch, resulting in a rocker-bottom foot. This often causes skin breakdown at the apex of the deformity.

Type 2 — Hindfoot (Fig. 7)

This region involves the subtalar, talonavicular and calcaneocubiod joints. It is the second most common site for Charcot's Arthropathy to develop, accounting for up to 20% of cases.

Type 3 (Fig. 8)

a) Ankle Joint
b) Posterior Calcaneus

Type 3 occurs mainly in the ankle and accounts for 10% of cases.

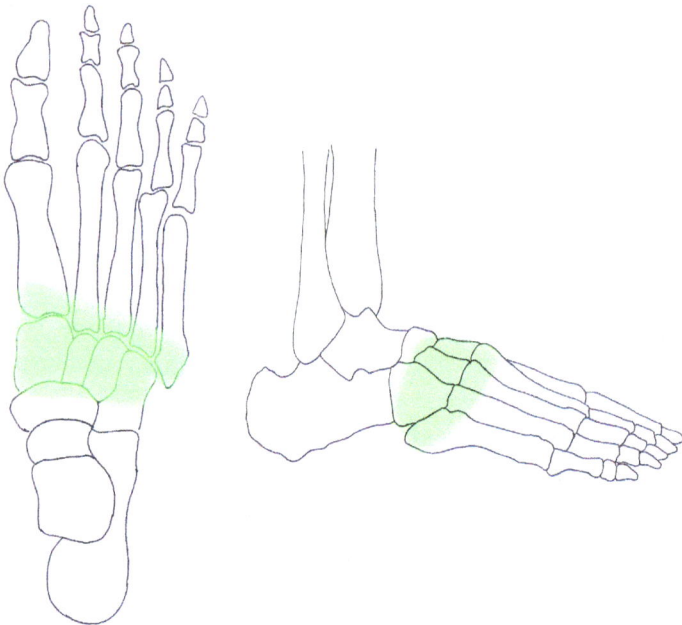

Figure 6a.   Brodsky's Classification Type 1

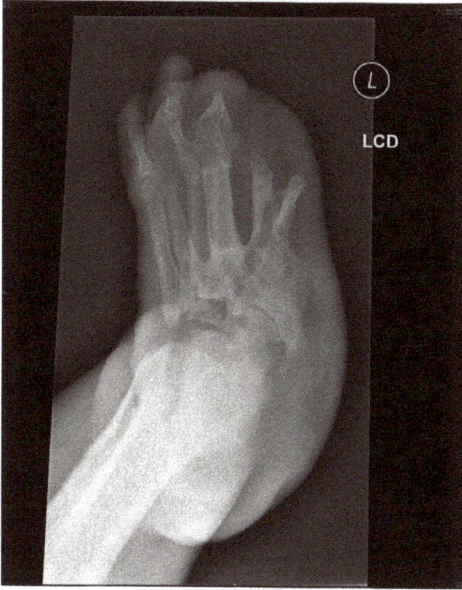

Figure 6b. X-ray of patient showing Brodsky Type 1

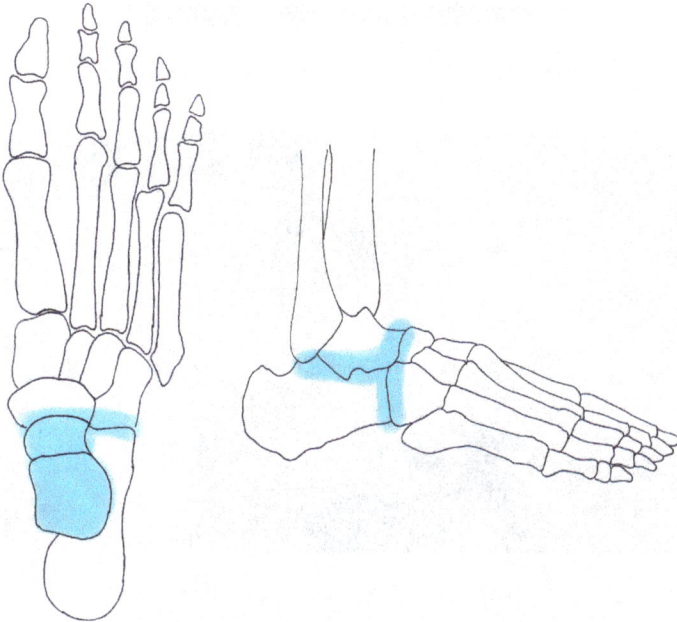

Figure 7a. Brodsky's Classification Type 2

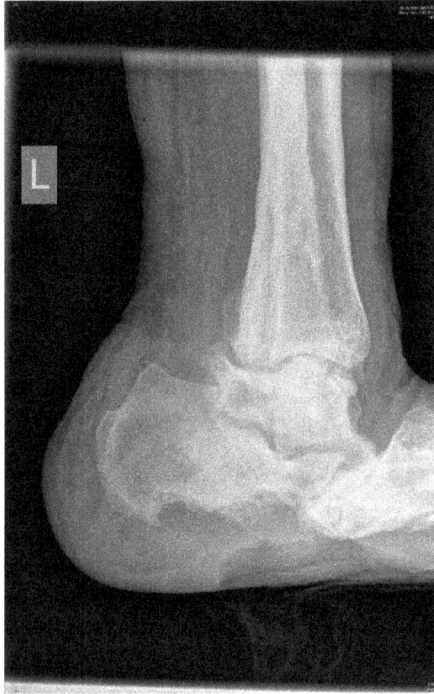

Figure 7b.　X-ray of patient showing Brodsky Type 2

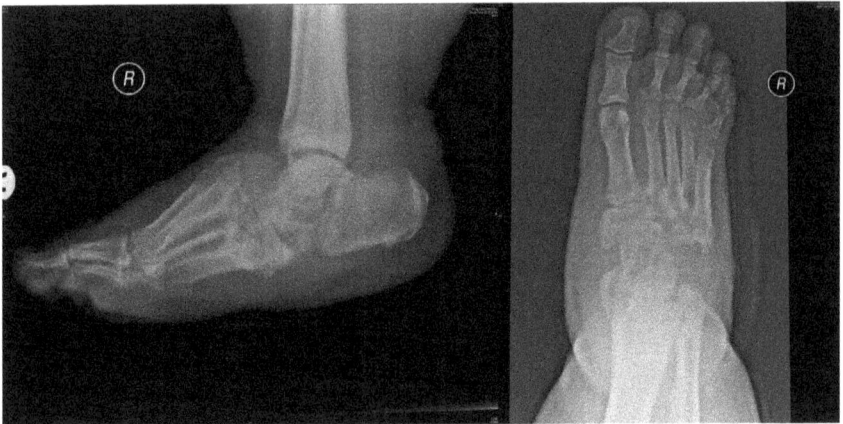

Figure 7c.　Radiographs of another patient with Brodsky Type 2

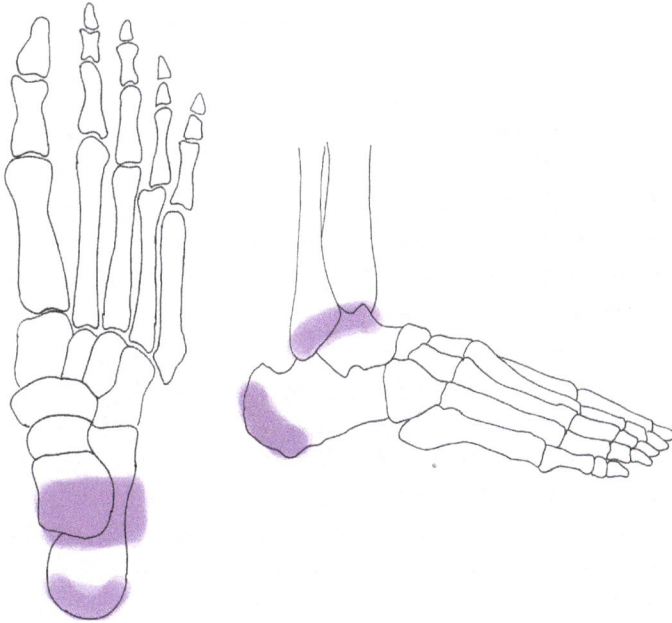

Figure 8. Brodsky's Classification Type 3a and 3b

Type 4 — Multiple Regions

Each region may be at a different stage of the Eichenholtz Classification System.

Type 5 — Forefoot (Fig. 9)

This region is an uncommon site of Charcot's Arthropathy.

Saunders' and Mrdjencovich's System of Classification[9]

Another anatomical classification system is described by Saunders and Mrdjencovich. It is similar to that described by Brodsky. It classifies CJD into 5 different patterns.

Pattern 1 (Fig. 10)

Pattern 1 involves the forefoot joints, including the interphalangeal joints, the phalanges, and the metatarsophalangeal joint. Common radiographic changes include osteopenia, osteolysis, juxta-articular cortical bone defects, subluxation and destruction. Pattern 1 accounts for 15% of cases of CJD.

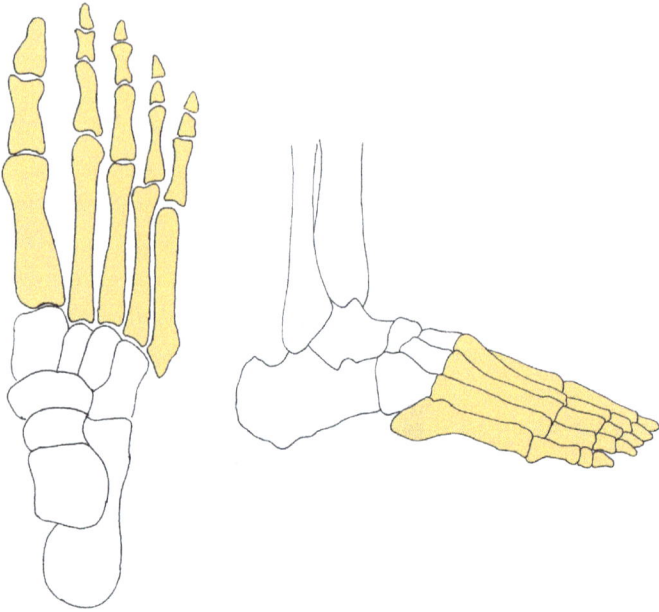

Figure 9. Brodsky's Classification Type 5

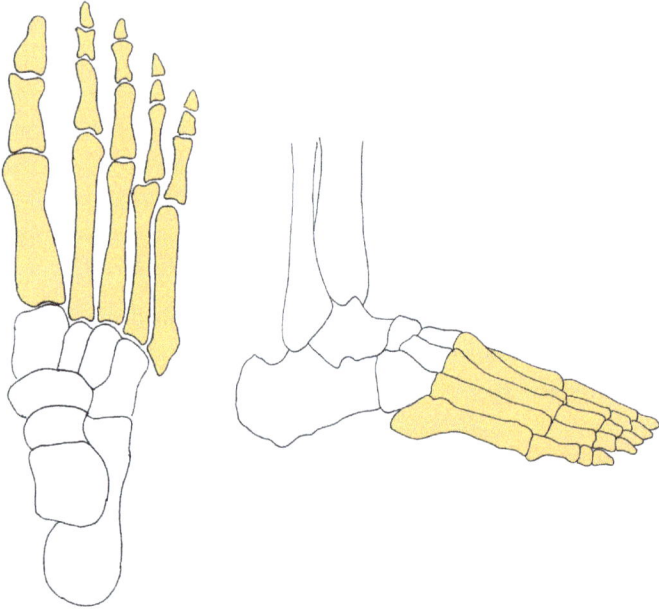

Figure 10. Saunders' and Mrdjencovich's Pattern 1

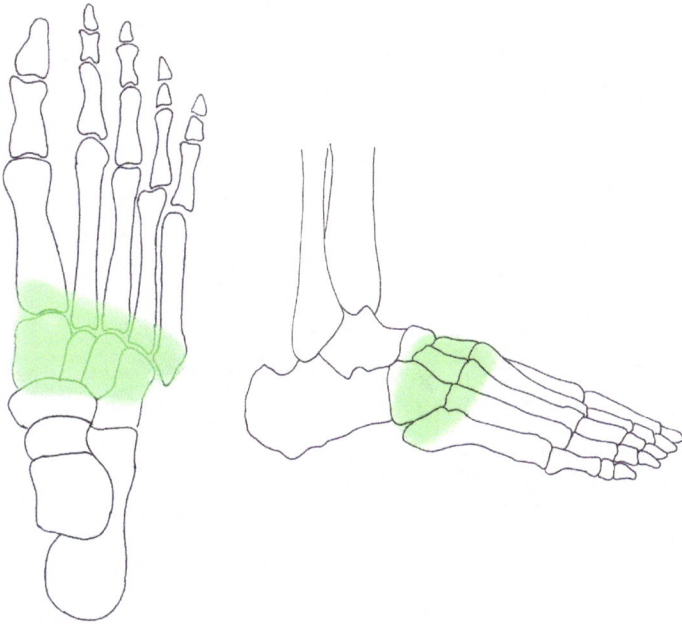

Figure 11. Saunders' and Mrdjencovich's Pattern 2

Pattern 2 (Fig. 11)

Pattern 2 involves the tarsometatarsal joints (Lisfranc's Joints), including the metatarsal bases, cuneiforms and cuboid. Involvement at this site may present as subluxation, fracture or dislocation. This typically results in the classic rocker bottom foot deformity. It accounts for 40% of all cases.

Pattern 3 (Fig. 12)

Pattern 3 involves the naviculocuneiform, talonavicular, and calcaneocuboid joints. Radiographic changes frequently show osteolysis of the naviculo-cuneiform joint (Chopart's Joint). There is also fragmentation and osseous debris dorsally and plantarly. It accounts for 30% of CJD cases.

Pattern 4 (Fig. 13)

Pattern 4 involves the ankle joint. Radiographs reveal erosion of bone and cartilage with extensive destructive of the joint. This may result in dislocation

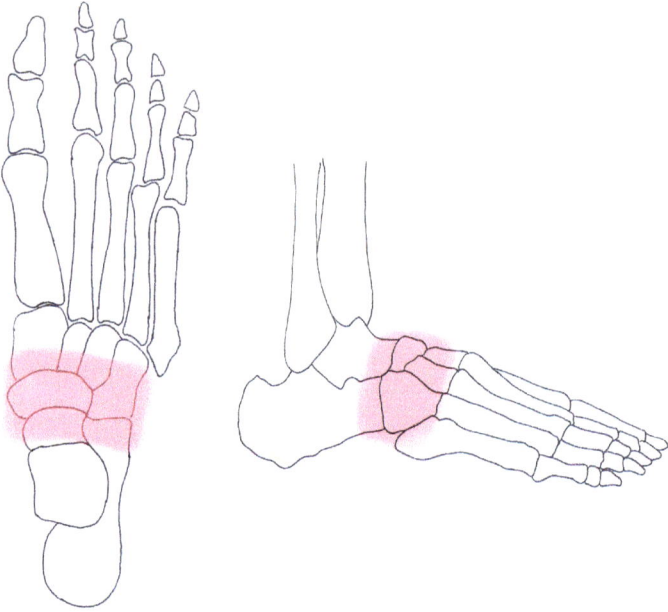

Figure 12. Saunders' and Mrdjencovich's Pattern 3

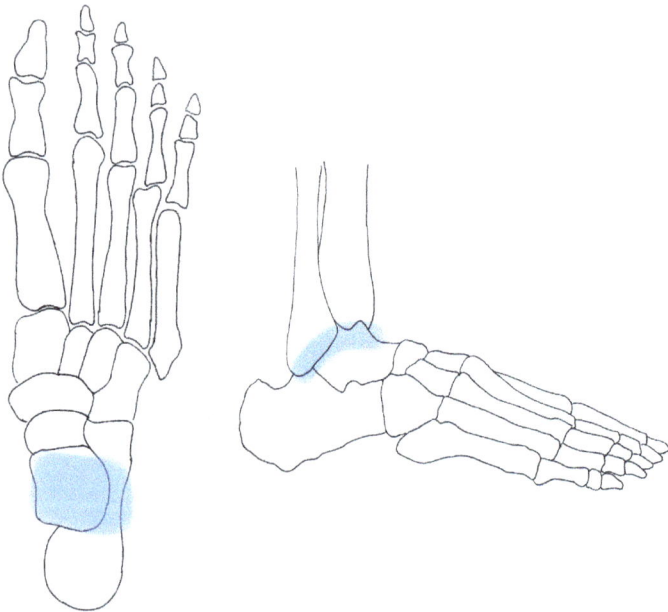

Figure 13. Saunders' and Mrdjencovich's Pattern 4

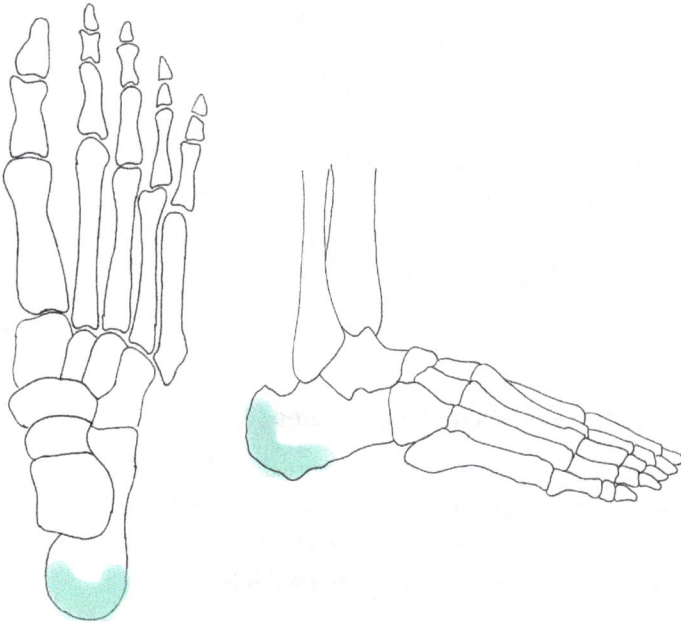

Figure 14.   Saunders' and Mrdjencovich's Pattern 5

or complete collapse of the joint. This pattern usually results in severe instability. Pattern 4 accounts for 10% of all cases.

Pattern 5 (Fig. 14)

Pattern 5 involves the posterior calcaneus. It accounts for only 5% of cases of CJD.

The most common levels of involvement were found to be in Pattern 2 tarsometatarsal joints (40%) and in Pattern 3 (30%) intertarsal joints. These patterns are often associated with plantar ulceration at the apex of the deformity.

Clinical Examination

The most important tool in diagnosis is to have a high index of clinical suspicion when a neuropathic patient presents with a swollen or deformed foot.

A complete physical examination of CJD of the foot must include neurological and vascular examination. The neurological examination must assess the severity of neuropathy. Pin prick, cotton wool and tuning fork are often used to assess sensory neuropathy. However, assessment of vibration sensation (with a biothesiometer) and touch sensation (with 5.07 Semmes-Weinstein Monofilament) is more objective and reproducible. The risk of developing a neuropathic ulcer is much higher if the patient has a biothesiometer reading of greater than 26 volts.

Investigations

Hematological and biochemical studies

Blood tests should be performed to measure the full blood count, serum urea and electrolytes. White blood cell counts are not raised except when infection is present. C-reactive protein (CRP) levels and Erythrocyte Sedimentation Rate (ESR) are also raised with superimposed infection.

Tissue biopsy

Tissue biopsy is the most specific method (gold standard) for diagnosing CJD. In cases where the diagnosis is in doubt, definitive diagnosis of CJD can be made with a synovial tissue biopsy, which will contain shards of bone and cartilage embedded deep into the synovium.[10]

Radiographs

Plain radiographs are usually used in the diagnosis of CJD because they are easily available and are not costly. Radiographs should consist of the weight-bearing antero-posterior, lateral and oblique views of the foot. However, plain radiographs are not sensitive or specific enough to differentiate changes resulting from Charcot's arthropathy and those due to an infection. They instead provide anatomic information that should be evaluated for disorganization related to the stage of arthropathy.[11]

Conservative Treatment of CJD

The treatment of CJD is largely non-operative. Treatment depends on the phase of CJD.

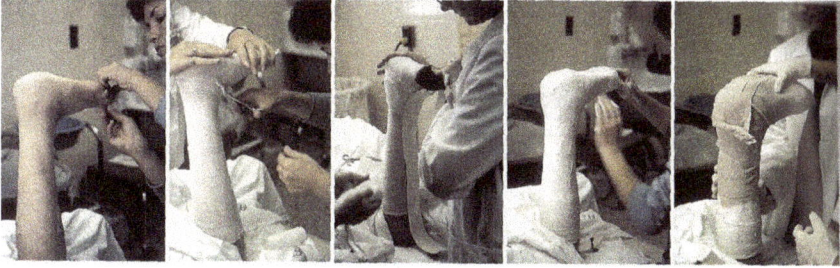

Figure 15.   Application of a total contact cast

Acute Phase

Early immobilisation and off-loading are critical in treatment of Acute CJD.

Immobilisation

The affected lower extremity is immobilised with a short below-knee full cast. The total contact cast is currently the gold standard for prolonged immobilisation (Fig. 15). It is designed to conform exactly to the shape of the affected foot and ankle. It distributes weight and pressure over the entire plantar aspect of the foot. The total contact cast allows ulcers to heal by relieving bony prominent areas of pressure.

The rapid reduction of oedema due to application of the total contact cast causes limb volume to decrease. The cast must be changed at regular intervals of 1–2 weeks. Regular removal of the cast allows the foot to be evaluated. It also allows for debridement to be performed for all ulceration that may develop. Patients with insensitive feet risk developing sores under the cast.

Immobilisation aims to decrease swelling, provide skeletal stability and protect the soft tissues. The total contact cast is a very effective treatment. However, an important prerequisite is that the foot must have an adequate blood supply. Immobilisation is continued until the patient's fractures heal and the foot no longer requires protection.

Off-loading

Off-loading can be achieved with either a weight-bearing or non-weight-bearing cast to reduce stress on the affected foot. A short leg plaster or fiberglass non-weight bearing cast can be used for acute CJD in patients with non-infected ulcerations. Complete non-weight-bearing is obtained with the use of crutches during the initial acute period of CJD.[12] While total non-weight bearing is ideal for treatment, compliance to this treatment is often very poor.

Duration of Healing Process

The duration of immobilisation and off-loading depends on the joints affected and the degree of destruction. As a rule, the larger the joint, the longer the duration of immobilisation needed. Serial plain radiographs should be taken monthly during the acute phase to evaluate progress.

Healing time also varies according to the location of the disease. Pattern 1 disease of Saunders' classification (forefoot pathology) heals in about two-thirds the time of pattern 3 or 4 (hind foot and ankle pathology).

In general, treatment with non weight-bearing immobilisation is recommended for a minimum of 3 months, followed by a period of protected weight bearing.

Post-Acute Phase

Reduction in skin temperature and oedema occurs following a period of immobilisation and off-loading. At this stage, the patient progresses into the Post-Acute Phase of CJD. The patients are allowed to progress to protected weight-bearing with the aid of crutches. With appropriately applied total contact casts or other devices (such as Fixed Ankle Walker or Air Cast) (Fig. 16) most patients may safely ambulate while bony consolidation of fractures progresses.

Management following the removal of the cast includes lifelong protection of the involved extremity. Many types of protective modalities for the initial weight-bearing ambulation may be used, including a patellar tendon-bearing brace, accommodative footwear with a modified Ankle-Foot Orthosis (AFO), a Charcot Restraint Orthotic Walker (CROW),[13] a pneumatic walking brace and a double metal upright AFO. To improve compliance, these walking aids can be made non-removable in the initial phase by simply applying tape or a fiberglass cast roll around the body of the walker (Fig. 17).

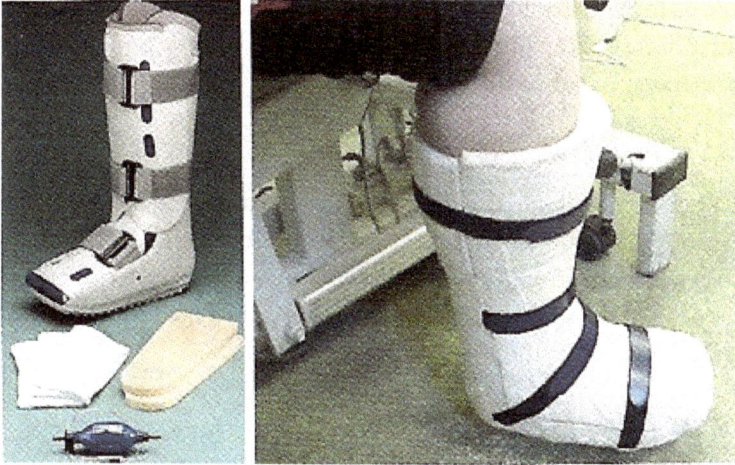

Figure 16. Aircast contains pneumatic envelopes inflated to ensure a precise fit. Ability to remove these devices means that patients may not wear them

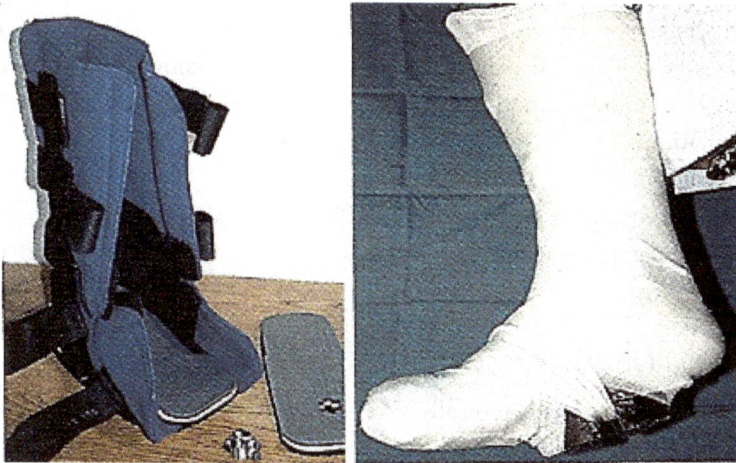

Figure 17. Wrapping the removable cast walker with a fibreglass cast roll

Braces

Many types of braces may be used to provide ankle stability especially since CJD often involves the ankle. Ankle Foot Orthosis (AFO) and high-top therapeutic shoes are beneficial for moderately unstable ankles. A severely unstable or maligned ankle requires a Patellar Tendon-bearing Brace (PTB). The latter decreases the mean rearfoot peak forces by at least 32%. PTB can be incorporated into a custom-made shoe.[14]

Custom footwear

When protective walking aids are no longer required, the patients needs to wear custom-made full-length inserts and comfort or extra-depth shoes with rigid soles and a plastic or metal shank.[15] If ulcers are present, a rocker-bottom sole can be used. In addition, Plastazote inserts can be used for insensate feet. This treatment can be stopped after 6–24 months.

Adjunctive therapy

Bisphosphonates

Bisphosphonates, a potent inhibitor of bone resorption, has been recently used as adjunctive therapy to expedite the conversion of the acute process to the quiescent, reparative stage.[16] In bones, homeostasis is maintained by osteoblasts that produce bone and osteoclasts that destroy bone. Bisphosphonates inhibit the osteoclastic activity of bone breakdown by encouraging osteoclasts to undergo apoptosis. They also promote healing and decrease local inflammation.

Pamidronate, a type of bisphophonate, alters the cycle of bone formation and breakdown in the body. Jude et al 2001 found that a single intravenous infusion of pamidronate led to a reduction in bone turnover, symptoms and disease activity in diabetic patients with active Charcot neuroarthropathy.[17]

Duration of healing process

The total healing process typically takes one to two years. Preventing further injury, noting temperature changes, checking feet every day, looking out for trauma, and receiving professional foot care are also important tenets of treatment. Patient education and professional foot care on a regular basis are important for lifelong foot protection.

Operative Treatment of CJD

The treatment of CJD is largely non-operative. If neuroarthropathy is identified in its early stages and immobilisation and off-loading are initiated, surgery is usually unnecessary. Surgery in the acute phase of CJD is generally non-advisable due to the extreme hyperaemia, osteopenia, and oedema present.

The main indications of surgery are persistently in infected ulcerations and instability. Infected ulcers due to CJD are managed in the same way as diabetic ulcers without CJD — drainage, debridement, ray amputations etc. Post-operatively, off-loading is required for the ulcers to heal. In addition, other bony prominences need off-loading as well to prevent the formation of new ulcers.

Classification System for Diabetic Foot Surgery

A system to classify different types of diabetic foot surgery (including surgery for CJD) has been developed by Armstong and Frykberg.[18] This classification aims to define distinct classes of surgery in an order of theoretically increasing risk for high-level amputation:

Class I: Elective Foot Surgery

This is performed to treat a painful deformity in a patient without loss of protective sensation.

Class II: Prophylactic Foot Surgery

This is performed to reduce risk of ulceration or re-ulceration in patients with loss of protective sensation but without open wound. These procedures involve correcting an underlying tendon, bone, or joint deformity. Prophylactic surgery for Charcot foot include exostectomy, digital arthroplasty, sesamoidectomy, single or multiple metatarsal head resection, joint resection or partial calcanectomy.

Class III: Curative Foot Surgery

This is performed to assist healing of an open wound.

Class IV: Emergent Foot Surgery

This is performed to arrest or limit progression of acute infection.

Complications

The most common complication is foot and ankle deformity which can occur even following early and appropriate treatment. Significant bone and joint

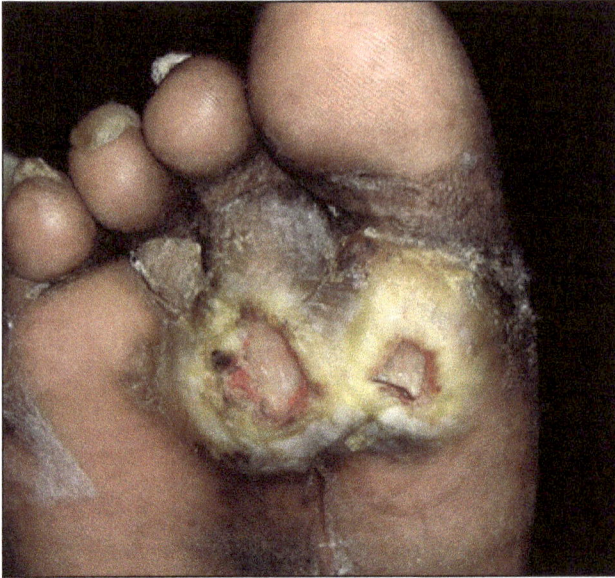

Figure 18.   Plantar callosities with ulcers over the first and second metatarsal heads

destruction lead to the disruption of the functional integrity of the foot causing deformity and instability. Ambulation becomes very difficult unless the foot and ankle are immobilised with appropriate stabilising devices.

Abnormal bony prominences appear as a result of foot deformity producing chronic callosities (Fig. 18) and ulcerations. The ulceration can result in a severe infection, which may lead to amputation of the extremity.

Another complication of CJD is collapse of the arch of the foot leading to formation of a rocker-bottom foot deformity (Fig. 19).

Other complications include the ossification of ligamentous structures, the formation of intra-articular and extra-articular exostoses, and the development of osteomyelitis.

Outcome

Outcomes depend on when the diagnosis is made and treatment instituted. A more favorable outcome occurs when joints are treated within two weeks of injury and when there is strict adherence to weight-bearing precautions.

Location of the disease also affects the outcome. Forefoot osteoarthropathy heals faster than midfoot, hindfoot, or ankle arthropathy.

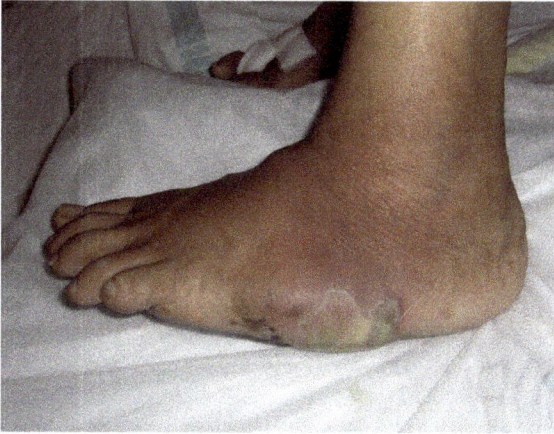

Figure 19. Early rocker bottom foot deformity with an abscess in the plantar area

Surgical treatment prolongs healing time.

The extent of the injury to bone and soft tissue in CJD also affects healing time. The more severe the Charcot changes, the longer it takes to heal, and the greater the likelihood of developing a permanent deformity. It generally takes 1–2 years to completely heal a Charcot Joint.

References

1. J. M. Charcot, Sur quelaquesarthropathies qui paraissentdependerd'une lesion du cerveauou de la moeleepiniere, *Arch. Des. Physiol. Norm. Path.* **1**:161–71 (1868).
2. W. R. Jordan, Neuritic manifestations in diabetes mellitus, *Arch. Int. Med.* **57**:307–66 (1936).
3. B. M. Perrin, M. J. Gardner, A. Suhaimi and D. Murphy, CJD of the foot, *Aust. Fam. Physician* **39**(3):117–9 (2010).
4. J. T. Johnson, Neuropathic fractures and joint injuries, *J. Bone Joint Surg.* **49**(A):1–30 (1967).
5. S. Meyer, The pathogenesis of diabetic Charcot joints, *Iowa Orthop. J.* **12**:63–70 (1992).
6. T. Yochum and L. Rowe, Neuropathic arthropathy. In: *Yochum and Rowe's Essentials of Skeletal Radiology*, 2nd Edition (William & Wilkins, Baltimore, USA), pp. 842–9 (1987).
7. S. N. Eichenholz. In: C. Charles (ed.), *In Charcot Joints* (Thomas, Springfield, 1966), pp. 1–20.
8. J. W. Brodsky, The diabetic foot. In: M. J. Coughlin and R. A. Mann (eds.), *Surgery of the Foot and Ankle*, 7th Edition (Mosby, St. Louis, MO), pp. 895–969 (1999).
9. L. J. Saunders and D. Mrdjencovich, Anatomical patterns of bone and joint destruction in neuropathic diabetics, *Diabetes* **40**:529A (1991).
10. L. Lee, P. Blume and B. Sumpio, CJD in diabetes mellitus. *Ann. Vasc. Surg.* **17**(5):571–80 (2003).

11. L. C. Schon, S. B. Weinfeld, G. A. Horton and S. Resch, Radiographic and clinical classification of acquired midtarsus deformities. *Foot Ankle Int.* 19(6):394–404 (1998).
12. R. G. Frykberg, T. Zgonis, D. G. Armstrong, *et al.* Diabetic foot disorders. A clinical practice guideline (2006 revision). *J. Foot Ankle Surg.* Sep–Oct, 45(5 Suppl):S1–66 (2006).
13. J. A. Mehta, C. Brown and N. Sargeant, Charcot restraint orthotic walker, *Foot Ankle Int.* 19:619–23 (1998).
14. S. T. Guse and F. G. Alvine, Treatment of diabetic foot ulcers and Charcot neuroarthropathy using the patellar tendon-bearing brace, *Foot Ankle Int.* 18:675–7 (1997).
15. J. M. Giurini, Applications and use of in-shoe orthoses in the conservative management of Charcot foot deformity, *Clin. Podiatr. Med. Surg.* 11:271–8 (1994).
16. R. G. Frykberg, Charcot foot: an update on pathogenesis and management. In: A. J. M. Boulton, H. Connors and P. R. Cavanagh (eds.), *The Foot in Diabetes*, 3rd Edition (John Wiley, London, 2000), pp. 235–60.
17. E. B. Jude, P. L. Selby, J. Burgess, P. Lilleystone, E. B. Mawer, S. R. Page, M. Donohoe, A. V. Foster, M. E. Edmonds and A. J. Boulton, Bisphosphonates in the treatment of Charcot neuroarthropathy: a double-blind randomised controlled trial, *Diabetologia* 44:2032–7 (2001).
18. D. G. Armstrong and R. G. Frykberg. Classifying diabetic foot surgery: toward a rational definition. *Diabet. Med.* 20(4):329–31 (2003).

16

Necrotising Fasciitis

Aziz Nather and Amy Pannapat Chanyarungrojn

Department of Orthopaedic Surgery
Yong Loo Lin School of Medicine
National University of Singapore

Introduction

Necrotising fasciitis (NF) is an infection located in the deep fascia which results in necrosis of the subcutaneous tissues[1] (Fig. 1). It is one of the most dangerous conditions that could develop in a limb. NF causes severe infection that spreads rapidly and can be fatal. It is also commonly known as the "killer bug disease" or "flesh-eating bacterial infection".

NF can be caused by various types of bacteria and fungi. The infection can be a result of a single pathogen or can be polymicrobial. The bacterial group A beta-haemolytic streptococci (*Streptococcus pyogenes*) is the most common cause of NF.[2]

Given the rapid progression of the disease, patients with NF should be treated as an emergency. However, NF can be difficult to diagnose in its early stage. A high index of suspicion is important. Once the infection reaches the connective tissue, the spread can be so fast that it can get out of control, even with both antibiotics and debridement surgery. In certain cases, the spread can be so fast that it may be fatal within 48 hours.

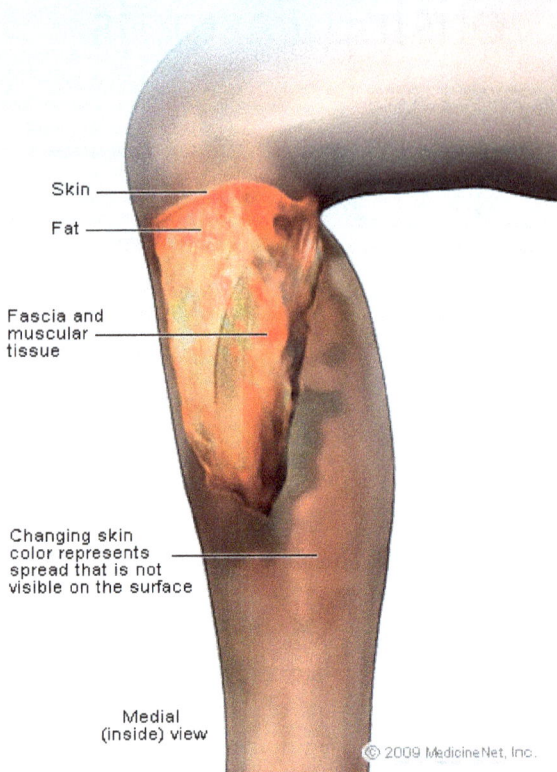

Figure 1. Showing necrotising fasciitis involving deep fascia
Source: C.P. Davis and M.C. Stöppler, 2012. http://www.medicinenet.com/necrotising_
fasciitis/article.htm

Types of NF

The types of NF[3] are:

- Type I ■ Polymicrobial NF
            ■ Can be mistaken for a simple wound cellulitis
            ■ Usually occurs after a trauma or surgery

- Type II   ▪ Group A streptococcal NF
          ▪ Known as the "flesh-eating" bacterial infection

Necrotising fasciitis refers to Type I or Type II. A third type described — Type III — usually refers to Gas Gangrene, which is an infection involving the skeletal muscle. This is quite different from NF, an infection of the deep fascia.

History
Profile of Patients

NF is not uncommon in Singapore. Wong *et al.* (2003)[4] reported 89 patients in Changi General Hospital alone over a 7-year period from January 1997 to August 2002. The mean age of patients with NF was found to be about 56 years.

Predisposing Factors

NF is common in immunocompromised patients. These include patients with diabetes, cancer, alcoholism, vascular insufficiency (impaired blood flow), organ transplants and Human Immunodeficiency Virus (HIV) infection.

Comorbidities

Comorbidities are common in patients with NF. Wong *et al.* (2003)[4] found diabetes mellitus to be the most common comorbidity, present in 70.8% of patients, peripheral vascular disease in 22.5%, chronic liver disease in 3.4% and cancer in 2.2%.

Liu *et al.* (2005)[5] in a study of 87 consecutive patients of NF from 1999 to 2004 also found diabetes mellitus to be the most common comorbidity — 53.2%.

History

NF can develop following trauma, around foreign bodies in surgical wounds or after surgical procedures including cardiac catheterisation.

Pathophysiology

Bacteria spread from the subcutaneous tissue along the superficial and deep fascial planes (Figs. 2a and 2b). The bacterial enzymes and toxins they produce facilitate the rapid spread of the disease.

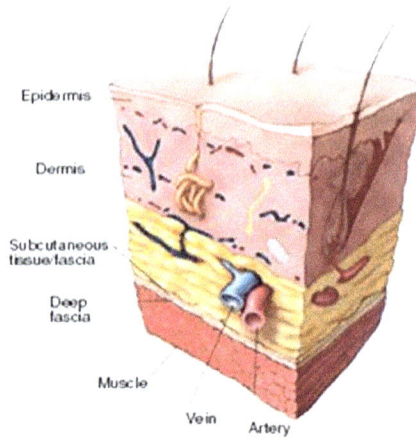

Figure 2a.   Normal skin
Source: E.K. Fishman, 2012. http://www.ctisus.com/learning/illustrations/musculoskeletal/605000067/4841373

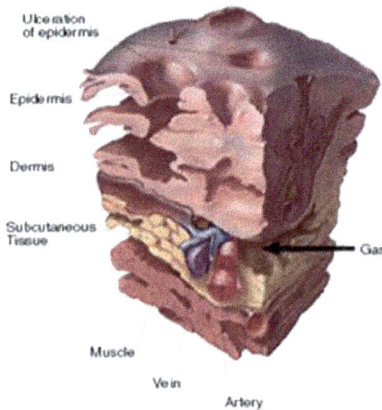

Figure 2b.   Necrotising fasciitis with necrosis of skin and vascular thrombosis
Source: E.K. Fishman, 2012. http://www.ctisus.com/learning/illustrations/musculoskeletal/605000067/4841375

Streptococcal pyogenic exotoxins (SPEs) A, B, and C are directly toxic. The pyogenic exotoxins, together with Streptococcal superantigen (SSA), lead to the release of cytokines and produce clinical signs such as hypotension. The poor prognosis in NF has been linked to infection with certain Streptococcal strains.

In NF, Group-A Haemolytic Streptococci and *Staphylococcus aureus* alone or in synergism are frequently the initiating infecting bacteria. Other aerobic and anaerobic pathogens include Bacteroides, Peptostreptococcus, Enterobacteriaceae, coliforms, Proteus, Pseudomonas and Klebsiella.

Most necrotising soft tissue infections have anaerobic bacteria present, usually in combination with aerobic gram negative organisms. They proliferate in an environment of local tissue hypoxia in patients with trauma, recent surgery or in patients who are immunocompromised. *Bacteroides fragilis* is usually present as part of a mixed flora in combination with *Escherichia coli* (Maynor *et al.*).[1]

Some cases of NF can be caused by *Vibrio vulnificus*. This organism is seen more often in patients with chronic liver dysfunction and often follows the consumption of raw seafood.

Wong *et al.* (2003)[4] found polymicrobial infection (NF Type I) to be the most common (53.9%) with Streptococci and Enterobacteriaceae being the most common pathogens. Group A Streptococcus was the most common pathogen of monomicrobial NF (Type II). They found diabetes mellitus to be the most common associated comorbidity (70.8%).

Examination

Clinical Findings

In the early phase, patients complain of severe pain that is out of proportion to their seemingly minor skin changes. He can also present with fever, chills, dehydration and tachycardia. A detailed history of the patient should be taken to find out about any recent illness, injury or exposure to seawater.

The patient's condition can deteriorate very quickly. After 1–2 days, there is an onset of severe pain, swelling and erythema at the site of trauma or recent surgery. This is often mistaken for cellulitis, as the necrosis of the deep fascia under the skin is not visible. However, unlike cellulitis, tenderness extends beyond the site of infection.

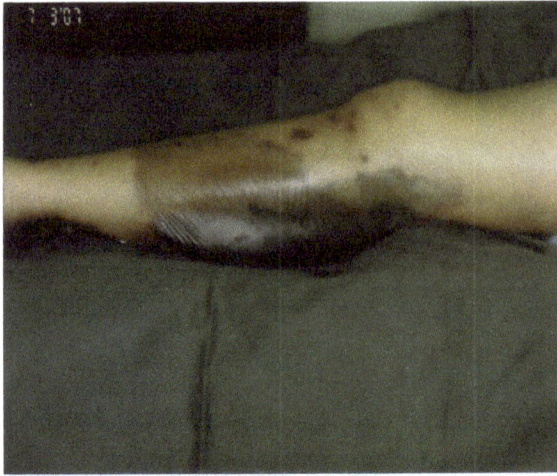

Figure 3a. Large blister on the medial side of the left leg

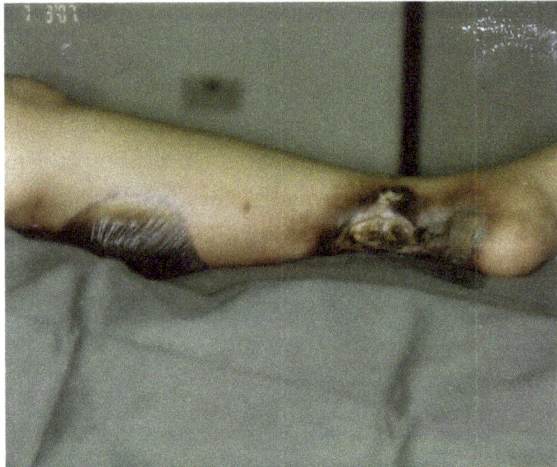

Figure 3b. Ulcer over Tendo-Achilles posteriorly, blister of skin containing brownish fluid over the back of calf

After 2–4 days, the patient develops swelling of the skin. Other changes include skin ulceration, supralesional vesiculation or bullae formation (formation of blisters) (Fig. 3a), necrotic eschars (black scabs) and gas formation in the tissue. A dusky or purplish skin discolouration can be observed (Fig. 3b).

Palpation can reveal crepitus (crackling or grating sounds under the skin) due to the formation of subcutaneous gas from the bacteria.

After 4–5 days, hypotension (low blood pressure) and septic shock (life-threateningly low blood pressure due to overwhelming infection) develop. Patients become confused, and if the NF is not kept under control, the results could be fatal.

Investigations

- Blood tests
  A full blood count and urea/electrolytes should be performed.
  Pointers to necrotising fasciitis[4,6] include:
  o C-Reactive protein   >16 mg/dL
  o White cell count   >15 x 10^9/L
  o Haemoglobin   <13.5 g/dL
  o Sodium   <135 mmol/L
  o Creatinine   >141 μmol/L
  o Glucose   >10 mmol/dL
  o Creatine kinase   >600 U/L
  o Urea   >18 mg/dL

  Wong *et al.* (2004)[7] developed a novel diagnostic scoring system to distinguish NF from other soft tissue infections based on laboratory tests routinely performed for evaluation of soft tissue infections: the Laboratory Risk Indicator for Necrotising Fasciitis (LRINEC) Score based on a study of 140 patients with NF and 309 patients with severe cellulitis or abscess in 2 institutions in Singapore. The six laboratory indicators were: total white cell count, haemoglobin, sodium, glucose, serum creatinine, and C-reactive protein (Table 1). Patients with a LRINEC Score of more than 6 should be carefully evaluated for the presence of NF.

- Microbiological tests
  Gram staining and culture should be conducted on blood cultures, exudates (fluid from the site of infection) by a wound swab and biopsied tissue. The results obtained can be useful in determining the organism(s) responsible for the infection. A fungal culture can also be obtained from patients who are immunocompromised and those who have a history of trauma.

Table 1. LRINEC score

Variable, Units	β	Score
C-Reactive protein, mg/L		
<150	0	0
≥150	3.5	4
Total white cell count, per mm^3		
<15	0	0
15–25	0.5	1
>25	2.1	2
Haemoglobin, g/dL		
>13.5	0	0
11–13.5	0.6	1
<11	1.8	2
Sodium, mmol/L		
≥135	0	0
<135	1.8	2
Creatinine, μmol		
≤141	0	0
>141	1.8	2
Glucose, mmol/L		
≤10	0	0
>10	1.2	1

Wong *et al.* (2003)[4] found polymicrobial synergistic infection to be the most common (53.9%), with Streptococci and Enterobacteriaceae being the most common pathogens identified. Group-A streptococcus was the most common cause of monomicrobial NF. Brook and Frazier (1995)[8] found polymicrobial infection with mixed-aerobic-anaerobic floras in 68%. Aerobic bacteria were recovered in only 10% of patients and anaerobic bacteria in only 22%.

- Radiological tests
Local radiographs can show the presence of gas in the subcutaneous fascial planes (Figs. 4a and 4b). This is characteristic of NF. MRI can be used to reveal the extent of surgical debridement required. However, clinical signs showing severe tenderness at fascial level coupled with presence of gas on plain radiographs are sufficient to indicate the presence and extent of NF.

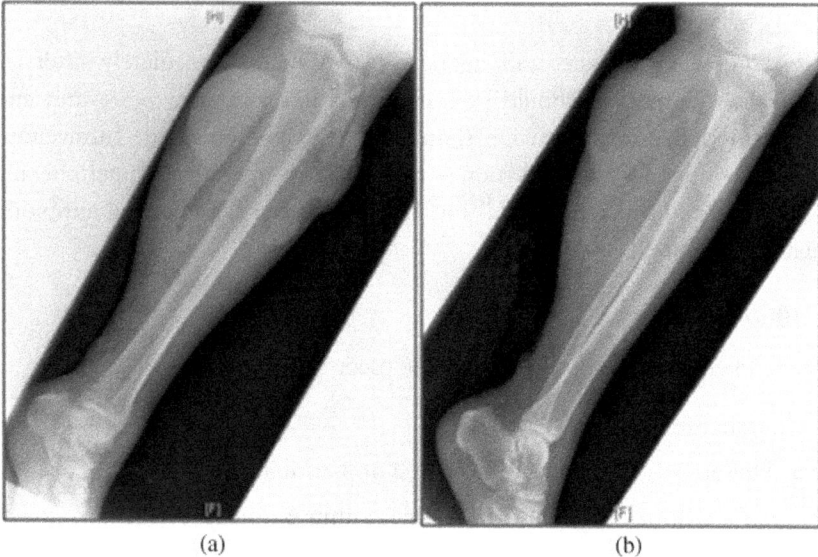

(a)   (b)

Figure 4.   Gas shadow seen in the calf of the same patient described in Fig. 1

Urgent preparations for surgery should not be delayed by time-consuming arrangements for MRI.

• Bedside finger test

This is carried out under local anaesthesia. It involves probing the deep fascia with a gloved index finger through a 2 cm incision. Lack of bleeding, the presence of "dishwasher pus" and non-contracting muscles after the blunt finger dissection are indicative of NF.[9]

A family conference must be convened as soon as possible to inform the family of the gravity of the situation. Mortality is high (between 20–25%). Severe morbidities can develop. These include hypotensive shock and acute renal shutdown. The need for urgent surgical debridement and post-operative care in an intensive-care unit must be emphasised. The patient and his family must also be informed that the chances of a second debridement is high (about 50%) and further closure of the wound with split skin grafting might be needed. The immediate dressing of the operative wound with negative pressure dressing must also be explained. If the debridement attempt is unable to adequately reduce the bacterial load, an amputation may be needed. The risk of major amputation is 10–20%.

Treatment

NF requires immediate and aggressive treatment immediately after its diagnosis. The patient should be hospitalised in an intensive care unit and his haemodynamic parameters should be closely monitored. Intravenous antibiotics must be started as soon as possible. Post-operatively, a peripherally inserted central catheter (PICC) line must be inserted. Prolonged antibiotic therapy is required.

Antibiotics

The following antibiotic regimes can be used.

- Combination therapy.
    o This approach involves the use of 2 or 3 antibiotics
        ■ Crystaline Penicillin (eg. 2–4 mega units 8 hourly) plus Clindamycin to cover aerobes (usually gram-negative organisms)
        ■ If the patient is allergic to Penicillin, give Meropenem plus Clindamycin or
        ■ Clindamycin plus Ciprofloxacin plus Metronidazole

These are regimes based on UK hospital guidelines.[6]
Note:

- Use high, intravenous doses.
- Treatment should be discussed with the local consultant microbiologist, and should be adjusted once culture results have returned.
- For suspected *Vibrio* spp., include a tetracycline and third-generation cephalosporin (e.g. Doxycycline plus Ceftazidime); Ciprofloxacin may be an alternative.

Medical Treatment

- Nutritional support is required from day one, owing to the high protein and fluid loss from the wound (similar to major burns). In severe cases, patients may need twice their basal caloric requirements. Nasogastric feeding may be helpful.
- Intravenous immunoglobulin may be a useful adjunct in severe streptococcal infections (to neutralise streptococcal toxins).
- Hyperbaric oxygen therapy for NF is controversial.[6]

Surgery

Surgical debridement must be performed as soon as possible, for higher chances of survival. The first surgery is the most important. To ensure that the debridement is extensive, the surgical incisions should be deep and should extend beyond the areas of necrosis until viable tissue is reached. This ensures that no infected tissue is left behind. Debridement is best done through 2 incisions — one on the medial side of the limb and the other on the lateral side of the limb. All necrotic fat, unhealthy tissue and necrotic fascia must be surgically excised. If the exposed underlying muscle is necrotic and non-viable, this must also be debrided until healthy, pink, contractile muscle is left behind.

A sample of tissue is sent for culture and sensitivity. The extensive wound is then flushed with hydrogen peroxide and with 2–3 litres of normal saline using jet lavage. Haemostasis is carefully and meticulously secured. A negative-pressure dressing is then applied.

The negative pressure dressings must be changed and the wound must be inspected every 2 days. If further pus, slough or necrosis is seen, a second or even third debridement must be performed. Once the infection markers have improved, the wound culture is negative and healthy granulation tissue is seen in the wound bed, a split skin grafting is performed.

In advanced cases of NF, an amputation may need to be performed due to the progression of the disease resulting in irreversible necrosis and gangrene. Lim *et al.*[10] showed that primary amputation should be considered in a patient with advanced NF. Amputation is done to completely remove the sepsis in the limb and reduces the need for repeated procedures involving general anaesthesia. This may be necessary for patients with multiple comorbidities including heart disease, as multiple operations puts the patient under significant risk.

Complications

- Necrotising fasciitis carries a significant mortality rate, particularly if marine organisms (above) are involved.
- Septic or toxic shock (the latter due to Streptococcal endotoxin production).
- The deep tissue infection may lead to vascular occlusion, ischaemia and tissue necrosis. There may be nerve damage and muscle necrosis.
- Large areas of tissue loss may require skin grafting, reconstructive surgery or amputation.[6]

In a study of 451 patients with NF involving both the upper and lower limb, Angoules *et al.* (2007)[11] found 22.3% underwent amputation or disarticulation of a limb following failure of multiple debridements.

Mortality

The poor prognosis in NF has been linked to infection with certain streptococcal strains. The mortality rate can be as high as 20–25%. Angoules *et al.* (2007)[11] found a mortality rate of 21.9%, while Shimizu and Tokuda (2010)[12] found it to be 25%.

Wong *et al.* (2003)[4] found that factors such as advanced age, two or more associated comorbidities and a delay in surgery of more than 24 hours adversely affected the outcome. Multivariate analysis showed that a delay in surgery of more than 24 hours was correlated with increased mortality ($p < 0.05$; relative risk $= 9.4$). They concluded that early operative debridement must be done to reduce mortality.

A high index of suspicion is very important in view of the paucity of specific cutaneous findings in the early course of the disease. Liu *et al.* (2005)[5] found multivariate logistic regression analysis showed that factors such as thrombocytopenia (abnormally low amount of platelets), anaemia, 2 or more associated comorbidities, a delay of more than 24 hours from onset of symptoms to surgery and age greater than 60 were independently associated with mortality.

Case Study

A 54-year-old Chinese male with Diabetes Mellitus of 10 years duration was admitted on 6/1/12 with severe pain and swelling of the front of the right thigh of 4 days duration. He had fever with chills and rigors over the last 2 days. Comorbidities included chronic Hepatitis B infection and liver cirrhosis.

Examination revealed severe tenderness over the anterior and medial aspects of the thigh. There was crepitus felt over the front of the thigh.

Radiographs done revealed gas shadows in the subcutaneous plane in the thigh (pathognomonic of NF) (Fig. 5). MRI was performed which revealed increased fluid seen in the interfascial plane between the rectus femoris, vastus lateralis and vastus medialis. Thin silver of fluid is also seen between the sartorius and the adductor longus (Figs. 6a and 6b). These changes, together with fascial thickening, are characteristic of NF.

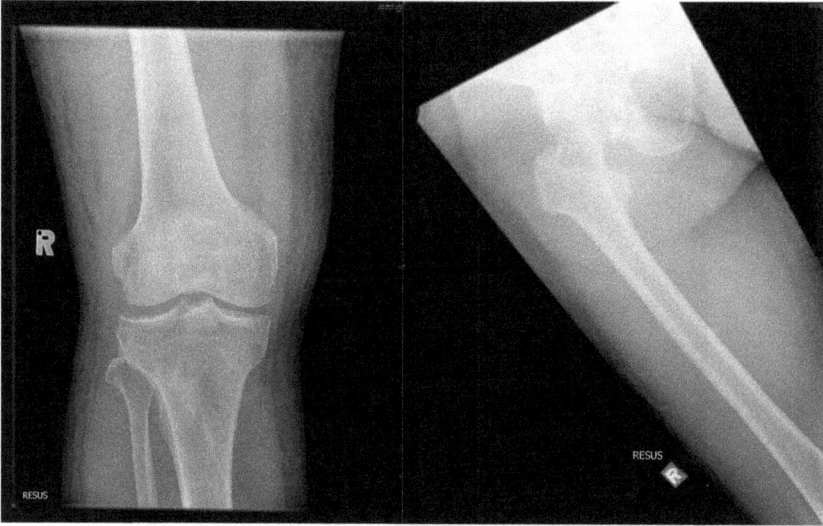

Figure 5. Plain radiographs showing gas shadows in the subcutaneous plane of the right thigh and knee

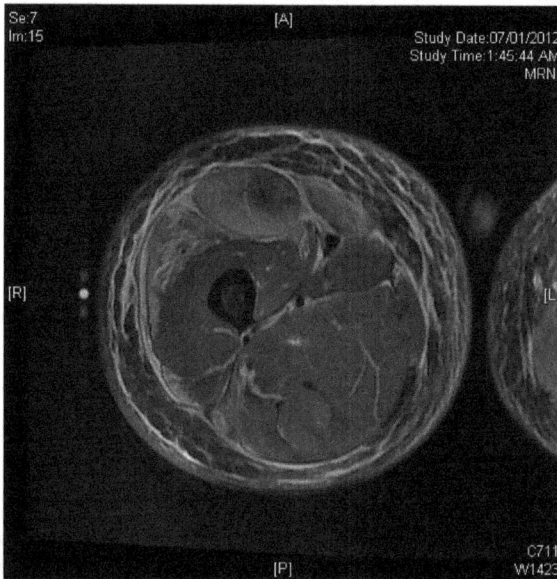

Figure 6a. Cross-section of MRI of the thigh showing increased fluid in the interfascial plane between the muscles and thickening of the deep fascia characteristic of NF. No abscess in the muscles

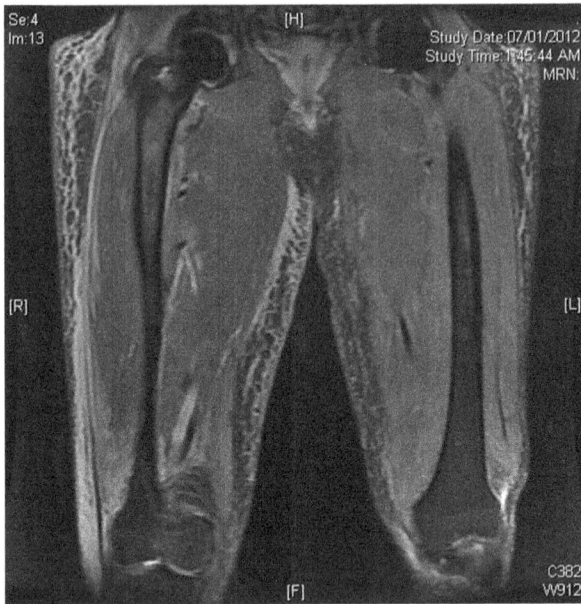

Figure 6b. AP view of MRI showing increased space due to fluid collection between the deep fascia and the subcutaneous tissue

Blood investigations revealed: HbA1c 8.3, Hb 12.5, Total white cell count 6.82, Platelets 41, CRP 180, Urea 9.2, Cr 161, Na 35, K 6 (mild lysis), CO2 14, Chloride 106, Gluc 18.2, AG 21, Alb 30, Bil 27, ALP 120, ALT 10, AST 44, LDH 695. Blood cultures were taken. The patient was treated in a high-dependency unit with intravenous antibiotics. Wound cultures were positive for Pseudomonas *aeruginosa*. The patient was treated with intravenous Ceftazidine and Clindamycin.

Extensive debridement was done under general anaesthesia on 7/1/12. Exploration revealed necrosis of subcutaneous tissue, thickening of the deep fascia and the presence of serosanguineous fluid superficial to the deep fascia. The thickened and unhealthy deep fascia and other necrotic tissues were excised. The debridement extended over the front and medial aspect of the thigh (Figs. 7a and 7b). The wounds were flushed with normal saline using jet lavage and the large wound was covered with a negative pressure dressing.

The patient had a stormy post-operative period and went into septic shock. He was resuscitated and Dopamine was administered. A second re-look

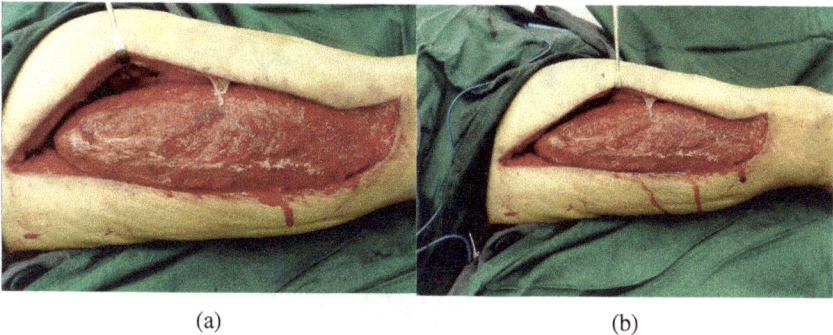

(a) (b)

Figure 7. Seropurrulent fluid and unhealthy deep fascia. Radical debridement done to excise all unhealthy tissues

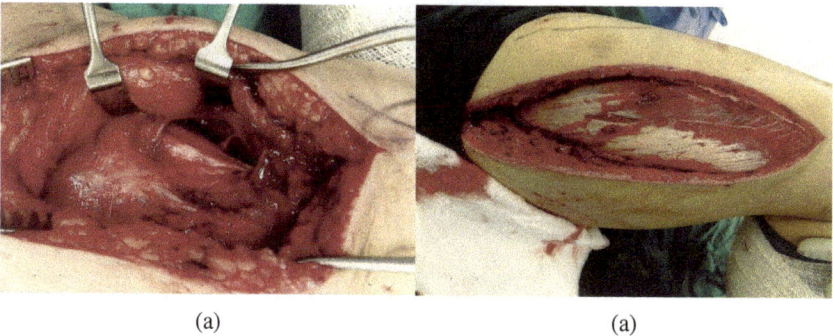

(a) (a)

Figure 8. More unhealthy and necrotic tissues excised during 2nd debridement

debridement was performed on 10/1/12. Debridement of necrotic tissues was performed on the medial side of the thigh including excision of necrotic fascia (Figs. 8a and 8b). VAC dressings were applied to the wounds, and were changed every 2 days.

A third wound debridement was carried out on 16/1/12 involving the large right anterolateral thigh wound, further excising all necrotic muscles and tissue (Fig. 9). VAC dressings were reinstituted over both the medial and lateral wounds, and were changed every 2 days.

The patient underwent a right thigh split skin grafting on 2/2/12 after the third debridement and was put on VAC dressing. To help improve wound healing, Hyperbaric Oxygen Therapy (HBOT) was administered daily for 2 weeks (until 4/2/12).

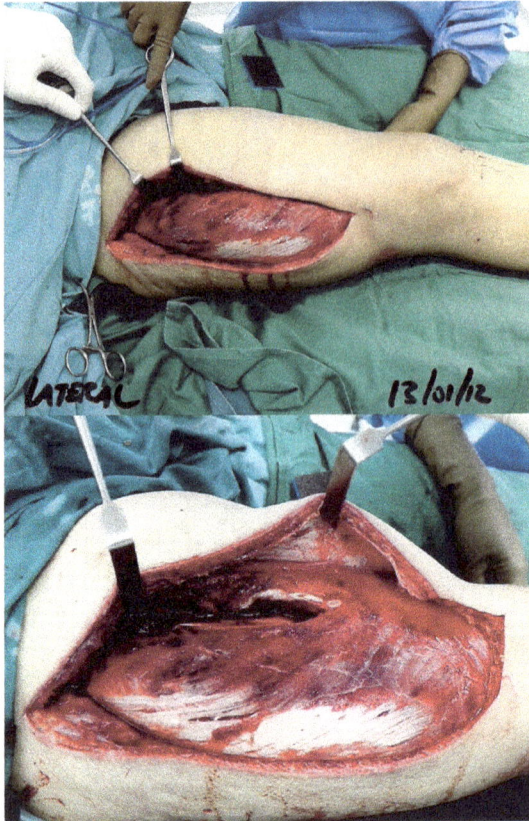

Figure 9.   More necrotic muscles and tissue excised during 3rd debridement

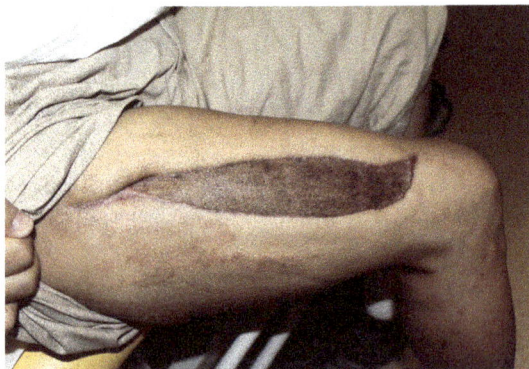

Figure 10a.   Healed SSG on the lateral aspect of the thigh 3 months later

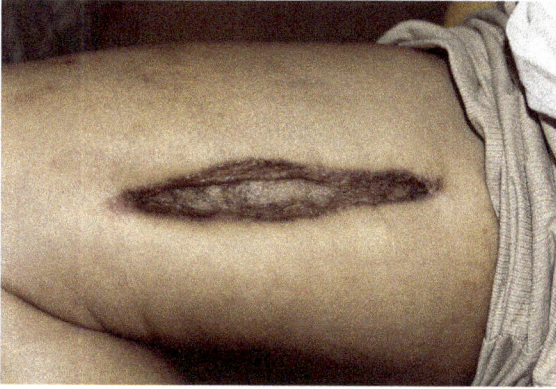

Figure 10b. Healed SSG on the medial aspect of the thigh 3 months later

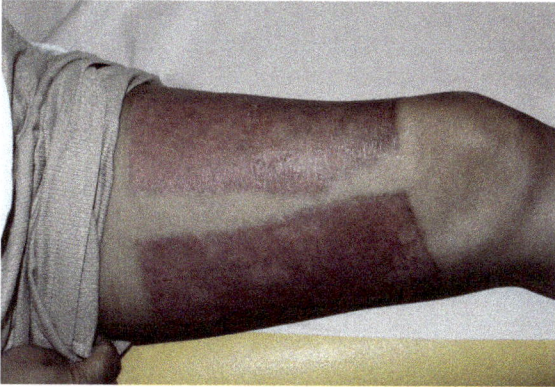

Figure 10c. Healed donor site on the left thigh

He was discharged from the ward non-weight bearing with a pair of crutches on 7/2/12. When seen in the outpatient clinic 3 months later, his wounds have completely healed (Figs. 10a to 10c) and he has returned to work.

References

1. M. Maynor, E. Kardon, F. Talavera, E.L. Weiss, J. Halamka and J. Adler, http://www. emedicine.com/emerg/topic332.htm
2. R. A. Schwartz and R. Kapila, Necrotising fasciitis, Emedicine (2007), http://www.emedi cine.com/derm/topic743.htm
3. C. P. Davis and M. C. Stöppler, Necrotising fasciitis, *MedicineNet.com* (2012), http://www.medicinenet.com/necrotising_fasciitis/article.htm

4. C. H. Wong, H. C. Chang, S. Pasupathy, L. W. Khin, J. L. Tan and C. O. Low, Nectrotizing fasciitis: clinical presentation, microbiology and determinants of mortality, *J. Bone Joint Surg. Am.* **85**:1454–60 (2003).

5. Y. M. Liu, C. Y. Chi, M. W. Ho, C. M. Chen, W. C. Liao, C. M. Ho, P. C. Lin and J. H. Wang, Microbiology and factors affecting mortality in necrotising fasciitis, *J. Microbiol. Immunol. Infect.* **38**(6):430–5 (2005).

6. N. Hartree, Necrotising fasciitis, *Egton Medical Information Systems* (2011), http://www.patient.co.uk/doctor/Necrotising-Fasciitis.htm

7. Y. J. Lim, F. C. Yong and A. B. H. Tan, Necrotising fasciitis and traditional medical therapy — dangerous liaison, *Ann. Acad. Med.* **35**:270–3 (2006).

8. I. Brook and E. H. Frazier, Clinical and microbiological features of necrotising fasciitis, *J. Clin. Microbiol.* **33**(9):2382–7 (1995).

9. T. J. Andreasen, S. D. Green and B. J. Childers, Massive infectious soft-tissue injury: diagnosis and management of necrotising fasciitis and purpura fulminans, *Plast. Reconstr. Surg.* **107**(4):1025–35 (2001).

10. C. H. Wong, L. W. Khin, K. S. Heng, K. C. Tan and C. O. Low, The LRINEC (Laboratory Risk Indicator for Necrotising Fasciitis) score: a tool for distinguishing necrotising fasciitis from other soft tissue infections, *Crit. Care Med.* **32**(7):1535–41.

11. G. Angoules, G. Kontaki, E. Drakoulakis, G. Vrentzos, M. S. Granick and P. V. Giannoudis, Necrotising fasciitis of upper and lower limb: a systematic review, *Injury* **38**(S5):S19–S26 (2007).

12. T. Shimizu and Y. Tokuda, Necrotising fasciitis, *Int. Med.* **49**:1051–7 (2010).

Section 5

Treatment of Diabetic Foot

17

Value of a Team Approach in Managing Diabetic Foot Problems

Chin Yu Xuan and Aziz Nather

Department of Orthopaedic Surgery
Yong Loo Lin School of Medicine
National University of Singapore, Singapore

Introduction

Multidisciplinary team approaches adopted in various countries to manage diabetic food problems have been shown to be highly effective.[1–7] The guidelines and recommendations entitled "Diabetes and Foot Care: Time to Act" published by the International Diabetes Ferderation and International Working Group on Diabetic Foot also showed a 60% reduction in amputation rate achieved through a combination of a multidisciplinary team approach and education in foot care and foot wear.[8]

A Multidisciplinary Team

Members

A multidisciplinary diabetic foot team includes the following health professionals with the following roles:

- Orthopaedic surgeon — performs operations when needed including debridements and amputations

- Vascular surgeon — perform revascularization surgery to achieve limb salvage
- Infectious diseases specialist — decides the choice of the appropriate antibiotics to be used to combat infections
- Endocrinologist — manage endocrine control for all patients with diabetic foot problems
- Podiatrist — assesses foot of patient for vasculopathy and immunopathy, provides insoles for off-loading, and provides appropriate footwear
- Wound nurse — provides wound care for the foot, performs foot screening
- Case manager — manage the holistic care of DFP patients from their hospital admission to outpatient follow-ups
- Medical social worker — help DFP patients and their families cope with social and emotional issues
- Pharmacist — ensures that therapeutics are given in right dosage and rate, and manages drug complications
- Dieticians — educate DFP patients on appropriate diets

Some teams also include other professionals like shoemakers and orthotists to make special shoes and orthoses for diabetic patients to prevent foot ulcers and injuries.[3,4,9,10]

Ward Rounds

Teams generally conduct combined ward rounds to allow interactive discussions between various specialists to decide on the optimal mode of treatment.

Some teams conduct joint ward rounds for inpatient care. Trautner *et al.* ruled that surgery can only be performed after indication rounds with diabetologists and surgeons.[11] After surgery, problem rounds followed. Sakka *et al.* conducted weekly joint diabetes, vascular and podiatry ward rounds.[4] The NUH team in Singapore also used weekly grand ward rounds for endocrine control, implementing antibiotic regimens and decision making for surgical intervention or podiatric treatment including footwear recommendations.[12]

Diabetic Foot Clinic

Teams also conduct weekly clinics in the presence of specialists from the various disciplines — an orthopaedic surgeon, endocrinologist, and podiatrist.

Teaching Sessions

Multidisciplinary teaching sessions are also held monthly to educate all members of the team. Topics covered all relevant disciplines, including endocrine control, bacteria, orthopaedic aspects, wound care, podiatric care etc.

Patient Education

Various team approaches also highlight the need for patient education on foot care and diabetes control.[1,3,4,6,9] Park and Ahn's team[6] provided individualized teaching whereby a patient has a session with an endocrinologist, nurse, dietician, pharmacist and social worker. The NUH team utilized ward rounds as the foundation for nurses and podiatrists to provide all patients with individualized education sessions on diabetes and foot care as well as footwear.[12]

Clinical Pathway — Sustaining the Team Approach

A strategic progression of the team system was the implementation of a clinical pathway for DFP patients. The case manager implemented and monitored the pathway. There must be full compliance by all house officers and medical officers.

Outcomes of a Team Approach

A multidisciplinary team approach minimizes the delay in treatment of a patient due to referrals from one discipline to another. This allows patients to receive much needed treatment in time before deterioration of their Diabetic Foot Problem. Hence, the major amputation rate, complication rate and readmission rate are reduced while limb salvage rate increased. The average length of stay and hospitalization cost will also fall. Total economic cost also decreases due to shorter hospitalization periods of DFP patients.

Major Amputation Rate

Many studies have revealed the reduced major amputation rate to be the most beneficial outcome of the team approach. Comprehensive multidisciplinary foot care programs were shown to increase quality of care and reduce amputation rates by 36% to 86%.[4,9,11,13–21]

The NUH team decreased the incidence of major amputations significantly (p = 0.022) from 31% in 2002 to 11% in 2007. Faglia *et al.* also showed that a "foot team" running a "foot clinic" also reduced the major amputation rate from 40.5% to 23.5%.[22] Similarly, Driver *et al.*'s "specialized foot care clinic" decreased the amputation rate dramatically from 9.9 per 1000 to 1.8 per 1000 over 5 years.[9] Larsson *et al.* also showed that a multidisciplinary team approach decreased the incidence of major amputations by 78%.[16] Apelqvist *et al.*, Van Damme *et al.*, Levin and Zandman *et al.* all reported a 50% reduction in amputation rate following the team approach.[23–25]

Lavery *et al.* reported a 47.4% decrease in amputation incidence from 12.89 per 1000 diabetics per year to 6.18 after implementing a multidisciplinary management programme.[26] Krishnan *et al.* also showed a 62% reduction in major amputations and 40% decrease in all amputations for 11 years after implementing a dedicated multidisciplinary diabetic-foot-care service.[15]

In particular, Martinez *et al.* showed that implementation of a clinical pathway on top of the team approach resulted in fall in rate of major amputations from 17.4% to 9.7%.[27] Therefore, a team approach, coupled with its extension in the form of a clinical pathway, is highly effective in reducing the major amputation rate. This in turn reduces the emotional and financial problems associated with amputations for patients and their families.

Limb Salvage Rate

Alexandrescu *et al.* revealed that comparison between limb salvage rates before and after initiating the multidisciplinary team approach showed a significant difference (p = 0.040, CI: 1.040–5.311, HR: 235, Chi Square = 4.22) with better results in the latest interval of the study.[28] This was largely due to a more integrated system of information that enabled earlier consultation and treatment under the team approach.

Complication Rate and Readmission Rate

The NUH diabetic foot team reported a significantly lower complication rate of about 6.1 to 7.3% after the team's formation as compared to 19.7% prior to the team's formation. Increasing evidence also suggested that implementing the team approach could reduce foot complication rates. The readmission rate also decreased by 6.35% during the implementation of the team approach (not statistically significant). This was supported by Martinez *et al.* who also reported that the rate of readmission in 30 days diminished from 9.3% to 6.5% (not statistically significant).[27]

Average Length of Stay (ALOS)

Following the formation of the NUH team, the ALOS for DFP patients admitted was reduced by 6 days (not statistically significant). While Martinez *et al.* also did not report any significant reduction in the ALOS,[27] Lavery *et al.* reported a significant reduction from 4.75 to 3.72 days (21.7%). Gibbons *et al.* showed reductions in overall length of stay instead.[29]

Hospitalisation Cost and Total Economic Cost

The NUH team found a reduction of SGD$1187 in mean cost of hospitalization following implementation of the team approach (not statistically significant). However, Reiber and Gibbons *et al.* found that adoption of the team approach led to statistically significant reductions in cost of care.[29,30]

Total economic cost is also reduced due to the fall in amputation rate as its related cost in terms of loss of productivity, disability and premature mortality is reduced. Ollendorf *et al.*'s model also estimated that a multidisciplinary team approach could avoid 47% of amputations which could translate into US$750,000 in potential savings in 1 year and US$2900 to US$4442 in per-patient costs.[31]

Conclusion

A two-pronged strategy is used by NUH to combat diabetic foot problems:

1. The primary strategy is prevention to ensure that all patients diagnosed with diabetes must undergo annual foot screening. This will prevent complications from developing.
2. When foot complications do occur, they are best treated by a multi-disciplinary diabetic foot team. Such a team will achieve maximal limb salvage and reduce hospitalization costs and length of stay, as well as reduce complication rates.

References

1. R. Anichini, F. Zechinni, I. Cerretini, G. Meucci, D. Fusilli, L. Alviggi, *et al.*, Improvement of diabetic foot care after the implementation of the International Consensus on the Diabetic Foot (ICDF): results of a 5-year prospective study, *Diabetes Res. Clin. Pract.* **75**:153–8 (2007).

2. R. J. Canavan, N. C. Unwin, W. F. Kelly and V. M. Connolly, Diabetes- and nondiabetes-related lower extremity amputation incidence before and after the introduction of better organised diabetes foot care, *Diabetes Care* **31**:459–63 (2008).

3. V. Dargis, O. Pantelejeva, A. Jonushaite, L. Vileikyte and A. J. M. Boulton, Benefits of multidisciplinary approach in the management of recurrent diabetic foot ulceration in Lithuania, *Diabetes Care* **22**:1428–31 (1999).

4. M. E. Edmonds, M. P. Blundell, M. E. Morris, L. T. Cotton and P. J. Watkins, Improved survival of the diabetic foot: the role of a specialized foot clinic, *Q. J. Med.* **60**:763–71 (1986).

5. C. Hedetoft, A. Rasmussen, J. Fabrin and K. Kolendorf, Four-fold increase in foot ulcers in type 2 diabetic subjects without an increase in major amputations by a multidisciplinary setting, *Diabetes Res. Clin. Pract.* **83**:353–7 (2008).

6. J. S. Park and C. W. Ahn, Educational program for diabetic patients in Korea — multidisciplinary intensive management, *Diabetes Res. Clin. Pract.* **77S**:S194–8 (2007).

7. K. E. Sakka, N. Fassiadis, R. P. S. Gambhir, M. Halawa, H. Zayed, M. Doxford, *et al.*, An integrated care pathway to save the critically ischaemic diabetic foot, *Int. J. Clin. Pract.* **60**:667–9 (2006).

8. K. Bakker, A. Foster, W. Van Houtum and P. Riley, *Diabetes and Foot Care: Time to Act* (International Diabetes Federation, Belgium, 2005), p. 34.

9. V. R. Driver, J. Madsen and R. A. Goodman, Reducing amputation rates in patients with diabetes at a military medical centre, *Diabetes Care* **28**:248–53 (2003).

10. G. Rose, F. Duerkson, E. Trepman, M. Cheang, J. N. Simonsen, J. Koulack, *et al.*, Multidisciplinary treatment of diabetic foot ulcers in Canadian aboriginal and non-aboriginal people, *Foot Ankle Surg.* **14**:74–81 (2008).

11. C. Trautner, L. M. Gatcke, B. Haastert, G. Giani and P. Mauckner, Reduced incidence of lower-limb amputations in the diabetic population of a German city, 1990–2005, *Diabetes Care* **30**:2633–7 (2007).

12. A. Nather, S. B. Chionh, K. L. Wong, X. V. Chan, L. Shen, P. A. Tambyah, A. Jorgensen and A. Nambiar, Value of team approach combined with clinical pathway for diabetic foot problems: a clinical evaluation, *Diabet. Foot Ankle* **1**:5731 (2010).

13. J. K. Davidson, M. Alogna, M. Goldsmith, *et al.*, Assessment of program effectiveness at Grady Memorial Hospital-Atlanta. In: G. Steiner and P. A. Lawrence (eds.), *Educating Diabetic Patients* (Springer Publishing Co, New York, 1981), p. 329.

14. P. Holstein, N. Ellitsgaard, B. B. Olsen, *et al.*, Decreasing incidence of major amputations in people with diabetes, *Diabetologia* **43**:844–7 (2000).

15. S. Krishnan, F. Nash, N. Baker, *et al.*, Reduction in diabetic amputations over 11 years in a defined U.K. population: benefits of multidisciplinary team work and continuous prospective audit, *Diabetes Care* **31**:99–101 (2008).

16. J. Larsson, J. Apelqvist, C. D. Agardh, *et al.*, Decreasing incidence of major amputation in diabetic patients: a consequence of a multidisciplinary foot care team approach?, *Diabet. Med.* **12**:770–6 (1995).

17. D. K. Litzelman, C. W. Slemenda, C. D. Langefeld, *et al.*, Reduction of lower extremity clinical abnormalities in patients with non-insulin-dependent diabetes mellitus: a randomized, controlled trial, *Ann. Intern. Med.* 119:36–41 (1993).
18. G. Rayman, S. T. Krishnan, N. R. Baker, *et al.*, Are we underestimating diabetes-related lower-extremity amputation rates? results and benefits of the first prospective study, *Diabetes Care* 27:1892–6 (2004).
19. C. J. Schofield, N. Yu, A. S. Jain, *et al.*, Decreasing amputation rates in patients with diabetes: a population-based study, *Diabet. Med.* 26:773 (2009).
20. W. H. van Houtum, J. A. Rauwerda, D. Ruwaard, *et al.*, Reduction in diabetes-related lower-extremity amputations in The Netherlands: 1991–2000, *Diabetes Care* 27:1042–6 (2004).
21. C. C. Van Gils, L. A. Wheeler, M. Mellstrom, *et al.*, Amputation prevention by vascular surgery and podiatry collaboration in high-risk diabetic and nondiabetic patients: the Operation Desert Foot experience, *Diabetes Care* 22:678–83 (1999).
22. E. Faglia, F. Favales, A. Aldeghi, P. Calia, A. Quarantiello, P. Barbano, M. Puttini, B. Palmieri, G. Brambilla, A. Rampoldi, E. Mazzola, L.Valenti, G. Fattori, V. Rega, A. Cristalli, G. Oriani, M. Michael and A. Morabito, Change in major amputation rate in a center dedicated to diabetic foot care during the 1980s: prognostic determinants for major amputation, *J. Diabetes Complications* 12(2):96–102 (1998).
23. J. Apelqvist and J. Larsson, What is the most effective way to reduce incidence of amputation in the diabetic foot?, *Diabetes Metab. Res. Rev.* 16(Suppl 1):S75–S83 (2000).
24. H. Van Damme and R. Limet, The diabetic foot, *Rev. Med. Liege* 60(5–6):516–25 (2005).
25. M. E. Levin, Foot lesions in patients with diabetes mellitus, *Endocrinol. Metab. Clin. North. Am.* 25(2):447–62 (1996).
26. L. A. Lavery, R. P. Wunderlich and J. L. Tredwell, Disease management for the diabetic foot: effectiveness of a diabetic foot prevention program to reduce amputations and hospitalizations, *Diabetes Res. Clin. Pract.* 70(1):31–7 (2005).
27. D. A. Martinez, J. Aguayo, G. Morales, M. Aguiran and F. Illan. Impact of a clinical pathway for the diabetic foot in a general hospital, *An. Med. Interna.* 21(9):420–4 (2004).
28. V. Alexandrescu, G. Hubermont, V. Coessens, Y. Philips, B. Guillaummie, *et al.*, Why a multidisciplinary team may represent a key factor for lowering the inferior limb loss rate in diabetic neuro-ischaemia wounds: application in a departmental institution, *Acta Chir. Belg.* 109(6):694–700 (2009).
29. G. W. Gibbons, E. J. Maraccio Jr., A. M. Burgess, *et al.*, Improved quality of diabetic foot care, 1984 vs 1990: reduced length of stay and costs, insufficient reimbursement, *Arch. Surg.* 128:576–81 (1993).
30. G. E. Reiber, Diabetic foot care. Financial implications and practice guidelines, *Diabetes Care* 15(Suppl 1):29–31 (1992).
31. D. A. Ollendorf, J. G. Kotsanos, *et al.*, Potential economics benefits of lower-extremity amputation prevention strategies in diabetes, *Diabetic Care* 21:1240–5 (1998).

18

Role of Revascularization in Management of Diabetic Foot Problems

Jackie Ho Pei

Consultant Vascular and Endovascular Surgeon
Department of Cardiac, Thoracic and Vascular Surgery
National University Hospital

Introduction

Foot ulcer is the leading cause of limb loss in our diabetic patient population. The underlying aetiology of diabetic foot ulceration is usually multi-factorial. It includes deformity, sensory neuropathy, peripheral arterial disease, unhealthy skin condition and infection. Cohort studies showed peripheral arterial disease (PAD) was found to be an important factor in nearly half of all the diabetic foot ulcers.[1,2] Foot ulcer in the presence of PAD is considered as critical limb ischemia. Ischemia due to arterial occlusive disease, nonetheless is one of the most reversible conditions. Various bypass surgeries and endovascular interventions with rapidly advancing technology enable effective revascularization of obstructed arteries of diabetic patients. The international working group on the diabetic foot (www.iwgdf.org) recommended 4 principles of management of diabetic foot ulcer as below

- treatment of any associated infection
- revascularization if possible and feasible

- off-loading in order to minimise trauma to the ulcer site
- management of the wound and wound bed in order to promote healing

Accurate diagnosis of peripheral arterial disease and prompt revascularization are the key factors in healing diabetic ischemic ulcers.

Diagnosis of peripheral arterial disease in diabetic foot patients

Based on the high prevalence of peripheral arterial disease in diabetic patients with foot ulcers, arterial assessment in the form of clinical examination and ankle brachial pressure index should be routinely carried out for all diabetic foot ulcers (including those with gangrene as well) on the very first evaluation. Arterial system examination of the lower limb includes careful palpation of all the lower limb pulses namely femoral, popliteal, dorsalis pedis and posterior tibial. Trophic changes including loss of hair, thinning of skin and deformed toe nail are commonly observed. The temperature of the foot and toe region will be lower compared to the thigh or the contralateral non-diseased limb. However, this feature may be masked by arterio-venous shunting, abnormal vasodilatation or presence of infection. The color of the sole and the toes may be paradoxically red in a dependent position and will turn pale upon elevation of the foot from supine position (Buerger's test).

Ankle brachial pressure index (ABPI) is the ratio between ankle arterial pressure (both dorsalis pedis and posterior tibial) and the highest brachial arterial pressure. The normal range is between 0.9 to 1.1. A low ABPI confirms the presence of arterial obstruction in the lower limb accurately. However, a normal ABPI does not exclude peripheral arterial disease. Falsely normal or high ABPI in diabetic patients is not uncommon because many have calcified hard tibial arteries. Some patients have abnormally high ABPI (>1.4) and they are associated with adverse cardiovascular events.[3] Thus the ABPI result should always be interpreted together with clinical information and with caution.

Alternatively, one can measure the toe pressure or toe pressure index (TPI) with special toe pressure cuff (Fig. 1). The normal toe pressure is between 90–100 mmHg and normal TPI is about 0.8. It is considered as abnormal when toe pressure ≤ 80 mmHg or TPI ≤ 0.6. Wound healing is unlikely if the toe pressure drop to <30 mmHg.

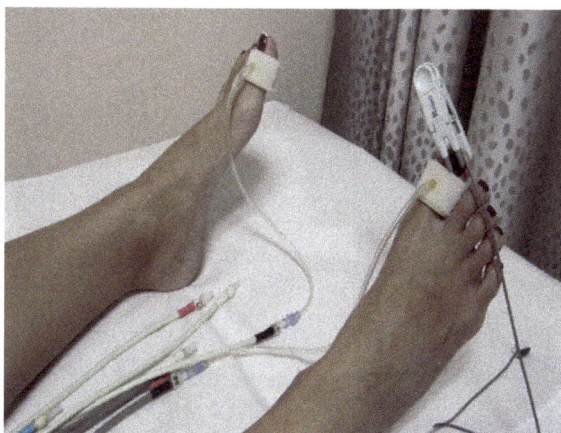

Figure 1.

Diabetic foot ulcer patients with either clinical feature or pressure study suggestive of PAD should be referred promptly to vascular specialists for further arterial investigation so that revascularization can be provided to appropriate patients in a timely manner.

Imaging modalities for arterial evaluation

The aim of performing imaging study on patients with suspected PAD disease is to i) confirm the diagnosis, ii) assess the severity of disease and most importantly iii) help formulate revascularization strategy. A proper arterial study should cover from the lower abdominal aorta to the ankle and foot arteries.

Duplex Ultrasound, a combination of real-time B mode image and pulsed Doppler flow study, is a useful tool to detect arterial obstructive lesion. It provides both anatomical as well as flow information. It also has the merit of being non-invasive and does not require contrast agent. Many of diabetic patients have pre-existing renal disease. A contrast free arterial study eliminates the worry of further impairing the renal function. A better way to show the result of a lower limb arterial duplex study is to illustrate the degree of obstruction as a diagram (Fig. 2). One important point to note: the quality of the arterial duplex scan is highly machine and performer dependent. An experienced vascular sonographer is the key to an accurate arterial duplex study. Even in an expert's hand, a thorough arterial duplex require 30 to 60 minutes

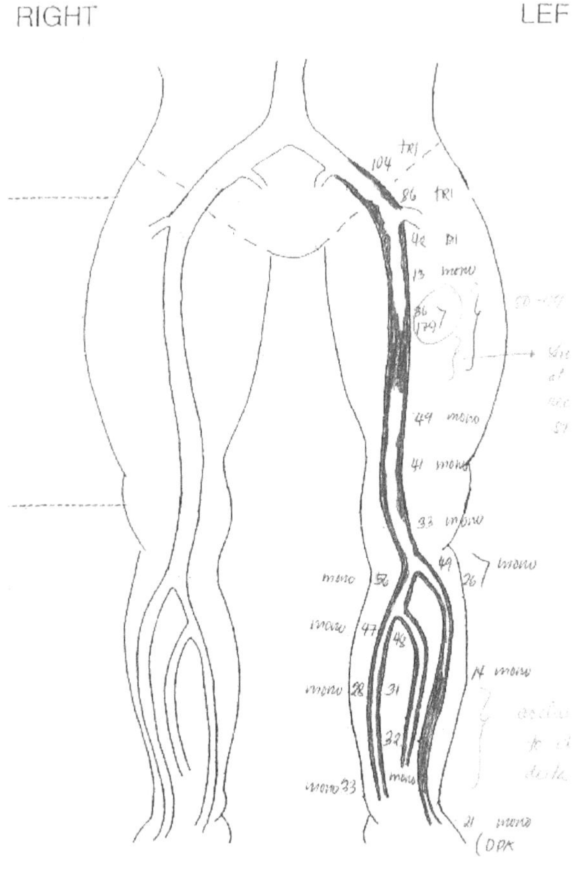

Figure 2.

to complete. Duplex ultrasound study becomes more challenging in the presence of arterial wall calcification and impossible with circumferential heavy calcification. Obese body habitus, severe lower limb oedema and uncooperative patients all cause scanning difficulty.

Computed tomography angiogram (CTA) is another commonly adopted imaging modality to assess lower limb arterial system. Iodine based contrast reagent injection is required to provide a meaningful image. After the acquisition of basic axial images, post-processing analysis including 3-dimensional reconstruction and bone elimination are needed to provide user-friendly information. Heavy calcification of vessel wall, not uncommon in diabetic patients, again poses severe interference to the image quality.

Magnetic resonance angiogram (MRA) with contrast (gadolinium) enhancement provides good lower limb arterial system information. Although gadolinium is much less nephrotoxic than iodine based contrast, risk of nephrogenic systemic fibrosis[4] has limited the use of MRA in renal impairment and failure patients. Some dedicated centres had shown a compatible accuracy of contrast-free un-enhanced MRA compared to contrast-enhanced MRA.[5] The development of this new technique will enable a wider use of MRA in diabetic PAD patients.

Nowadays, lower limb anteriogram is seldom performed for diagnostic purpose only but rather as part of intervention. A systemic review comparing the three imaging modalities[6] showed similar sensitivity and specificity for detecting arterial stenosis 50% or more with contrast enhanced MRA demonstrating higher accuracy. The choice of imaging modality as arterial assessment tool is mostly determined by the availability of expertise and resources in individual institution. The author's preference is arterial duplex ultrasound as the primary choice of imaging. MRA or CTA will be used in patients with obese body habitus or those unable to tolerate duplex scanning.

Pattern of arterial obstruction

The atherosclerotic disease of diabetic patients can affect all regions of lower limb arterial system but more frequently affects smaller size arteries (tibial, peroneal and pedal arteries) than non-diabetics. Nonetheless, multi-level arterial occlusive disease is commonly found in diabetic patients. Study also showed a higher incidence of arterial total occlusion rather than stenosis in diabetes.[7] Another special feature of diabetic PAD patients is the calcification of the media of artery. This alone will not cause obstruction to the artery. However, the calcification will increase the impedance of the artery, affect the value of ankle brachial index, impair image quality of arterial duplex and CTA, and render bypass surgery more difficult to perform. All these features are more prominent in patients with both diabetes and renal insufficiency[8]

Revascularization

The revascularization option and method for arterial disease in diabetic patients is similar to PAD patients without diabetes. The small vessel predominance and presence of medial calcification make revascularization for diabetic PAD patients more challenging. The modalities for revascularization are surgical bypass, endovascular intervention or a combination of both. Both surgical bypass and endovascular intervention have its merits, risks and limitations (see Table 1).

In centers with dedicated revascularization program, good limb salvage results for diabetic foot ulcer patients were achieved both with bypass surgery[9] (Fig. 3) and endovascular intervention[10,11] (Fig. 4). Long term limb salvage rate can be as good as 78.2% to 82%.[12–14] Failed revascularization, poor runoff score[15] and renal failure on dialysis[11] were poor prognostic factors for limb salvage.

It is still controversial regarding whether revascularization modality should be the first approach for diabetic critical limb ischemia patients. Currently there is only one multi-center randomized control trial (RCT) comparing endovascular first and surgical bypass first approach in severe limb ischemia patients with infra-inguinal arterial diseases — The BASIL study.[16,17] 452 patients with severe limb ischemia (life-style limiting claudication, rest pain and tissue loss) due to infra-inguinal arterial occlusive disease were randomized to either endovascular first or bypass first approach for revascularization. This RCT did not include patients with aorto-iliac disease and was not specific for diabetic patients only. The early result of BASIL study showed that the endovascular intervention first and bypass surgery first groups showed similar amputation-free survival and overall survival up to 2 years, although bypass first group had significantly more morbidity and higher cost in the short term.[16] But for those patients surviving more than 2 years, bypass first group is associated with better ischemic pain relief, ulcers healing, major amputation rate, quality of life and survival.[17] Nonetheless, only 42% of the BASIL subjects were diabetic with a predominance of femoro-popliteal disease. The trial result may not be directly applicable to diabetic patients with mainly below the knee disease. Comparative or randomized control trial on the revascularization strategy for diabetic PAD patients is wanting.

In the real-world clinical practice, a trend of more clinicians adopting endovascular revascularization for diabetic patients was observed.[18] Over the

Table 1. Comparison of surgical bypass to endovascular intervention

	Surgical bypass	Endovascular intervention
Body tissue trauma	Significant	Minimal
Anesthesia	Regional or general anesthesia	Local or regional anesthesia
Treatment easy to repeat	No	Yes
Wound complication	Possible (could be a concern in distal artery bypass if the surgical wound is close to the ulcer area)	Minimal
Arterial access problem	Minimal	Possible (hematoma, pseudoaneurysm)
Vessel patency	Longer (but depends on run off condition and quality of conduit)	Comparatively less durable (Also depends on severity of disease of target vessel as well as run off condition)
Arterial dissection and embolization	Minimal	Possible
Prerequisite	Patent proximal and distal artery to the diseased segment Reasonable size vein harvested as conduit	Better to have patent distal runoff vessel, but it is acceptable to open into collateral vessels Calcified but patent distal runoff artery is not a limitation
Limitations	Very small caliber or severely calcified distal landing artery is not suitable for bypass Patients with multiple severe medical co-morbidities bear high risk of anesthesia and surgery Distal bypass usually only target on one of the ankle arteries	Difficult to achieve a satisfactory vessel lumen if the arterial obstruction is heavily calcified Risk of progressing to renal failure will increase if patient has pre-existing poor renal function Endovascular intervention can be performed to all three crural arteries depending on the severity of the lesion

last two decades, there was tremendous improvement in the technique and devices used for endovascular intervention for PAD. The profile and material of angioplasty balloon had been improved. Stent material had been changed from stainless steel to majority nitinol which can conform better to the artery. New designs of stent structure were made to withstand torsion force in the

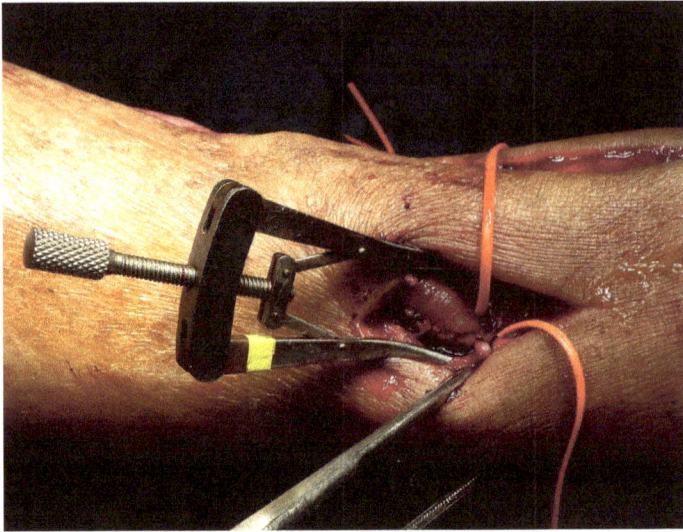

Figure 3.

superficial femoral artery during movement. Drug eluted stents were used for femoro-popliteal artery[19] with preliminary favourable result. For chronic total occlusion lesions, some used low profile, or hydrophilic catheter to provide extra support to the guidewire, and specially designed guidewires were made for crossing the occlusion. Some adopted subintimal approach[20] for crossing. In difficult conditions, devices like OUTBACK catheter (Cordis) and Pioneer catheter (Medtronic, Inc) can facilitate interventionists to re-enter from the subintimal plain into the true lumen distally. Others used a device with micro-dissection forceps over the tip (Frontrunner catheter, Cordis) to negotiate through the occlusion. Laser was also being applied for penetrating the calcified cap of total occlusive lesion. Besides simple ballooning to open up the lumen of an artery, various atherectomy devices (SilverHawk, Covidien) (Diamondback 360° PAD System, Cardiovascular Systems, Inc) worked by excising or debulking the atherosclerotic plaque away from the vessel to increase the luminal diameter. Cryotherapy (PolarCath, Boston Scientific) was applied by using nitrous oxide to inflate the angioplasty balloon so as to induce apoptosis of the arterial smooth muscle cells. Several studies reported favorable results of these newer devices for lower limb revascularization.[21–23] However most of them were single arm study or small

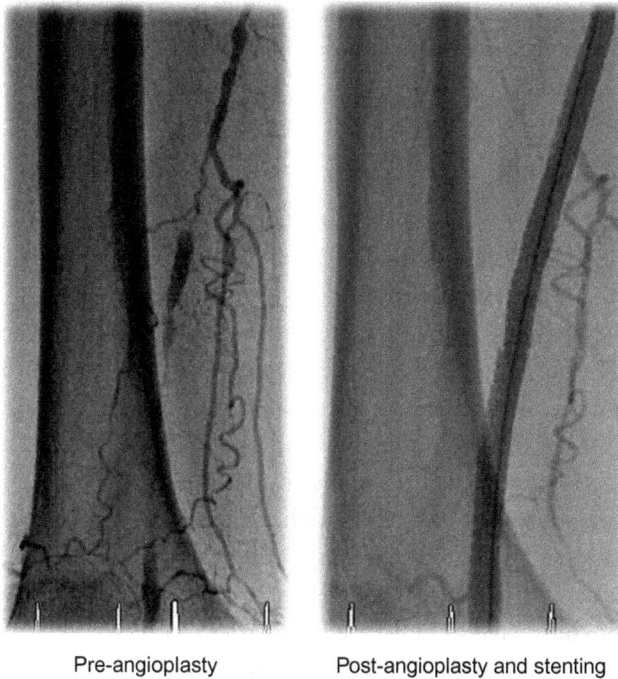

Pre-angioplasty   Post-angioplasty and stenting

Figure 4.

scale RCT.[24] Recently drug coated angioplasty balloon had become the focus of interest with several randomized control studies suggesting advantageous patency over simple angioplasty balloon.[25,26] However, these early RCT trials recruited mainly claudicants with relatively less severe arterial obstruction. Its role in endovascular intervention for diabetic patients with critical limb ischemia required further studies. Nevertheless, with all these advances, the procedural success rate of endovascular intervention for all regions of the lower limb artery was much improved.

Endovascular intervention and surgical bypass are not mutually exclusive. Diabetics with PAD affecting multiple regions of the lower limb artery may require a combination of revascularization modalities. There are reports on successful revascularization and limb salvage with various combinations of endovascular and open surgery eg superficial femoral artery angioplasty together with popliteal to tibial artery bypass.[27] Endovascular intervention can also be applied to salvage failing or failed bypass conduit.[28] The combination of the two treatment modalities increases the versatility of revascularization for patients with different arterial disease condition and co-morbidity status.

Angiosome concept

One important concept in revascularization of the lower extremity is "Angio-some". Taylor and Palmer first described the angiosome concept in 1987 where 3-dimensional vascular territories were being drawn up according to its predominant feeding artery. In the foot and ankle region, 6 angiosomes were identified. The medial side of heel, medial and lateral planter region are mainly supplied by posterior tibial artery and its branches. The dorsum of the foot is mainly supplied by dorsalis pedis artery and its branches. The lateral ankle and the lateral heel region are mainly supplied by peroneal artery. Revascularization of the crural artery that directly supplies the angiosome where the foot ulcer or lesion situated considered as direct revascularization. In contrast, revascularization of the artery that does not directly supply the corresponding angiosome is considered as indirect revascularization. Studies reviewing both lower limb bypass surgeries[29] and endovascular interventions[30] confirmed that the chance of wound healing and limb salvage is significantly better for direct revascularization than indirect revascularization. This knowledge provides important guidance for clinicians to select and prioritize which crural artery to treat for patients with foot ulcer.

Timing of revascularization and minor surgical amputation or debridement

Diabetic patients with foot ulcer and PAD are considered having critical limb ischemia. Revascularization should be provided as soon as the condition is identified to avoid further tissue loss and irreversible limb loss.[31]

If the tissue loss at presentation is minor, many of these patients only require proper wound dressing for healing after the revascularization. For more extensive tissue loss, minor amputation or debridement of non-viable tissue would be necessary to facilitate wound healing. These surgical procedures are preferably performed immediately after or shortly after the revascularization. This approach will facilitate the clinician to determine how much tissue to remove based on the status of tissue perfusion. Moreover, this also ensures that at the time of amputation or debridement, tissues over the incision site already have improved perfusion so as to provide the best chance of healing. An exception to this is the presence of active infection of the foot lesion that causes significant systemic sepsis. Urgent surgical removal of infected tissue can reduce the spread of infection and improve the general condition of the patient. Nevertheless, revascularization procedure should be followed as soon as possible together with proper aggressive antibiotic treatment. The risk of inducing infection to the stent or the artery during revascularization in the presence of infected foot ulcer is low. However, this risk will be higher for bypass surgery using synthetic graft.

Beyond revascularization

Usually there are multiple underlying causes for diabetics to develop foot ulcer even though arterial obstruction is one of the very reversible causes. Diabetic patients with ischemic foot ulcers also suffer significant systemic atherosclerosis that increases their cardiovascular risk. Thus besides revascularization of the lower limb, lots of effort are needed to improve their medical health and nutrition, eradicate infection, remove non-viable tissue, correct high pressure areas, and stimulate wound healing. A dedicated multi-disciplinary team would be a better service structure to provide comprehensive care for this group of patients.[31,32]

Conclusion

Diabetic foot ulcer is a limb threatening condition with nearly half of the situations related to arterial disease. Current revascularization technology provides good chance of healing for the ischemic diabetic ulcers and prevents limb loss. Universal arterial assessment for all diabetics with foot ulcer and early referral of those with ischemic component for revascularization are the key to successful limb salvage.

References

1. L. Prompers, M. Huijberts, J. Apelqvist, *et al.*, High prevalence of ischaemia, infection and serious comorbidity in patients with diabetic foot disease in Europe. Baseline results from the Eurodiale study, *Diabetologia* **50**(1):18–25 (2007).
2. M. A. Gershater, M. Löndahl, P. Nyberg, *et al.*, Complexity of factors related to outcome of neuropathic and neuroischaemic/ischaemic diabetic foot ulcers: a cohort study, *Diabetologia* **52**(3):398–407 (2009).

3. L. Pasqualini, G. Schillaci, M. Pirro, *et al.*, Prognostic value of low and high ankle-brachial index in hospitalized medical patients, *Eur. J. Intern. Med.* **23**(3):240–4 (2012).
4. J. C. Weinreb and A. K. Abu-Alfa, Gadolinium-based contrast agents and nephrogenic systemic fibrosis: why did it happen and what have we learned?, *J. Magn. Reson. Imaging* **30**(6):1236–9 (2009).
5. P. A. Hodnett, E. V. Ward, A. H. Davarpanah, *et al.*, Peripheral arterial disease in a symptomatic diabetic population: prospective comparison of rapid unenhanced MR angiography (MRA) with contrast-enhanced MRA, *AJR Am. J. Roentgenol.* **197**(6): 1466–73 (2011).
6. R. Collins, J. Burch, G. Cranny, *et al.*, Duplex ultrasonography, magnetic resonance angiography, and computed tomography angiography for diagnosis and assessment of symptomatic, lower limb peripheral arterial disease: systematic review, *BMJ* **334**:1257–61 (2007).
7. E. Faglia, Characteristics of peripheral arterial disease and its relevance to the diabetic population, *Int. J. Low. Extrem. Wounds* **10**(3):152–66 (2011).
8. N. Diehm, S. Rohrer, I. Baumgartner, *et al.* Distribution pattern of infrageniculate arterial obstructions in patients with diabetes mellitus and renal insufficiency — implications for revascularization, *Vasa* **37**(3):265–73 (2008).
9. F. Pomposelli, N. Kansal, A. Hamdan, *et al.*, A decade of experience with dorsalis pedis artery bypass: analysis of outcome in more than 1000 cases, *J. Vasc. Surg.* **37**(2):307–15 (2003).
10. E. Faglia, L. Dalla Paola, G. Clerici, *et al.*, Peripheral angioplasty as the first-choice revascularization procedure in diabetic patients with critical limb ischemia: prospective study of 993 consecutive patients hospitalized and followed between 1999 and 2003, *Eur. J. Vasc. Endovasc. Surg.* **29**(6):620–7 (2005).
11. E. Faglia, G. Clerici, J. Clerissi, *et al.*, Early and five-year amputation and survival rate of diabetic patients with critical limb ischemia: data of a cohort study of 564 patients, *Eur. J. Vasc. Endovasc. Surg.* **32**(5):484–90 (2006).
12. P. Schneider, M. Caps, D. Ogawa, *et al.*, Intraoperative superficial femoral artery balloon angioplasty and popliteal to distal bypass graft: an option for combined open and endovascular treatment of diabetic gangrene, *J. Vasc. Surg.* **33**(5):955–62 (2001).
13. R. Ferraresi, M. Centola, M. Ferlini, *et al.*, Long-term outcomes after angioplasty of isolated, below-the-knee arteries in diabetic patients with critical limb ischaemia, *Eur. J. Vasc. Endovasc. Surg.* **37**(3):336–42 (2009).
14. A. Lazaris, A. Tsiamis, G. Fishwick, *et al.*, Clinical outcome of primary infrainguinal subintimal angioplasty in diabetic patients with critical lower limb ischemia, *J. Endovasc. Ther.* **11**(4):447–53 (2004).
15. M. Daniel, M. Ihnat and M. Joseph, Current assessment of endovascular therapy for infrainguinal arterial occlusive disease in patients with diabetes, *J. Vasc. Surg.* **52**:92S–5S (2010).
16. D. J. Adam, J. D. Beard, T. Cleveland, *et al.*, Bypass versus angioplasty in severe ischaemia of the leg (BASIL): multicentre, randomised controlled trial, *Lancet* **366**:1925–34 (2005).
17. A. W. Bradbury, D. J. Adam, J. Bell, *et al.*, Bypass versus angioplasty in severe ischaemia of the leg (BASIL) trial: an intention-to-treat analysis of amputation-free and overall survival in patients randomized to a bypass surgery-first or aballoon angioplasty-first revascularization strategy, *J. Vasc. Surg.* **51**(Suppl):S5–17S (2010).

18. P. P. Goodney, A. W. Beck, J. Nagle, *et al.*, National trends in lower extremity bypass surgery, endovascular interventions, and major amputations, *J. Vasc. Surg.* **50**:54–60 (2009).
19. M. Dake, G. Ansel, M. Jaff, *et al.*, Paclitaxel-eluting stents show superiority to balloon angioplasty and bare metal stents in femoropopliteal disease: twelve-month Zilver PTX randomized study results, *Circ. Cardiovasc. Interv.* **4**(5):495–504 (2011).
20. A. Lazaris, A. Tsiamis, G. Fishwick, *et al.*, Clinical outcome of primary infrainguinal subintimal angioplasty in diabetic patients with critical lower limb ischemia, *J. Endovasc. Ther.* **11**(4):447–53 (2004).
21. M. Basco, F. Schlösser, B. Muhs, *et al.*, Lower extremity limb salvage with cryoplasty: a single-center cohort study, *Vascular* **20**(1):36–41 (2012).
22. J. McKinsey, L. Goldstein, H. Khan, *et al.*, Novel treatment of patients with lower extremity ischemia: use of percutaneous atherectomy in 579 lesions, *Ann. Surg.* **248**(4):519–28 (2008).
23. F. Serino, Y. Cao, C. Renzi, *et al.*, Excimer laser ablation in the treatment of total chronic obstructions in critical limb ischaemia in diabetic patients. Sustained efficacy of plaque recanalisation in mid-term results, *Eur. J. Vasc. Endovasc. Surg.* **39**(2):234–8 (2010).
24. N. Shammas, D. Coiner, G. Shammas, *et al.*, Percutaneous lower-extremity arterial interventions with primary balloon angioplasty versus Silverhawk atherectomy and adjunctive balloon angioplasty: randomized trial, *J. Vasc. Interv. Radiol.* **22**(9):1223–8 (2011).
25. G. Tepe, T. Zeller, T. Albrecht, *et al.*, Local delivery of paclitaxel to inhibit restenosis during angioplasty of the leg, *N. Engl. J. Med.* **358**:689–99 (2008).
26. M. Werk, S. Langner, B. Reinkensmeier, *et al.*, Inhibition of restenosis in femoropopliteal arteries. Paclitaxel-coated versus uncoated balloon: femoral paclitaxel randomized pilot trial, *Circulation* **118**:1358–65 (2008).
27. J. Lantis, M. Jensen, A. Benvenisty, *et al.*, Outcomes of combined superficial femoral endovascular revascularization and popliteal to distal bypass for patients with tissue loss, *Ann. Vasc. Surg.* **22**(3):366–71 (2008).
28. G. Carlson, J. Hoballah, W. Sharp, *et al.*, Balloon angioplasty as a treatment of failing infrainguinal autologous vein bypass grafts, *J. Vasc. Surg.* **39**(2):421–6 (2004).
29. R. Neville, C. Attinger, E. Bulan, *et al.*, Revascularization of a specific angiosome for limb salvage: does the target artery matter?, *Ann. Vasc. Surg.* **23**(3):367–73 (2009).
30. O. Iida, Y. Soga, K. Hirano, *et al.*, Long-term results of direct and indirect endovascular revascularization based on the angiosome concept in patients with critical limb ischemia presenting with isolated below-the-knee lesions, *J. Vasc. Surg.* **55**:363–70 (2012).
31. M. Lepäntalo, J. Apelqvist, C. Setacci, *et al.*, Chapter V: diabetic foot, *Eur. J. Vasc. Endovasc. Surg.* **42**(Suppl 2):S60–S74 (2011).
32. H. Zayed, M. Halawa, L. Maillardet, *et al.*, Improving limb salvage rate in diabetic patients with critical leg ischaemia using a multidisciplinary approach, *Int. J. Clin. Pract.* **63**(6):855–8 (2009).

19

Antibiotics for Diabetic Foot Infections

Hey Hwee Weng Dennis and Aziz Nather

Department of Orthopaedic Surgery
Yong Loo Lin School of Medicine
National University of Singapore

Introduction

Infection is a common diabetic foot problem. Nather *et al.* (2008)[1] showed that infection occurred in 122 out of a cohort of 202 patients (60.4%). Of these, 63 (31.2%) had monomicrobial infections and 59 patients (29.2%) had polymicrobial infections.

Choosing the Antibiotic Regime

Four major factors must be considered before selecting the appropriate empirical antibiotic:

1. Local microbiological data
2. Gram stain results and previous cultures
3. Severity of the infection (as shown by PEDIS Classification)[2]
4. Patient Profile (drug allergy, kidney and liver dysfunction, immune-compromise, recent hospitalization)

Empirical antibiotics should be guided by local microbiological data. In another study, Nather *et al.*[3] analysed a cohort of 100 patients treated for diabetic foot infections. The most common infection were abscess (32%), wet gangrene and infected ulcers (19%); 13% of cases had osteomyelitis.

48% of infections were monomicrobial and 52% were polymicrobial. With monomicrobial infections, the most common pathogens were *Staphylococcus aureus* (31.3%), methicillin- resistant *S. aureus* (MRSA) (16.7%) and *Pseudomonas aeruginosa* (16.7%). With polymicrobial infections, the most common organisms were Staphylococcus aureus (48.1%), Bacteroides fragilis (46.2%) and Pseudomonas aeruginosa (34.6%). With both mono- and polymicrobial infections combined, the most common pathogens were Staphylococcus aureus (39.7%), Bacteroides fragilis (30.3%), *Pseudomonas aeruginosa* (26.0%) and *Streptococcus agalactiae* (21.0%).

In Singapore, treatment must therefore be mainly directed against Staphylococcus aureus, Bacteroides fragilis, Pseudomonas aeruginosa and Streptococcus agalactiae. A combination of antibiotics against Staphylococcus aureus and gram-positive cocci (i.e. cloxacillin and/or 2nd–3rd generation cephalosporin would be appropriate.[4-6])

Specimen Collection

Diabetic foot infection is diagnosed on the basis of presence of purulent discharge and at least two of the cardinal signs of inflammation (redness, warmth, swelling, pain).

Microorganism can contaminate or infect the wound. It is therefore important to collect a good specimen for deciding what antibiotic to give. Tissue specimens are preferred to swabs. They should be taken aseptically from the debrided floor of the infected ulcer. Swabbing of undebrided ulcers should be avoided. The microorganisms obtained are likely to be contaminants or colonisers of the wound rather than being true pathogens. Needle aspirations under aseptic conditions may also be done to collect pus. Blood culture should also be performed for all diabetics.

The Future

Recently, there has been great concern about the increased incidence of MRSA and less commonly, vancomycin-resistant Enterococci (VRE).[7] There is also the concern for the emergence of vancomycin-intermediate Staphylococcus aureus (VISA) and vancomycin-resistant Staphylococcus aureus (VRSA)[8] among patients with diabetes.

Newer antibiotics which have been approved by international regulatory agencies in the past few years, for treating diabetic foot infections, include: Linezolid, daptomycin, tigecycline and ertapenem. Both linezolid and daptomycin have activity against MRSA and VRE. Tigecycline has a good spectrum of activity against Gram-positive cocci including bacilli and additional anaerobic coverage.[9] Ertapenem has good Gram-positive (excluding MRSA), Gram-negative and anaerobic coverage but no activity against *Pseudomonas aeruginosa* or *Acinetobacter baumannii*.[10]

However, cost is a major consideration with the use of these newer antibiotics. They should only be prescribed in consultations with an infectious disease specialist. It must also be noted that none of these newer agents have been shown to have superiority in proper randomized clinical trials against conventional agents such as amoxicillin clavulanate or ciprofloxacin and clindamycin.

Conclusion

Diabetic foot infections are a growing problem not only in Asia, but also globally. They are best managed by a multi-disciplinary approach and the judicious use of appropriate antibiotics. The emergence of resistant microbes is a growing problem globally as well. Solutions must be found in the near future if we are to reduce the morbidity and mortality of infections in our very vulnerable diabetic population.

References

1. A. Nather, S. B. Chionh, Y. H. Chan, L. J. Chew, C. B. Lin, S. H. Neo, E. Y. Sim, Epidemiology of diabetic foot problems and predictive factors for limb loss, *J. Diabetes Complications* **22**:77–82 (2008).
2. International Working Group on the Diabetic Foot, International Diabetes Foundation, Brussels (May 2003).
3. Z. Aziz, K. L. Wong, A. Nather and C. Y. Huak, Predictive factors for lower extremity amputations in diabetic foot infections, *Diabet. Foot Ankle* **2**:7463 (2011).
4. E. J. Goldstein, D. M. Citron and C. A. Nesbit, Diabetic foot infections: bacteriology and activity of 10 oral antimicrobial agents against bacteria isolated from consecutive cases, *Diabetes Care* **19**:638–41 (1996).
5. V. Urbanic-Rovan and M. Gubina, Bacteria in superficial diabetic foot ulcers, *Diabet. Med.* **17**:814–5 (2000).
6. National University Hospital Antibiotics Guidelines (2007).
7. A. Hartemann-Heutier, J. Robert, *et al.*, Diabetic foot ulcer and multi-drug resistant organisms: risk factors and impact, *Diabet. Med.* **21**:710–5 (2004).

8. Centers for Disease Control and Prevention, Vancomycin-resistant *Staphylococcal aureus.* Pennsylvania, 2002, *MMWR* **51**:902 (2002).

9. Prescribing Information, Tigecycline (Tygacil), (Wyeth, 2006).

10. Prescribing Information, Ertapenem (Invanz), (Merck, 2007).

20

Role of Chinese Medicine in Managing Diabetic Foot Ulcers

Ping-Chung Leung

Institute of Chinese Medicine
The Chinese University of Hong Kong, HKSAR

INTRODUCTION

The incidence of diabetes mellitus is increasing globally.[1] Patients with diabetes have a 12–25% lifetime risk of developing a foot ulcer.[2,3] Foot ulcers have become a major and increasing public health problem; the morbidities, impairment of the quality of life of patients, and the implied costs for management have attracted the attention of health policy providers.[4,5]

In spite of their rising importance, the management provided for foot ulcers is often inadequate, resulting in delayed healing and, eventually, the possibility of amputation[6,7]

If a wound has received a wide range of treatments yet has failed to heal, alternative treatment is an option. Different modalities are frequently tried, from the old traditional herbal treatment (topical or systemic) to more innovative ultrasonic therapy.[8,9] Many reports are available in Chinese language medical journals, describing the effectiveness of herbal combinations in ulcer healing. However, these reports are not validated by proper clinical trials.

In Hong Kong, a comprehensive investigation has just been completed on a popular herbal formula. In the laboratory, the formula has been studied, looking at its effects on fibroblast culture, and wound healing through granulation formation and angiogenesis, and so far the outcome has been very positive.[9] A randomised placebo controlled trial was conducted on 80 patients with non-healing diabetic ulcers occurring in legs which had been listed for major amputation, using the same herbal formula. 85% of the legs were salvaged and the herbal treatment group revealed better granulation, more rapid healing, better surface oxygen tension and microcirculation.[10]

This chapter is prepared to give a brief account of the laboratory research which attempts to work out the mechanisms of action of the herbal formula with reference to its tissue healing effects, followed by a simple report about the clinical trials that have been completed and those that are still going on.

THE HERBAL FORMULA

Using herbal preparations as means to heal chronic ulcers must have enjoyed hundreds of years of application in Folk practices among village dwellers. Such practices have remained popular among those who have failed to get their ulcers healed in spite of all conventional therapies. Under most circumstances, the herbal preparations are applied as topical agents.

The practice of Chinese Medicine in Chinese Communities is taking a divergent form. The tradition of herbal treatment favours oral intake of broths of medical herbs as much as topical applications since it is believed that the chronic ulcers result not only from local and regional hazards, but also occur as a consequence of the loss of internal harmony, which needs to be ameliorated with a systemic preparation.

We started to use herbal medicine in an attempt to heal chronic ulcers of diabetic patients when we learned that such ulcers were treated with herbal formulae in a Shanghai hospital and reports claimed that the results were very good. A personal visit to the Shanghai Hospital was followed by a pilot study using exactly the same preparations in Hong Kong. The use of herbal formulae was rather complicated. One anti-infection formula was used in the initial stage of treatment, followed by another formula to achieve harmonizing effects and then lastly, when granulations became obvious, the final formula of tissue growth was administered. We believed that since we used potent antibiotics in the initial stage to combat infection, we could skip the first formula and use the second and third formulae.

The pilot study was done in year 2002 on 30 patients and 40 legs with chronic ulcers. 35 legs treated with the herbal formulae were salvaged. Of the 35 feet rescued from amputation, 27 took less than 10 weeks to heal, the rest took 11 to 30 weeks.[11]

By that time, we had completed our laboratory studies on the herbal formulations and understood the essential biological effects of the individual herbs and their combinations. Since the formulae used contained more that ten herbs, we wanted to reduce the number and at the same time, use only one formula, rather than the staged use of two (Fig. 1).

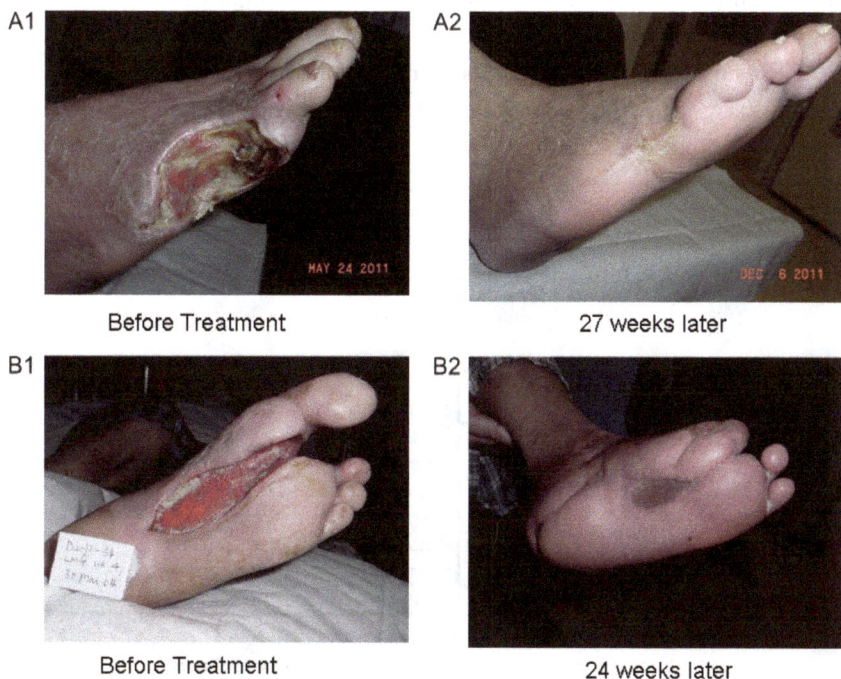

A1

Before Treatment

A2

27 weeks later

B1

Before Treatment

B2

24 weeks later

Figure 1. Raw herbs of *Radix Astragali, Radix Rehmanniae* and the simplified 2-herb formula sachet

LABORATORY STUDIES

The complicated herbal combinations forming the Shanghai treatment regime were derived from a popular ancient formula of six herbs that was designated to be an effective preparation that "strengthens muscles and controls swelling".

This formula contains six Chinese medical herbs, including *Radix Astragali, Radix Rehmanniae, Rhizoma Smilacis Chinensis, Rhizoma Atractylodis Macrocephalae, Radix Polygoni Multiflori Preparata, and Radix Stephania Tetrandrae.* The objective of the laboratory study was to use an interdisciplinary approach to test the hypothesis that the formula and its components influence tissue and systemic glucose homeostasis. The results of *in vitro* studies indicated that all herbal extracts can modify cellular glucose homeostasis.

Subsequent studies on the individual herbs indicated that two of them, viz. *Radix Rehmanniae* (RR) and *Radix Astragali* (RA), had the most impressive effects on both *in vitro* and *in vivo* platforms of wound healing. It was therefore envisaged that a simple 2-herb formula could be created as a novel replacement of the cumbersome ancient formulae. The newly composed formula would need laboratory confirmation and clinical trials to prove its efficacy.[12]

This simplified 2-herb formula (NF3) comprising of RA and RR in the ratio of 2:1 was used for further *in vivo* studies. It was examined for its ulcer healing effect in diabetic rats, after its mechanisms of action in fibroblast proliferation, angiogenesis and anti-inflammation have been studied *in vitro* (Fig. 2a).

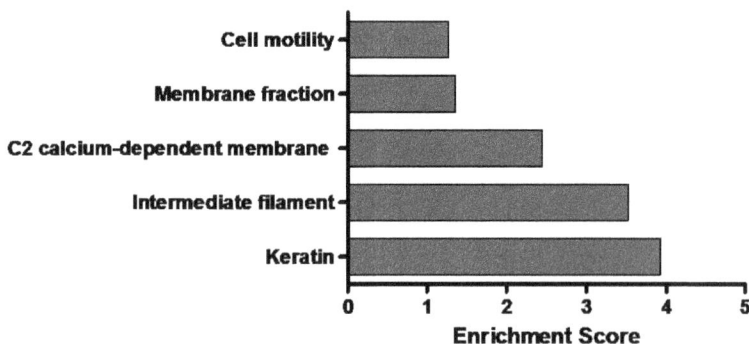

Figure 2. Diabetic rats showing healing of an artificially produced ulcer. Healing was faster with the 2-herb formula (NF3) consumption

The *in vivo* results demonstrated a significant reduction of wound area at Day 8 in two-herb formula NF3 (0.98 g/kg) group as compared to control (p < 0.01) (Fig. 2b).

CLINICAL TRIALS

After the pilot study was completed in year 2002, an extension trial started in 2004 using a single modified herbal formula composed of six herbs.

The study was conducted in two orthopaedic units of two different hospitals. The patients selected from the orthopaedic wards were all suffering from extensive ulcerations, complicated with infection, or gangrenous parts. Amputation was already the recommended treatment from the orthopaedic teams. The study protocol was properly screened and approved by the Clinical Research Ethics Committees of the Chinese University of Hong Kong. All patients were required to give written informed consent before registration.

The objective of the study was to see whether simple wound care together with standard diabetic and infection control, supplemented by a herbal drink, could promote ulcer healing in the diabetic patients, in an attempt to avoid major amputation.

The study was a double-blinded, randomized placebo-controlled trial. Based on the reported result of 85% successful limb salvage, a total of 80 patients formed the cohort of study. Safety of the herbal formula being used was ascertained through a thorough literature search which confirmed that the herbs had perfect safety records. Laboratory screening of the preparations were also done to rule out toxic contaminants like heavy metals, insecticides, and biological agents, according to guidelines of health product production set by the Department of Health in Hong Kong.[13]

The primary outcome measure was ulcer healing with no major amputation. Secondary outcomes included skin temperature, surface oxygen consumption, quality of life measures and liver/renal functions to ensure the detection of adverse effects.

Treatment consisted of standard diabetic control measures and standard courses of antibiotic treatment as required. Either the herbal drink or placebo was given after randomisation. Treatment continued for three to four weeks while close monitoring on the ulcer size and ulcer bed was performed. If after three to four weeks of blind treatment (either using the herbal formula or placebo), did not bring obvious improvement, the patient would be given the herbal option irrespective of whether he/she belonged to the placebo group. No unblinding was necessary at this stage of conversion to open treatment.

Other routine treatment consisted of: daily local wound care, i.e. antiseptic bathing, cleaning and dressing; weekly or biweekly debridement of necrotic tissues; limited removal of gangrenous toes and soft tissues. Wound assessments were done carefully. In the worst situation, uncontrolled wound deterioration might lead to major amputation. Treatment continued for a maximum of 24 weeks during which some ulcers healed and a few received skin grafting to facilitate the closure.

The different herbs used were listed in Table 1.

Results

From January 2004 to April 2006, eighty diabetic patients were admitted into the orthopaedic units because of non-healing foot ulcers which satisfied the selection criteria and were recruited into the study. Expert orthopaedic opinion advised major amputation at below-knee level because of the chronic nature of

Table 1.   List of herbs contained in the herbal formula

	Name in Chinese medicine	Description of used parts and botanical origins	Raw herb proportions
1	*Radix Astragal*	Dried root of *Astragalus membranaceus* (Fisch.) Bge. in the family Leguminosae	40 g
2	*Radix Rehmanniae*	Dried rhizome derived from *Rehmannia glutinosa* Libosch. in the family Scrophulariaceae	21 g
3	*Rhizoma Atractylodis Macrocephala*	Dried rhizome of *Atractylodes macrocephala* Koidz. in the family Compositae	9 g
4	*Radix Stephaniae Tetrandrae*	Dried root tuber of *Stephania tetrandra* S. Moore in the family Menispermaceae	9 g
5	*Radix Polygoni Multiflori Preparata*	Dried root tuber of *Polygonum multiflorum* Thunb. in the family Polygonaceae	9 g
6	*Rhizoma Smilacis Chinensis*	Dried rhizome of *Smilax china* L. in the family Smilacaceae	9 g

the ulcers, together with obvious infection in most of these diabetic patients. 86% of the recruited patients were above 65 years of age.

The patients gave full consent to the clinical trial of ulcer healing using a herbal formula in an attempt to limb salvage, and were randomized into the herbal treatment group and placebo group. The demographic data of the two groups and their clinical conditions were listed under (Table 2).

Clinical Outcome

Early deterioration and amputation

All patients were eager to retain their ulcerated limb but the outcome was dependent on the clinical behaviour of the ulcers. If rapid deterioration and/or life-threatening infection happened, amputation had to be done. When the condition showed no progress in the first 4 weeks, and yet remained stable, only herbal treatment was allowed without unblinding, so as to offer the best opportunity to limb salvage unless improvement was not achieved.

Six patients underwent amputation (3 herbal, 3 placebo) because of rapid deterioration within the initial 4 weeks. Another 18 patients (6 herbal, 12 placebo) continued with herbal treatment after the first 4 weeks. All ulcers in the herbal group healed, while 6 of the initial placebo group required leg amputation. The difference between the two groups was statistically significant (p = 0.048). Table 3 gives a summary of the results (Fig. 3).

Table 4 gives the duration taken by the two different groups for granulation maturation. Among patients healing within the 24-week period, the mean time to healing was shorter in the herbal group compared with the placebo group.(5.91 ± 1.36 vs. 9.15 ± 1.90)

Other healing parameters

Local circulation state

Surface circulation around the chronic ulcers improved with gradual healing due to the control of infection, good ulcer care and bed rest.

Cytokine study

Serum cytokine could be studied to assess the state of inflammatory responses. Tumor necrotising factor TNF α was taken as an effective marker indicating

Table 2. Baseline demographic characteristics of 80 patients treated with herbal treatment or placebo

	Herbal treatment	Placebo	Herbal vs. placebo
No. of patients	40	40	
Sex			
Male	25/40	22/40	0.496
Female	15/40	18/40	
Age (years)	66.3 ± 12.6	68.5 ± 11.1	0.408
Range	40–85	49–86	
Diabetes, duration (years)	8.4 ± 7.6	12.4 ± 8.8	0.034
Ulcer duration (week)	7.8 ± 8.2	12.9 ± 24.6	0.296
Ulceration size (cm^2)	28.7 ± 31.3	26.7 ± 27.3	0.789
Diabetes types			
Type I	5/40(13%)	9/39(23%)	0.218
Type II	35/40(88%)	30/39(77%)	
Diabetes current medication			
Oral hypoglycemic	28/40(70%)	26/40(65%)	0.891
Insulin injection	7/40(18%)	8/40(20%)	
Diet control	5/40(13%)	6/40(15%)	
Diabetes control			
Good (blood check steady)	19/37(51%)	17/35(49%)	0.321
Fair (blood check occasional fluctuate)	14/37(38%)	17/35(49%)	
Poor (blood check fluctuate)	3/37(8%)	1/35(3%)	
Smoking			
Smoking experience (3 cigarettes per week)	13/40(33%)	16/40(40%)	0.485
Non-smoker	27/40(68%)	24/40(60%)	
Ulcer bed			
Infected with slough	28/35(80.0%)	30/36(83.3%)	0.171
Edematous with patchy	6/35(17.1%)	0	
Relatively clean	1/35(2.9%)	2/36(5.6%)	
Gangrenous tissue			
Dry	12/38(32%)	8/31(26%)	
Wet	19/38(50%)	12/31(39%)	
None	7/38(18%)	11/31(35%)	
Nutrition state			
Body weight (kg)	59.1 ± 12.3	61.2 ± 12.3	0.601
Serum albumin(g/L)	317 ± 45	322 ± 42	0.647

Table 3. Outcome of cases with poor responses

	Amputation because of rapid deterioration in first 4 weeks	No improvement in first 4 weeks	Shift to open herbal treatment	Limb salvaged after herbal treatment	Amputation in spite of herbal treatment	Total no. of amputation
Herbal treatment	3	6		6	0	3
Placebo	3	12		6	6	9
Total	6	18		12	6	12

the active state of inflammation. A decline of TNF α level indicated an improvement of inflammatory processes which was mandatory for good healing. Patients treated with herbal treatment showed a significant gradual decline of TNF α when compared with placebo (Table 5).

Analysis of the clinical trial

In the first 4 weeks of blinded management, some ulcers deteriorated rapidly in spite of treatment, while others gradually improved and started to show granulations. 18 patients were thus detected as not responding to treatment and were transferred to the herbal treatment group to make sure that the best offer was given. 12 of the 18 patients thus transferred for open-label treatment were from the placebo group. Once changed to herbal treatment, 6 patients of this group showed gradual improvement and limb salvage was subsequently successful. 6 others did not improve and later received below-knee amputation. In the treatment group patients either responded satisfactorily, initially or subsequently after a longer duration of the treatment. However 6 patients did not do well and eventually required a major amputation.

The most exciting finding was the decline of serum tumor necrosis factor alpha (TNF α). The inflammation cytokine increased by 2.11 (pg/mL) in the placebo group while for the treatment group it decreased by 0.039 in the treatment group (p = 0.034).

The clinical study might be not impressive, very much related to the limited recruitment, however the parallel study on biomarkers and molecular targeting illustrated clearly the effect of the herbs on anti inflammation

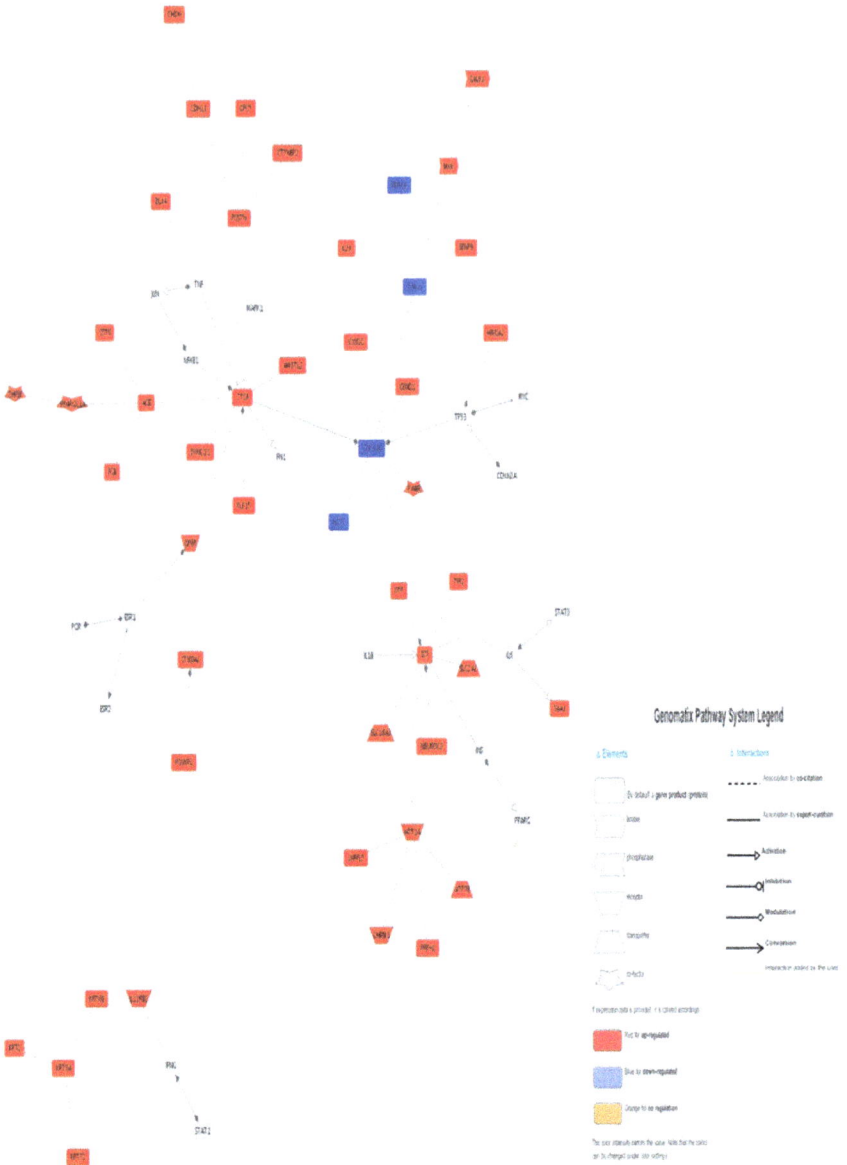

Figure 3. Diabetic foot ulceration of two patients before and after herbal treatment.

Table 4.   Time taken for granulation maturation (before skin grafting)

Group	Healing time (week)
Herbal treatment (n = 32)	
Mean	5.91 ± 1.36
Median	3.43
Placebo (n = 32)	
Mean	9.15 ± 1.90 (↑76%)
Median	6.86 (↑100%)
p-value	0.147

Table 5.   Change of TNF-α after at each visit of 80 patients

Visit	Week 0 (Baseline)	Week 2	Week 4	% change at Week 4
Herbal treatment	48.42 ± 16.34	35.60 ± 75.95	28.25 ± 61.83	−41.7
Placebo	43.86 ± 83.35	40.59 ± 68.46	39.46 ± 63.82	−10.0
p-value	0.841	0.433	0.703	

Comparing the two groups in percentage change from baseline to week 4 by paired- t test, p-value is 0.037.

(TNF-α) and that the herbs were acting on the genes related to inflammation, angiogenesis and cell proliferation.[14]

DISCUSSION

For chronic ulcers with extreme chronicity, one expects a very slow progress of healing if possible at all. Our simple herbal formula has been effective in helping to heal those ulcers. Our laboratory results have demonstrated their combined multiple target effects, including anti-inflammation, cell proliferation and angiogenesis. Ulcer formation is the result of multiple risk factors combined. Using *Rehmanniae* and *Astragalus* as a simple combined formula, it has been found to be capable of initiating ulcer healing, probably at the tissue level involving cellular and molecular activities.

In spite of scattered clinical reports, one must realise that growth factors, and stem cell therapy remain, as yet, experimental. If the ischaemic state is really so bad that even the marginal nutritional needs for all tissues is not satisfied, the outcome is still tissue necrosis and gangrene irrespective of any form of topical or regional treatment.

The herbal formula might be affecting the molecular changes via multiple channels in a concerted effort to initiate ulcer healing.

This chapter has introduced an alternative option to aid in the healing of a chronic ulcer. The positive results of the herbal treatment have gone through the evidence based studies, under both clinical settings and laboratory platforms. The ancient formula composed of many herbs has gradually been reduced to a simple twin-herb formula.

The innovative development has taken over ten years. The process started with the identification of the difficult problem of chronic ulcers failing to respond to conventional treatment. A search on herbal classics showed the possibility of using combinations to help the healing. A pilot study showed that the chosen herbs did work. However the effective formula looked too clumsy and too old. There should be scientific ways to modify the formula to make it simpler and more effective. The rationale of change and the details of modification were provided in the laboratory. The twin-herb formula was the result of repeated *in vitro* and *in vivo* experiments, eventually also proven effective clinically.

Chinese Medicine works on a supportive, harmonizing principle. The effects are achieved only gradually. If one compares the results of treatment with modern pharmaceuticals, one might be disappointed. Not only is the speed taken to gain evidence of improvement slow, but the extent, though accumulative, could be fragmented and of small scale. With a simple twin-herb formula, it is easier to continue with the research which might eventually adopt a drug discovery direction. However, given the complexity and cost demand for drug discovery, an innovative herbal formulation might be as good as a new drug, provided that the health claim is evidence-based.[15] After all, the current attitude of the intelligent public, is that preventive measures provided in Alternative Medicine, can be more seriously considered, as long as it is evidence-based.

Acknowledgments

This study was supported by the University Grants Council of Hong Kong and is part of a project entitled Area of Excellence in the Study and Development of Chinese Medicine.

References

1. G. E. Reiber, Epidemiology of foot ulcers and amputation in the diabetic foot. In: J. H. Bowker and M. A. Pfeifer (eds.), *Levin and O'Neal's The Diabetic Foot* (Mosby, Inc., St. Louis, 2001), pp. 13–32.
2. C. A. Abbott, A. P. Garrow, A. L. Carrington, J. Morris, E. R. van Ross and A. J. Boulton, Foot ulcer risk is lower in South-Asian and African-Caribbean compared with European diabetic patients in the UK: the North-West diabetes foot care study, *Diabetes Care* **28**:1869–75 (2005).
3. S. D. Ramsey, K. Newton, D. Blough, D. K. McCulloch, N. Sandhu, G. E. Reiber and E. H. Wagner, Incidence, outcomes and cost of foot ulcers in patients with diabetes, *Diabetes Care* **22**:382–7 (1999).
4. T. G. Ragnarson and J. Apelqvist, Health-economic consequences of diabetic foot lesions, *Clin. Infect. Dis.* **39**(Suppl 2):S132–9 (2004).
5. D. J. Margolis, L. Allen-Taylor, O. Hoffstad and J. A. Berlin, Diabetic neuropathic foot ulcers and amputation, *Wound Repair Regen.* **13**:230–6 (2005).
6. D. J. Margolis, J. Kantor and J. A. Berlin, Healing of diabetic neuropathic foot ulcers receiving standard treatment: a meta-analysis, *Diabetes Care* **22**:692–5 (1999).
7. D. J. Margolis, L. Allen-Taylor, O. Hoffstad and J. A. Berlin, Healing diabetic neuropathic foot ulcers: are we getting better?, *Diabet. Med.* **22**:172–6 (2005).
8. P. K. Mukherjee, K. Mukherjee, M. Rajesh Kumar, M. Pal and B. P. Saha, Evaluation of wound healing activity of some herbal formulations, *Phytother. Res.* **17**:265–8 (2003).
9. W. J. Ennis, P. Foremann, N. Mozen, J. Massey, T. Conner-Kerr and P. Meneses, Ultrasound therapy for recalcitrant diabetic foot ulcers: results of a randomised, double-blind, controlled, multicenter study, *Ostomy Wound Manage.* **51**:24–39 (2005).
10. P. C. Leung, W. N. Wong and W. C. Wong, Limb Salvage in extensive diabetic foot ulceration: an extended study using a herbal supplement. *Hong Kong Med. J.* **14**:29–33 (2008).
11. M. W. Wong, P. C. Leung and W. C. Wong, Limb salvage in extensive diabetic foot ulceration — a preliminary clinical study using simple debridement and herbal drinks, *Hong Kong Med. J.* **7**:403–7 (2001).
12. T. W. Lau, D. S. Sahota, C. H. Lau, C. M. Chan, F. C. Lam, Y. Y. Ho, K. P. Fung, C. B. S. Lau and P. C. Leung, An *in vivo* investigation on the wound-healing effect of two medicinal herbs using an animal model with foot ulcer, *Eur. Surg. Res.* **41**:15–23 (2008).
13. Department of Health Hong Kong, *Regulations on Medicinal Herbal Preparations* (Department of Health, Hong Kong, 2004).
14. R. Lobmann, G. Schultz and H. Lehnert, Proteases and the diabetic foot syndrome: mechanisms and therapeutic implications, *Diabetes Care* **28**:461–71 (2005).
15. J. P. Aggett, J. M. Antoine, N. G. Asp, F. Bellisle, L. Contor, J. H. Cummings, J. Howlett, D. J. F. Muller, C. Persin, L. T. J. Pijls, G. Rechkemmer, S. Tuijtelaars and H. Verhagen, PASSCLAIM — Consensus on Criteria, *Eur. J. Nutr.* **44**:I/5–1/30 (2005).

21

Reducing the Pain of Diabetic Neuropathy: What Works

Mary Suma Cardosa

INTRODUCTION

Diabetic peripheral neuropathy (DPN) affects up to 50% of patients with diabetes; the prevalence of painful diabetic peripheral neuropathy (PDPN) has been reported in 8 to 34% of diabetics, with those with type 2 diabetes having a higher risk of developing PDPN.[1−3] More than 80% of those with PDPN report having moderate to severe pain and those with PDPN had poorer quality of life.[2−4]

PDPN, like other types of neuropathic pain, is poorly treated. In a study of 55,686 patients with painful peripheral neuropathies (10.8% of whom had PDPN) it was found that 54% were treated with opioids, 40% were treated with non steroidal anti-inflammatory drugs or cyclo-oxygenase 2 inhibitors, 21% with benzodiazepines, 14% with SSRIs, 11% anticonvulsants 11% tricyclic antidepressants and almost a quarter had no treatment at all.[5]

PATHOPHYSIOLOGY, SYMPTOMS AND SIGNS

Development of neuropathic pain follows complex and heterogenous events involving changes in both the peripheral and central nervous systems, leading to an increased sensitivity to stimuli and decreased inhibitory controls, which results in abnormal generation and conduction of impulses along nerves, spinal cord and to the brain.[6,7]

Pain may be continuous (usually described as burning or deep pressure pain) or intermittent (usually described as shooting, lancinating or electric shock-like) and may be spontaneous (not evoked by any particular event or movement). Other positive sensory symptoms are tingling, hyperalgesia (an increased response to a painful stimulus) or allodynia (pain in response to a non-painful stimulus) or dysaesthesias (unpleasant abnormal sensations). In addition, patients may have negative sensory symptoms like numbness, loss of balance and loss of sensation.[8,9]

MANAGEMENT

Like other forms of chronic neuropathic pain, painful diabetic peripheral neuropathy should be managed using a multimodal, multidisciplinary approach, based on the biopsychosocial model of understanding chronic pain. Management begins with a full assessment to confirm the diagnosis as well as explore the impact of the pain on the patient's mood, function and quality of life.

Assessment

Evaluation of a patient may include the use of screening questionnaires to determine whether the pain is neuropathic. Examples of screening questionnaires used are shown in Tables 1 and 2.

History:

The characteristics of neuropathic pain are typically described as burning, stabbing, shooting or electric shock-like, and patients with PDPN typically have numbness or loss of sensation as well. In addition to the above, they may also have hyperalgesia, allodynia or dysaesthesias.

History should also include information on blood sugar control. Assessment of the impact of the pain on the patient's function and quality of life should include the effect on sleep, presence of anxiety and depression, and problems with work and relationships, as all of these may arise due to the

Table 1. ID pain[10]

Question	Score	
	Yes	No
1. Did the pain feel like pins and needles?	1	0
2. Did the pain feel hot/burning?	1	0
3. Did the pain feel numb?	1	0
4. Did the pain feel like electrical shocks?	1	0
5. Is the pain made worse with touch of clothing or bed sheet?	1	0
6. Is the pain limited to your joints?	−1	0

Minimum total score $= -1$, maximum total score $= 5$
| −1 | Neuropathic pain not likely | 2–3 | Consider neuropathic pain |
| 0–1 | Neuropathic pain less likely | 4–5 | Strongly conisder neuropathic pain |

Table 2. DN4 neuropathic pain diagnostic questionnaire[11]

Interview of patient		Yes	No
Question 1	Does the pain have one or more of the following characteristics?		
	1. Burning	1	0
	2. Painful cold	1	0
	3. Electric shock	1	0
Question 2	Is the pain associated with one or more of the following symptoms in the same area?		
	4. Tingling	1	0
	5. Pins and needles	1	0
	6. Numbness	1	0
	7. Aching	1	0
Examination of patient			
Question 3	Is the pain located in an area where the physical examination may reveal one or more of the following characteristics?		
	8. Hyperaesthesia to touch	1	0
	9. Hypoaesthesia to prick	1	0
Question 4	In the painful area, can the pain be caused or increased by:		
	10. Brushing	1	0

A "YES" score of (more than or equal to 4) is diagnostic of Neuropathic Pain

persistent pain and themselves may also exacerbate the pain and, if present, need to be addressed in the holistic management of the patient.[12]

Physical Examination:

Neurological examination usually reveals a peripheral sensory deficit of the typical "glove and stocking" distribution. Assessment of vibration and position sense may reveal involvement of these modalities. Assessment of autonomic function (e.g. test for postural hypotension, sudomotor axon reflex test and ECG to determine heart rate variability) should also be carried out so as to detect autonomic neuropathy which may occur in addition to the peripheral neuropathy.

Management Modalities

The goals of management are to reduce or eliminate pain (if possible), to improve physical function, reduce psychological distress and to improve the overall quality of life. Management includes the following modalities:

1. Pharmacotherapy — Four drug classes have consistently demonstrated efficacy against various types of neuropathic pain in randomized, controlled clinical trials; these include anticonvulsants, antidepressants, opioids and local anaesthetics. NSAIDs have not been found to be effective and should not be used for the treatment of neuropathic pain.
2. Physical therapy — this includes stretches to maintain flexibility, strengthening exercises as well as aerobic exercises (e.g. brisk walking, swimming) to maintain general fitness.
3. Psychological therapy — this includes relaxation and cognitive therapy and also application of pain management strategies like distraction, planning and activity pacing.

Clear goals of treatment should be set and the patient should have realistic expectations of the therapy. As complete pain relief is difficult to achieve, the goal of pharmacological treatment should be a reduction in pain with acceptable side effects. Patient education about the cause of the pain, explanation about the mechanism of neuropathic pain and emphasis on the importance of non-pharmacological techniques including exercise, relaxation, stress management, sleep hygiene and other self-management techniques are critical in the management of patients with PDPN. In addition, patients must

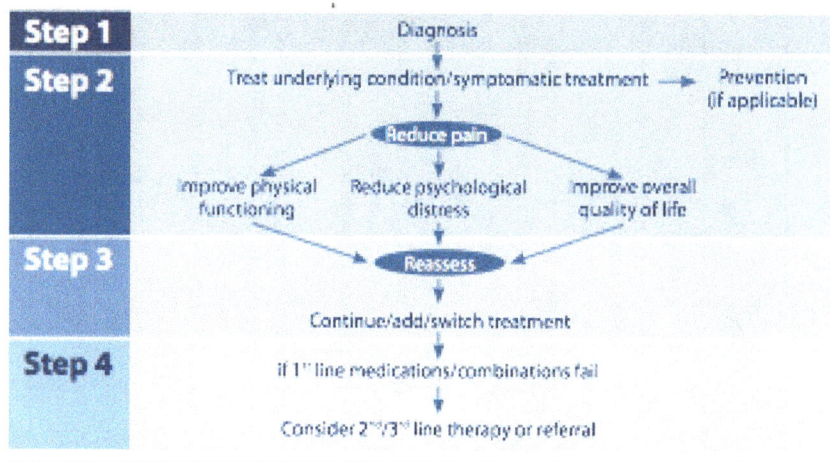

Figure 1. Stepwise approach to the management of neuropathic pain[13]

also be advised to maintain a healthy balanced diet and to keep their blood sugar well controlled in order to prevent exacerbation of the peripheral neuropathy.

Pharmacotherapy[13,14]

This should be done in a stepwise manner with the goal of not just reducing pain but also improving function, reducing distress and improving overall quality of life, as shown in Fig. 1 above.

Pharmacotherapy can be initiated with any of the following antineuropathic agents

1. A secondary-amine tricyclic antidepressant [TCA] (amitriptyline, nortriptyline) or a serotonin– norepinephrine reuptake inhibitor [SNRI] (duloxetine, venlafaxine)
2. A calcium channel α2-d ligand, either gabapentin or pregabalin
3. Topical lignocaine may also be used alone or in combination with one of the other first-line therapies

After initiation of pharmacotherapy, allowing for gradual increase in the dose to the maximum indicated or tolerated, reassess pain and health-related quality of life.

— If substantial pain relief (e.g. average pain score reduced to $\leq 3/10$) with tolerable adverse effects, continue treatment.

Table 3. Antineuropathic agents

Drug	Starting dose	Dose titration/maximum dose	Duration of adequate trial	Potential adverse effects
Amitriptyline	10–25 mg daily at bedtime	Increase by 10 to 25 mg weekly, up to maximum of 75 mg daily (single dose at bedtime)	3 months at maximum tolerated dosage	Dry mouth, sweating, sedation, disturbed vision, cardiotoxicity, palpitations, postural hypotension, urinary retention, constipation, drowsiness
Duloxetine	30 mg/day	Increase to 60 mg/day after 1 week, up to maximum of 120 mg/day (60 mg bid)	4 wks	Nausea/vomiting, dry mouth, constipation, GI distress, decreased appetite, insomnia, dizziness, somnolence, blurred vision, increased sweating, fatigue
Pregabalin	150 mg/day as 75 mg bid	Increase to 300 mg daily after 3–7 days, then by 150 mg/d every 3–7 days as tolerated, up to maximum of 600 mg daily (300 mg bid)	4 wks	Dizziness, somnolence, weight gain, blurred vision, dry mouth, constipation, peripheral oedema, euphoric mood, disturbed attention, increased appetite, unsteady gait
Gabapentin	Day 1, 300 mg at bedtime; Day 2, 300 mg bid; Day 3, 300 mg tid	Increase by 300 mg tid every 1–7 days as tolerated up to maximum of 3,600 mg daily (1200 mg tid or 900 mg qid)	3–8 wks for titration plus 2 wks at maximum tolerated dosage	Dizziness, somnolence, weight gain, blurred vision, dry mouth, constipation, peripheral oedema, euphoric mood, disturbed attention, increased appetite, unsteady gait
Tramadol	50 mg daily or bid	Increase by 50–100 mg daily in divided doses every 3–7 days as tolerated, up to maximum of 400 mg daily	4 wks	Dizziness, dry mouth, nausea, constipation, somnolence; risk of seizures/ epilepsy; risk of serotonergic syndrome if combined with SSRIs

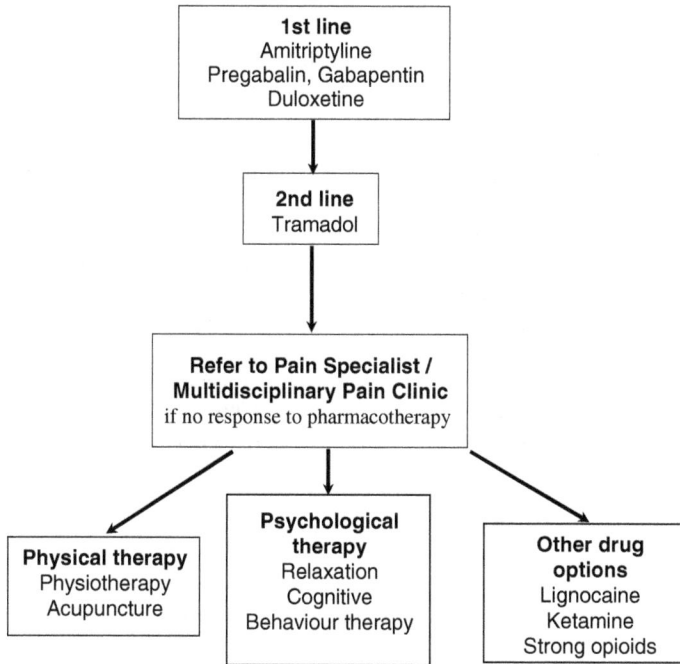

Figure 2. Summary of management of painful diabetic peripheral neuropathy

— If partial pain relief (e.g. average pain remains $\geq 4/10$) with tolerable side effects, ***add*** one of the other first-line medications.

— If no or inadequate pain relief (e.g. $<30\%$ reduction in pain score) and/or if side effects are intolerable, ***switch*** to another of the first-line medications.

If trials of first-line medications alone and in combination fail, consider second- and third-line medications or referral to a pain specialist or multidisciplinary pain center.

2nd line medications include opioids (morphine, oxycodone, methadone) and tramadol.

3rd line medications include carbamazepine, lamotrigine, topiramate, valproaic acid, NMDA receptor antagonists (ketamine) and topical capsaicin.

Table 3 below gives details of the drug dosages, side effects and precautions.

References

1. C. A. Abbott, R. A. Malik, E. R. van Ross, J. Kulkarni and A. J. Boulton, Prevalence and characteristics of painful diabetic neuropathy in a large community-based diabetic population in the U.K., *Diabetes Care* **34**(10):2220–4 (2011).

2. M. Davies, S. Brophy, R. Williams and A. Taylor, The prevalence, severity, and impact of painful diabetic peripheral neuropathy in type 2 diabetes, *Diabetes Care* **29**(7):1518–22 (2006).

3. E. Q. Wu, J. Borton, G. Said, T. K. Le, B. Monz, M. Rosilio and S. Avoinet, Estimated prevalence of peripheral neuropathy and associated pain in adults with diabetes in France, *Curr. Med. Res. Opin.* **23**(9):2035–42 (2007).

4. K. Van Acker, D. Bouhassira, D. De Bacquer, S. Weiss, K. Matthys, H. Raemen, C. Mathieu and I. M. Colin, Prevalence and impact on quality of life of peripheral neuropathy with or without neuropathic pain in type 1 and type 2 diabetic patients attending hospital outpatients clinics, *Diabetes Metab.* **35**(3):206–13 (2009).

5. A. Berger, E. M. Dukes and G. Oster, Clinical characteristics and economic costs of patients with painful neuropathic disorders, *J. Pain* **5**(3):143–9 (2004).

6. R. H. Dworkin, M. Backonja, M. C. Rowbotham, *et al.*, Advances in neuropathic pain. Diagnosis, mechanisms and treatment recommendations, *Arch. Neurol.* **60**: 1524–34 (2003).

7. N. Harden and M. Cohen, Neuropathic pain: from mechanisms to treatment strategies. Unmet needs in the management of neuropathic pain, *J. Pain Symptom Manage.* **25**:S12–7. (2003).

8. R. H. Dworkin, An overview of neuropathic pain: syndromes, symptoms, signs, and several mechanisms, *Clin. J. Pain* **18**:343–9 (2002).

9. J. Serra, Overview of neuropathic pain syndromes, *Acta Neurol. Scand. Suppl.* **173**:7–11 (1999).

10. R. Portenoy, Development and testing of a neuropathic pain screening questionnaire: ID pain, *Curr. Med. Res. Opin.* **22**:1555–65 (2006).

11. D. Bouhassira, N. Attal, H. Alchaar, *et al.*, Comparison of pain syndromes associated with nervous or somatic lesions and development of a new neuropathic pain diagnostic questionnaire (DN4), *Pain* **114**:29–36 (2005).

12. K. Meyer-Rosberg, A. Kvarnstrom, E. Kinnman, *et al.*, Peripheral neuropathic pain — a multidimensional burden for patients, *Eur. J. Pain* **5**:379–89 (2001).

13. R. Vijayan, K. J. Goh, M. S. Cardosa and E. M. Khoo, *Malaysian Guidelines: Management of Neuropathic Pain*, 2nd Edition (Malaysian Association for the Study of Pain, Kuala Lumpur, 2012).

14. N. Attal, G. Cruccu, R. Baron, M. Haanpaa, P. Hansson, T. S. Jensen and T. Nurmikko, EFNS guidelines on the pharmacological treatment of neuropathic pain: 2010 revision. *Eur. J. Neurol.* **17**(9):1113–23 (2010).

Section 6

Guide to Operative Surgery

22

Major Amputations in Diabetics

Aziz Nather, Gurpal Singh, Amy Pannapat Chanyarungrojn and Andrew Hong Choon Chiet

Department of Orthopaedic Surgery
Yong Loo Lin School of Medicine
National University of Singapore

INTRODUCTION

In diabetic patients, major amputations include:

- Below knee amputation (BKA)
- Through knee amputation (TKA)
- Above knee amputation (AKA)

More proximal amputations such as Hip Disarticulation and Hind-Quarter Amputation are seldom performed for diabetic foot surgery. The mortality rate of such procedures is high — more than 50%.

THE BELOW KNEE AMPUTATION (BKA)

Below knee amputation (BKA) is one of the most commonly performed amputations in diabetic patients.

Indications

- Infection extending up to ankle
- Severe ischaemia/gangrene involving the whole foot
- Both dorsalis pedis and posterior tibial pulses are not palpable

- ABI < 0.5, TBI < 0.5
- Presence of rest pain in the foot or lower part of the leg
- Gangrene or ulcer of the heel, not salvageable by a flap

Pre-operative workup

- Full Blood Count (FBC), Erythrocyte Sedimentation Rate (ESR), C-Reactive Protein (CRP)
- Urea and electrolytes
- HbA1C
- Chest X-ray (CXR), Electrocardiogram (ECG)
- **Group and Cross Match:** Haemoglobin must be kept above 10 g/dL pre-operatively to provide sufficient oxygen for wound healing.
- **Total proteins:** Albumin level must be kept above 38 g/L by a high protein diet pre-operatively to provide sufficient nutrition for wound healing.
- Blood Thinners such as Plavix and Aspirin must be stopped at least 3 days before operation.
- **Cardiac Assessment:** Must be performed by cardiologist for a patient with history of acute myocardial infarction (AMI) or ischaemic heart disease (IHD). This includes a 2-D Echocardiogram.
- **Risk of mortality** of the operation must be communicated to the patient based on his Ejection Fraction results:
  - 55–70%   Normal
  - 40–54%   Low Risk
  - 35–39%   Moderate Risk
  - <35%   High Risk
- **Risk of morbidity** of the operation must also be discussed. Chances of wound healing must be communicated, based on vascularity of the tissue at the level of amputation
  - ≥70%   Good
  - 51–69%   Fair
  - ≤ 50%   Poor
- A patient conference must be convened by the Consultant. All potential anaesthetic risks and surgical complication risks must be explained in detail. The risk of a second operation (10–20%) must also be discussed. This involves a higher level of amputation (TKA or AKA) when the below knee

stump fails to heal. The risk of revision surgery is higher in patients with concomitant renal failure.

- Note that the risk of mortality in a BKA is 5–10% in diabetic patients with no previous medical history or comorbidity. This must be communicated to the patient. The risk of infection of the below knee stump is about 10%.

Anaesthesia

- Use general or regional anaesthesia. The latter includes spinal or femoral nerve block for a high risk case. Regional anaesthesia cannot be performed when a patient is on Plavix or Aspirin and these have not been removed 3 days prior to the operation.
- Continue giving intravenous antibiotics started in the ward.

Patient positioning

- The patient is placed in the supine position.
- Place a sandbag underneath the buttock on the side of the amputation.
- A pneumatic tourniquet is applied on the thigh but not inflated.

Operative procedure

There are two commonly practiced methods of doing BKA — the Burgess long posterior flap[1] and the Skew Flap.[2] The authors favour the use of the long posterior myocutaneous (Burgess) flap technique.

1. Skin flaps are marked using a marker pen. The level of tibial osteotomy (Fig. 1a) must be at least 1 hand's breadth below the tibial tuberosity. 2 points (A, B) are marked at this level on the leg, medially and laterally (Fig. 1b).

2. A short anterior flap is drawn, connecting points A and B at least 2 cm distal to the level of tibial osteotomy. A long posterior myocutaneous flap (Fig. 1c) is drawn connecting the points A and B again. The posterior flap is approximately one and a half times the circumference of the leg at the level of amputation. It is always better to mark the flaps slightly longer than required as longer flaps can be trimmed or refashioned during closure. However, if the flap is too short, the tension on closure will prevent the wound from healing. More bone would then need to be cut. This is a bad and unsatisfactory situation.

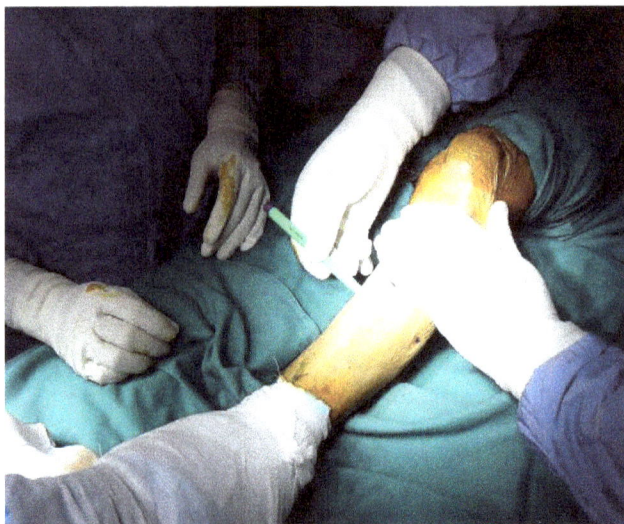

Figure 1a. Level of tibial osteotomy

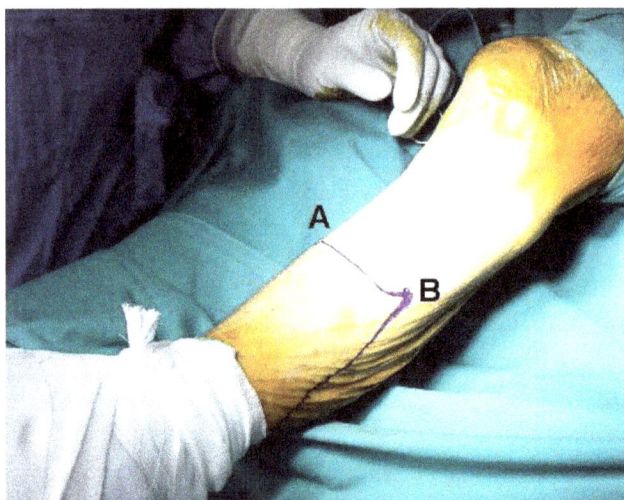

Figure 1b. Anterior skin flap

3. The skin in both marked flaps is then cut down to the deep fascia (Fig. 2a). Medially, the great saphenous vein (Fig. 3) is clamped, divided and ligated. Posteriorly, the small saphenous vein (Fig. 3) is clamped, divided and ligated.

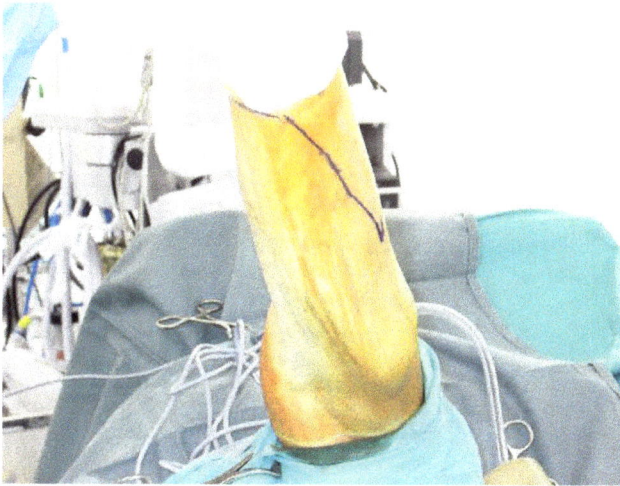

Figure 1c. Posterior skin flap

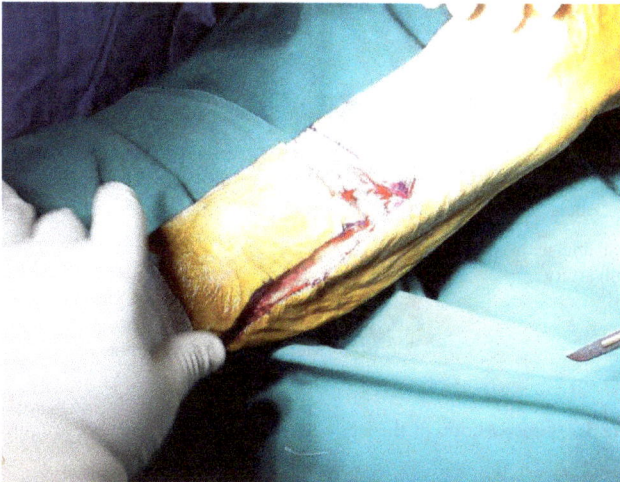

Figure 2a. Dissection to deep fascia

4. The leg is placed on a kidney dish covered by a steridrape. The pressure of the leg against the dish prevents venous bleeding from the posterior flap (tamponade effect) (Fig. 2b).

5. The periosteum on the medial aspect of the tibia is then cut at the level of the flap and stripped upward with a periosteal elevator (Fig. 4).

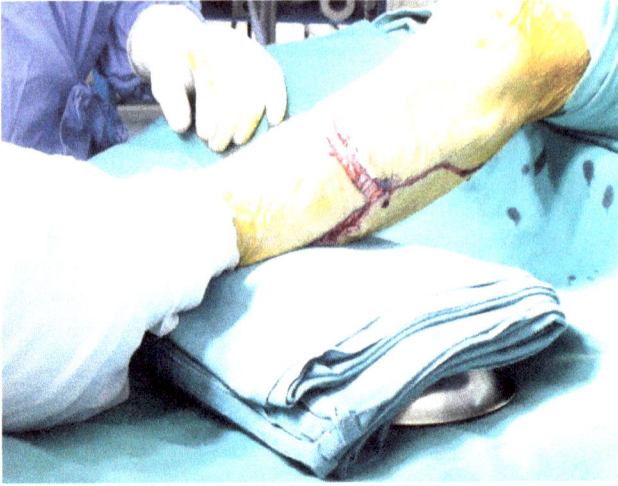

Figure 2b.   Use of kidney dish for tamponade effect

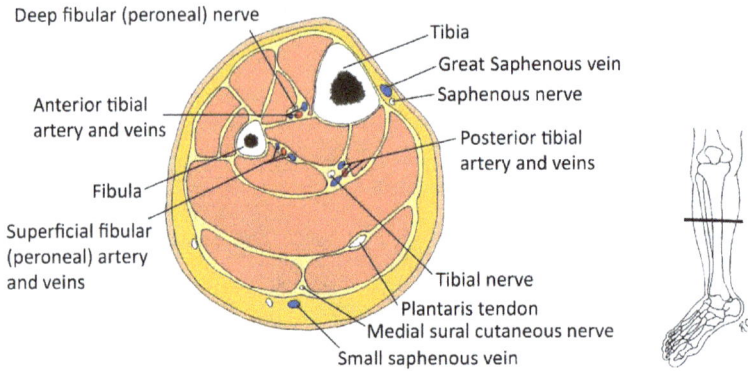

Deep fibular (peroneal) nerve

Tibia

Great Saphenous vein

Saphenous nerve

Anterior tibial
artery and veins

Posterior tibial
artery and veins

Fibula

Superficial fibular
(peroneal) artery
and veins

Tibial nerve

Plantaris tendon

Medial sural cutaneous nerve

Small saphenous vein

Figure 3.   Cross-section of the leg, at the level of the below knee amputation

6. The extensor muscles are stripped off the lateral surface of the tibia using a periosteal elevator. The extensor muscles and vessels are also stripped off the interosseous membrane.

7. The periosteal elevator is then inserted from the tibial border to the fibula, lifting off the extensor muscles (Fig. 5a). A scalpel is then used to cut the muscles layer by layer. Cutting diathermy should not be used. Any vessels encountered are clamped, divided and ligated.

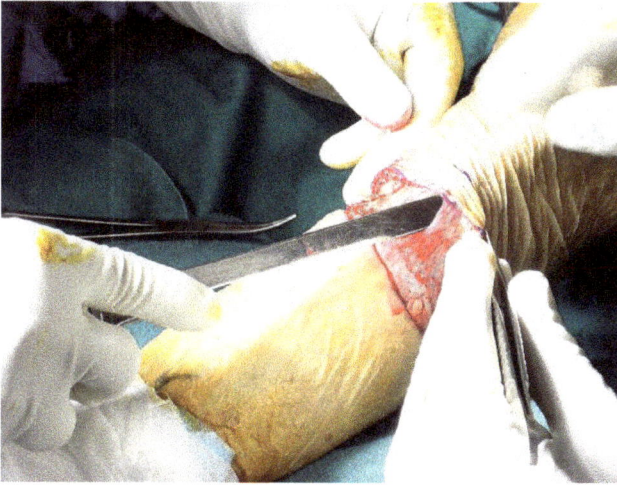

Figure 4. Use of periosteal elevator on medial aspect of tibia

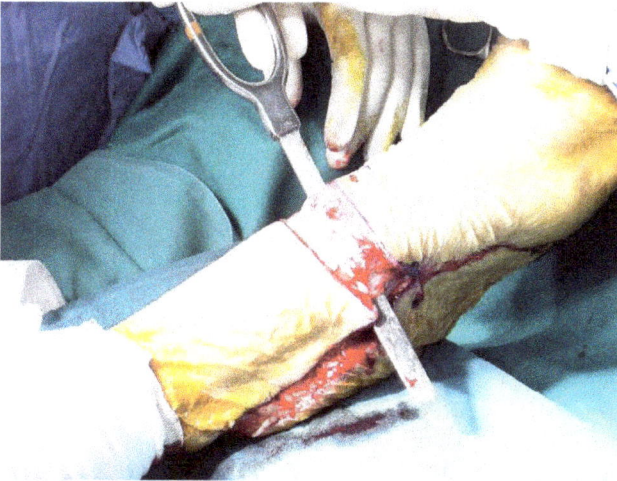

Figure 5a. Periosteal elevator lifting extensor muscles

8. The anterior tibial vessels (Fig. 3) are clamped, divided and double ligated using 2 strands of 0-silk sutures (Fig. 5b).

9. The peroneal muscles are stripped from the periosteal surface of the fibula and cut layer by layer with a scalpel. The peroneal vessels are also clamped, divided and ligated using 0-silk sutures.

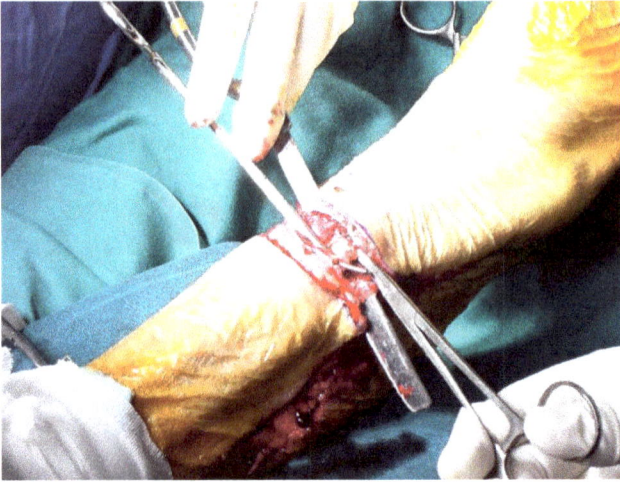

Figure 5b.   Clamping the anterior tibial artery

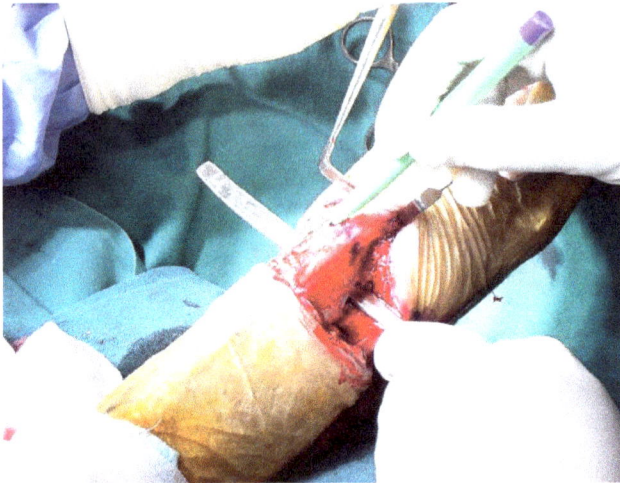

Figure 6a.   Marking level of tibial osteotomy

10. The level of the tibial bone osteotomy (one hand's breadth below the tibial tuberosity) is marked using a marker pen (Fig. 6a).
11. An oscillating saw is then used to cut the tibia (Fig. 3) at this level (Fig. 6b).

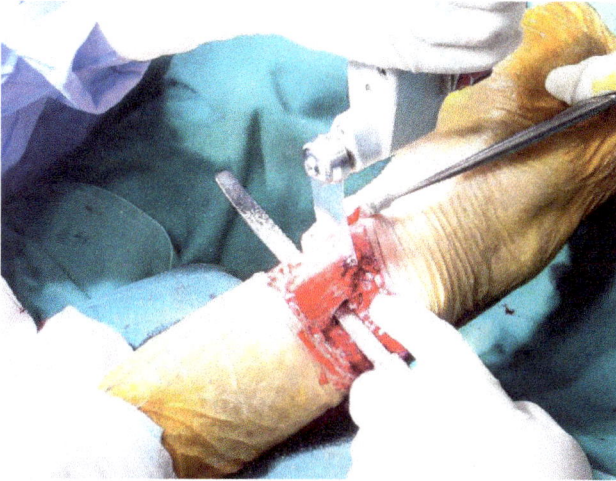

Figure 6b. Oscillating saw to cut tibia

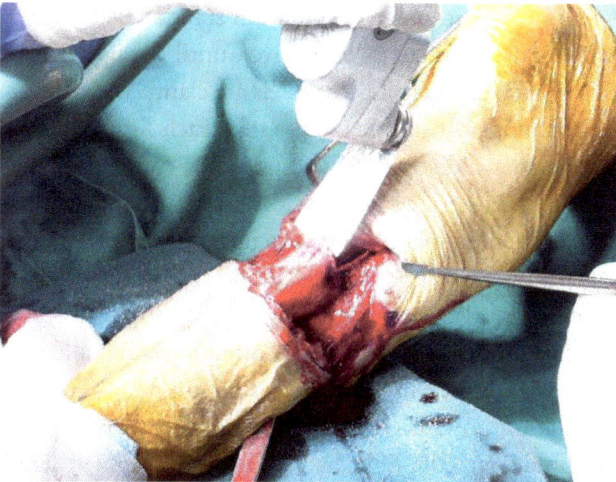

Figure 7. Anterior bevelling of tibia

12. The anterior end of the tibial stump is then bevelled (Fig. 7) with the anterior tibial edge cut at an angle of 30 degrees. A bone file is then used to smoothen all the bone edges and surface.

13. The fibula (Fig. 3) is then exposed using a periosteal elevator. A bone cutter is then inserted and the fibula is cut at least 1 cm proximal to the tibial cut (Fig. 8).

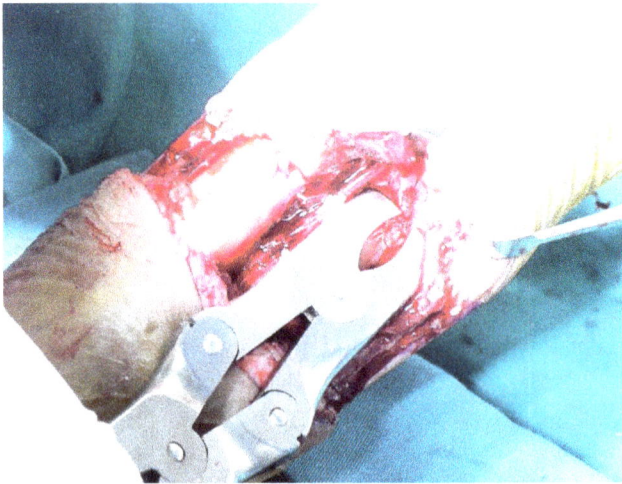

Figure 8. Use of bone cutter to cut fibula

14. The leg is then placed on an amputation stand. The posterior compartment muscles are then cut layer by layer, until the posterior tibial artery and veins (Fig. 3) are seen. These vessels are clamped, divided and doubly ligated. 2 strands of 0-silk tie are used for each ligature. Sutures are cut slightly long to avoid slippage. The posterior compartment muscles are cut close to the posterior surface of the tibia and fibula. A bone hook is used to pull the proximal tibial stump upwards (Fig. 9) and Langenback retractors are used to retract the distal tibia and fibula downwards.

15. The posterior tibial nerve (Fig. 3), which lies adjacent to the posterior tibial artery and veins, is pulled, transected flush and allowed to retract. This is essential to prevent neuroma formation.

16. The amputation knife is then placed behind the distal portions of the tibia and fibula with the right hand (Fig. 10a). The left hand holds the long posterior flap in the palm. The muscles are then cut with one swift stroke of the amputation knife to exit at the posterior flap incision.

17. The amputated leg is then passed to the circulating nurse for disposal (biohazard waste) or for return to the patient for burial (if requested, and for Muslims).

18. The below knee stump is then repositioned on the amputation stand. Haemostasis is secured (Fig. 10b), and any bleeding vessels are clamped, divided and ligated using 0-silk ties.

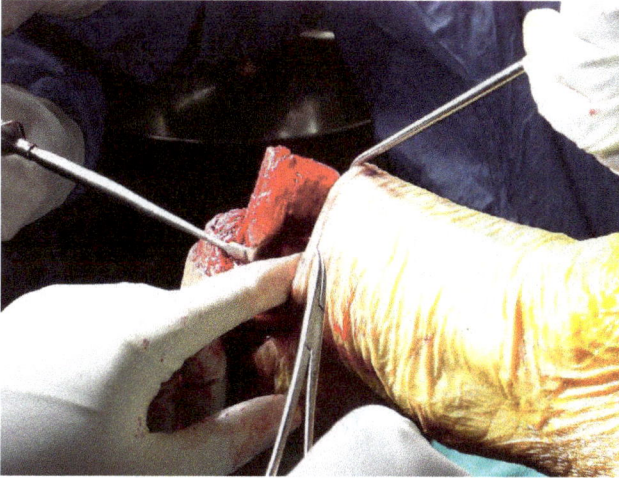

Figure 9. Use of bone hook to retract tibia

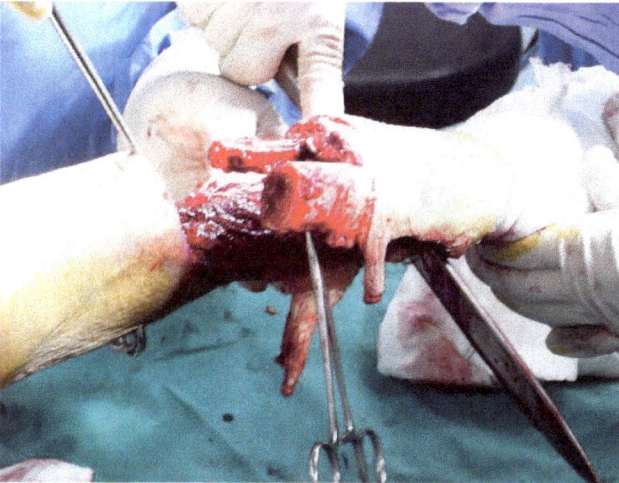

Figure 10a. Use of amputation knife

19. Two litres jet lavage is then used to irrigate the wound (Fig. 11). Normal saline is used for the lavage.
20. A drain is then placed, exiting at the lateral side of the wound (Fig. 12), as the long saphenous vein lies on the medial side. The drain is anchored

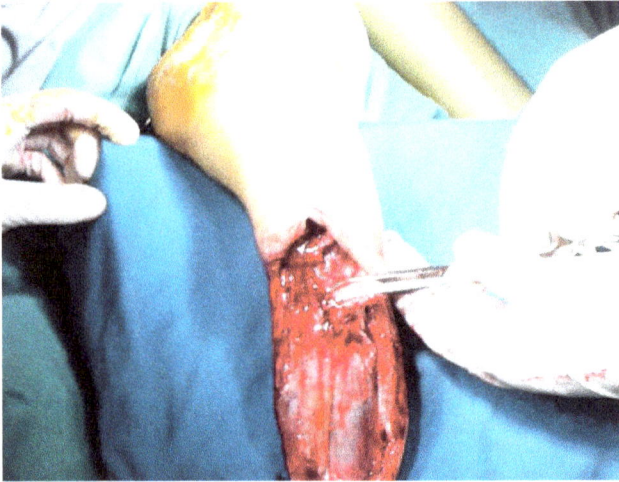

Figure 10b. Securing haemostasis in posterior flap

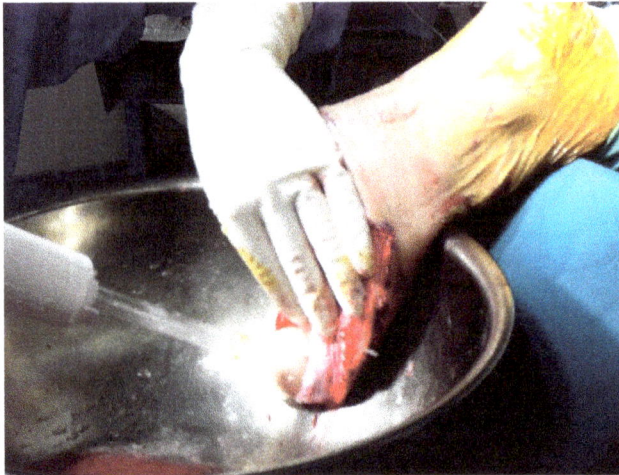

Figure 11. Jet lavage

with a 2-0 silk suture. In the posterior flap, the sural nerve is pulled, cut flush and allowed to retract.

21. The middle of the deep fascia posteriorly is opposed to the periosteum of the anterior tibial crest using 1-0 vicryl stitch — the centering stitch (Fig. 13). On either side of this centering stitch, the deep fascia is apposed

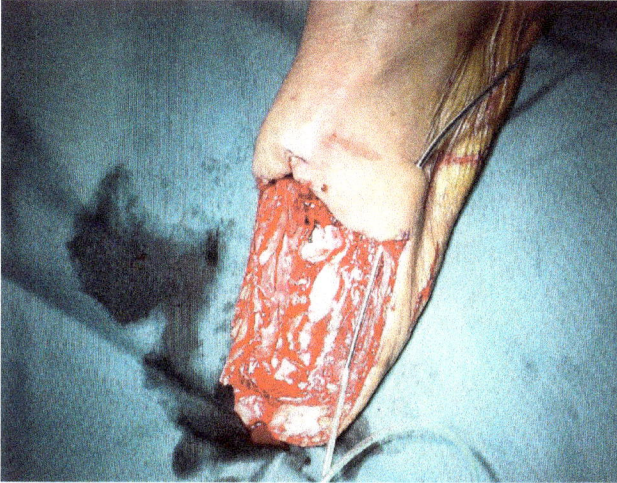

Figure 12. Exiting drain laterally

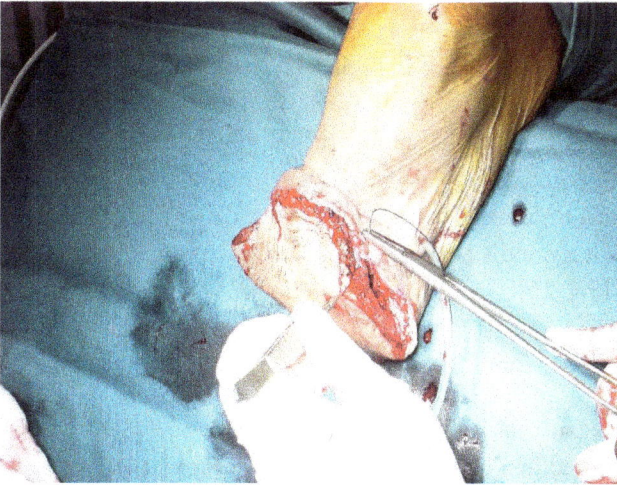

Figure 13. Centering stitch

to each other using 3–4 interrupted sutures. No tooth forceps should be used to handle the tissues.

22. The skin is tagged using 3-0 prolene vertical mattress sutures, starting with a centering skin stitch. 3–4 interrupted vertical mattress sutures are

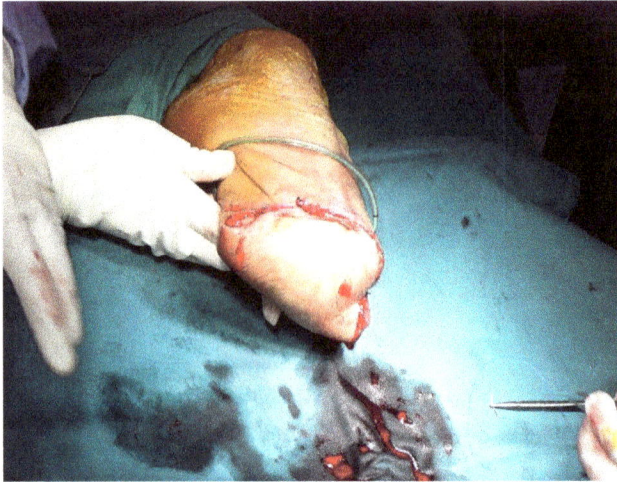

Figure 14. Closure of fascial layer

placed on either side of the centering stitch (Fig. 14). These sutures are placed far apart and care is taken to ensure that they are not too tight to prevent strangulation of the skin.

23. Tulle Gras (TG) dressing, followed by primapore is applied to the wound. Gauze and cotton wool pad is then applied. The dressing is completed with a six inch crepe bandage wrapped around the stump in a figure-of-8 fashion. The dressing must extend above the knee. Care is taken to ensure the drain is not dislodged. A stockinette is then applied and drain secured again. (Fig. 15)

Post-operative care and monitoring

1. High-risk patients with co-existing medical problems such as IHD should be monitored in a high-dependency ward or intensive care unit.
2. Hourly parameters for 24 hours — blood pressure, heart rate, respiratory rate, arterial oxygen saturation (SaO_2).
3. The drain must be monitored and if drain volumes exceed 300 ml per day in the first post-operative day, the drain should be clamped. The consultant should be called to review the patient regarding the need for re-exploration of the amputation stump for haemostasis. The drain is removed on the third post-operative day, provided the drainage is less than 50 ml.

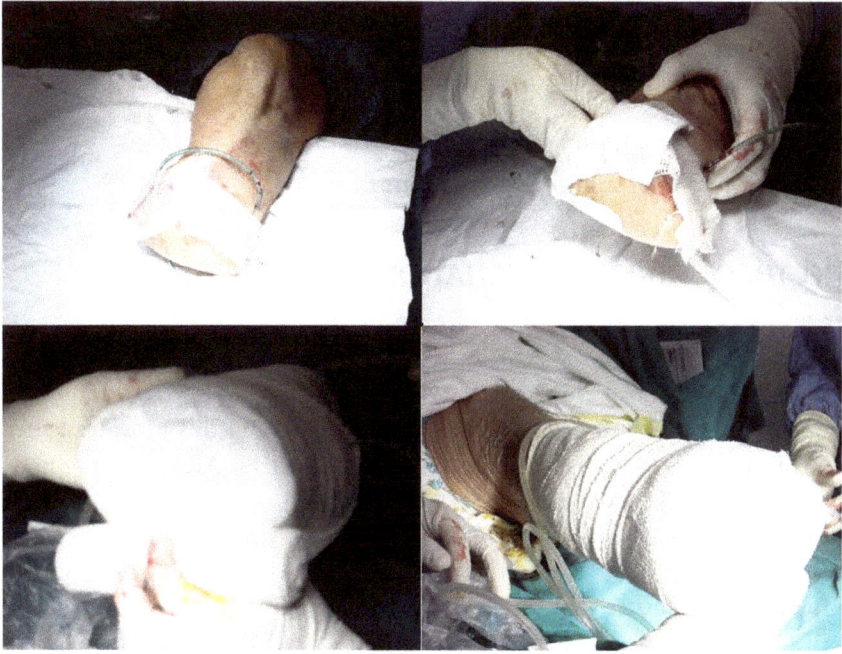

Figure 15.   Application of TG dressing, gauze, cotton wool padding and crepe bandage

4. An above knee thermoplastic splint is applied the day after operation to protect the stump and to prevent flexion contracture of the knee.

5. Post-operative haemoglobin is checked on first post-operative day. If the haemoglobin is less than 10 g/dL, blood transfusion(s) must be performed.

6. The wound is inspected on third post-operative day, where the dressings are lightened and the drain is removed. The next wound inspection is done on the seventh post-operative day.

7. Intravenous antibiotics are continued until the wound has healed.

Complications

1. Early

   a. Reactive haemorrhage
   b. Haematoma of BKA stump
   c. Wound dehiscence

d. Necrosis of flaps — requires revision of BKA

e. Infection of BKA stump — requires revision of BKA

2. Late

a. Phantom limb pain

b. Ulceration of stump post prosthetic fitting

THE THROUGH-KNEE AMPUTATION (TKA)

Indications

1. TKA is performed in a patient with a previous AKA performed in the other limb. A TKA gives a longer stump length and this provides better balance than another AKA. A patient with bilateral AKA has very poor body balance.
2. A failed below knee amputation

Operative procedure

1. Skin flaps (shorter anterior and longer posterior flap) are marked as shown (Figs. 16a and 16b).
2. Skin flaps are cut down to level of deep fascia (Fig. 16c).

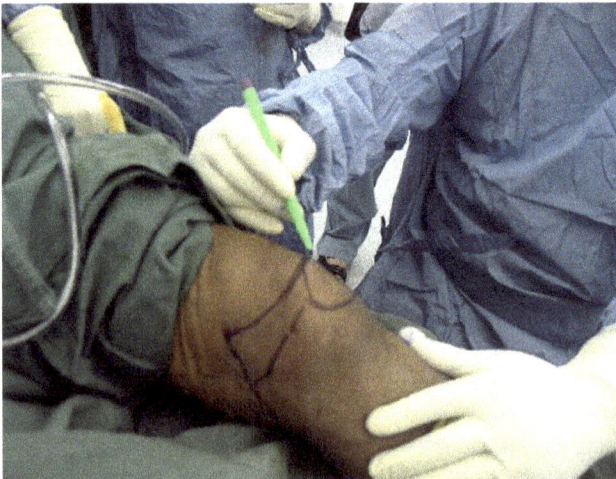

Figure 16a. Skin flaps (lateral view)

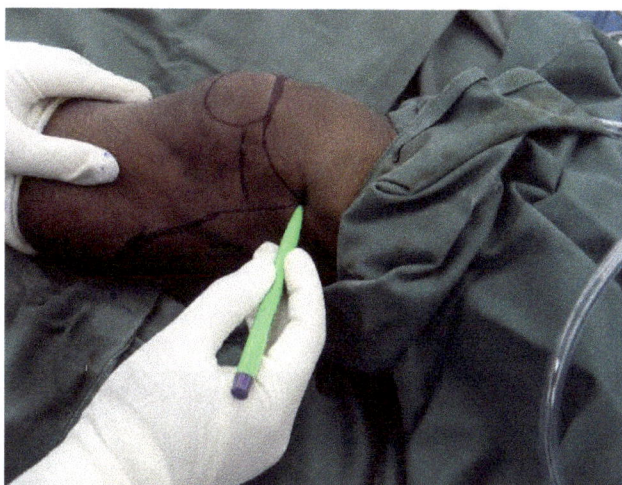

Figure 16b. Skin flaps (medial view)

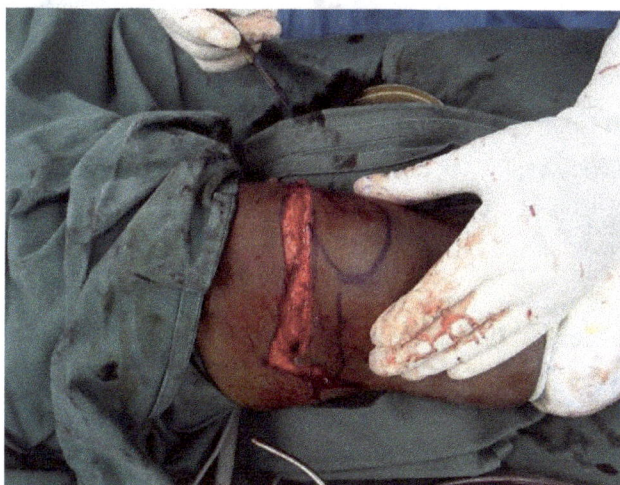

Figure 16c. Dissection to deep fascia

3. A kidney dish with a steridrape is placed under the leg. The pressure of the leg against the dish provides tamponade effect and prevents oozing from the posterior flap.
4. Anterior dissection — the rectus femoris and lateral patellar retinaculum (Fig. 17) are cut (Fig. 18a) at the upper border of patella (Fig. 17).

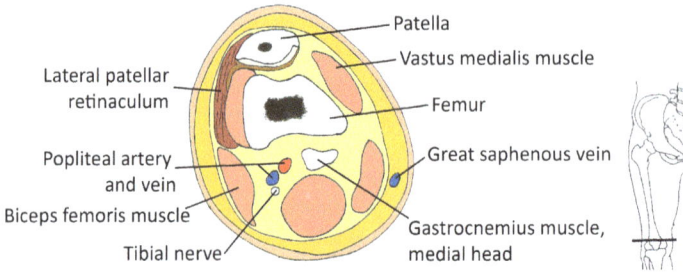

Figure 17. Cross section of the knee through the patella and distal end of the femur

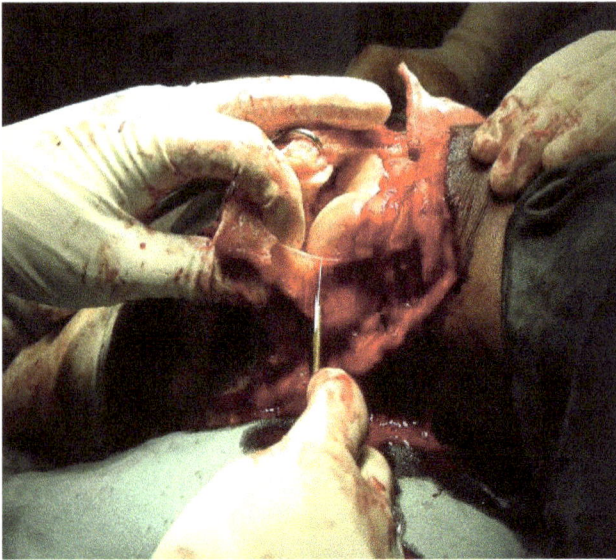

Figure 18a. Dividing the lateral retinaculum

The lateral collateral ligament is cut (Fig. 18b). The patella is reflected upwards (Fig. 18c) and excised together with the ligamentum patellae, which is divided from its attachment on the tibial tuberosity. The anterior and posterior cruciate ligaments are divided (Fig. 18d). The medial collateral (Fig. 18e) ligament is cut. The posterior capsule is dissected carefully (Fig. 18f). The popliteal vessels (Fig. 17) are identified, clamped, divided and double ligated using 2 strands of 0-silk sutures (Fig. 19). Note that the popliteal artery and vein are very close to the posterior surface of the femur and tibia (Fig. 17).

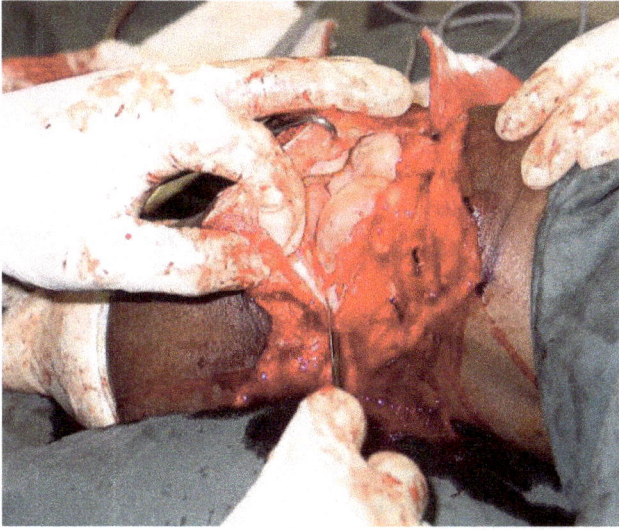

Figure 18b. Cutting the lateral collateral ligament

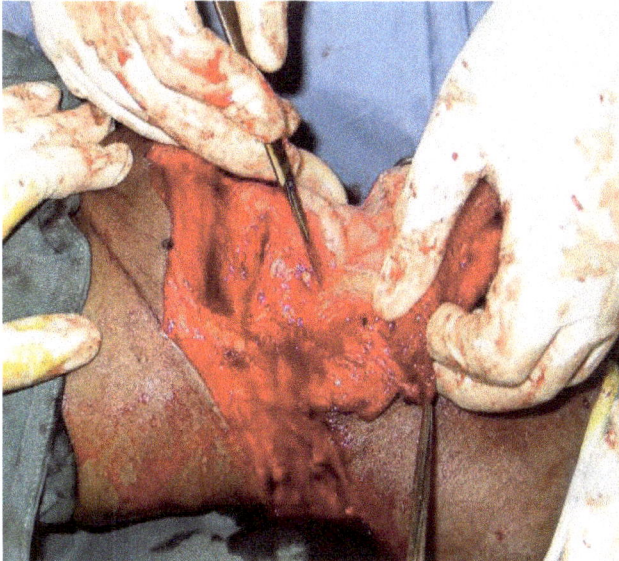

Figure 18c. Patella reflected upwards

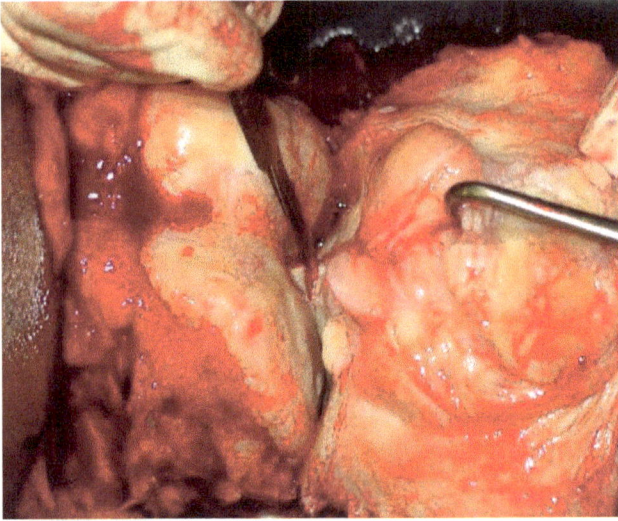

Figure 18d.　Dividing the cruciate ligaments

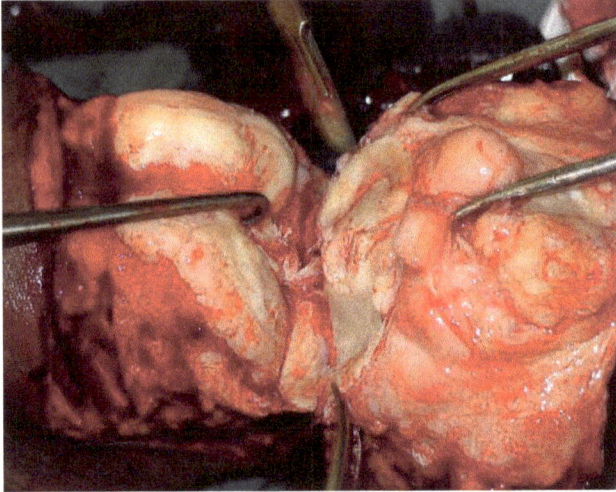

Figure 18e.　Cutting the medial collateral ligament

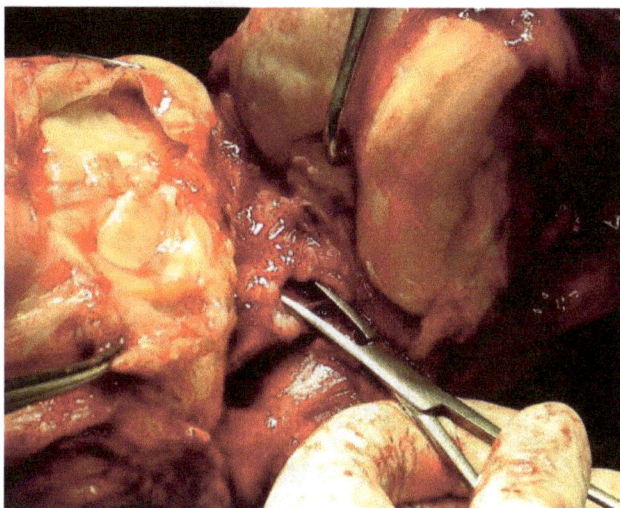

Figure 18f. Dissection of posterior capsule

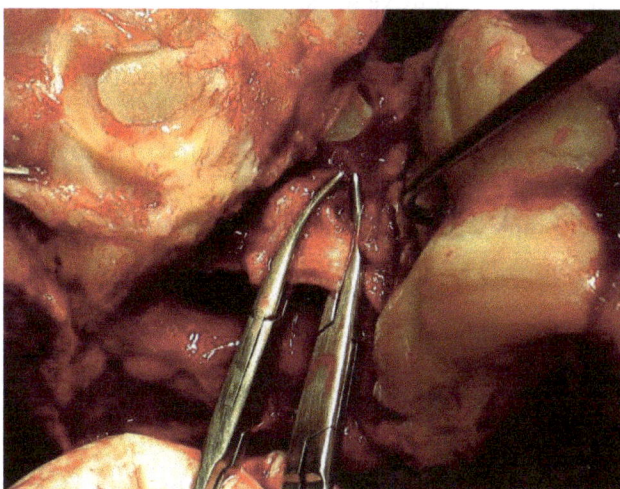

Figure 19. Clamping the popliteal artery

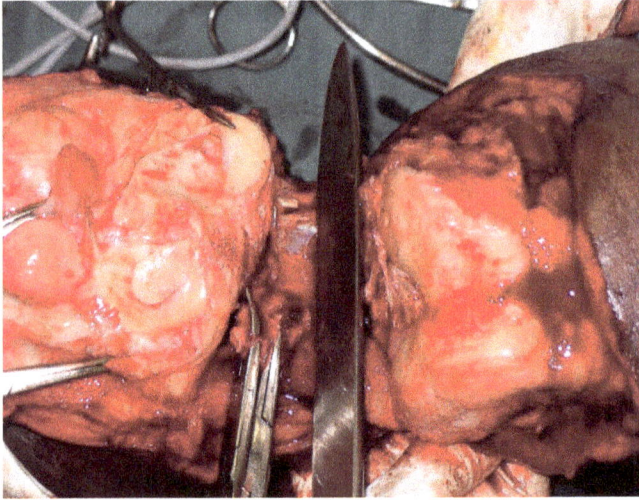

Figure 20. Use of an amputation knife as illustrated

5. An amputation knife is then used with the left hand holding the posterior flap and the knife in the right hand (Fig. 20), to cut the posterior muscles, layer by layer. Any bleeding vessels are ligated.
6. An oscillating saw is then used to cut the femur (Fig. 21) just above the level of the condyles. All four surfaces (anterior, posterior, medial and lateral) are bevelled smooth.
7. Haemostasis is secured and jet lavage with 2 litres of normal saline is used to wash the wound.
8. The centre of the deep fascia of the posterior flap is stitched to the centre of the deep fascia of the anterior flap using a vertical mattress suture using 1-0 vicryl.
9. The flaps were then closed in the same fashion as described for a BKA — using a drain exiting laterally, a centering stitch and closure in 2 layers with 1-0 vicryl sutures for the deep fascia and 3-0 prolene sutures for the skin.

Post-operative care and monitoring

Post-operative care is similar to that of the below knee amputee, as described above.

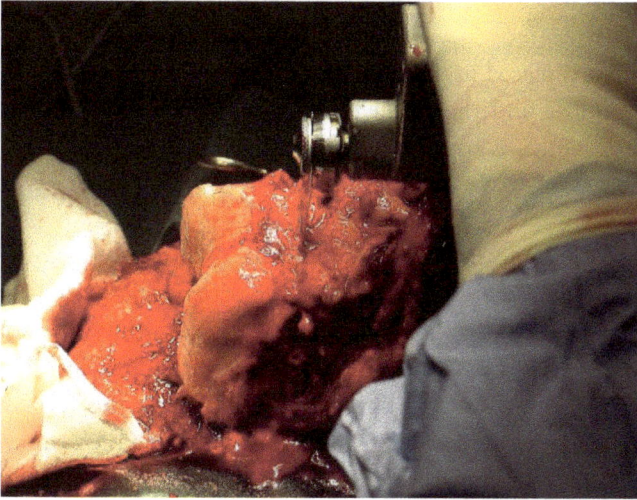

Figure 21. Use of an oscillating saw for femoral osteotomy

THE ABOVE KNEE AMPUTATION (AKA)

An above knee amputation gives a higher probability of wound healing because there is better vascularity of the muscles at this level of amputation. However, an AKA requires a higher level of energy expenditure for ambulation compared to a BKA prosthesis.

Indications

1. Infection of the foot extending into the middle of the leg — Unable to preserve minimal stump length of 7 cm below tibial tuberosity by BKA.
2. Ischaemia extending to the middle of the leg.
3. Flexion contracture of the knee in a patient with diabetic foot problem — with poor prognosis for ambulation.
4. Failed below knee amputation.

Anaesthesia

- Use general or spinal anaesthesia.
- Continue intravenous antibiotics started in the ward.

Patient positioning

- The patient is placed in the supine position.
- Place a sandbag underneath the buttock on the side of the amputation.
- A high tourniquet is applied but not pumped up.

Operative Procedure

The level of the bone transection should be as distal as possible. A longer stump will provide maximum balance to the patient. However, it should not be too distal. It should be above the supracondylar region of the femur. In the condylar region, the femur is surrounded by tendons and the region is relatively avascular. Wound healing would be poor at this level, above the patellar, the femur is surrounded by muscles. At this level, it is more vascular. Wound healing would be good.

1. Marking the skin flaps (Figs. 22a and 22b) — A fish mouth incision is fashioned distal to the level of bone transection. The anterior and posterior flaps are of equal length.
2. The level of bone cut is marked on the skin.
3. The skin flaps are then cut down to level of deep fascia (Fig. 22c) anteriorly and posteriorly.

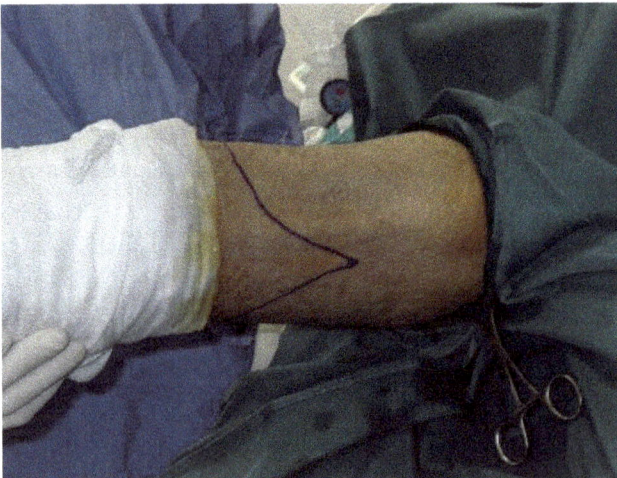

Figure 22a.   Medial skin flap marking

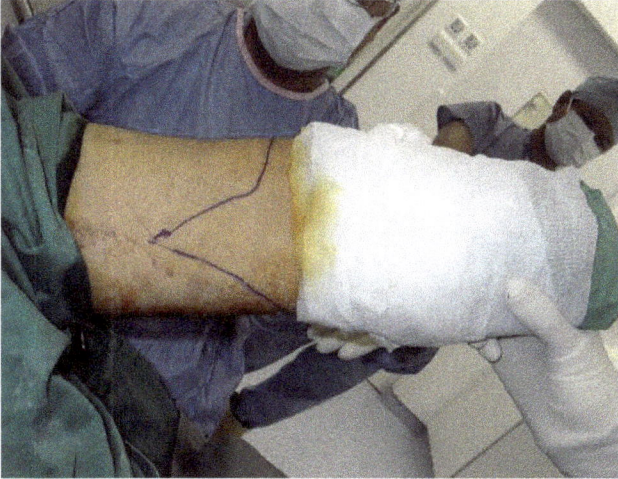

Figure 22b. Lateral skin flap marking

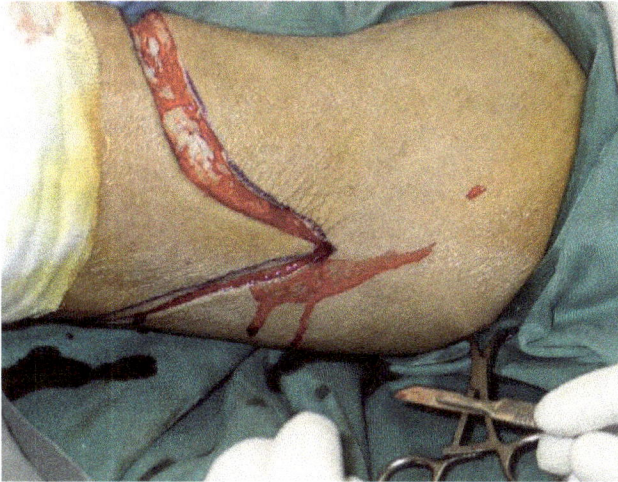

Figure 22c. Dissection to deep fascia

4. The leg is placed on a kidney dish covered by a steridrape. The pressure of the thigh against the dish prevents venous bleeding from the posterior flap (tamponade effect) (Fig. 23).

5. Anterior dissection — Medially, the great saphenous vein (Fig. 24) is clamped and ligated. A periosteal elevator is placed as shown (Fig. 25).

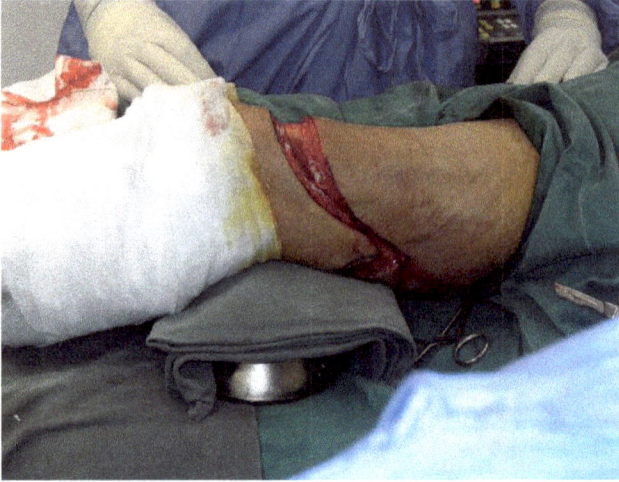

Figure 23.   Use of kidney dish for tamponade effect

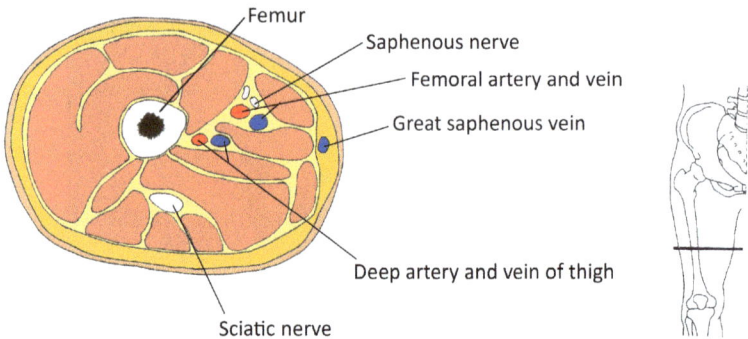

Figure 24.   Cross section of the thigh at the level of the amputation

Flexor muscles of the thigh and extensors of the knee are then cut with a
scalpel, layer by layer. Any vessels encountered are clamped with an artery
forceps, divided and ligated.

6. The femoral artery and vein (Fig. 24) are clamped (Fig. 26) and doubly
ligated with 2 strands of 0-silk tie. The profunda femoris artery and its
accompanying venae commitantes are also doubly clamped and ligated.
7. Muscle dissection is then continued anteriorly until the periosteal surface
of the femur (Fig. 24) is reached.

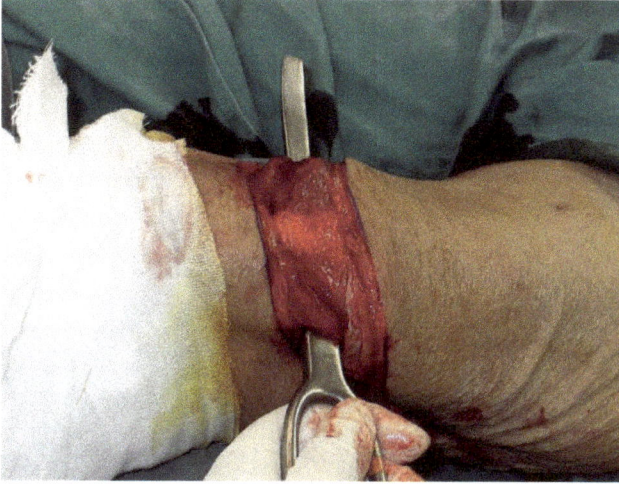

Figure 25. Periosteal elevator beneath quadriceps muscle

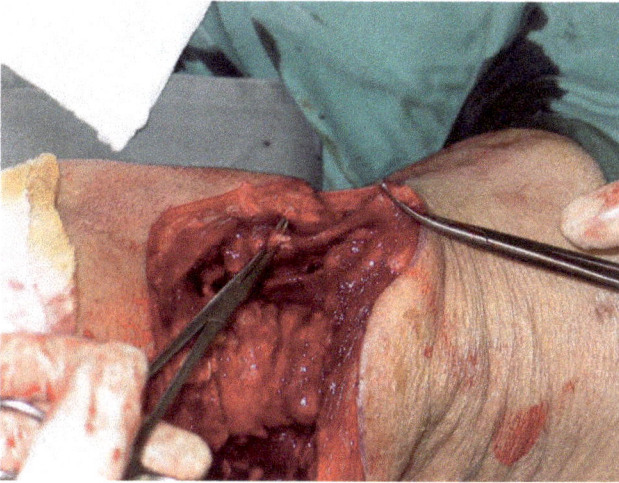

Figure 26. Clamping the femoral artery

8. The level of bone cut is then marked with a marker pen (Fig. 27a).
9. Using an oscillating saw, the femur is cut (Fig. 27b).
10. The sciatic nerve (Fig. 24) is identified, pulled and transected as high as possible, and allowed to retract. This is essential to prevent neuroma

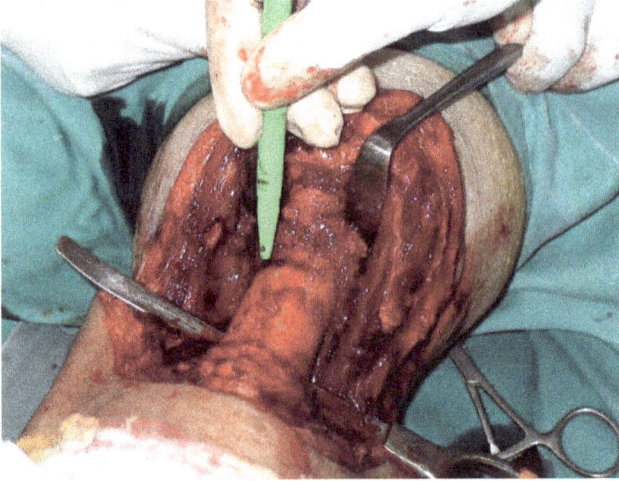

Figure 27a. Marking level of femoral osteotomy

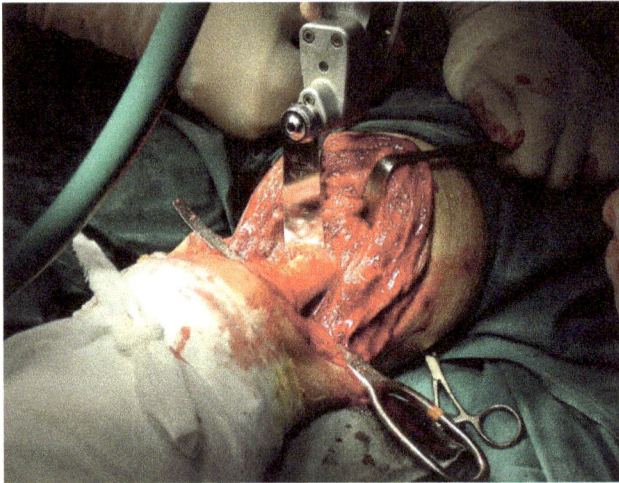

Figure 27b. Use of oscillating saw

formation. The short saphenous vein is clamped and ligated (in the posterior flap).

11. Using an amputation knife with the right hand and placing the posterior flap on the palm of the left hand, the posterior compartment muscles are then cut with one swift stroke of the amputation knife (Fig. 28).

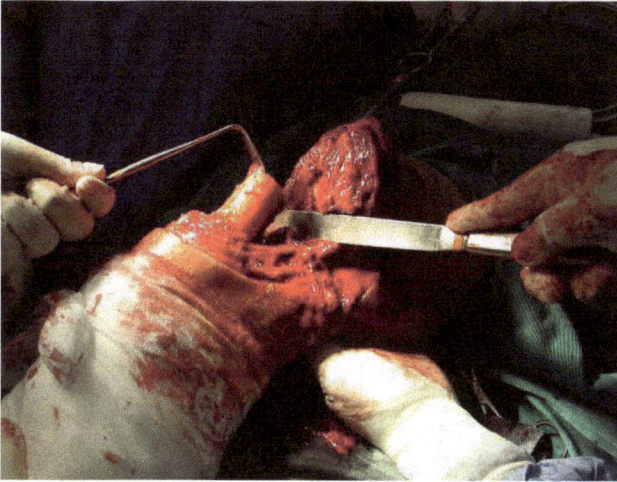

Figure 28. Use of amputation knife

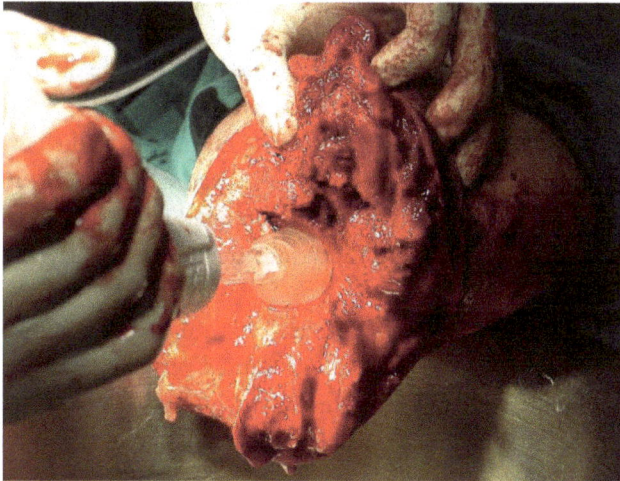

Figure 29. Jet lavage

12. The stump is then placed on the amputation stand. Haemostasis is secured, and any bleeding vessels are clamped and secured with ligatures.
13. Two litres of normal saline is the used to flush the wound using jet lavage (Fig. 29).

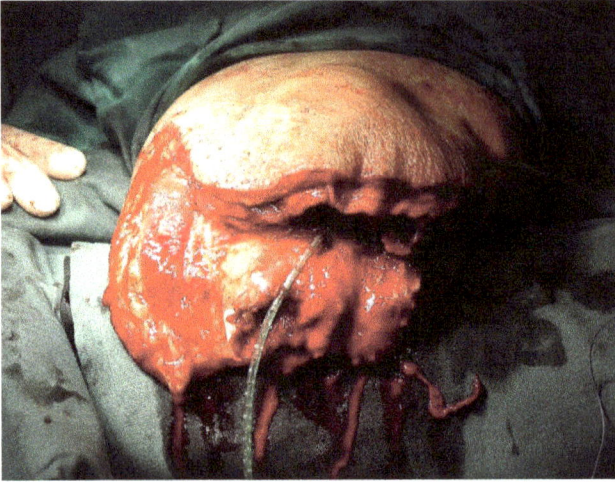

Figure 30.   Placement of drain

14. A drain is then placed, exiting at the lateral side of the wound (Fig. 30), as the great saphenous vein lies on the medial side. The drain is anchored with a silk suture (2-0 silk) to prevent slippage.

15. The middle of the deep fascia posteriorly is opposed to the periosteum of the femur using 1-0 vicryl stitch — the centering stitch. On either side of this centering stitch, the deep fascia is apposed to each other using about 3–4 interrupted sutures. No tooth forceps should be used to handle the tissues.

16. The skin is tagged using 3-0 prolene vertical mattress sutures, starting with a centering skin stitch. 3-4 interrupted vertical mattress sutures are placed on either side of the centering stitch. These sutures are placed far apart and care is taken to ensure that they are not too tight to prevent strangulation of the skin.

17. Tulle Gras dressing, followed by primapore is applied to the wound. Gauze and cotton wool padding is then applied and the dressing is completed with a six-inch crepe bandage wrapped around the stump in a figure-of-8 fashion. Care is taken to ensure the drain is not dislodged. A stockinette is then applied and the drain is secured again.

Post-operative care and monitoring

These are similar to the instructions for a patient who has undergone a below knee amputation.

References

1. E. M. Burgess, Interclinic information bulletin, *New York University Medical School* 8(4) (1969).
2. K. P. Robinson, Skew-flap below knee amputation, *Ann. R. Coll. Surg. Engl.* 73(3):155–7 (1991).

23

Minor Amputations

*Aziz Nather, Gurpal Singh, Teo Zhen Ling
and Francis Wong Keng Lin*

*Department of Orthopaedic Surgery
Yong Loo Lin School of Medicine
National University of Singapore*

In this chapter, the following operative procedures are described:

- Ray Amputation
- Transmetatarsal Amputation
- Syme's Amputation
- Modified Pirogoff Amputation

Introduction

A Below Knee Amputation is considered as a failure of limb salvage. The most proximal amputation that can achieve limb salvage is a Syme's or Pirogoff amputation. Other distal amputations with successful limb salvage include Chopart's amputation, Lisfranc's amputation, transmetatarsal amputation and ray amputation. A Syme's is considered successful limb salvage as the patient can be fitted with special Syme's shoes. The stump is also end-weight bearing.

Amputations through the ankle — Syme's,[1] Boyd's[2,3] or Pirogoff[4–8] are not commonly performed in surgery of the diabetic foot as they often lead to poor results. Selection of cases for these amputations must thus be performed carefully. The Ray amputation is the most common amputation performed for the diabetic foot. Toe disarticulation (through the metatarso-phalangeal joint) should not be performed in diabetics. It is well known to cause complications, leading to more proximal amputations such as Syme's or Below Knee Amputation.

Ray Amputation

Indications

- Wet or dry gangrene of toe
- Osteomyelitis of metatarsal head/proximal phalange
- Septic Arthritis of metatarso-phalangeal joint (MTPJ) of the toe.
- Gross infection of the toe
- Palpable dorsalis pedis and posterior tibial pulses. At least one distal foot pulse must be palpable.
- Ankle Brachial Index ≥ 0.8
- Toe Brachial Index ≥ 0.7

Pre-operative preparation

Ensure that these are in the normal range:

- Full Blood Count (FBC), Erythrocyte Sedimentation Rate (ESR), C-Reactive Protein (CRP)
- Urea and electrolytes
- HbA1C
- Chest X-ray (CXR), Electrocardiogram (ECG)
- Haemoglobin must be above 10 g/dL to provide sufficient oxygen for wound healing.
- Total proteins: Albumin level must be above 38 g/L by a high protein diet to provide sufficient nutrition for wound healing.
- Blood Thinners such as Plavix and Aspirin must be stopped at least 3 days before operation.
- Cardiac Assessment: It must be performed by a cardiologist for patients with a history of acute myocardial infarction (AMI) or ischaemic heart disease (IHD). This includes a 2-D Echocardiogram.
- **Risk of mortality** of the operation must be communicated to the patient based on his Ejection Fraction results:
  - 55–70%   Normal
  - 40–55%   Low Risk

- 35–39%   Moderate Risk
- <35%   High Risk

(1) **Risk of morbidity** of the operation must also be discussed. The chance of wound healing is based on the vascularity of the tissue at the level of amputation. This must be communicated to the patient.

- ≥70%   Good
- 51–69%   Fair
- ≤50%   Poor

(2) The Consultant must convene a patient conference. All potential anaesthetic risks and surgical complication risks must be explained in detail. The risk of a second operation (10–20%) must also be discussed. This involves amputation of adjacent toes or more proximal amputations — transmetatarsal, Chopart's or Syme's. The risk of more proximal amputation is higher in patients with concomitant renal failure.

Anaesthesia

- Use general or regional anaesthesia. The latter includes spinal or femoral nerve block in 'high risk' cases. Regional anaesthesia cannot be performed when a patient is on Plavix or Aspirin. These have to be removed 3 days prior to the operation.
- Continue intravenous antibiotics that were already started in the ward.

Patient positioning

- The patient is placed in the supine position.
- Place a sandbag below the buttock on the side of the amputation.
- A pneumatic tourniquet is applied on the thigh. Once the leg is cleaned, the tourniquet is inflated.

Operative technique

(1) The skin flaps are marked:

- Terminal Ray Amputation (first or fifth ray) —
  - For the big toe, the dorsal skin flap extends from the midline of the medial eminence (of first metatarsal) to the first web space. The plantar flap is marked, preserving as much plantar skin as possible.

This is to allow the larger plantar flap to be pulled up to cover the amputation wound after the amputation.

- For the fifth toe, the dorsal skin flap extends from the midline of the lateral eminence (of fifth metatarsal) to the 4th web space. The plantar flap is marked preserving as much plantar skin as possible. This is to allow the larger plantar flap to be pulled up to cover the amputation wound after the ray amputation.

- Non-terminal ray amputation (second, third or fourth ray) —

For the second toe (Fig. 1), an elliptical incision (Fig. 2) is marked from Point A (dorsum of the second metatarsal bone) passing downwards through the centre of the first web space to Point B (volar aspect of the second metatarsal bone). A similar elliptical incision is marked on the lateral side of the second ray from Point A to Point B passing through the centre of the second web space.

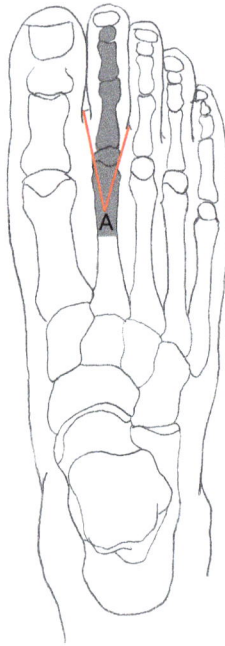

Figure 1.   Diagram showing the bones removed (shaded) in a second ray amputation

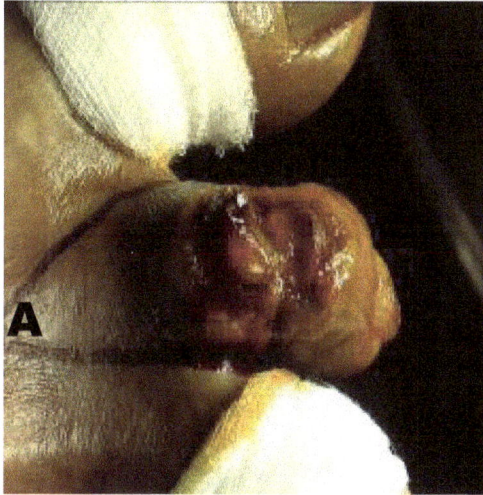

Figure 2. Dorsal view of the skin flaps

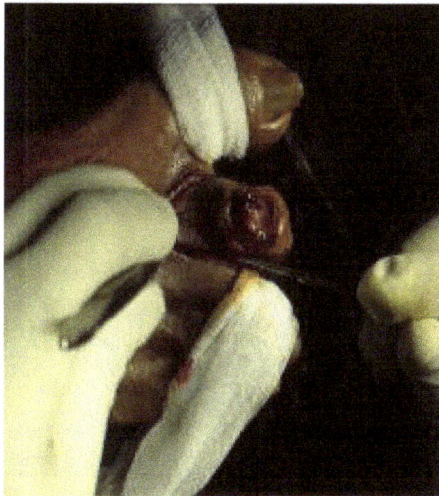

Figure 3. Cutting the skin flaps down to deep fascia

(2) Cut the medial and lateral flaps down to deep fascia (Fig. 3) to excise en-bloc the infected or gangrenous toe. This is essential to avoid contamination of the remaining healthy tissue.

(3) The second toe is disarticulated at the metatarso-phalangeal joint (Fig. 4). The toe is discarded (Fig. 5).

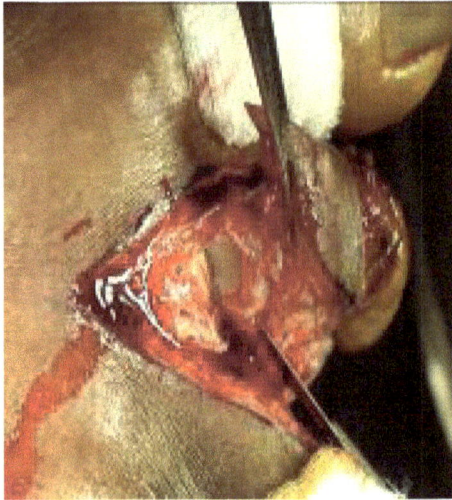

Figure 4. Disarticulation at the metatarsophalangeal joint

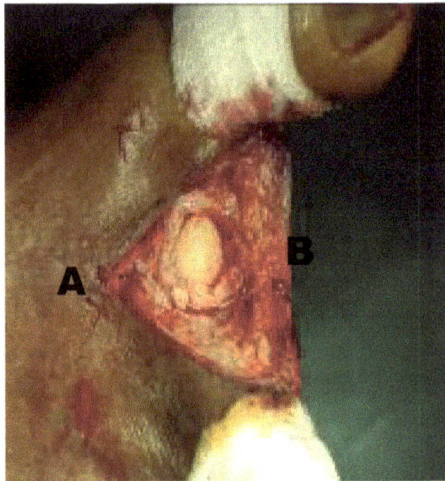

Figure 5. Infected toe has been discarded

(4) The distal part of the metatarsal is exposed. Small Hohmann retractors are used to expose the metatarsal on both the dorsal and volar side. A small oscillating saw or manual osteotome is used to osteotomise the metatarsal bone (Fig. 6). The distal metatarsal bone and its head are then resected (Figs. 7 and 8). A bone nibbler is then used to nibble the metatarsal bone

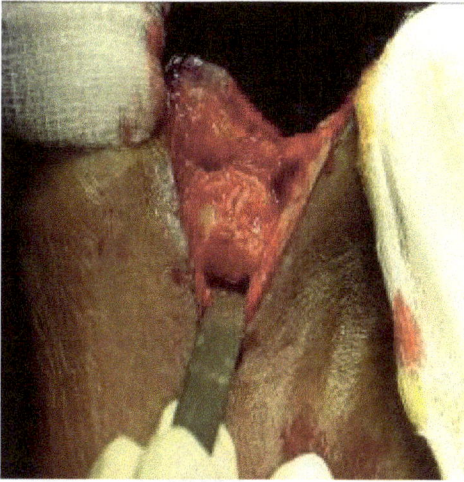

Figure 6. A manual osteotome is used to osteotomise the metatarsal head

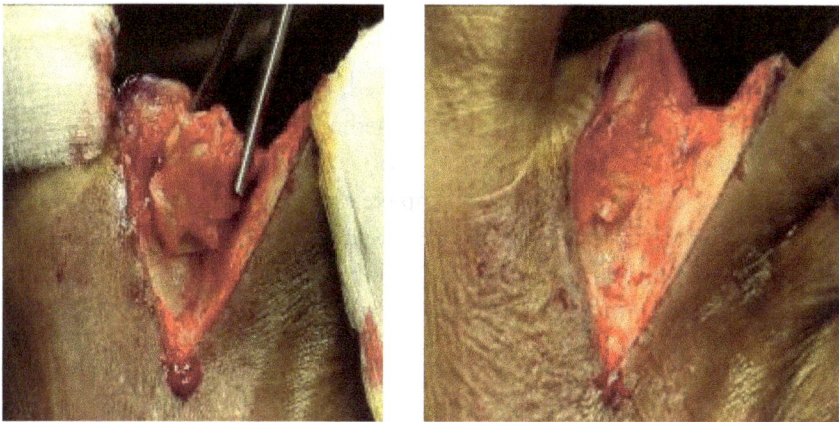

Figure 7 and 8. Resection of the terminal end of the second metatarsal bone

end, smoothening sharp edges. The edges of the wound must be healthy and show good capillary bleeding. If not, further debridement of the edge is needed.

(5) The wound is then flushed with hydrogen peroxide solution and normal saline.

(6) The tourniquet is released and hemostasis is secured.

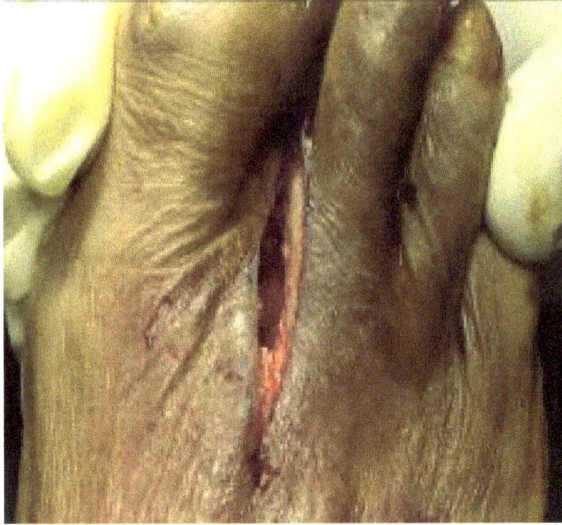

Figure 9. Closure of the wound

(7) If infected tissue is completely removed, primary closure is performed (Fig. 9). The skin edges are sutured together with interrupted 3-0 prolene vertical mattress sutures.

(8) If there is doubt regarding the complete excision of infection, the wound should be left open and dressed with Kaltostat and Tulle Gras dressing.

(9) Gauze and cotton wool is applied. Crepe bandage is then used to wrap and complete the dressing.

Post-operative care

- High-risk patients with co-existing medical problems such as ischaemic heart disease should be monitored in a high-dependency ward.
- For patients in ordinary wards, 4-hourly parameters — blood pressure, heart rate and respiratory rate, must be monitored for 24 hours.
- Post-operative haemoglobin is checked on post-operative day 1. If the haemoglobin is less than 10 g/dL, blood transfusion(s) must be performed.
- Wound inspection is carried out on post-operative day 3.
- Wound inspection is repeated on post-operative day 7.

- Stitches are removed on post-operative day 14.
- Diabetes Mellitus must be well controlled.
- Intravenous antibiotics are continued until the wound has healed.
- Offloading of the foot is required.

Transmetatarsal Amputation

Indications

- Wet or dry gangrene involving only the forefoot (Fig. 10)
- Infection involving only the forefoot
- Palpable dorsalis pedis and posterior tibial pulses. At least one distal foot pulse must be palpable.
- Ankle Brachial Index ≥ 0.8
- Toe Brachial Index ≥ 0.7

Pre-operative preparation

Follow the same preparation as for ray amputation.

Anaesthesia

Same as for ray amputation.

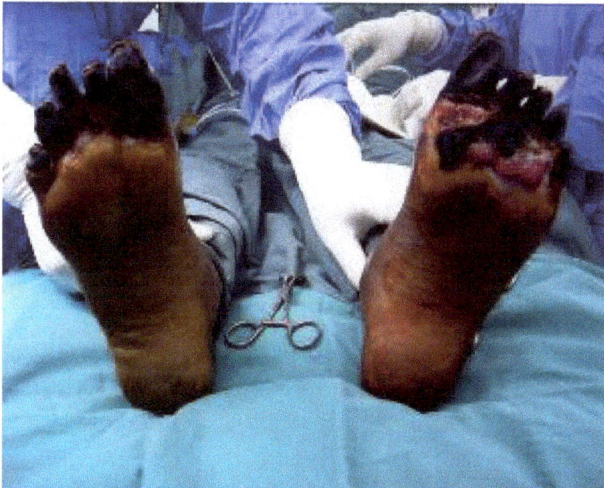

Figure 10.   Pre-operation photograph showing bilateral forefoot wet gangrene

Patient positioning

Same as for ray amputation.

Operative technique

(1) For a transmetatarsal amputation, skin flaps are marked giving a shorter dorsal and longer plantar flap (Figs. 11 to 14).

(2) The skin flaps are then cut down to deep fascia (Figs. 15 and 16).

(3) The saphenous vein is located between the first and second metatarsal, in the first dorsal webspace (Fig. 17). It is clamped, divided and ligated.

(4) The dorsalis pedis artery is identified. It lies on a deeper place in the same first dorsal webspace as the saphenous vein (Fig. 17). It is also clamped, divided and ligated.

(5) The extensor tendons (extensor hallucis longus, extensor digitorum longus and extensor digitorum brevis) are divided in the line of incision (Fig. 17).

(6) The flexor tendons are divided in the line of incision (Fig, 17).

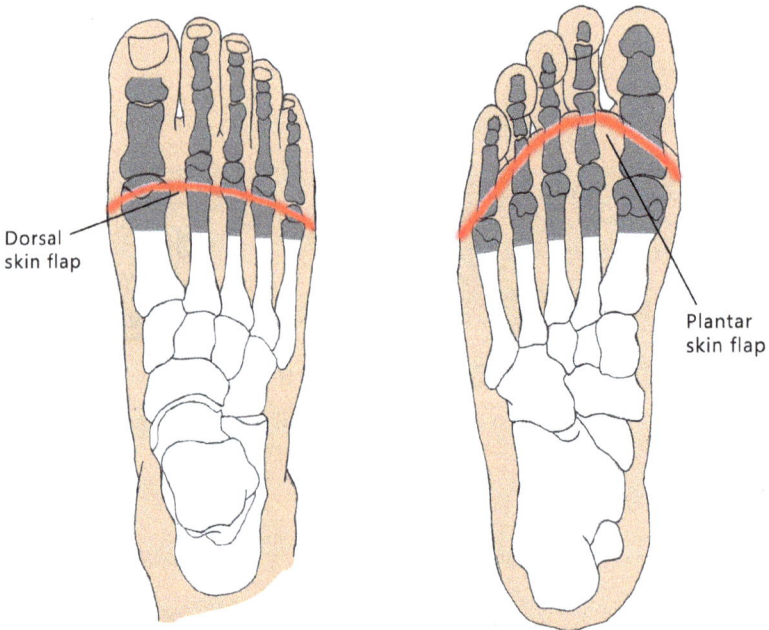

Dorsal skin flap

Plantar skin flap

Figures 11 and 12. Dorsal and plantar view of the foot showing the bones removed (shaded) and the dorsal and posterior skin flaps in a transmetatarsal amputation.

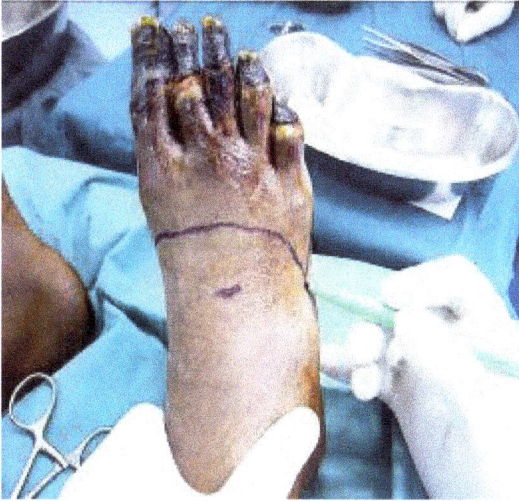

Figure 13. Marking the dorsal skin flap

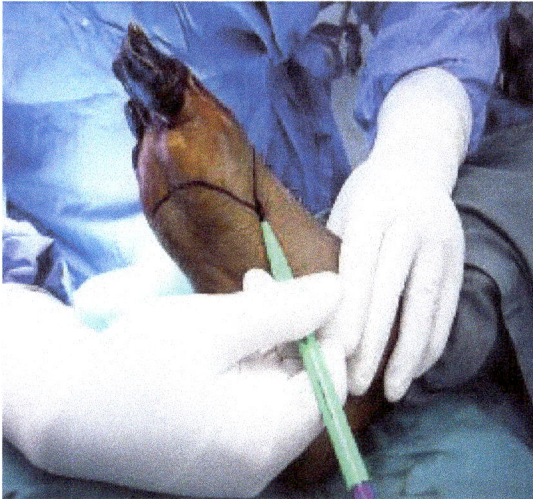

Figure 14. Marking the plantar skin flap

(7) A small oscillating saw is then used to cut through the middle of the metatarsal bones (Fig. 18). Care is taken to ensure that the saw does not damage the soft tissue of the posterior flap.

(8) The forefoot is removed and passed to the circulating nurse.

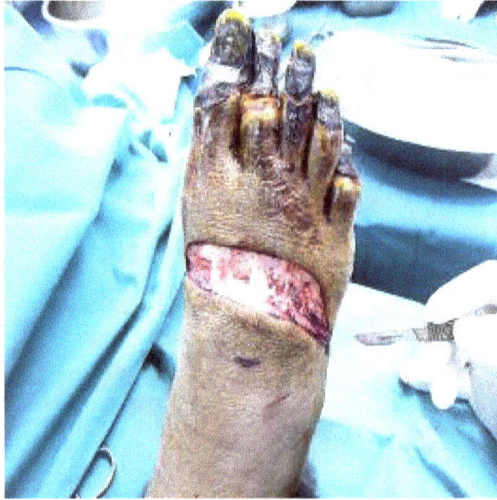

Figure 15. Dorsal skin flap is cut down deep fascia

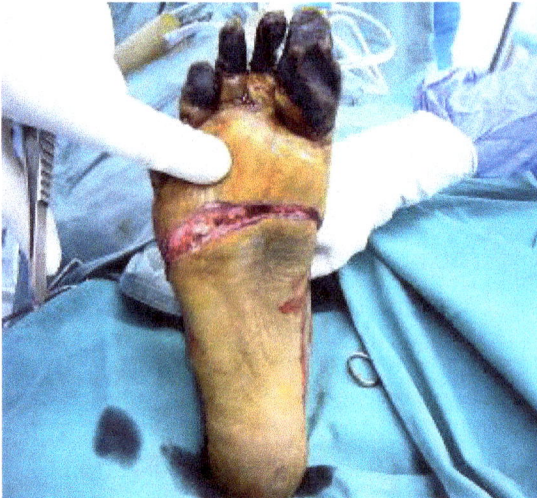

Figure 16. Plantar skin flap is cut down to deep fascia

(9) The flexor and extensor tendons are pulled, transected and allowed to retract (Fig. 19).

(10) The tourniquet is released and hemostasis is secured. The stump (Fig. 20) is flushed with normal saline using jet lavage.

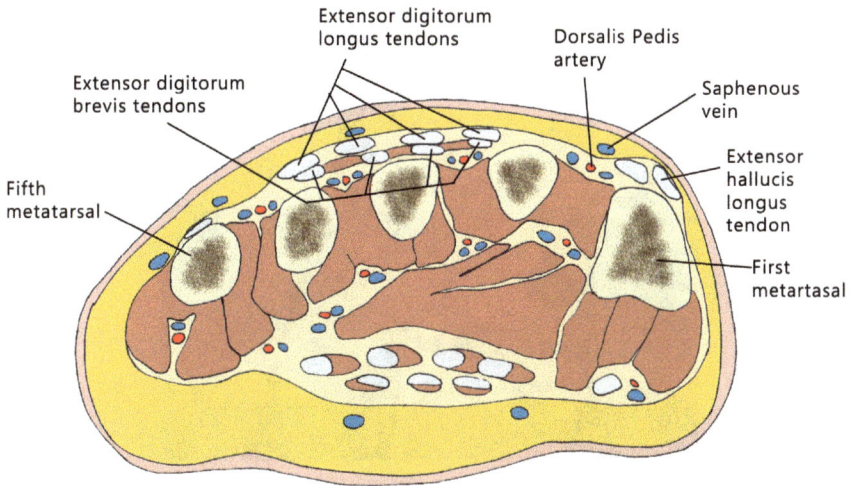

Figure 17. Crossection of the foot at the transmetatarsal level. It shows the structures encountered in a transmetatarsal amputation, including the dorsalis pedis artery and the saphenous vein

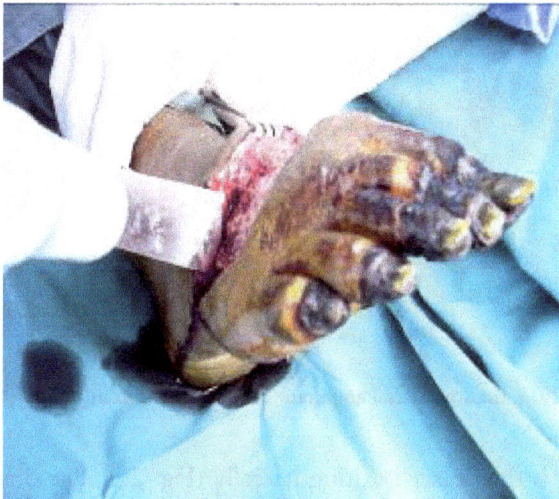

Figure 18. An oscillating saw is used to cut the metatarsal bones

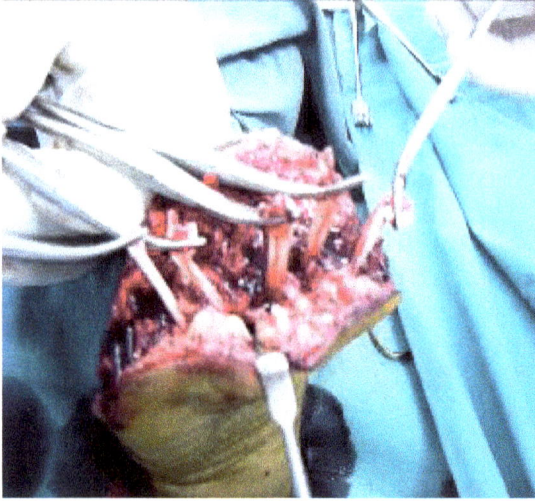

Figure 19. Pulling and division of flexor and extensor tendons

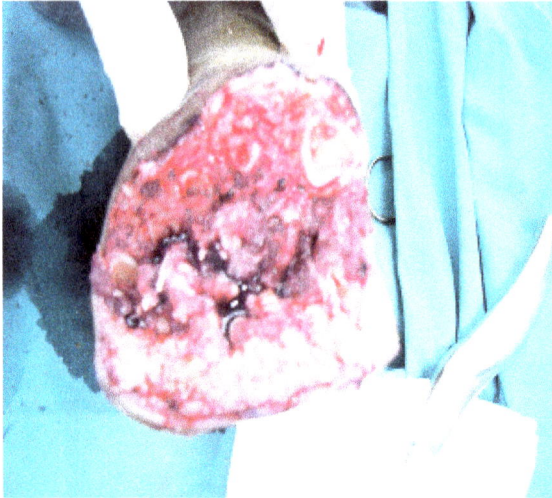

Figure 20. Transmetatarsal amputation stump after flushing with jet lavage

(11) A drain is then placed exiting laterally (Fig. 21). The drain is secured with a silk stitch.

(12) The deep fascia is then tagged together with absorbable vicryl 1 sutures. A centering stitch is placed to oppose the centre of the plantar flap to the

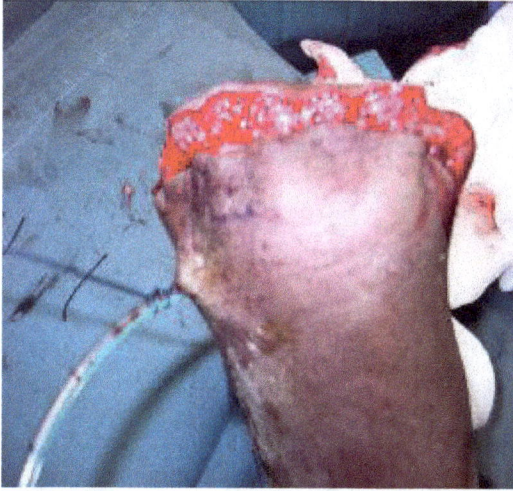

Figure 21. Stump with drain and absorbable vicryl 1 sutures

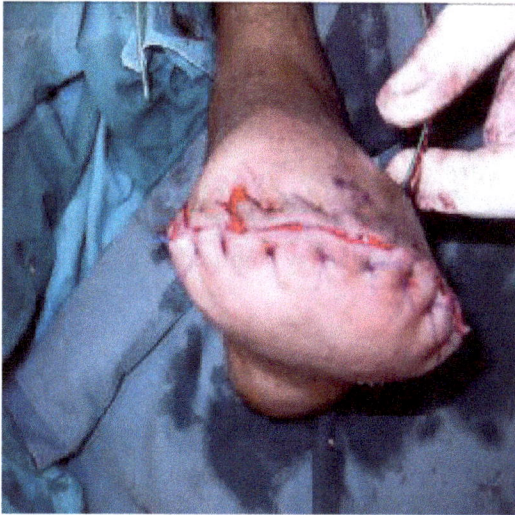

Figure 22. Wound closure using 3-0 prolene sutures

centre of the dorsal flap. Three to four interrupted more sutures are then placed on either side of the centering stitch (Fig. 21). The skin edges are then opposed with interrupted 3-0 prolene vertical mattress sutures (Fig. 22).

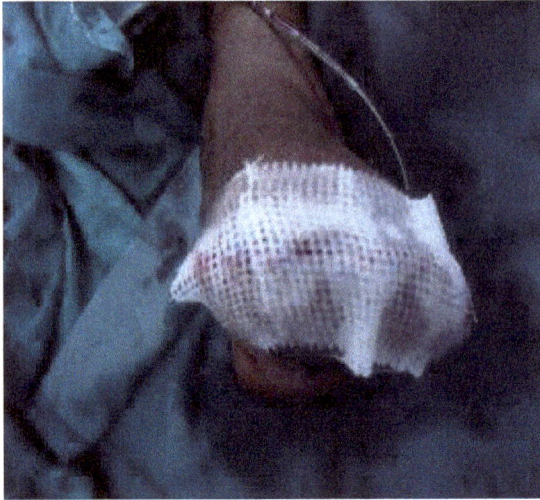

Figure 23. Application of tulle Gras dressing

(13) Tulle Gras dressing (Fig. 23), gauze and cotton wool are then applied. Crepe bandage is used to wrap and complete the dressing (Fig. 24). A stockinette is applied over the bandage.

Post-operative care

Post-operative care for a transmetatarsal amputation is the same as the post-operative care of a patient with a ray amputation.

Syme's Amputation

Indications

- Wet or dry gangrene of only the forefoot (Fig. 25)
- Infection of only the forefoot
- Palpable dorsalis pedis and posterior tibial pulses. The posterior tibial pulse must be strong and palpable.
- Ankle Brachial Index ≥0.8
- Toe Brachial Index ≥0.7

Pre-operative preparation

Follow the same preparation as for ray amputation.

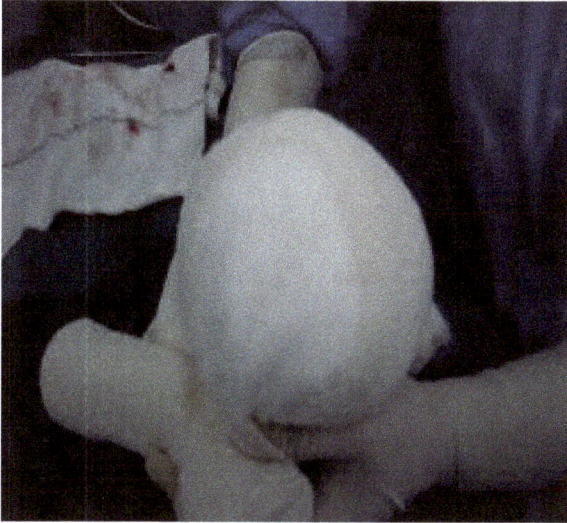

Figure 24. Bandaging the stump

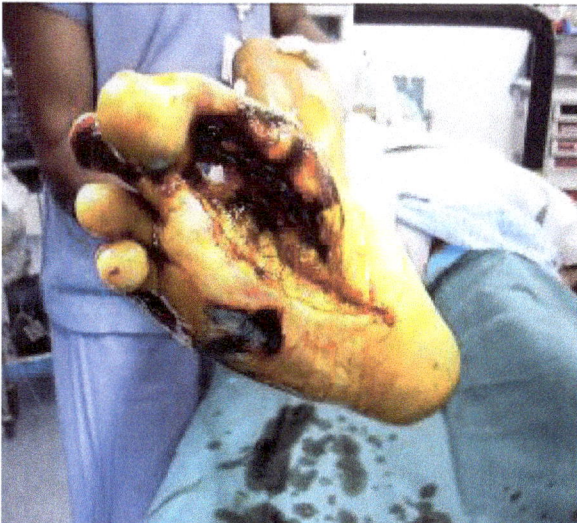

Figure 25. Pre-operation photograph showing wet gangrene of the forefoot

Anaesthesia

Same as for ray amputation.

Patient positioning

Same as for ray amputation.

Operative procedure

(1) Skin flaps are first marked. A long posterior heel flap is used to prevent tension when the wound is closed later.

(2) The anterior flap is marked from the distal tip of the lateral malleolus (Point A), passing across the anterior aspect of the ankle joint to a point one-finger breadth below the tip of the medial malleolus (Point B). The posterior flap runs vertically downwards from Point A to the sole of the foot. It continues horizontally across the sole of the foot to the lateral border of the foot. It runs vertically upwards to join Point B (Figs. 26 and 27).

(3) The skin flaps are then cut down to deep fascia and bone (Fig. 28).

(4) The saphenous vein is located in the subcutaneous plane, between the first and second metatarsal. It is divided and ligated. The dorsalis pedis artery

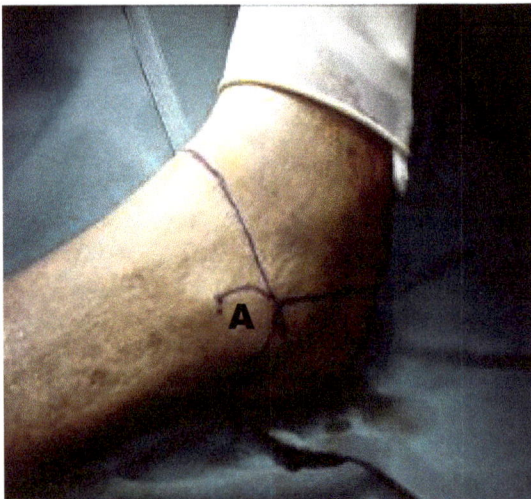

Figure 26.   Marking skin flap (lateral view)

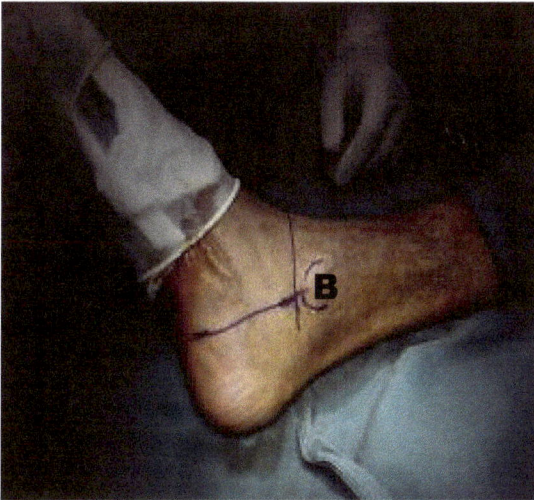

Figure 27.   Marking skin flap (medial view)

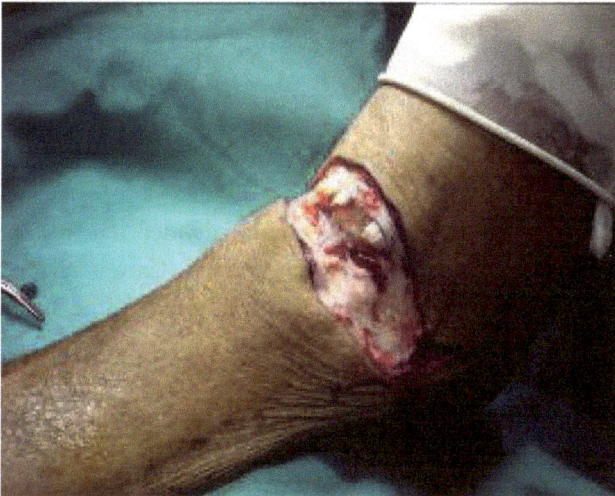

Figure 28.   The skin flap is cut down to deep fascia and bone

lies between the extensor hallucis longus and the extensor digitorum longus (Fig, 29). It is clamped, divided and ligated (Fig. 30). It. The extensor tendons are cut. Laterally, the peroneus longus and brevis tendons are cut.

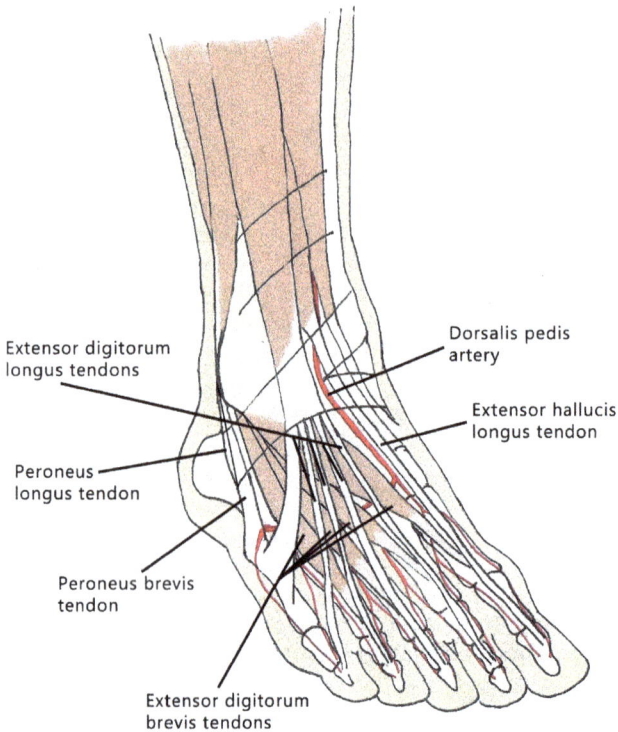

Figure 29.   Diagram showing structures encountered during Syme's amputation.

(5) The anterior capsule of the ankle joint is divided. The medial collateral ligament of the ankle joint is then divided. Care is taken to prevent damage to the posterior tibial artery. Laterally, the calcaneofibular ligament is also divided.

(6) A bone hook is then used to pull the talus forward and downward (Fig. 31). The soft tissue around the talus is divided. The talus is then excised (Fig. 32).

(7) The calcaneum is dissected subperiosteally, medially, laterally and posteriorly. The Tendo-achilles is incised close to its insertion. The calcaneum is then excised (Fig. 33).

(8) The calcaneo-cuboid joint is opened.

(9) The posterior flap is deepened to cut the flexor tendons.

(10) The distal foot containing the cuboid is amputated and passed to the circulating nurse.

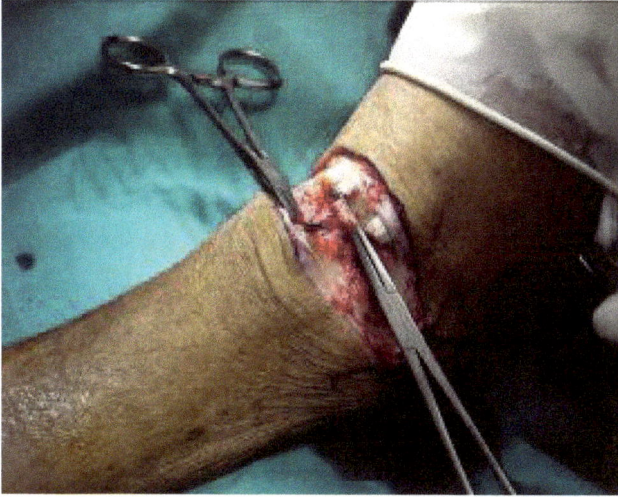

Figure 30. Clamping and dividing the dorsalis pedis artery

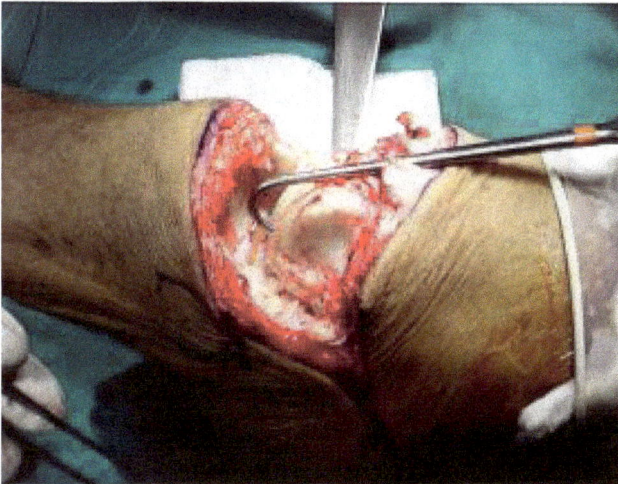

Figure 31. A bone hook is used to retract the talus

(11) An oscillating saw is used to cut the tibia just above the tibial plafond (Figs. 34 and 35). The medial malleolus is transected at the same level. The lateral malleolus is also osteotomised.

(12) The wound is then flushed using jet lavage (Fig. 36). The tourniquet is released and hemostasis is secured.

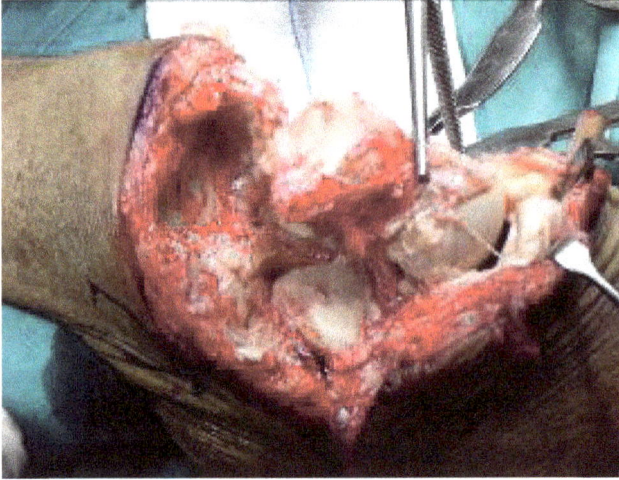

Figure 32.   Excision of talus

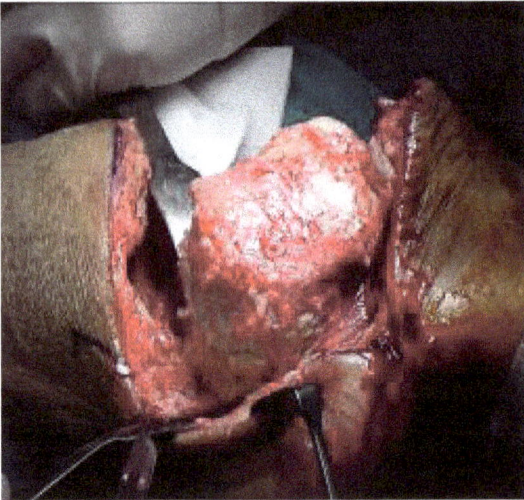

Figure 33.   Excision of the calcaneum

(13) The deep fascia of the posterior heel flap is then opposed to the periosteum of the tibia (Fig. 37). Two Kirschner wires are drilled from the centre of the heel flap upwards, into the centre of the tibia. This serves to anchor the posterior flap to the tibia to avoid floppiness of the heel pad.

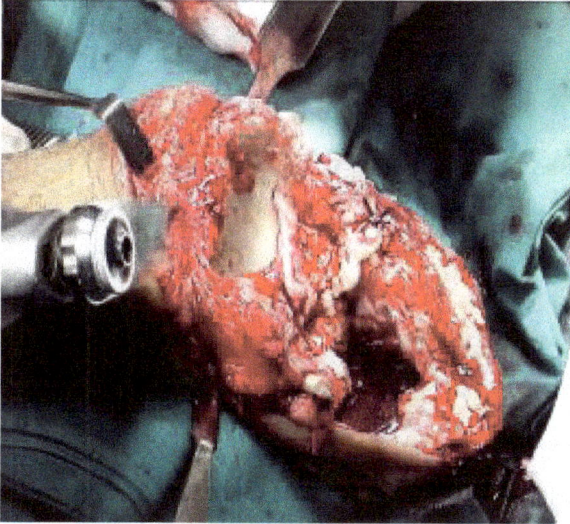

Figure 34. Tibial osteotomy

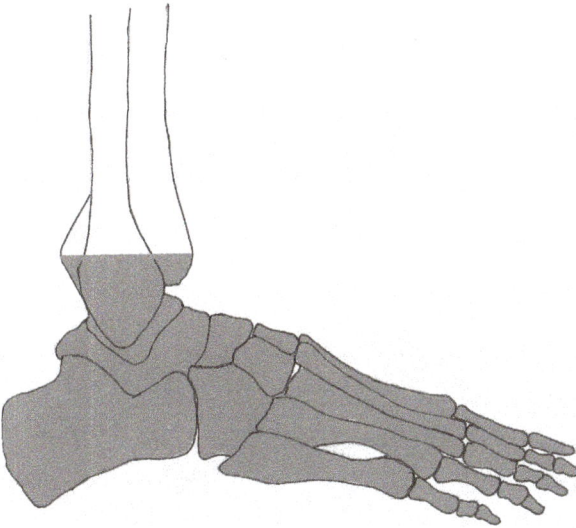

Figure 35. Diagram showing the bones removed (shaded) in a Syme's amputation. The tibial osteotomy just above the tibia plafond is also shown

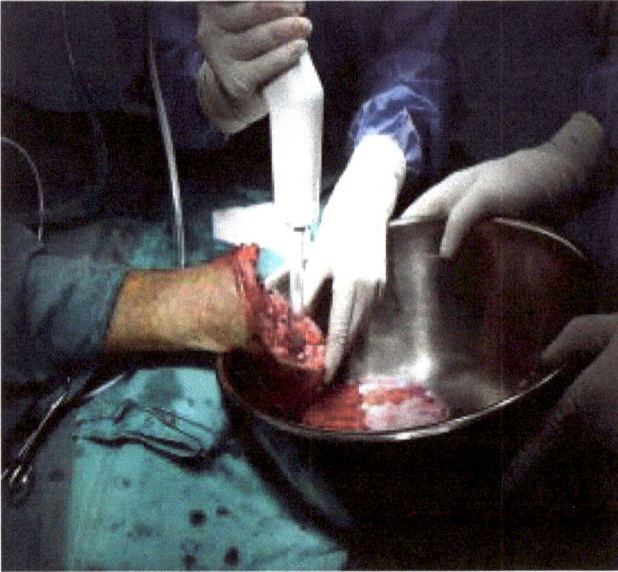

Figure 36. Jet lavage is used to flush the stump and wound

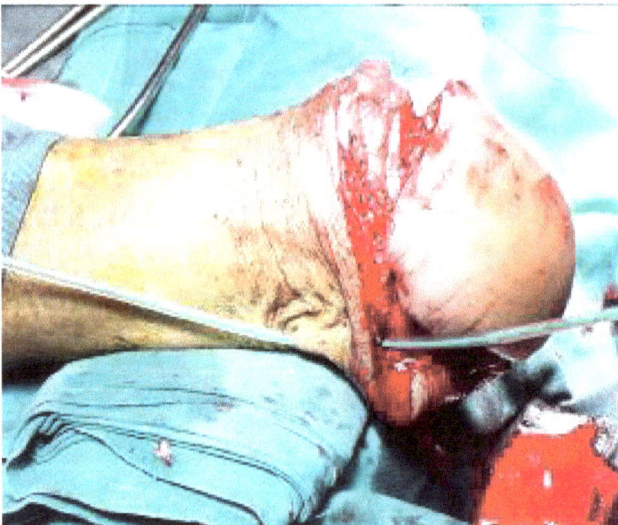

Figure 37. Opposition of anterior and posterior flaps

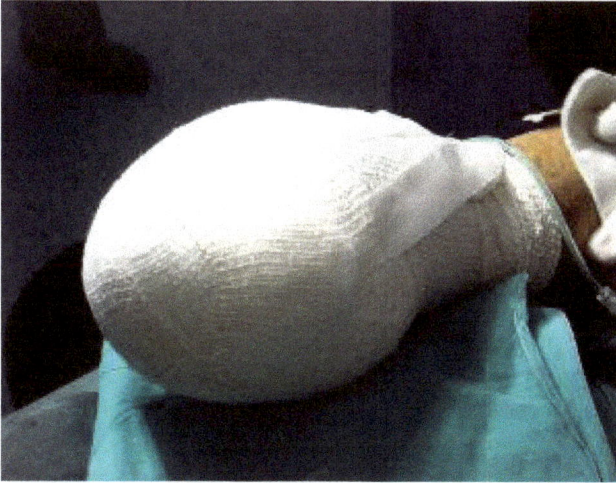

Figure 38. Crepe bandage is used to wrap the stump

(14) The deep fascia is tagged together with 1-0 vicryl sutures. Interrupted 3–0 prolene vertical mattress sutures are used to oppose the skin.

(15) Tulle Gras dressing and cotton wool are then applied. Crepe bandage is used to wrap and complete the dressing (Fig. 38). A stockinette is then applied.

Post-operative care

Post-operative care is similar to that of a patient with a ray amputation.

Modified Pirogoff Amputation

The author prefers a Pirogoff amputation to a Syme's amputation. In a Syme's amputation, the calcaneum is dissected from the heel flap. Doing so can devascularise the flap. No such dissection is required in a Pirogoff (Fig. 39). This is a major advantage, especially in a diabetic foot.

Boyd's Amputation has a similar advantage to a Pirogoff amputation in avoiding dissection of the calcaneum from the heel flap (Fig. 39). However, with Boyd's amputation, a larger flap is required to allow for calcaneo-tibial arthrodesis. With Pirogoff amputation, a smaller flap will suffice.

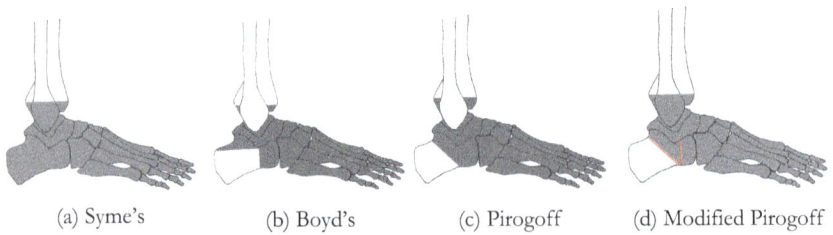

| (a) Syme's | (b) Boyd's | (c) Pirogoff | (d) Modified Pirogoff |

Figure 39. Diagrams comparing the bones removed (shaded) in a Syme's, Boyd's, original Pirogoff and modified Pirogoff amputation (from left to right)

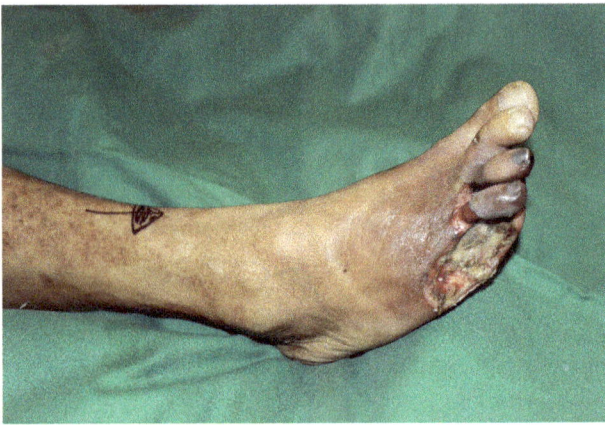

Figure 40. Pre-operation photograph showing wet gangrene of the 3rd and 4th right toes

Indications

- Wet or dry gangrene of only the forefoot (Fig. 40)
- Infection of only the forefoot
- Palpable dorsalis pedis and posterior tibial pulses. The posterior tibial pulse must be strong and palpable.
- Ankle Brachial Index ≥ 0.8
- Toe Brachial Index ≥ 0.7

Pre-operative preparation

Follow the same preparation as for ray amputation

Anaesthesia

Same as for ray amputation.

Patient positioning

Same as for ray amputation.

Operative technique

(1) Anterior and posterior skin flaps are marked (Figs. 41 and 42).
(2) The anterior flap runs from one-finger breadth below the distal tip of the medial malleolus (Point A) over the anterior aspect of the ankle to the tip of the lateral malleolus (Point B).

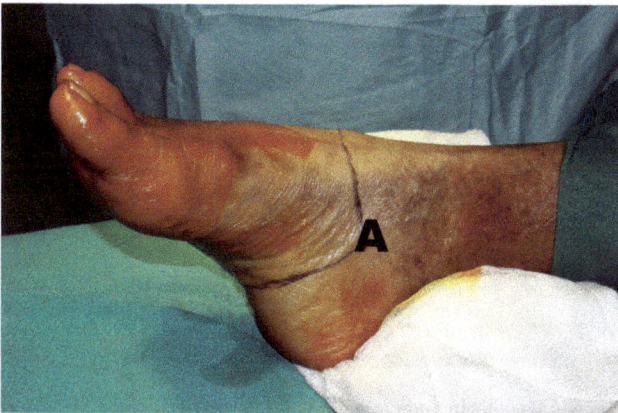

Figure 41.   Skin flaps are marked (medial view)

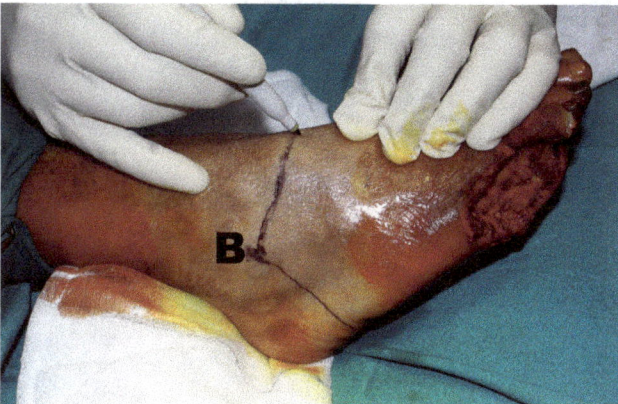

Figure 42.   Skin flaps are marked (lateral view)

(3) The posterior flap runs vertically downwards from Point A to the sole of the foot. It continues horizontally across the sole of the foot to the lateral border of the foot. It runs vertically upwards to join Point B.

(4) The skin flaps are incised down to the deep fascia (Fig. 43).

(5) Anteriorly, on the medial side, the long saphenous vein is divided and ligated (Fig. 44).

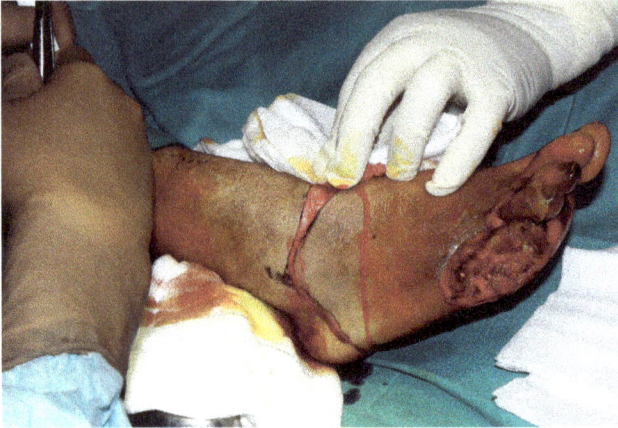

Figure 43. The incision is made along the marked anterior skin flap

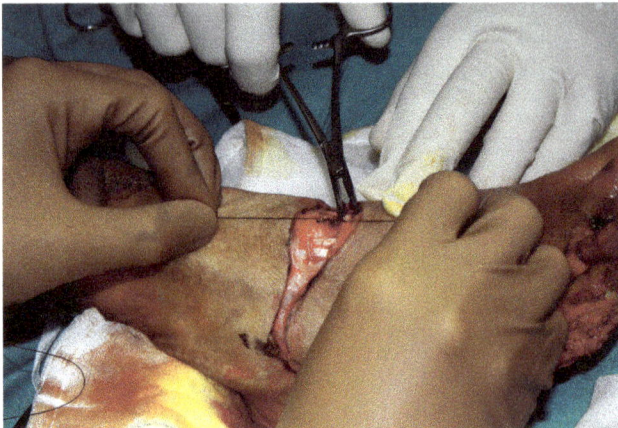

Figure 44. The saphenous vein is divided and ligated

(6) Lateral to the saphenous vein is the dorsalis pedis artery. It runs between the extensor hallucis longus and the extensor digitorum longus (Refer to figure 17 and 29). It is clamped, divided and ligated (Fig. 45).

(7) The extensor tendons (hallucis longus, digitorum longus and digitorum brevis) are cut along the line of incision.

(8) On the lateral side of the foot, the peroneus brevis (Fig. 46) and peroneus longus tendons are cut.

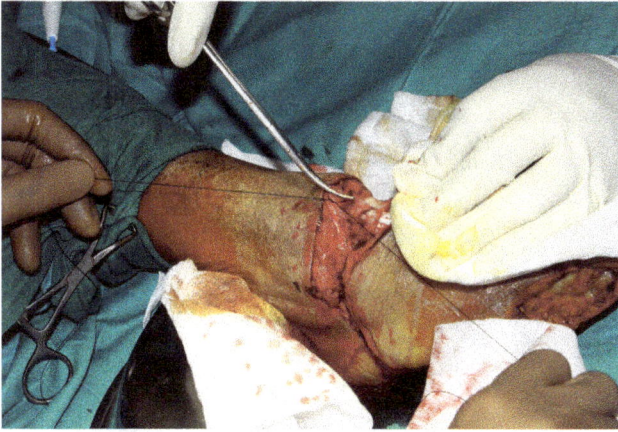

Figure 45. The dorsalis pedis artery is ligated

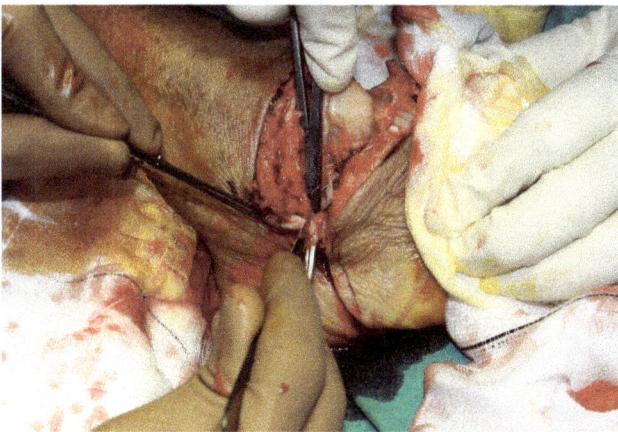

Figure 46. The peroneus brevis tendon is cut

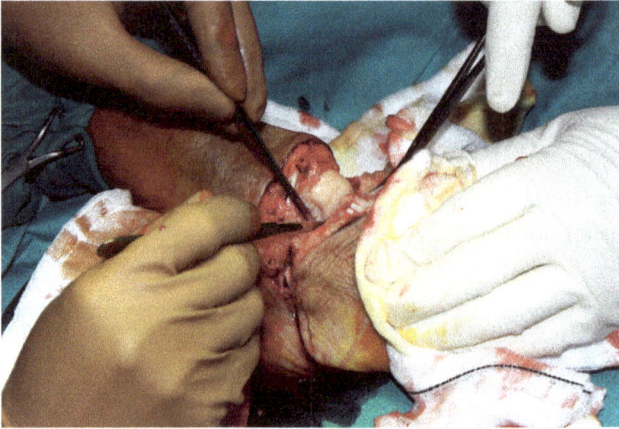

Figure 47. The anterior capsule is opened

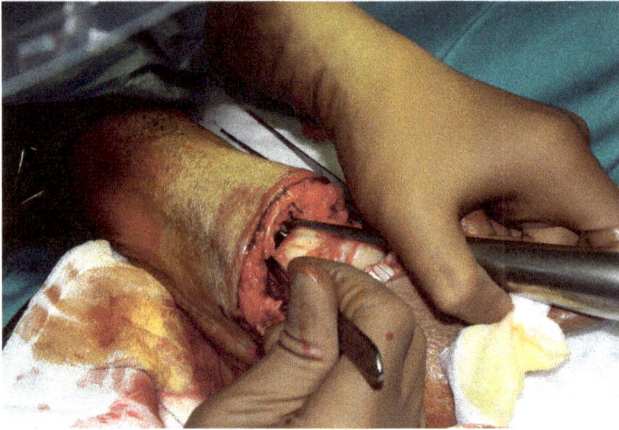

Figure 48. A bone hook is used on the talus to facilitate dissection

(9) The foot is placed in an equinus position. The anterior capsule is incised (Fig. 47) to expose the articular surfaces of the tibia and the talus.

(10) On the medial side, the deltoid ligament of the ankle is sectioned. Take care not to damage the posterior tibial artery.

(11) On the lateral side, the calcaneo-fibular ligament of the ankle is incised.

(12) A bone hook is used to pull the talus forward and upward (Fig. 48) for easy dissection of the talus from the underlying calcaneum. The talus is excised and removed (Figs. 49 and 50).

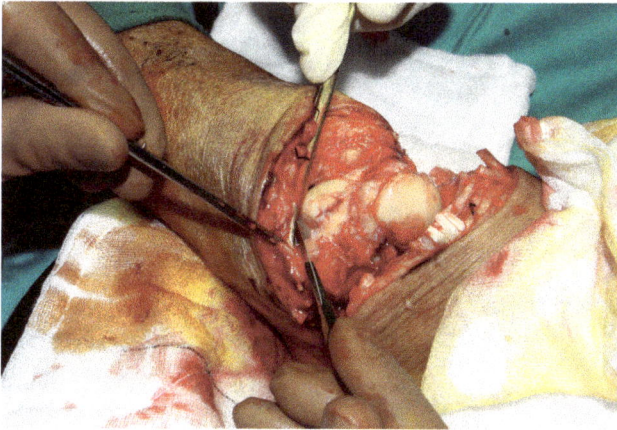

Figure 49. Dissection of the talus

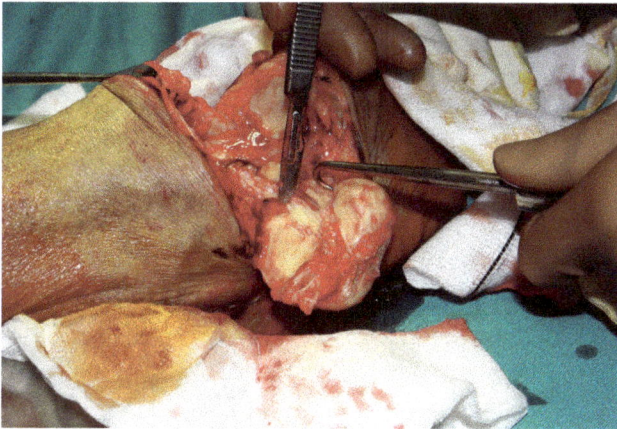

Figure 50. The talus is excised

(13) The anterior talar articular surface, middle talar articular surface and posterior talar articular surface of the calcaneum are exposed (Figs. 51 and 52).

(14) The incision on the sole is deepened. The flexor tendons are cut (Fig. 53).

(15) The calcaneo-cuboid joint is identified and its capsule incised on the lateral side of the foot (Fig. 54). The articular surface of the calcaneum for the cuboid bone (Fig. 52) is exposed.

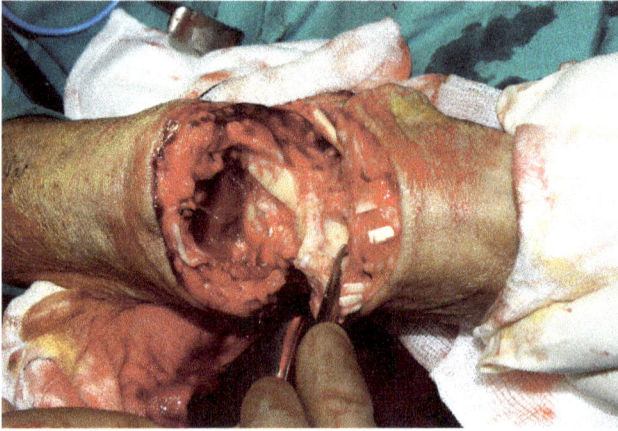

Figure 51. The anterior, middle and posterior talar articular surface of the calcaneum are exposed

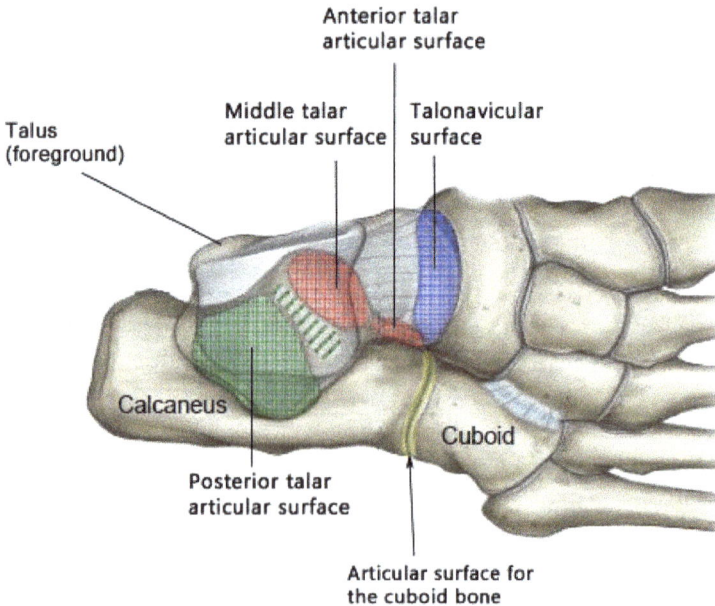

Figure 52. Superior view of the foot showing the surfaces of the calcaneum (*Diagram adapted from: www.cobocards.com*)

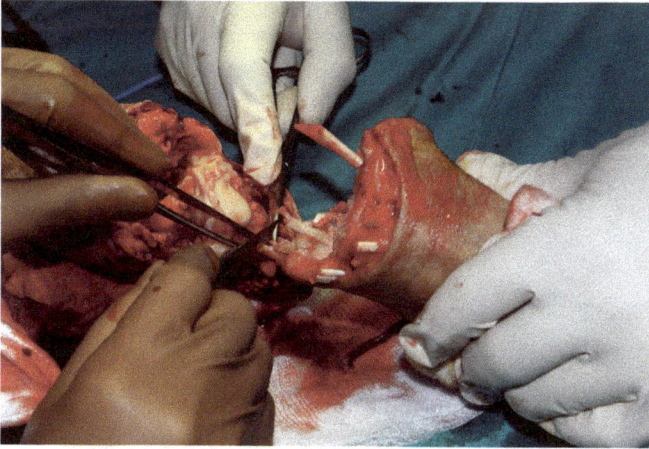

Figure 53. Dividing the flexor tendons

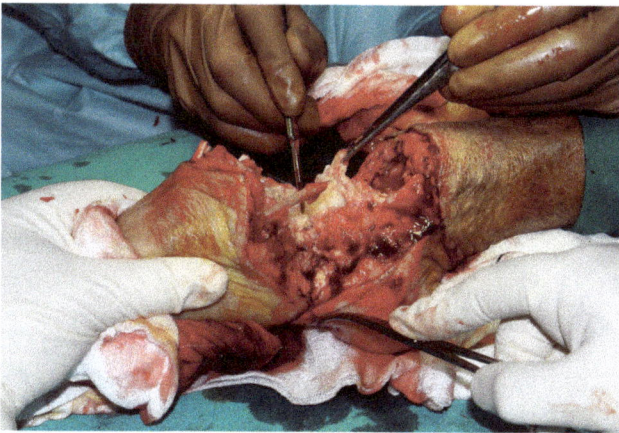

Figure 54. Cutting the calcaneo-cuboid joint

(16) The distal part of the foot containing the cuboid is excised, leaving the calcaneum in the plantar flap (Fig. 55).

(17) Using an oscillating saw, an osteotomy is performed on the calcaneum, just behind the anterior talar articular surface. The distal one quarter of the calcaneum is osteotomised (Figs. 56 to 58). The line of osteotomy (CD) is perpendicular to the calcaneum.

(18) An oblique osteotomy is then performed from Point D to Point E — the posterior border of the upper end of the calcaneum (Fig. 57). The wedge of bone osteotomised is removed. This osteotomy gives a 60-degree cut (Figs. 57 and 59) to the remaining calcaneum left behind in the flap.

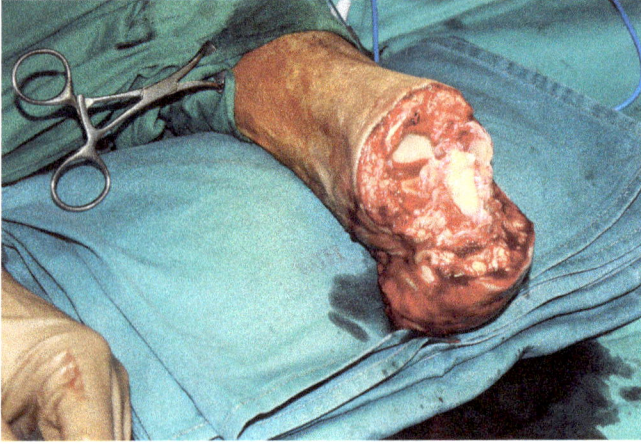

Figure 55. Stump with the calcaneum left on the posterior flap

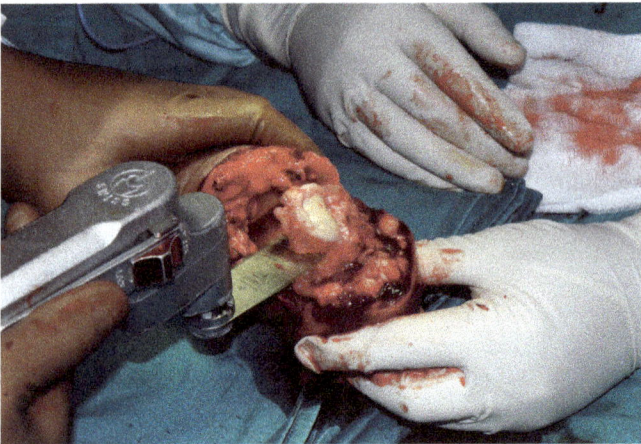

Figure 56. An oscillating saw is used to osteotomise the distal one quarter of the calcaneum

(19) The lower articular surface of the tibia is exposed using Hohmann retractors.

(20) Using an oscillating saw, the distal end of the tibia is osteotomised (Fig. 60). The line of osteotomy (line FG) is perpendicular to the tibia (Fig. 61). The medial malleolus (Point F) and the lower part of the fibula

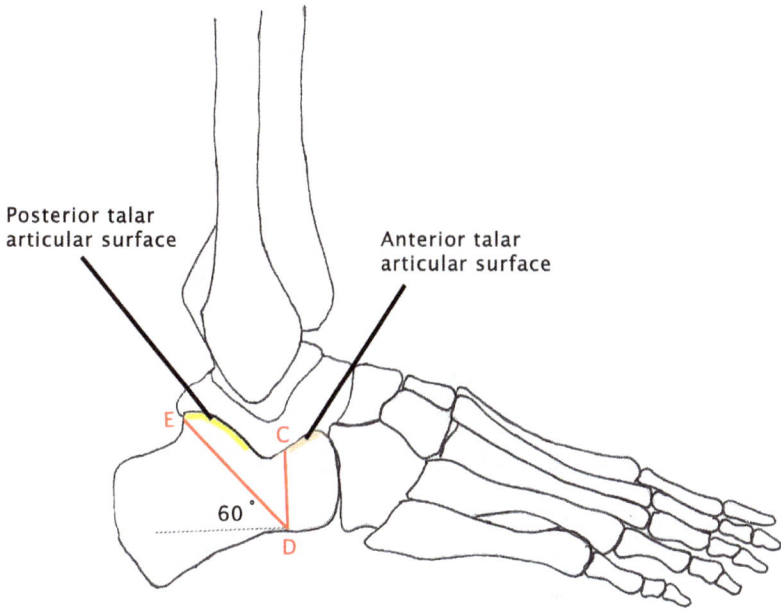

Figure 57. Lateral view of foot showing the 2 lines of osteotomy (CD and DE) at the calcaneum

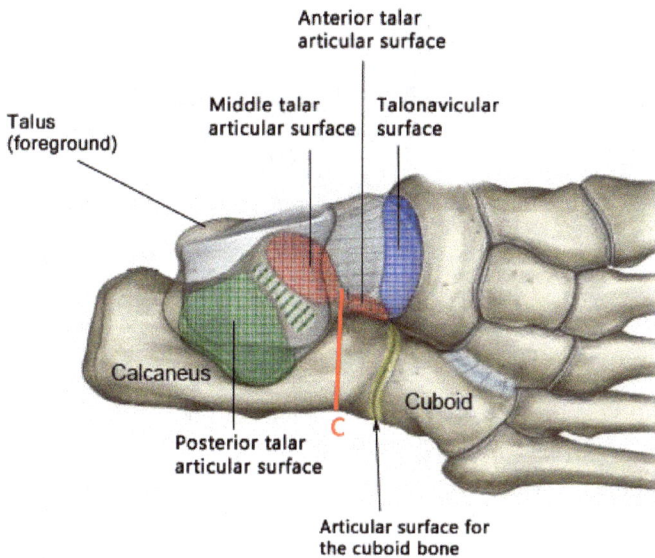

Figure 58. Superior view of the foot showing the line of incision (red) just behind the anterior talar articular surface
(*Diagram adapted from: www.cobocards.com*)

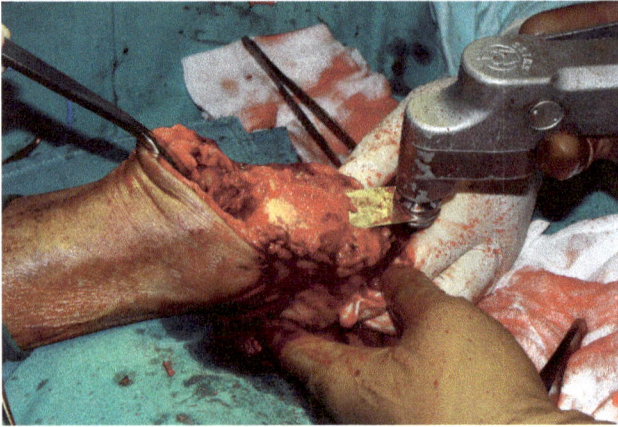

Figure 59. A 60-degree cut is made to the calcaneum

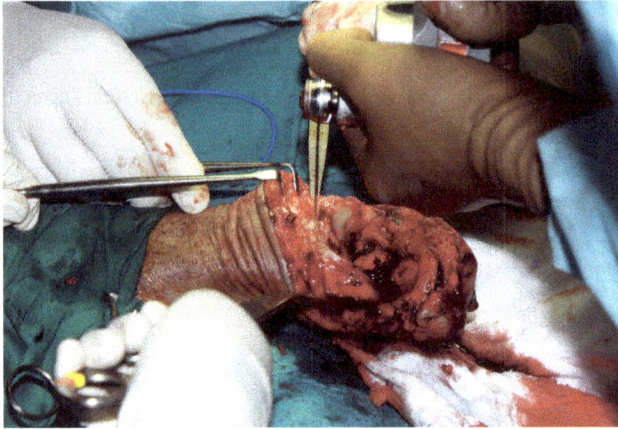

Figure 60. Tibial osteotomy: A 90-degree cut is made using the oscillating saw

(from Point G) are osteotomised along the line of the tibial osteotomy. The osteotomy removes the articular surface of the tibia (Figs. 62 and 63) and prepares a smooth bony surface (cortico-cancellous) to be opposed to the osteotomised calcaneum.

(21) Using jet lavage, the wound and the bone surfaces are flushed with normal saline.

(22) The tourniquet is released and hemostasis is secured.

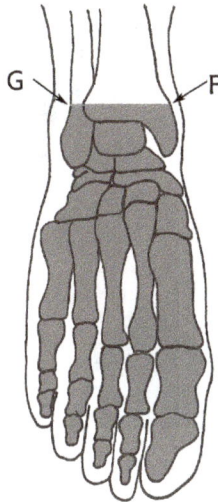

Figure 61. Diagram showing the line of tibial osteotomy (FG) and the bones removed (shaded) in a modified Pirogoff amputation

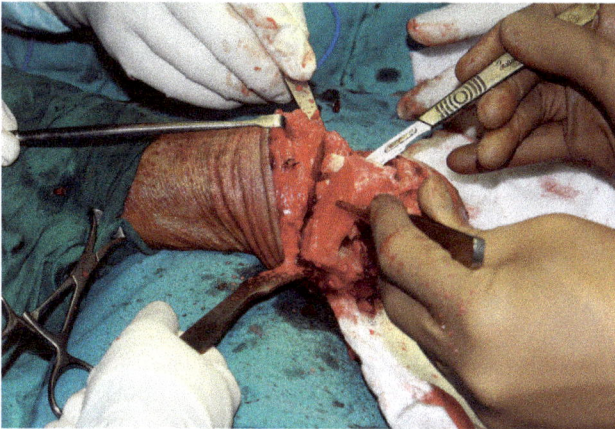

Figure 62. The distal portion of the tibia is excised

(23) The calcaneum is then apposed to the tibia. To avoid tension, the calaneum is positioned slightly posteriorly so that the distal part of the remaining calcaneum can be readily apposed to the tibia.

(24) After making small incisions in the calcaneal flap, two 2 mm Kirschner wires are inserted in a criss-cross fashion through the calcaneum to engage

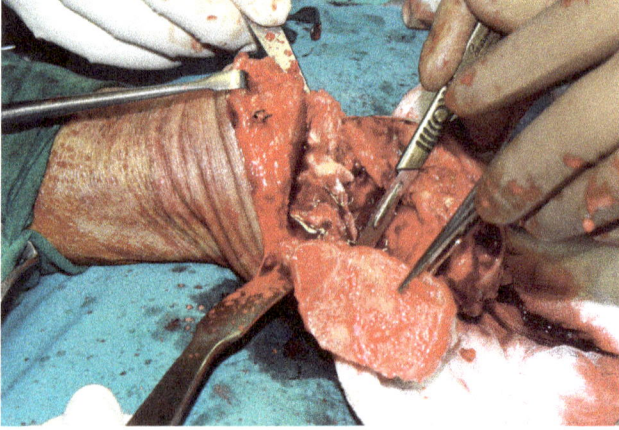

Figure 63. The distal portion of the tibia is excised

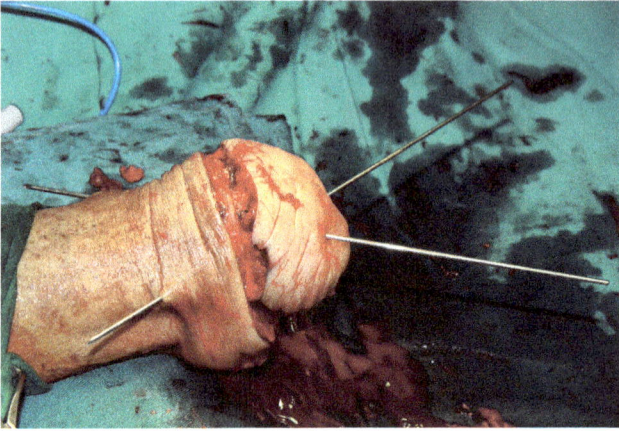

Figure 64. Two Kirschner wires are inserted through the stump in a criss-crossed manner

the tibial cortical surface (Fig. 64). The wires hold the raw surface of the tibia in good apposition with the calcaneum surface. The positions of the Kirschner wires are confirmed to be satisfactory using an image intensifier.

(25) The track of the Kirschner wires are then drilled and tapped with a 7.0 mm cancellous tap.

(26) Two 7.0 mm partially threaded cannulated hip screws are then inserted over the Kirschner wires. To achieve compression, partially threaded

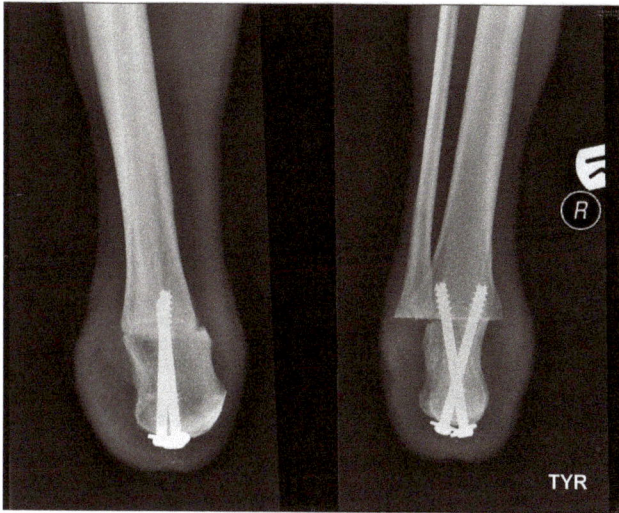

Figure 65. Lateral and AP views of radiographs showing compression of tibio-calcaneal surfaces by two partially threaded cannulated hip screws

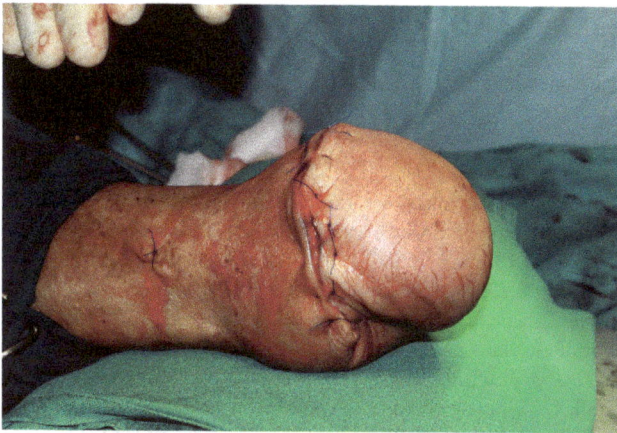

Figure 66. Final Pirogoff amputation stump with 3-0 prolene sutures

cancellous screws are inserted according to the lag-screw principle. The screws are tightened and their positions are confirmed to be satisfactory via image intensifier (Fig. 65).

(27) The anterior and posterior flaps are opposed with one single layer of 3-0 prolene sutures (Fig. 66).

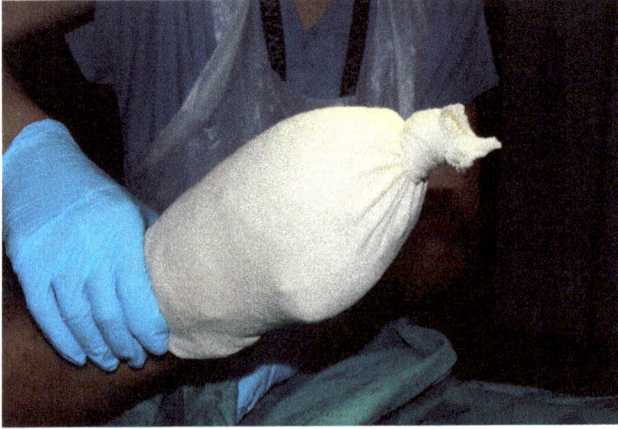

Figure 67. Pirogoff amputation stump wrapped in cotton wool, crepe bandage and stockinette

(28) Tulle-Gras dressing is applied over the wound. Gauze and cotton wool is then used to wrap the stump before crepe bandage is applied in a figure-of-8 fashion. A stockinette is then applied (Fig. 67).

Post-operative care

Post-operative care is similar to that of a patient with a ray amputation.

References

1. J. Syme, Amputation at the ankle joint, *London Edinburgh Monthly J. Med. Sci.* 2:93 (1843).
2. H. B. Boyd, Amputation of the foot, with calcaneotibial arthrodesis, *J. Bone Joint Surg.* 21: 997–1000 (October 1939).
3. M. Altindas and A. Kilic, Is Boyd's operation a last solution that may prevent major amputations in diabetic foot patients?, *J. Foot Ankle Surg.* 47(4):307–12 (July 2008).
4. N. L. Pirogoff, Resection of bones and joints and amputations and disarticulation of joints. 1864, *Clin. Orthop. Relat. Res.* 266:3–11 (May 1991).
5. N. L. Pirogoff, Osteoplastic elongation of the bones of the lower leg in conjunction with release of the foot from the ankle joint, *J. Military Med.* 63:83 (1854).
6. F. M. den Bakker, H. R. Holtslag and J. G. van den Brand, Pirogoff amputation for foot trauma: an unusual amputation level. A case report, *J. Bone Joint Surg. Am.* 92(14): 2462–2465 (October 2010).
7. A. R. Langeveld, R. J. Oostenbroek, M. P. Wijffels and M. T. Hoedt, The Pirogoff amputation for necrosis of the forefoot: a case report, *J. Bone Joint Surg. Am.* 92(4):968–72 (April 2010).
8. A. R. Langeveld, D. E. Meuffels, R. J. Oostenbroek and M. T. Hoedt. The Pirogoff amputation for necrosis of the forefoot: surgical technique, *J. Bone Joint Surg. Am.* 93(Suppl. 1):21–29 (March 2011).

24

Other Diabetic Foot Surgery

Aziz Nather, April Voon Siew Lian,
Amy Pannapat Chanyarungrojn, Lim Chin Tat
and Andrew Hong Choon Chiet

Department of Orthopaedic Surgery
Yong Loo Lin School of Medicine
National University of Singapore

Introduction

In this chapter, the following procedures will be described:

- Surgical debridement
- Split thickness skin grafting
- Surgery for osteomyelitis/septic arthritis
  — Excision arthroplasty of metatarso-phalangeal joint
  — Excision of lateral malleolus and ankle arthrodesis
  — Partial calcanectomy

The commonest procedure performed for diabetic foot surgery is surgical debridement. Another common procedure that must be mastered by all surgeons dealing with diabetic foot is split thickness skin grafting.

Surgical Debridement

Debridement is the excision of necrotic, devitalised or infected tissue from a wound, leaving healthy and vascular tissue behind. It is the most common surgical procedure performed for the treatment of a diabetic foot.[1] Registrars usually perform debridement as an emergency. This is often poorly done. Indeed, the most difficult operation to teach residents is how to do an adequate surgical debridement. Often, necrotic fascia and tendon are left behind, leading to the necessity for a re-debridement.

Why Debridement?

- Devitalised tissue in the wound floor prevents the clinician from adequately assessing the depth and nature of the wound. Concealed dead spaces could harbour bacteria and increase the risk of local infection.[2]
- Necrotic or devitalised tissue may mask signs of local wound infection.[3]
- The presence of necrotic tissue is a physical barrier to healing.[4] Bacterial colonies, which are often present in necrotic tissue, can produce proteases. The latter breaks down important constituents of the extracellular matrix and have a negative effect on the formation of granulation tissue and re-epithelisation.[5]
- Bacteria form a biofilm for their own protection. This is extracellular matrix that binds to the wound floor and may cause resistance to antibiotics instituted. This biofilm must be removed to allow the wound to heal properly.

Surgical Technique

Surgical debridement (also known as sharp debridement) makes use of a scalpel to cut necrotic, infected or devitalised tissue from a wound.

It is a fast way to remove debris and necrotic tissue from the wound bed. It is performed when there is an extensive amount of necrotic tissue in the wound.

Surgical debridement should result in minimal damage to the surrounding tissue. Minor bleeding following the procedure allows inflammatory mediators to reach the wound site. Inflammatory mediators release cytokines that assist in the wound repair process.

Debridement cannot be performed on patients who are on Plavix or Aspirin until the medication has been stopped for at least 3 days prior to the operation.

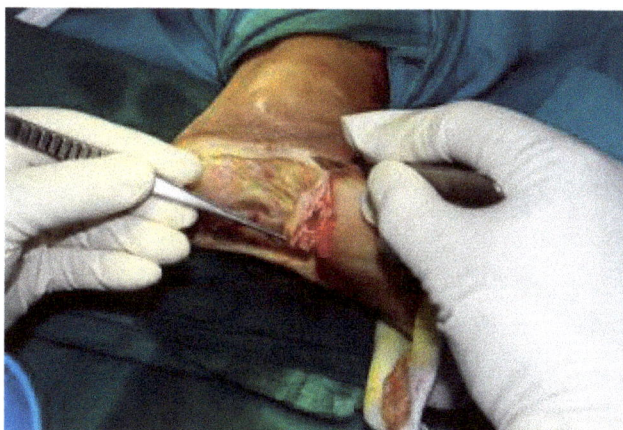

Figure 1.   Excision of infected and devitalized tissue

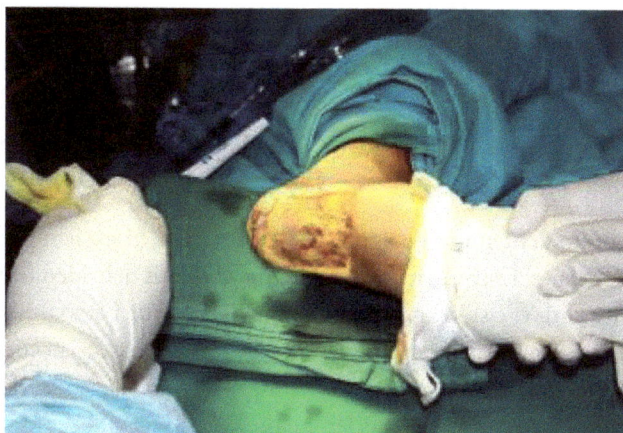

Figure 2.   Wound after flushing with saline

Principles of Surgical Debridement

The "sterile" surgical debridement is a 2-step technique:

- Step 1
  - Excise all infected and devitalised tissues until pink and healthy tissue is observed. Bleeding occurs in healthy tissue (Fig. 1).
  - Flush with 1–2 litres of normal saline using jet lavage (Pulsavac) (Fig. 2).

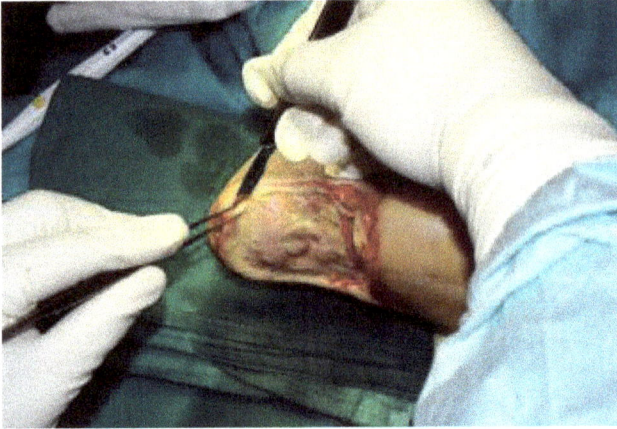

Figure 3.   Final debridement

- Step 2
    - Use new blades and forceps to perform a final debridement to remove more infected or devitalised tissue left behind (Fig. 3). The tissues are "excised" in the same manner as that used to excise a soft tissue malignancy.

Surgical debridement must be aggressive and radical in excising all infected and necrotic tissues. One must ensure that the wound is debrided from layer to layer, starting with the skin and the subcutaneous tissue. No exposed tendons should be left behind as any tendons left behind will necrose to become slough. Likewise, no fascia exposed can be left behind. This must also be debrided. If necrotic tendon, muscle or fascia is left behind, they will all become slough — a redebridement will then be needed.

Split Thickness Skin Grafting

Diabetic foot most commonly present with diabetic wounds or ulcers. Ulcers are treated with dressings or in some cases, negative pressure therapy is used to prepare the wound. Once healthy granulation tissue is present and the culture for sensitivity comes back negative, the wound is then ready for split skin grafting. Next to debridement and ray amputation surgery, split thickness skin grafting is the most common diabetic foot surgery performed.

Indications

- Ulcer over non-weight bearing portion of the foot — dorsum of foot, arch of foot, etc.
- Ulcer of leg or thigh following debridement for necrotising fasciitis
- Ulcer of leg following debridement for diabetic leg abscess

Specialised Instruments for Skin Grafting (Fig. 4)

- Zimmer Air Dermatome
- Zimmer 1-, 2-, 3- and 4-inch templates
- Tulle Gras as skin graft carrier
- 2 metal plates
- Zimmer Skin Mesher
- Marking pen
- Jet lavage

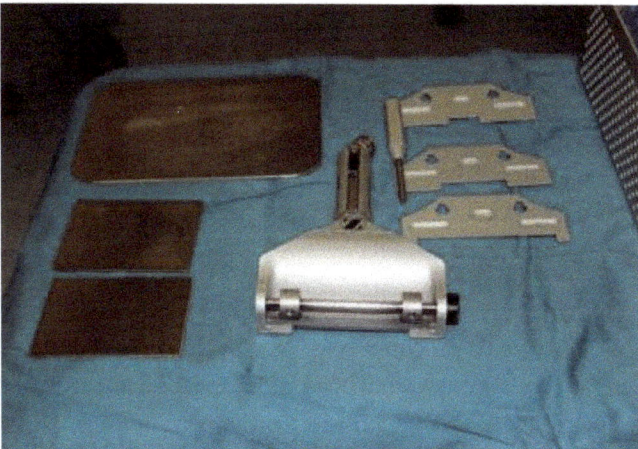

Figure 4. Specialised instruments for skin grafting

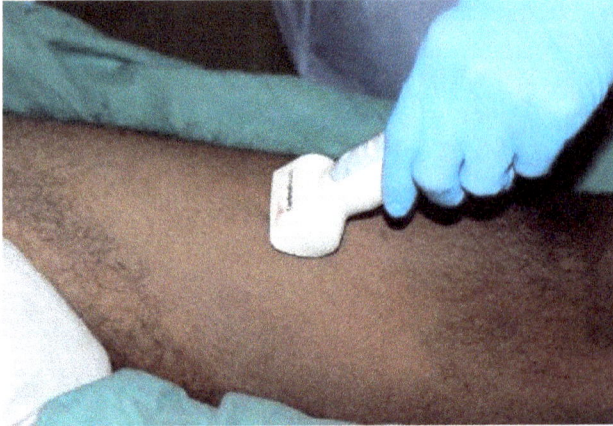

Figure 5.   Shaving hair on donor site

Patient Positioning

Patient is placed in the supine position. A sandbag is placed underneath the buttock on the side of the split thickness skin grafting.

The skin on the thigh (donor site) is cleansed with Cetrimide and normal saline. Hair on the thigh (donor site) is then shaved with an electric shaver (Fig. 5). The skin is covered with a layer of Cetrimide before cleansing for the operation.

A leg stand is used for suspension of the whole lower limb (Fig. 6) for easy cleansing with Cetrimide and Chlorhexidine. The donor skin is usually taken from the thigh of the same leg.

Operative Procedure

Recipient site

- The recipient site is carefully measured to determine the size of the skin graft that needs to be procured (Fig. 7). Care must be taken into account the increased size of the wound after surgical debridement.
- The recipient site is covered with wet gauze (with normal saline) to keep the wound moist.

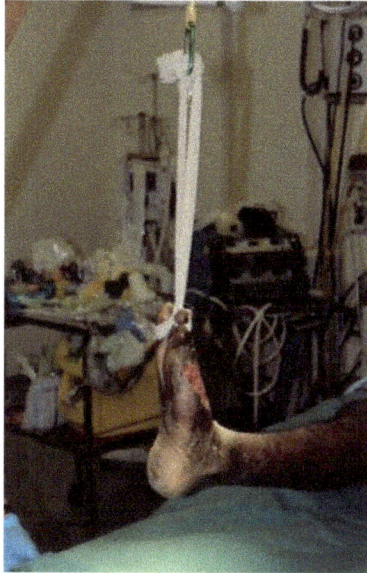

Figure 6. Leg stand to suspend the lower limb

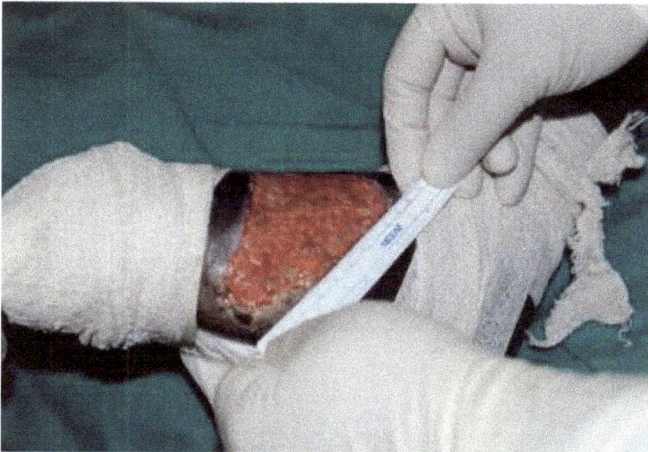

Figure 7. Measuring size of recipient site

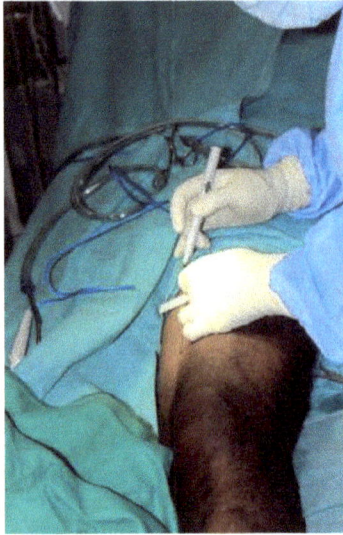

Figure 8. Marking donor site

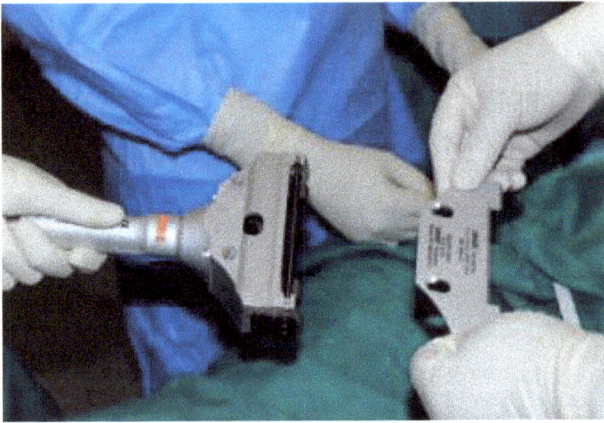

Figure 9. Choosing size of template

Donor site

- Mark the size and shape of the donor skin needed on the thigh (Fig. 8).
- The thigh donor skin is made tense by an assistant to present the thigh skin more readily for the dermatome.
- The size of the template is chosen based on the surgeon's assessment of the width of the skin that needs to be procured (Fig. 9).
- The dermatome blade is then inserted into the machine (Fig. 10).

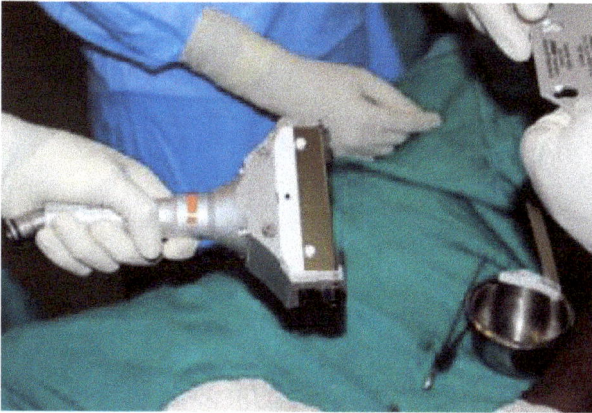

Figure 10. Blade inserted into dermatome

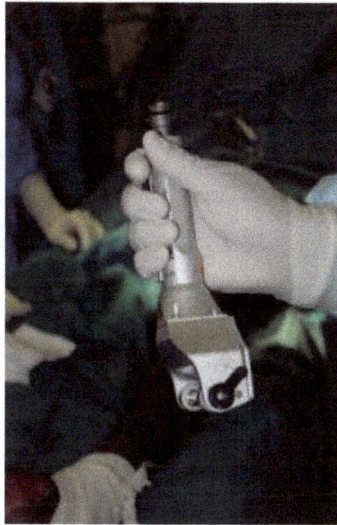

Figure 11. Choosing thickness of skin to be cut

- The chosen template is then placed on the blade and fixed in place using 2 screws, which are tightened to finger tightness of the non-dominant hand. Before tightening, some paraffin is applied on the blade and the template.
- The thickness of the skin that needs to be cut is also chosen (Fig. 11) — usually set at point 12 to 14 (12/1000 to 14/1000 of an inch) (Fig. 12).

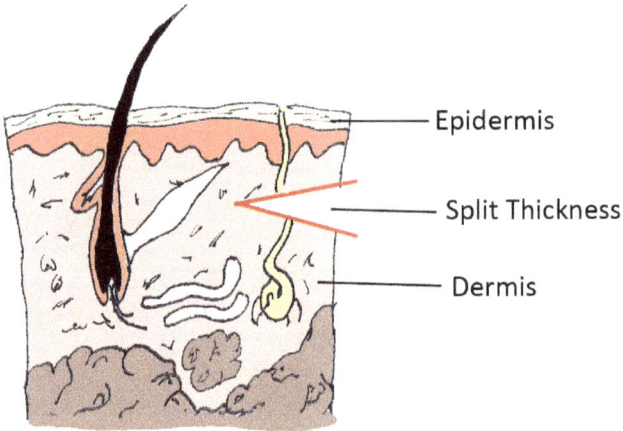

Figure 12.　Cross-section of skin showing level of cut of skin for split thicness

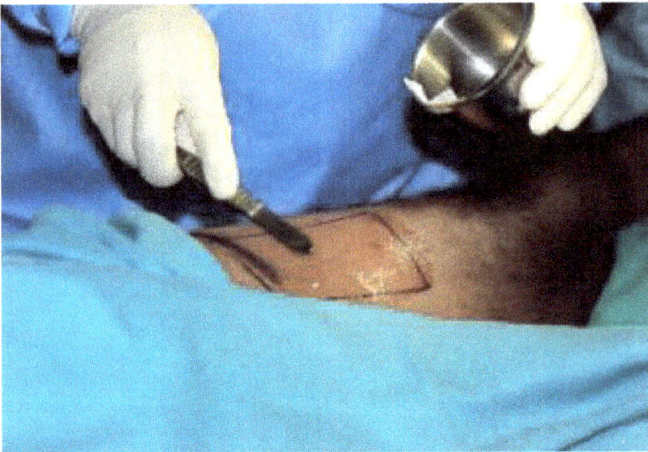

Figure 13.　Applying a layer of paraffin oil

- A layer of paraffin oil is applied evenly to the donor skin using a McDonald's dissector (Fig. 13) (gauze will usually absorb most of the oil and should not be used for this).
- A metal plate is applied to the thigh proximally and another plate distally to make the thigh skin tense (Fig. 14).

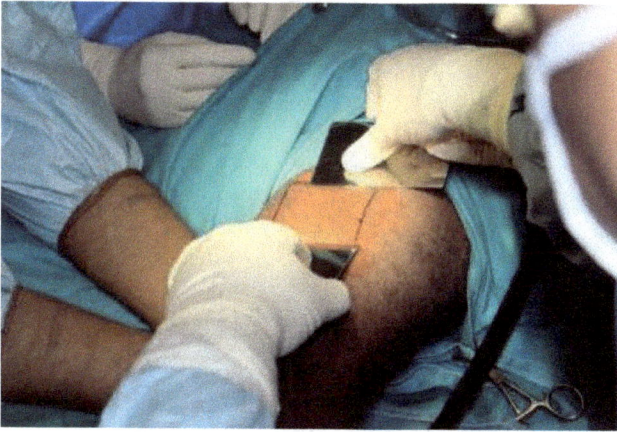

Figure 14. Making thigh skin tense

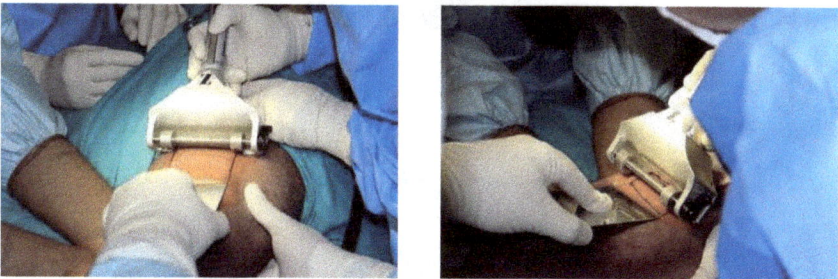

Figure 15. Using the dermatome

- The dermatome is then applied gently at an angle of 45° until contact is made with the skin. Move the dermatome downwards parallel to the donor skin with a steady and even pressure while the skin is under tension until the appropriate amount of donor skin has been procured (Fig. 15).
- The dermatome is slowly angulated upwards to release the skin from the site (Fig. 16). A pair of McIndoe scissors is then used to cut the lower end of the procured skin.
- The correct thickness of the skin procured is shown by punctate bleeding of the donor graft site (Fig. 17).

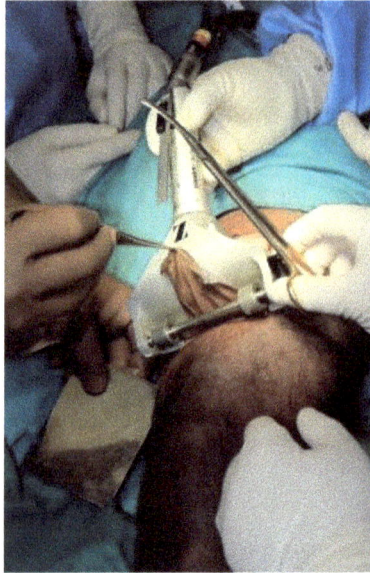

Figure 16. Releasing skin from donor site

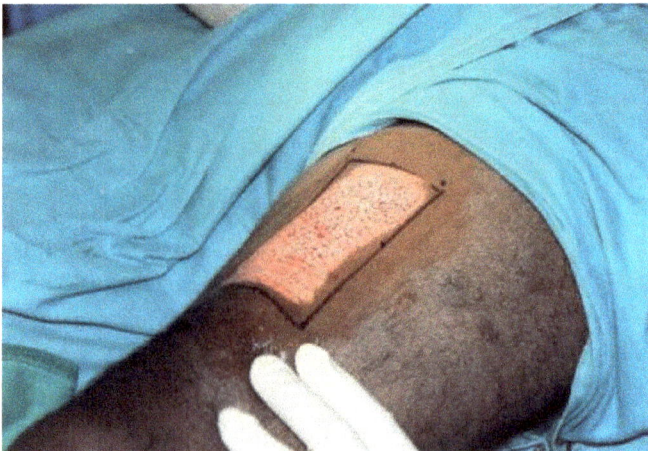

Figure 17. Donor site after skin procurement

- Kaltostat is applied to the raw wound on the thigh followed by Allevyn Dressing (Fig. 18).
- Gauze is applied and a 6-inch crepe bandage is used to complete the dressing.

Meshing of the skin

The skin procured is then meshed using the appropriate-sized carrier needed to give the necessary expansion. Usually, the 1.5:1 carrier is sufficient for split thickness skin grafting in the diabetic foot (Figs. 19a to 19e).

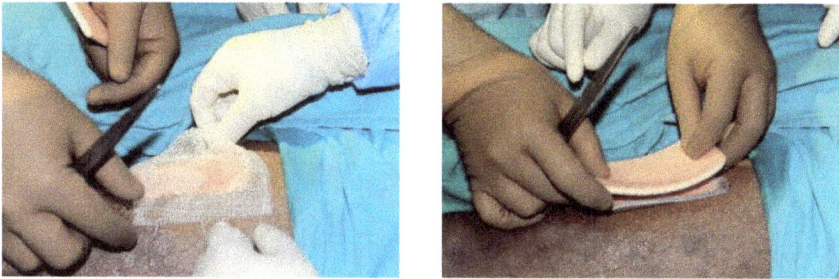

Figure 18. Applying Kaltostat then Allvyn dressings

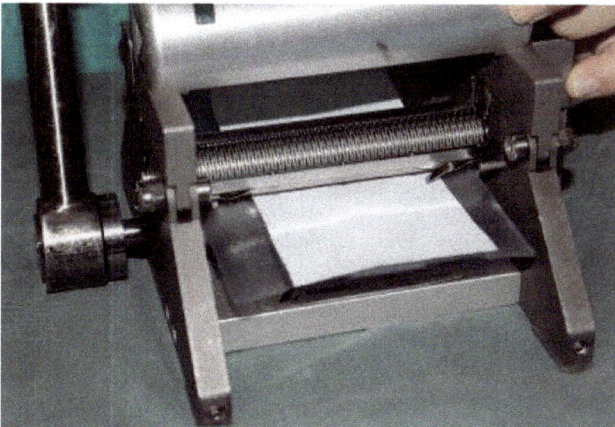

Figure 19a. Meshing machine assembled with the carrier in place

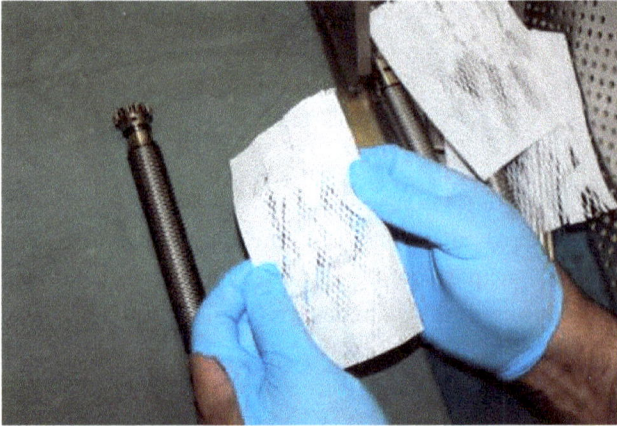

Figure 19b.   Carrier for 1.5:1 meshing

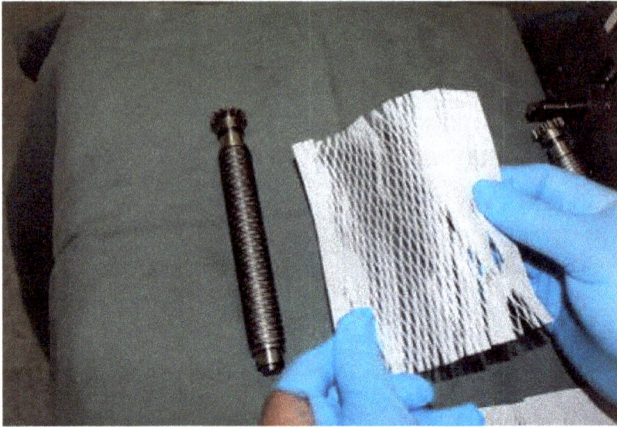

Figure 19c.   Carrier for 3:1 meshing

Preparation of the skin graft (when skin is not meshed)

- The nurse prepares to receive the graft by applying Tulle Gras over the larger metal plate.
- The procured graft is placed over the Tulle Gras layer with the outer surface downwards (Fig. 20). The inner surface of the graft (dermis) faces upwards.

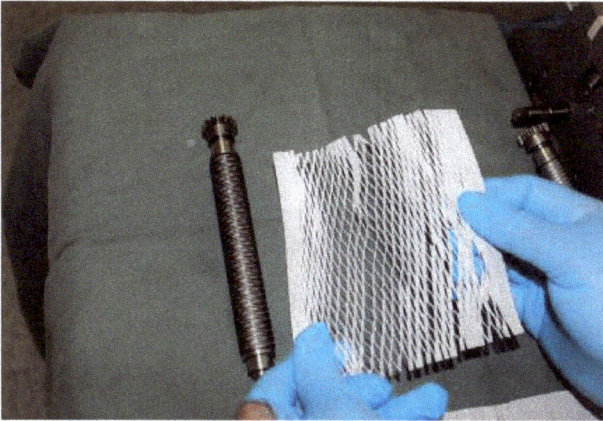

Figure 19d. Carrier for 6:1 meshing

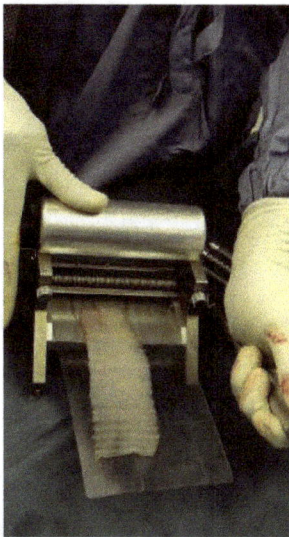

Figure 19e. The skin is placed on the plastic sheet with its cutaneous surface facing up, and pass through the meshing machine with the selected carrier in place

- Using a scalpel, small nicks are made on the skin (Fig. 21). These linear perforations allow any haematoma collecting in the recipient wound to drain.
- The extra Tulle Gras not covered by the graft is then cut around the borders of the skin with a pair of McIndoe scissors (Fig. 22).

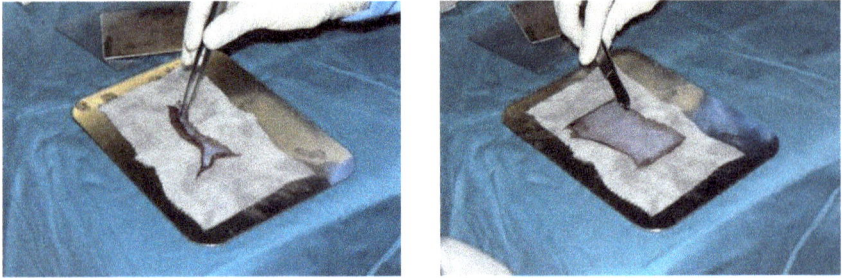

Figure 20. Procured graft placed over Tulle Gras layer

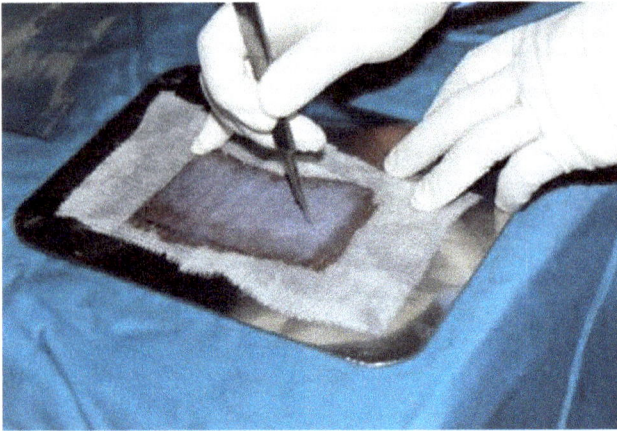

Figure 21. Making small nicks on procured skin

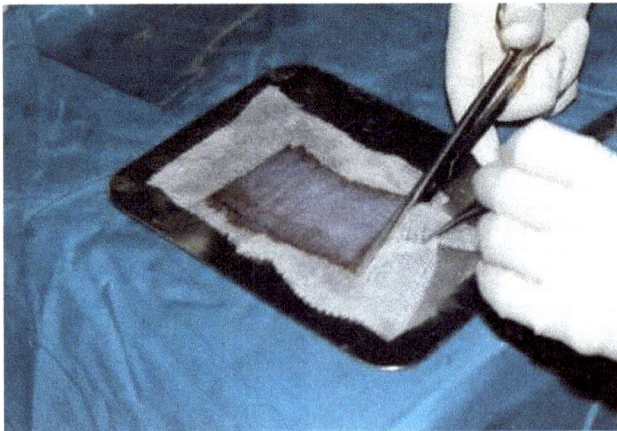

Figure 22. Cutting extra Tulle Gras

Preparation of recipient site

- Final debridement of the wound is done.
- The edge of the wound is excised leaving healthy skin edge.
- The floor of the wound is freshened until healthy granulation tissue — with slight bleeding — is seen.
- Haemostasis is secured. The wound is then flushed with normal saline.
- Hydrogen peroxide is also used (Fig. 23). This causes an exothermic reaction and helps to promote micro-haemostasis by coagulating fine capillaries.
- Final washing is done with normal saline (Fig. 24).

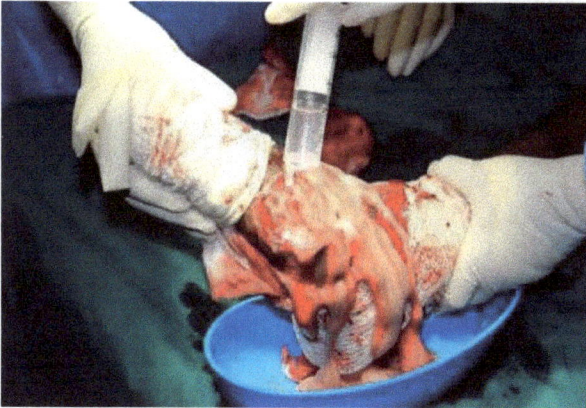

Figure 23. Flushing wound with hydrogen peroxide

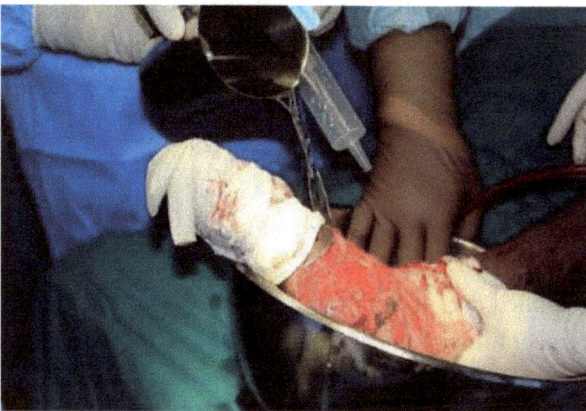

Figure 24. Final flushing of wound with normal saline

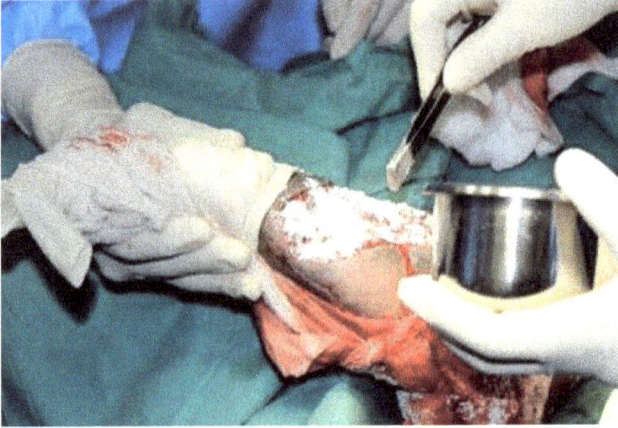

Figure 25. Antibiotic powder applied on recipient site

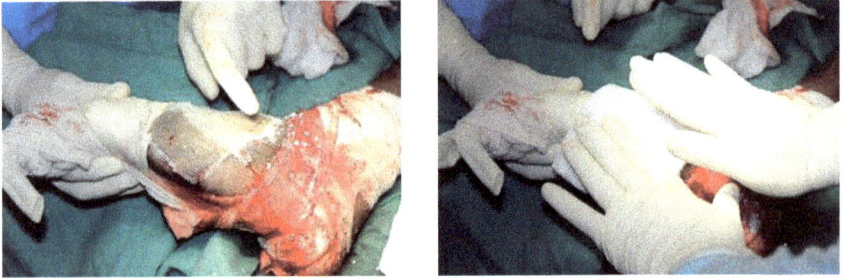

Figure 26. Applying prepared donor graft on recipient bed

- Antibiotic powder is applied on the recipient site (eg. Vancomycin powder) (Fig. 25).

Application of skin graft

- The prepared donor graft is applied on the recipient bed (Fig. 26).

Gauze technique

- Gauze is applied over the graft and is used to gently press the graft to fit the uneven contours of the wound.
- The skin graft is then stitched to the recipient site using 3-0 silk sutures (Fig. 27).

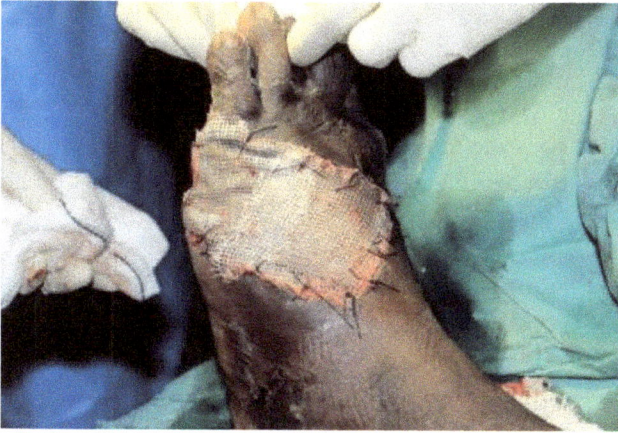

Figure 27. Stitching skin graft using 3-0 silk sutures

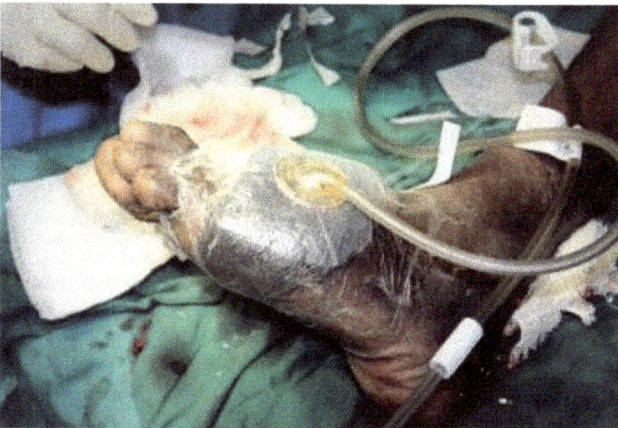

Figure 28. Applying VAC dressing

Application of VAC dressing for STSG

- VAC dressing is then applied (Fig. 28). When negative pressure is applied, the foam is sucked to fit the wound contours. This ensures that the skin is in close apposition to the wound bed.
- This technique is especially useful for large wounds or for wounds with uneven contours.

Post-operative Care

- A polyethylene ankle foot orthosis with the ankle in plantigrade position is applied
- Non-weight bearing must be strictly followed
- Wound is inspected on the 5th Post-Operative Day (POD)
- Tulle Gras dressing is applied

Excision of Osteomyelitic Bone

In diabetic foot, the most common bones involved with osteomyelitis are:

- Metatarsal head
- Proximal phalange
- Distal phalange
- Metatarsal base
- Calcaneum
- Lateral malleolus

For osteomyelitis involving the distal phalanx or the middle phalanx, it can be treated with a disarticulation of the toe — metatarso-phalangeal joint (MTPJ) disarticulation — if the infection has not spread to involve the soft tissue of the proximal phalanx.

Ray Amputation

Osteomyelitis commonly involves the metatarsal head or the proximal phalanx (Fig. 29). The first ray is commonly involved, followed by the fifth ray. There is pain over the metatarsal head on weight bearing. Changes can be seen on Radiographs, including periosteal reaction, radiolucency or area of bone destruction.

These are best treated by ray amputation, as described in the previous chapter. One must make sure that enough metatarsal bone is removed to ensure clearance of all infected tissue. Following the ray, where skin is available, closure is performed. It is good to plan the flaps so that volar skin can be preserved. Where skin loss is large, the ray amputation is left open.

Excision Arthroplasty of Metatarso-phalangeal Joint

In diabetic foot, septic arthritis most commonly involves the metatarso-phalangeal joint (MTPJ). The common sites involved are the ball of the

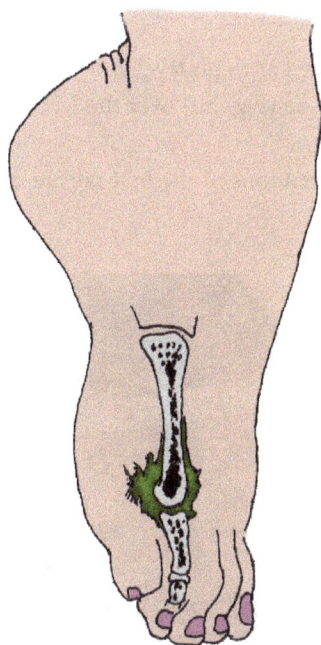

Figure 29.　Septic arthritis involving the 4th MTPJ

foot (first MTPJ) or the fifth MTPJ. Where the soft tissue infection is severe or advanced, one needs to do a ray amputation. However, for early MTPJ involvement without severe soft tissue infection, one can avoid a ray amputation and still get good results — by doing an excision arthroplasty of the joint involved. This is especially useful when patient refuses consent for a ray amputation. Most of our patients are not keen on losing even one digit, especially the big toe. In such a case, one could offer excision arthroplasty of the MTPJ of the big toe. For osteomyelitis involving the fifth toe, it is relatively easier to get consent for a fifth ray amputation.

Indications

- Septic arthritis involving MTPJ of the big toe or the little toe (1st MTPJ or 5th MTPJ)
- Presence of at least one palpable foot pulse (DP or PT)
- Patient refusing consent for a ray amputation

Operative Technique

1. A tourniquet is applied at thigh level and inflated.
2. The infected soft tissue (Fig. 30) over the MTPJ is debrided and excised (Fig. 31).
3. Extensor and flexor tendons of the first ray are excised.

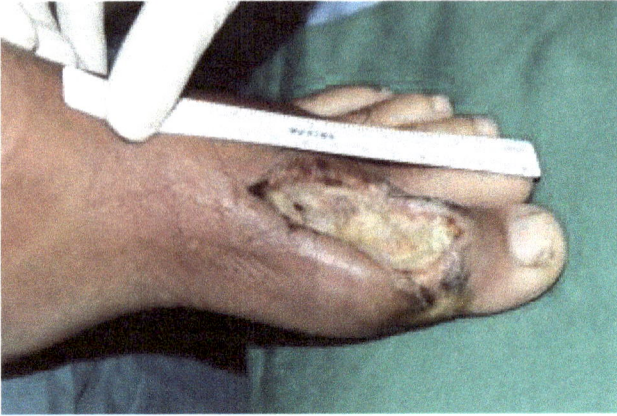

Figure 30.   Septic arthritis of MTPJ

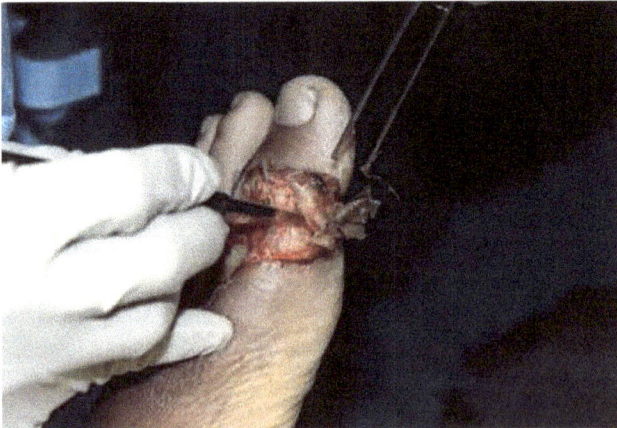

Figure 31.   Infected soft tissue and slough are radically debrided

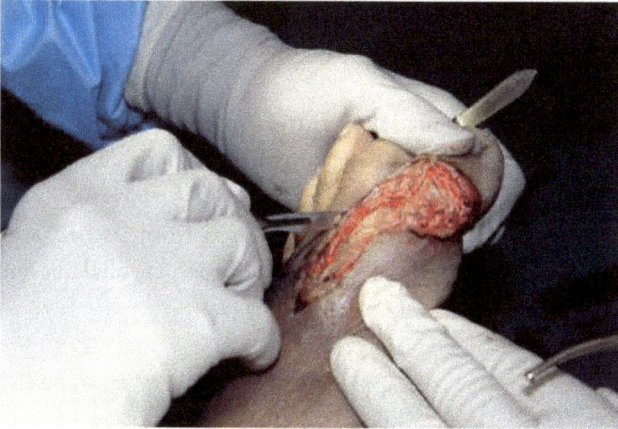

Figure 32. Healthy tissue remaining incised with a knife to expose metatarsal bone

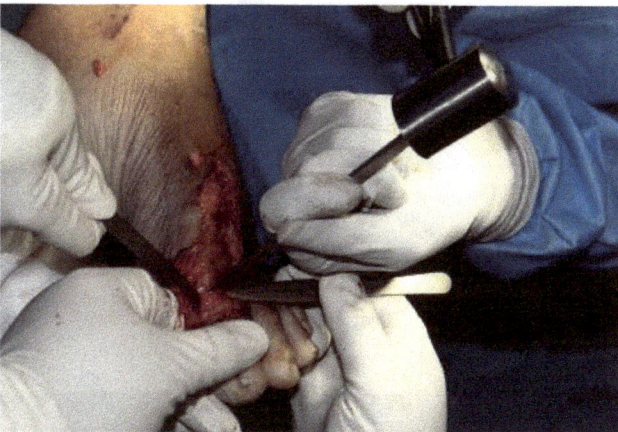

Figure 33. Osteotomy of the metatarsal bone using a small osteotome

4. Metatarsal bone is dissected and exposed (Fig. 32). The soft tissue on the medial and lateral side of the metatarsal bone is retracted using small Hohmann retractors.
5. Proximal osteotomy is made over the metatarsal bone, proximal to the site of osteomyelitis in the metatarsal head using a small osteotome (Fig. 33).

6. The proximal phalanx is dissected and exposed. The soft tissue on the medial and lateral side of the proximal phalanx is retracted using small Hohmann retractors.

7. Distal osteotomy is made over the proximal phalanx distal to the osteomyelitis in the base of the proximal phalanx using the osteotome (Fig. 34).

8. The distal part of the metatarsal is excised from its bed together with the MTPJ and the proximal part of the proximal phalanx and removed (Figs. 35a and 35b).

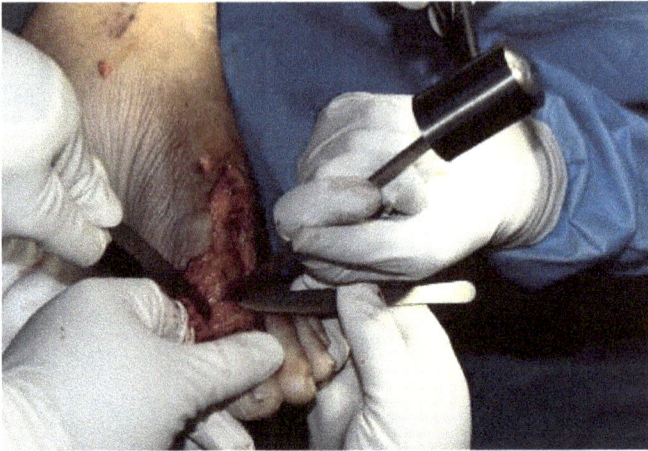

Figure 34.   Osteotomy of the proximal phalanx

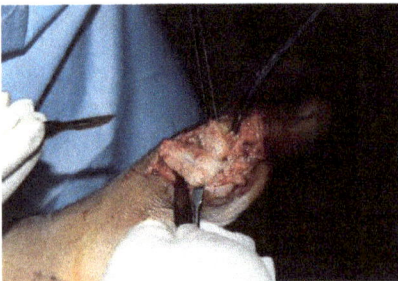

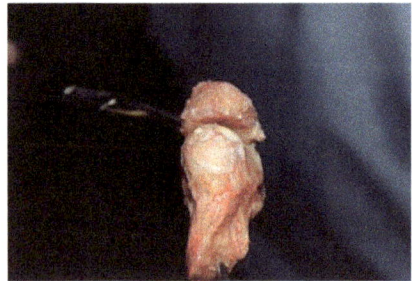

(a)   (b)

Figure 35.   (a) Metatarsal head MTPJ and proximal phalanx being excised. (b) Showing the metatarsal bone joint and proximal phalanx excised

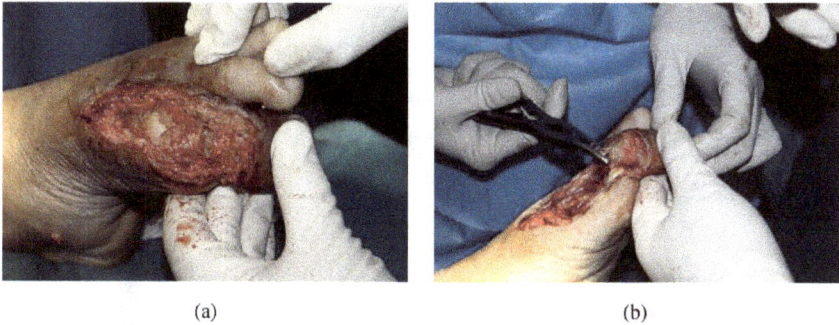

(a)

(b)

Figure 36. (a) Showing remnant metatarsal bone and proximal phalanx in wound bed. (b) Remaining metatarsal and proximal phalanx bone nibbled by a Bone Rongeur

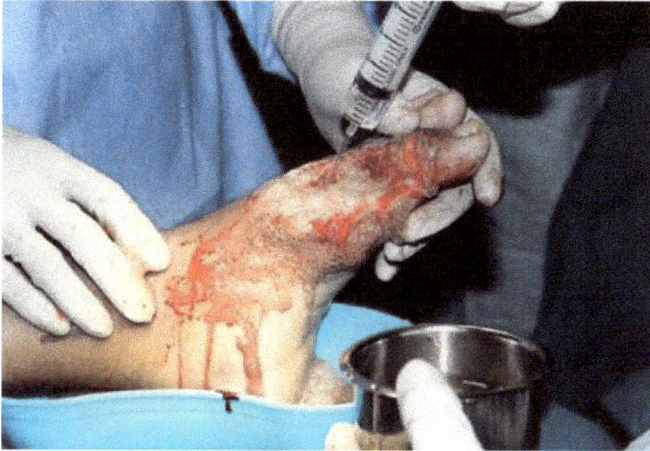

Figure 37. Wound bed is flushed with hydrogen peroxide, followed by saline

9. A piece of tissue from the infected bone and joint is sent for culture and sensitivity for aerobic and anaerobic organisms.
10. The bone edges of the metatarsal and the proximal phalanx left behind are nibbled or smoothened using a Bone Rongeur (Fig. 36b). Any other infected or devitalised tissue remaining is excised.
11. The wound bed is flushed with hydrogen peroxide and normal saline (Fig. 37). The tourniquet must be released at this point.
12. Good bleeding must be observed from the wound (Fig. 38). Haemostasis is secured.

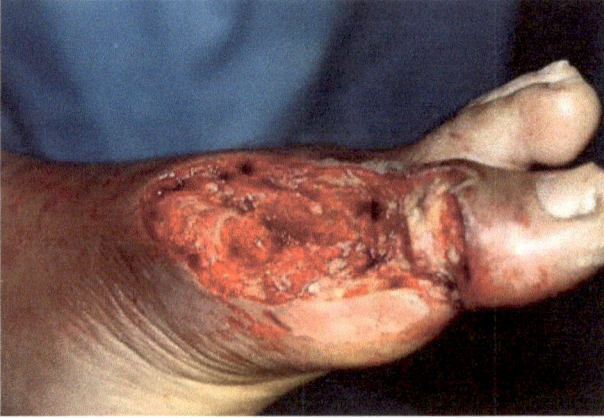

Figure 38.   Good bleeding from the wound bed after release of tourniquet

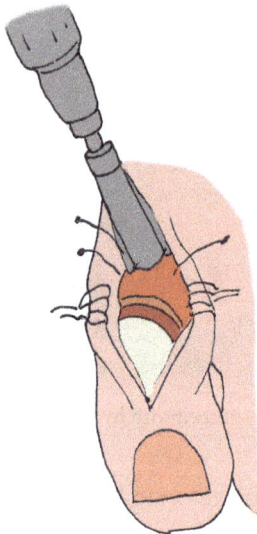

Figure 39a.   Osteotomy of metatarsal bone and proximal phalanx

13. Skin is closed with 3-0 Prolene.
14. Tulle Gras dressing is applied.

Below is an diagrammatic illustration of excision arthroplasty of the MTPJ (Figs. 39a to 39c).

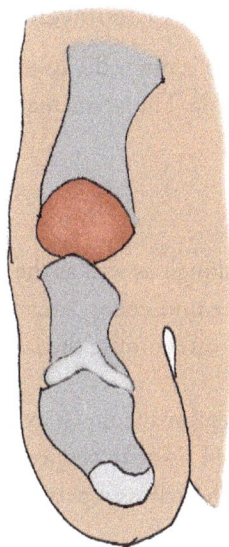

Figure 39b. Excision of MTPJ

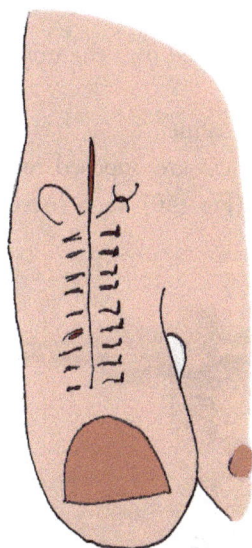

Figure 39c. Closure of the wound

Excision Lateral Malleolus for Osteomyelitis

Lateral malleolus osteomyelitis is often the result of a decubitus ulcer arising over the lateral aspect of the ankle. The lateral malleolus exposed has underlying osteomyelitis.

Procedure

1. The infected tissue and slough as well as the wound edge are excised and thoroughly debrided. The underlying lateral malleolus is exposed.
2. Use an oscillating saw to osteotomise the lateral malleolus well above the site of osteomyelitis.
3. The distal part of the lateral malleolus is excised.
4. Any infected or devitalised tissue in the wound is further excised.
5. The wound is flushed with hydrogen peroxide and saline. The tourniquet is removed at this point.
6. The ankle joint is usually exposed once the lateral malleolus is excised. This joint is compromised by infection and must be debrided.
7. Proximal osteotomy is performed over the lower end of the tibia to excise the articular surface.
8. Distal osteotomy is performed over the upper end of the talus to excise its articular surface.
9. The joint is flushed with saline.
10. The two raw bone surfaces are opposed to each other using Charnley Compression Clamps (Fig. 40) to achieve arthrodesis of the ankle (Fig. 41).

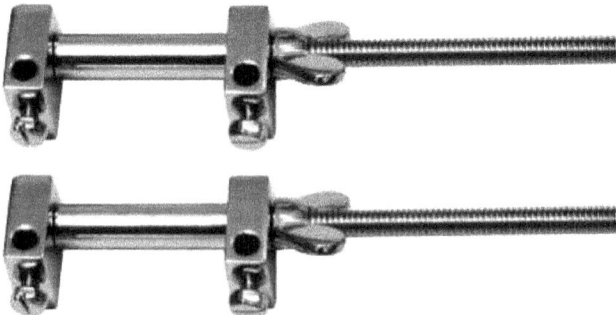

Figure 40. Charnley compression clamps

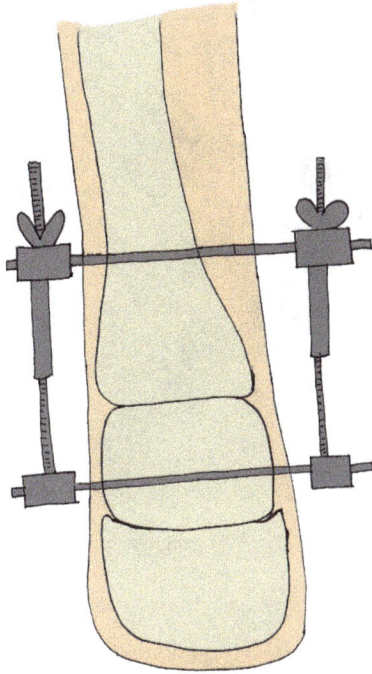

Figure 41. Ankle arthrodesis using charnley compression clamps

Partial Calcanectomy

This can be performed for:

- Wet or dry gangrene of the heel (Fig. 42)
- Osteomyelitis of calcaneum

Procedure

1. The infected tissue and ulcer are excised (Fig. 43).
2. The edge of the ulcer is completely excised to leave healthy skin edge.
3. All necrotic, infected or devitalised tissue is excised from the heel (Fig. 44).
4. The calcaneum is exposed (Fig. 45).
5. Using an oscillating saw, an oblique osteotomy is made above the osteomyelitic focus in the calcaneum (Figs. 46 and 47).
6. The infected calcaneum is then excised (Fig. 48).

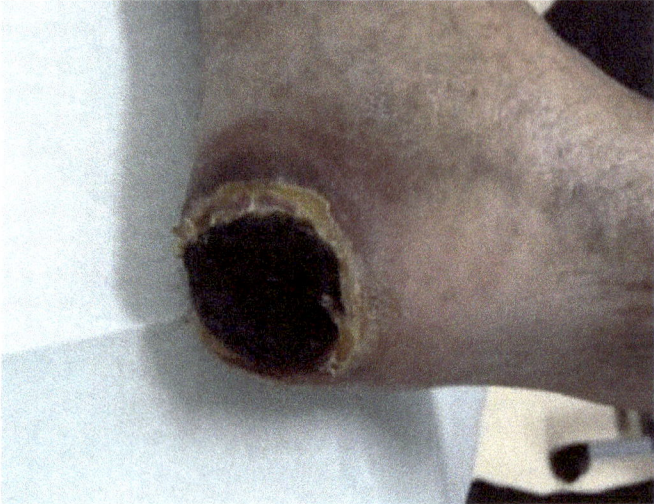

Figure 42. Wet gangrene of the heel

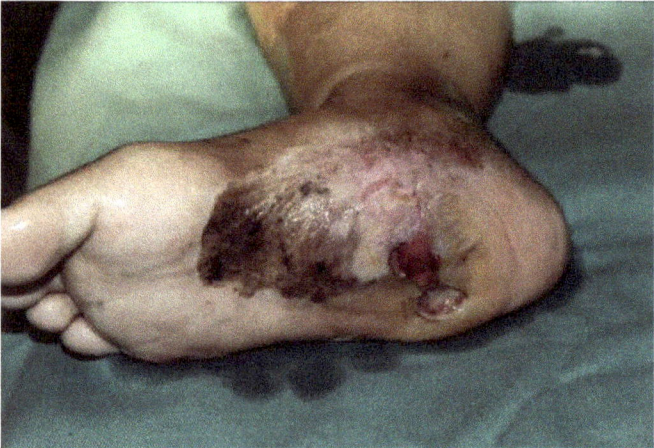

Figure 43. Charcot Joint Disease with infected ulcer and osteomyelitis involving the navicular and calcaneum bones

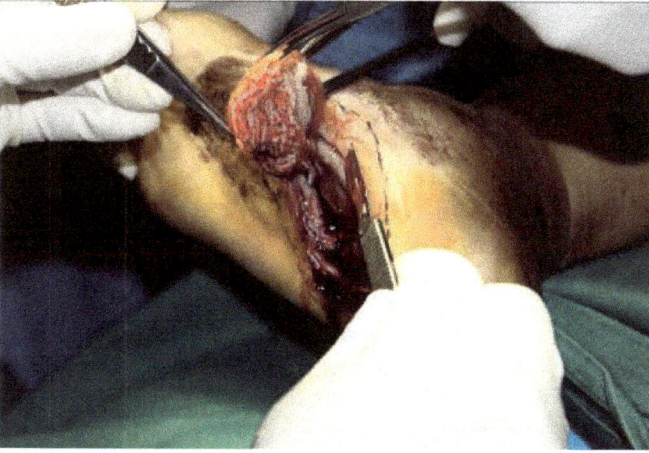

Figure 44. Excision of infected tissue

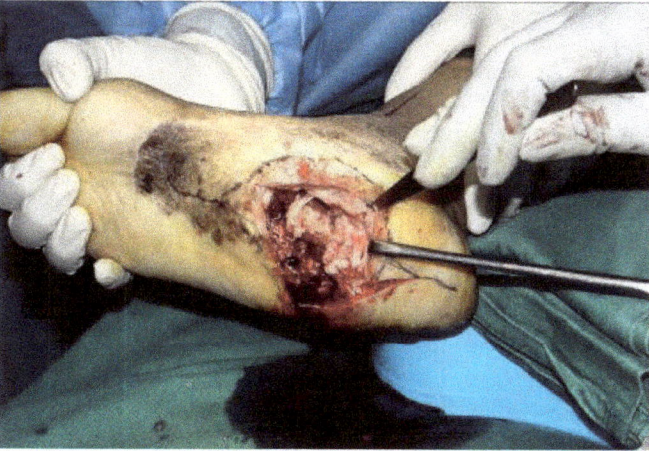

Figure 45. Calcaneum exposed

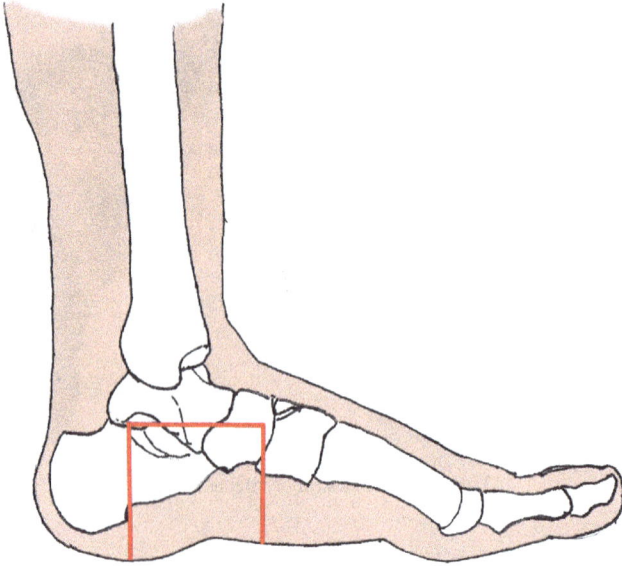

Figure 46. Osteotomy of calcaneum and navicular bone to remove the osteomyelitic focus

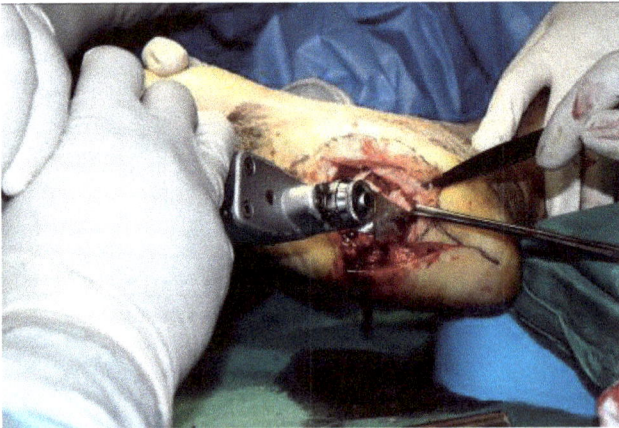

Figure 47. Making an oblique osteotomy

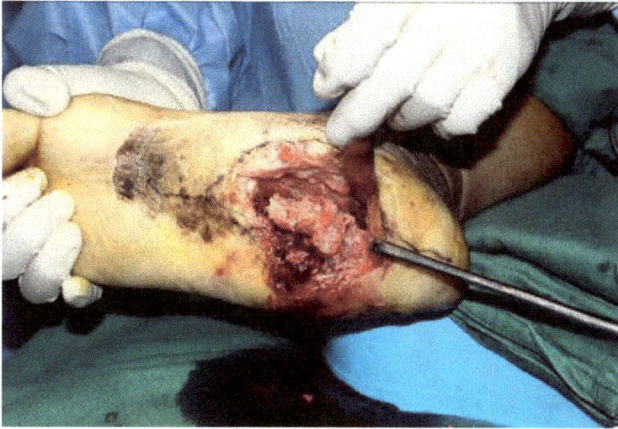

Figure 48. Excising infected calcaneum

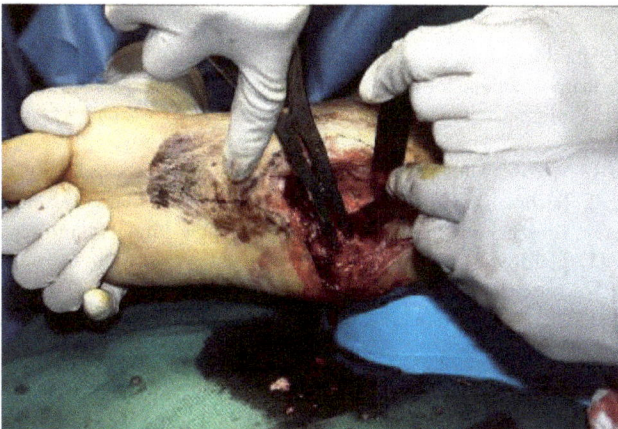

Figure 49. Nibbling bone edges with a Bone Rongeur

7. The wound is flushed with hydrogen peroxide and normal saline.
8. Torniquet is released and haemostasis is secured.
9. The edges of the bone are further nibbled using a Bone Rongeur (Fig. 49).
10. Where possible, the skin edges are loosely apposed (Fig. 50). Where not possible, VAC dressing is applied (wound prepared for later flap cover).

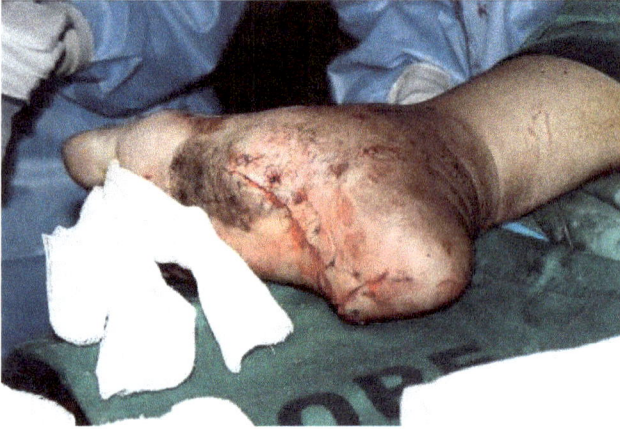

Figure 50. Skin edges loosely apposed

References

1. M. E. Edmonds, A. V. M. Foster and L. J. Sanders, *A Practical Manual of Diabetic Foot Care* (Blackwell Publishing, 2008).
2. D. Leaper, Sharp technique for wound debridement, *World Wide Wounds* (2002).
3. M. O'Brien, Exploring methods of wound debridement, *Br. J. Community Nurs.* **Dec**:10–18 (2002).
4. M. Kubo, L. Van de Water, L. C. Plantefaber, M. W. Mosesson, M. Simon, M. G. Tonnesen, L. Taichman and R. A. Clark, Fibrinogen and fibrin are anti-adhesive for keratinocytes: a mechanism for fibrin eschar and slough during wound repair, *J. Invest. Dermatol.* **117**(6):1369–81 (2001).
5. D. Weir, P. Scarborough and J. A. Niezgoda, Wound debridement. In: D. L. Krasner, G. T. Rodeheaver and R. G. Sibbald (eds.), *Chronic Wound Care: A Clinical Source Book for Health Professionals*, 4th Edition (HMP Communications, Pennsylvania, 2008).

Section 7

Wound Care

25

Assessment of Diabetic Wounds

Aziz Nather and Teo Zhen Ling

Department of Orthopaedic Surgery
Yong Loo Lin School of Medicine
National University of Singapore

Introduction

Good wound management is an important part of diabetic foot treatment. To effectively manage wounds, one must understand the basic science of wound healing. Appropriate treatment can only be provided after careful assessment has been completed.

Initial Wound Assessment

The wound is assessed according to the following:

- *Site*
- *Size*
- *Shape*
- *Edge of wound*
- *Floor of wound*
- *Contents of ulcer*
- *Condition of adjacent skin*

In addition, the foot must be assessed for:

- *Vasculopathy*

The key markers are:

- Capillary refill (>2 seconds)
- Temperature (cold)
- Colour (Pallor)
- Pulses:
    - Dorsalis Pedis (not palpable)
    - Posterior Tibial (not palpable)
- ABI: Ankle Brachial Index (<0.8)
- TBI: Toe Brachial Index (<0.7)
- Pulse oximeter readings

Is there sufficient perfusion to nourish the wound?

- *Sensory neuropathy*

The key markers are:

- 10 point SWNT (< 7/10)
- Vibration Perception Threshold (>25V)
- Position sense

Is there biomechanical loading?
An ulcer at a weight-bearing portion of the foot — over metatarsal head, must be off-loaded before it can heal.

- *Immunopathy*

Look for underlying deep infection:

- Abscess
- Osteomyelitis of metatarsal head
- Septic Arthritis

Look for radiological changes:

- Destruction of Bone: Osteomyelitis of Metatarsal Head
- Destruction of adjacent bones in a joint: Septic arthritis
- Gas in subcutaneous tissue: Necrotising Fasciitis

Assess the markers for infection:

➤ TWC: Total White cell count ($>10 \times 10^9$/L)
➤ ESR: Erythrocyte Sedimentation Rate (>100 mm/hr)
➤ CRP: C-Reactive Protein (>10 mg/L)

Assess the patient for renal failure:

Patients with renal failure are immunocompromised. In ensuring adequate nutritional uptake for wound healing, renal failure poses a big challenge. It gives a very poor prognosis. The indicators for renal failure are:

➤ Urea (>25 mg/dL)
➤ Creatinine (>2 mg/dL or $>177\,\mu$mol/L)

Types of Wounds

The wound can be classified as:

- Healthy
- Infected
- Ischaemic
- Infected and Ischaemic
- Neuropathic
- Decubitus

Healthy wound

A healthy wound (Figs. 1 and 2) is filled with granulation tissue. The wound edge and floor are pink or red in colour. It has a textured and shiny appearance and bleeds readily. There is no slough or pus.

Infected wound

An infected wound (Figs. 3 and 4) contains slough and pus or inflammatory exudate. The skin around the wound is inflamed.

Ischaemic wound

An ischaemic wound (Figs. 5 and 6) may present with a necrotic edge or necrotic tissue in the floor of the wound.

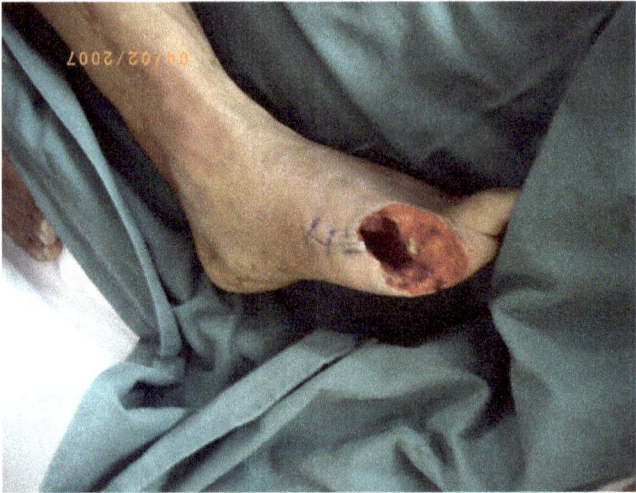

Figure 1.   Good healing of an open wound

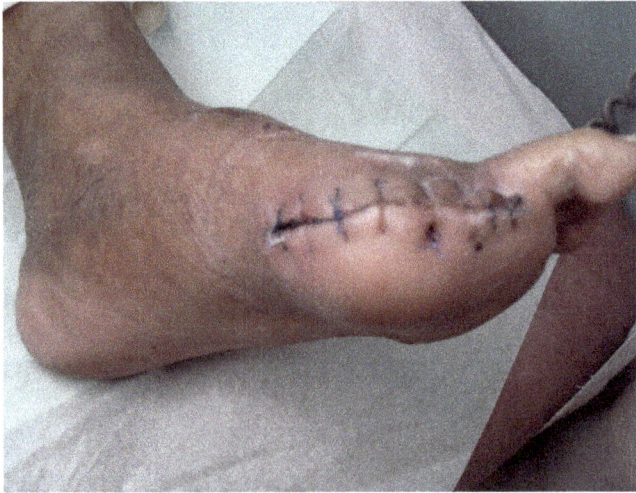

Figure 2.   Good healing of a closed wound

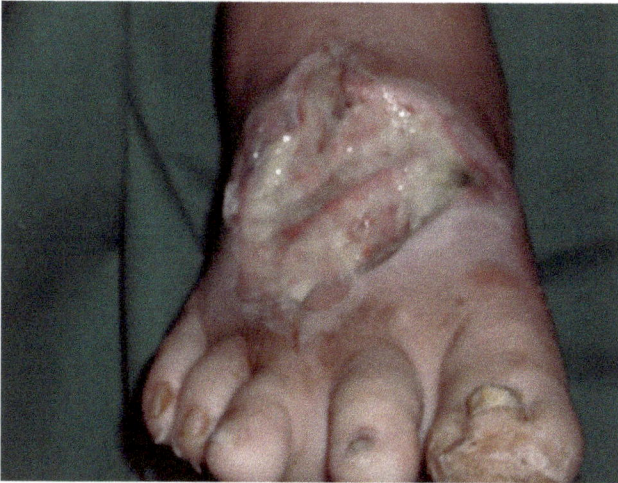

Figure 3. Ulcer at dorsum of foot, with slough and exudate

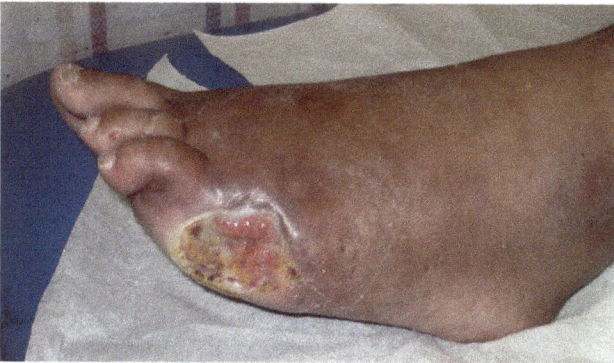

Figure 4. Ulcer over the 5th metatarsal head with slough. Cellulitis of the adjacent skin

Infected and ischaemic wound

In some wounds, both infection and ischaemia are present (Figs. 7 and 8).

Neuropathic ulcer[1]

A neuropathic ulcer (Figs. 9 and 10) has a callosity in the edge of the wound, caused by repetitive pressure. With sensory neuropathy, the patient does not

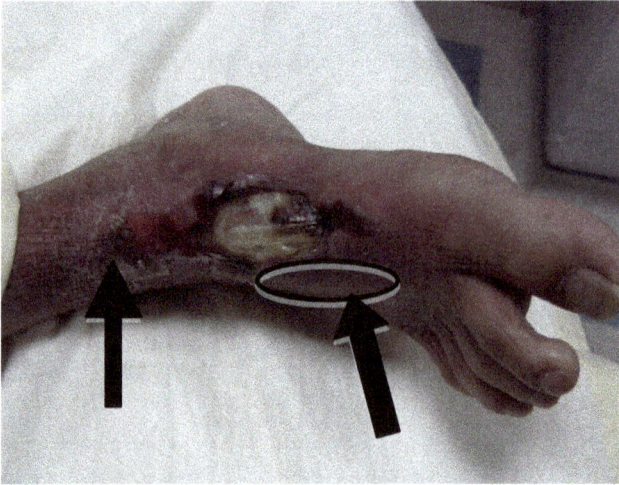

Figure 5. Ulcer over dorsum of foot and ankle. Necrotic edges and slough at wound floor present

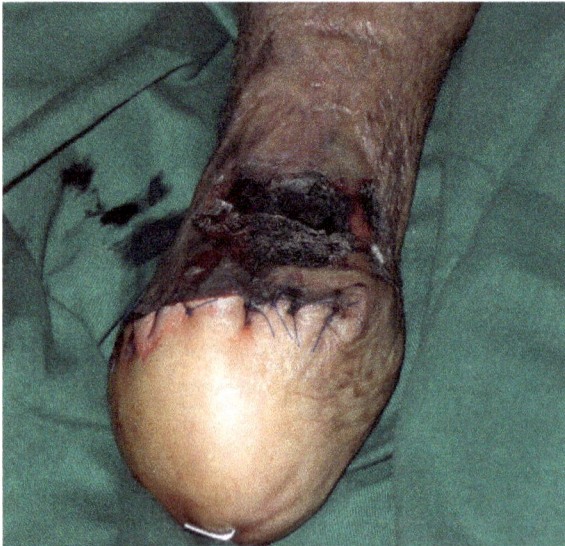

Figure 6. Necrosis of anterior part of Pirogoff's amputation stump

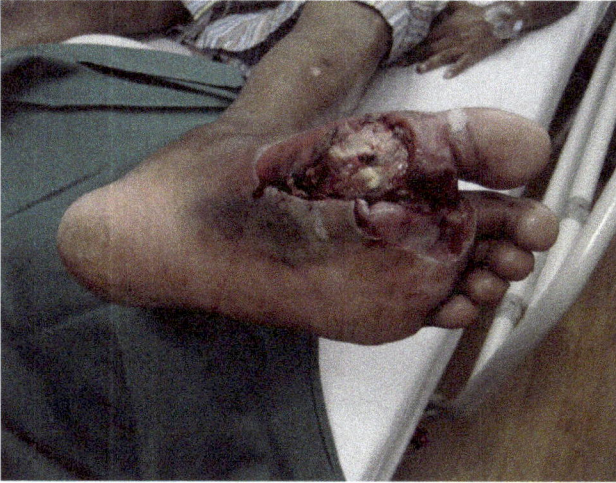

Figure 7. Ulcer at sole of foot with necrosis and slough

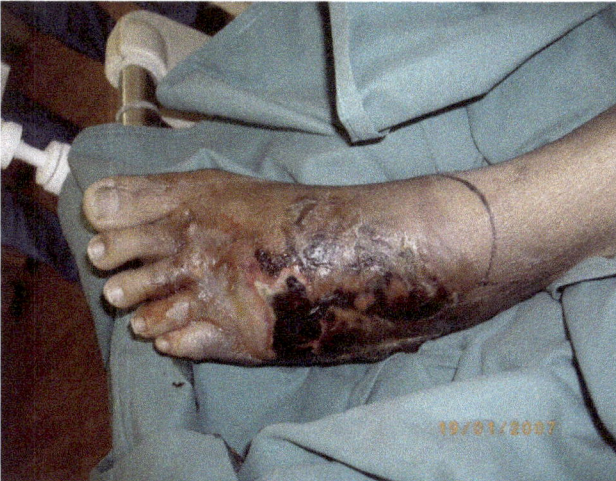

Figure 8. Necrosis of skin at dorsum of foot with cellulitis

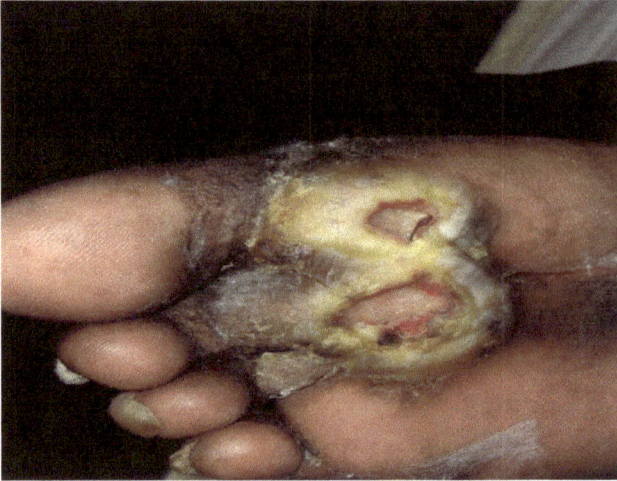

Figure 9. Callosity over head of 1st and 2nd metatarsal

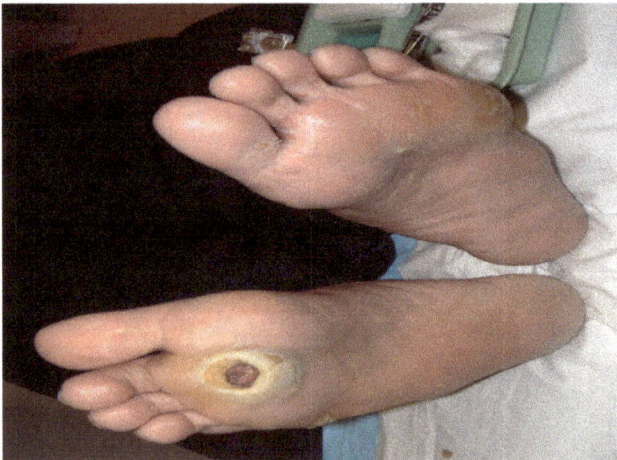

Figure 10. Callosity over 2nd metatarsal head

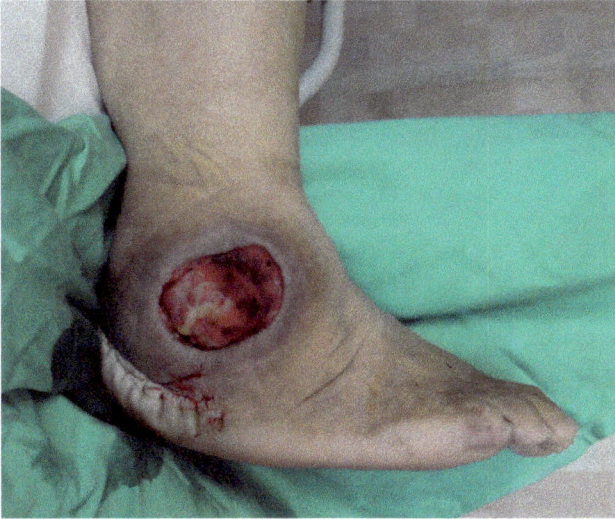

Figure 11. Decubitus ulcer over lateral malleolus

experience pain. A neuropathic ulcer is most commonly found in the sole of the foot.

Decubitus ulcer[2]

A decubitus ulcer is a pressure ulceration due to immobility. Decubitus ulcers are most commonly found over:

- Lateral malleolus (Fig. 11)
- Lateral aspect of base of 5th metatarsal (Fig. 12)
- The heel (Fig. 13)

Assessment of Nutrition

Good nutrition is vital for wound healing. The wound needs oxygen and nutrients such as proteins for healing. PEM[3] is often seen in elderly patients with chronic wounds.

The two markers for good wound healing are:

- Haemoglobin level
  — Hb levels must be more than 10.0 g/dL

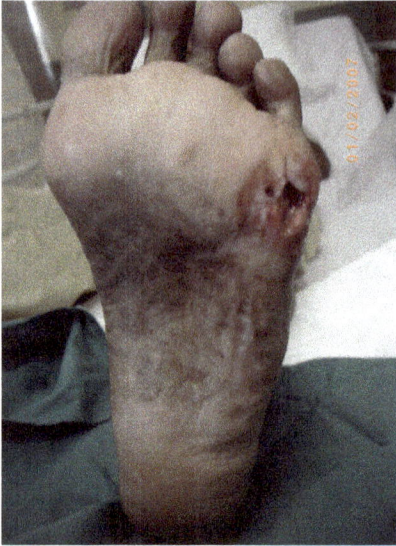

Figure 12. Decubitus ulcer over base of 5th metatarsal

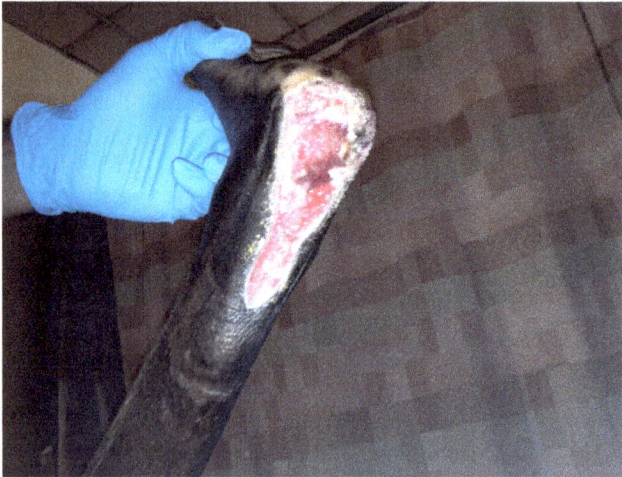

Figure 13. Decubitus ulcer over the heel

— Normal range:

> ➢ 13.8–17.2 g/dL (male)
> ➢ 12.1–15.1 g/dL (female)

- Albumin level

    — Albumin levels must be greater than 38 g/L
    — Normal range: 38–48 g/L

Assessment of Endocrine Control

Endocrine control is important as uncontrolled high blood glucose levels can impair wound healing. Hyperglycaemia can prolong the inflammatory phase of wound healing, thus delaying the phases of proliferation and maturation.

The 2 key indicators for endocrine control are:

- HbA1c

    — Normal range is 3.5–5.5 %

- Hypocount monitoring

    — Normal range is 4.0–7.8 mmol/L
    — Tds +10pm (readings taken 3 times daily + at 10pm)

Repeating Wound Assessment

The wound must be inspected daily to monitor the progress of wound healing.

Choosing the Right Antibiotic

After assessing the culture and sensitivity results, the appropriate antibiotics are selected. Common pathogens include:

Staphylococcus aureus: Thick, brownish-white, odourless discharge
Pseudomonas aeruginosa: Greenish discharge with a "rotten fruit" smell
Bacteroides fragilis: Faecal smelling discharge

These are the characteristics. One can start the appropriate antibiotics such as cloxacillin, ciprofloxacin and flagyl respectively, once the culture is taken. There is no need to wait for 3 days till the culture results become available.

Decision for Surgery

Upon completion of the assessment of the wound, the surgeon must decide whether surgery is needed. The type of surgery required includes:

- Surgical debridement of the wound (Fig. 14)
- Ray Amputation: 1 or more (Fig. 15)

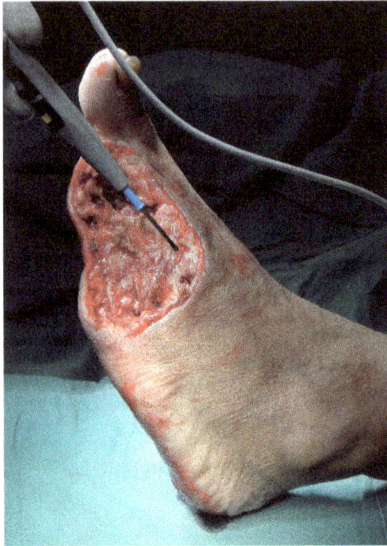

Figure 14. Surgical debridement of ulcer at dorsum foot

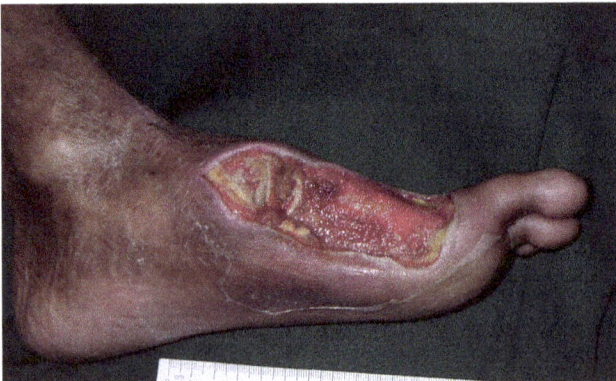

Figure 15. 1st and 2nd ray amputation

➢ At least 1 distal pulse must be palpable for the amputation wound to heal

• Excision Arthroplasty of the Metatarso-phalangeal joint (MTPJ)
• Transmetatarsal/Midfoot amputation

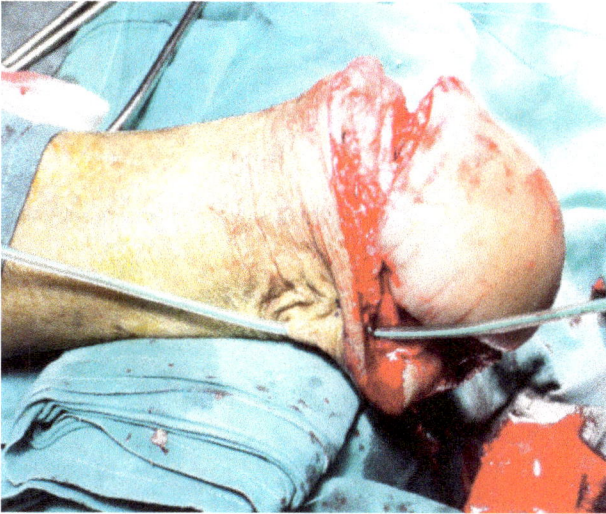

Figure 16. Pirogoff amputation

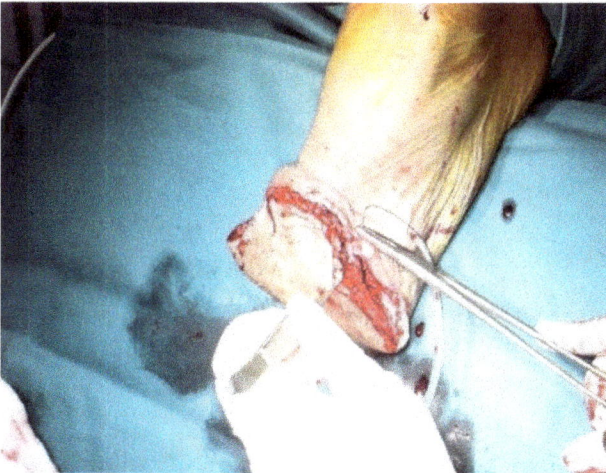

Figure 17. Below knee amputation

- ➤ At least 1 distal pulse must be palpable
- Syme's/Pirogoff's/ Boyd's (Fig. 16)
  - ➤ At least 1 Distal pulse must be palpable
- Major amputation needs to be performed when both distal pulses are not palpable and revascularisation surgery is not possible.
  - ➤ BKA (Fig. 17)

References

1. M. E. Levin, Management of the diabetic foot, *South Med. J.* **95**(1):article 426899_4 (2002, Medscape news).
2. D. Bluestein and A. Javaheri, Pressure ulcers: prevention, evaluation and management, *Am Fam Physician* 78(10):1186–94 (2008).
3. R. H. Demling and L. DeSanti, Protein energy malnutrition and the non-healing cutaneous wound, Article 418377 (2003, Medscape Education).

26

Types of Dressings for Diabetic Foot Ulcers

Tiffany Tsao

Senior Podiatrist
Head of Podiatric Department
Rehabilitation Medicine Department
National University Hospital

Introduction

The concept of using a wound dressing to heal wounds started in 1960. It is believed that wound healing is achieved by keeping the wound dry to form crust and skin scab.[1] This concept has evolved and changed in the last few decades through evidence-based practice. Wound healing achieved its optimal stage by maintaining a moisture-balanced environment. Moisture-balanced environment is essential for a wound to heal and to prevent scar formation. This is achieved by application of a good wound dressing. An ideal wound dressing should have the following properties:

(a) absorb wound exudate;
(b) maintain a balanced environment moisture;
(c) protect viable tissue;
(d) provide thermal insulation;
(e) provide a barrier against bacteria (Fig. 1).

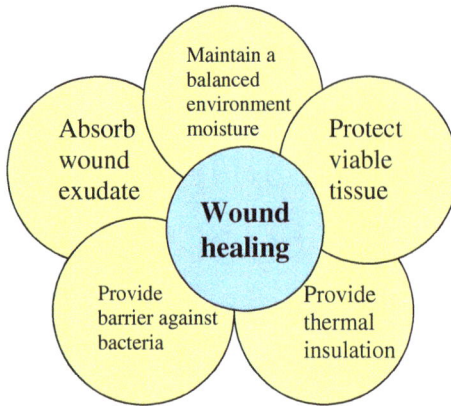

Figure 1.   Five important components to aid wound healing

Dressing Type

Several wound dressings are available in Singapore. Many people asked whether it is important to have all kinds of dressing on hand before starting a practice for wound care. The answer depends on whether the institute has the budget, and the professional training of the personnel managing the wound.

Common Wound Healing Products in Singapore

There are 6 types of wound dressings:

- Transparent films
- Hydrocolloids
- Foams
- Absorptive cavity wound fillers
- Hydrogels
- Collagens
- Antimicrobials

The types of dressings in each group commonly used are listed in Table 1.

Transparent Films (Fig. 2)

This dressing is inexpensive and commonly used in an inpatient setting. It is not absorbent and provides total occlusion to the wound. It can be used

Table 1. Types of dressings

Group	Product	Company
Transparent films	Opsite	Smith & Nephew
	Tegaderm	3M
	Mepore	Molnlycke
Hydrocolloids	Duoderm	ConvaTec
	Intrasite	Smith & Nephew
	Tegasorb	3M
Foams	Allevyn	Smith & Nephew
	Biatain	Coloplast
	Lyofoam	ConvaTec
	Mepilex	Molnlycke
	Polymem	Ferris
	Tielle	Systagenix
Absorptive cavity wound fillers	AlgiSite M	Smith & Nephew
	Comfeel SeaSorb	Coloplast
	Kaltostat	ConvaTec
	Melgisorb	Molnlycke
	Aquacel	ConvaTec
	Mesalt	Molnlycke
Hydrogels	Purilon gel	Coloplast
	DuoDerm Hydroactive	ConvaTec
	NuGel	Systagenix
Collagens	Prisma	Systagenix
	Fish Collagen	Origin
Antimicrobials	Acticoat	Smith & Nephew
	Acticoat Flex	
	Acticoat Absorbent	
	Iodosorb	Smith & Nephew
	Aquacel Ag	ConvaTec
	Seasorb Ag	Coloplast
	Mepilex Ag	Molnlycke

to perform autolytic debridement for wound bed preparation.[2] Transparent films provide a good skin protection and allow visual assessment. They are waterproof, flexible and easy to apply. The indication is for dry to minimal exudating wounds. Contraindications include infected wounds, heavy wound exudate and wounds over bony prominence.

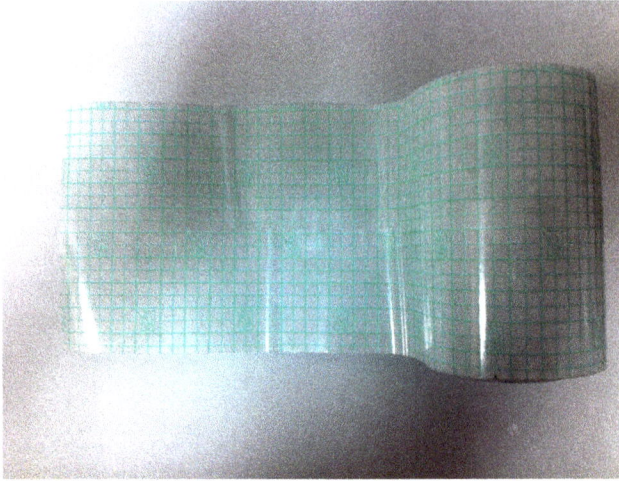

Figure 2.   Transparent film

Hydrocolloids (Fig. 3)

Hydrocolloid dressing is often used as a waterproof barrier and as a wafer to protect the wound from exogenous bacteria or friction. The active ingredient interacts with the wound exudate or fluid and forms a gel to maintain moisture and hydration level. Gelatin, pectin or carboxymethylcellulose are often seen as the main components in hydrocolloid dressing.[3] Hydrocolloids are indicated for low to moderate exudating wounds and for prevention of tissue hydration. Contraindications include wounds with heavy fluid and possible sinus tracking or infection.

Foams

Foam dressing (Fig. 4) is the most versatile dressing for wound care management. It is highly absorbent, flexible and protects the wound for up to 7 days upon application. Foam dressing is indicated for mild to heavy exudating wounds. The technology uses polyurethane as the ingredient, which allows high moisture vapor transmission rate and prevents tissue from undergoing hypoxia.[4,5] It is contraindicated in dry wounds. Such a dressing has strong absorbency ability and may cause trauma and friction on fragile skin upon dressing removal. Foam dressing is one of the most common dressings used.

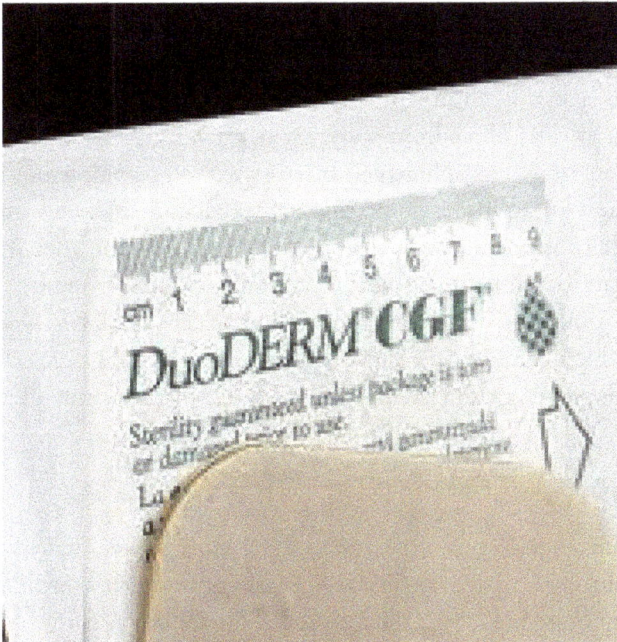

Figure 3. Hydrocolloids

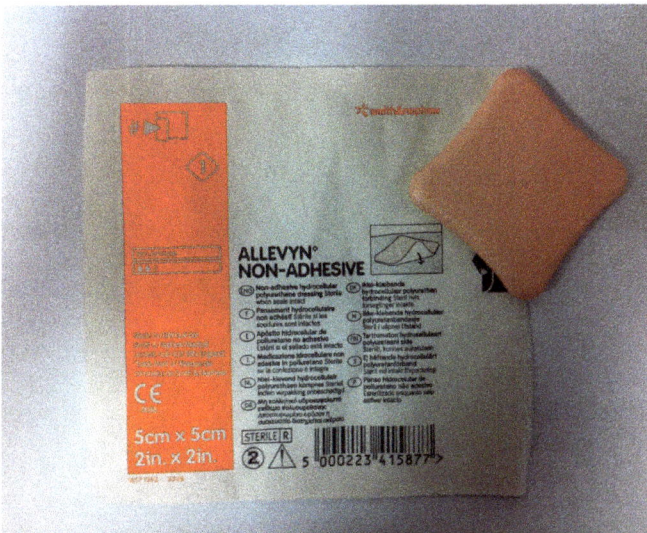

Figure 4. Foam dressing

Absorptive Cavity Wound Fillers (Fig. 5)

Absorptive wound filler, or sometimes referred to as Alginate Calcium Dressing, is a highly absorbent, biodegradable dressing. Alginate Calcium Dressing derives its fibres from seaweed. It provides a high absorbency rate and forms a strong hydrophilic gel. It limits wound secretion and minimises possible bacterial contamination. Alginate Calcium Dressing maintains a physiologically moist micro-environment, which promotes wound healing and stimulates granulation tissue formation in chronic wounds. It can also be used for prothrombotic coagulation and platelet activation in wound care.[6] It contains high content of calcium ions linked to mannuronic or guluronic groups. This provides good haemostasis to stop the wound from bleeding after surgery.

Collagens

Collagen dressings (Fig. 6) are commonly used in United States of America and Australia. There are only limited number of products available locally as the costs are quite high. The collagen dressings are derived from fish, bovine or porcine sources from human placenta. Some products incorporate alginate, hydrogel or silver ingredients. Studies have claimed that adding exogenous

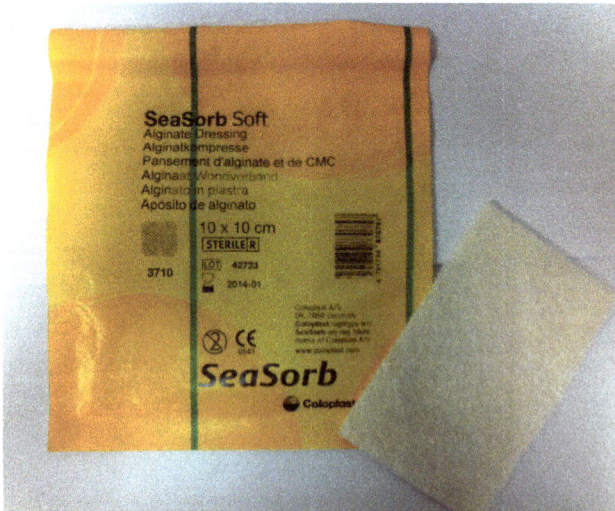

Figure 5.   Absorptive cavity wound filler

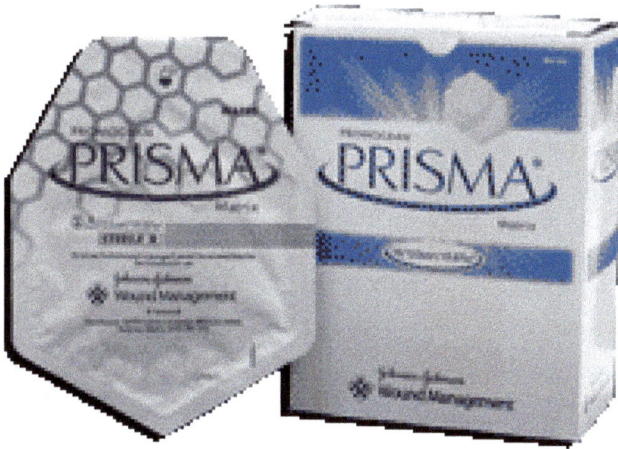

Figure 6. Collagen dressing

collagen to a wound promotes both haemostasis and chemotasis. Collagen dressing acts as matrices for new cells to grow into thereby promoting wound healing.[7] Collagen dressing also provides a high absorbency to the wound. It is indicated for wounds that are clean and not containminated. It is best used post surgical debridement or ultrasonic debridement. The dressing is only used as a primary dressing and needs to have an absorbent secondary dressing. It may be used for up to seven days.[8]

Antimicrobials

Antimicrobials (Fig. 7), also known as silver dressings are ideal to use for heavily contaminated and infected wounds.[9] The dressing is used for reducing the number of bacterial counts and controls the bacterial burden in the wound. When an antimicrobial dressing is in contact with the wounds, it starts to absorb fluid. It unlocks the silver content from the dressing and slowly releases silver ions into the wound to kill bacteria. Antimicrobial dressing contains silver ions with a broad-spectrum activity against many microorganisms. Pathogens such as the two common super bugs, which are Methicillin-Resistant *Staphylococcus Aureus* (MRSA) and Vancomycin-Resistant Enterococci (VRE).[10] Antimicrobial dressing is indicated for infected wounds. However all patients with infection should also be treated primarily with systemic antibiotic therapy in addition to adequate surgical debridement.

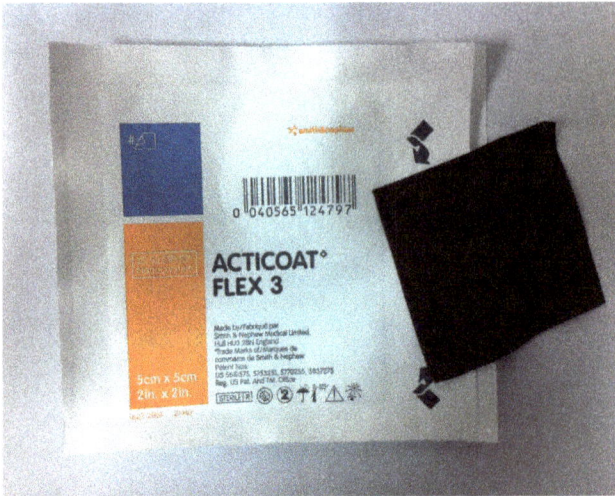

Figure 7.   Antimicrobial dressing

In summary, the ideal dressing should provide adequate absorption rate, provide a moisture balance wound environment, eliminate dead space; does not harm the wound; and lastly provides thermal insulation and a barrier to the wound against bacteria. Selection of the appropriate dressing is critical for optimal wound healing. Wound dressing can only be used as an adjunct in treatment plan. Treating the underlying problem is still the most essential part to achieve optimal wound healing.

References

1. C. Y. Cho and J. S. Lo, Dressing the part, *Dermatol. Clin.* **16**(1):25–47 (1998).
2. M. Mulder, The selection of wound care products for wound bed preparation, *Prof. Nurs. Today* **15**(6):30–6 (2011).
3. L. G. Ovington, The well-dressed wound: an overview of dressing types, *Wounds* **10**(Suppl A):1A–11A (1998).
4. G. D. Mulder, Standardizing wound treatment procedures for advanced technologies, *J. Am. Podiatr. Med. Assoc.* **92**:7–11 (2002).
5. S. Palamand, R. A. Brenden and A. M. Reed, Intelligent wound dressings and their physical characteristics, *Wounds* **3**:149–56 (1992).
6. T. Gilchrist and A. M. Martin, Wound treatment with Sorbsan — an alginate fibre dressing, *Biomaterials* **4**(4):317–20 (1983).
7. O. J. Lorenzetti, B. Fortenberry, E. Busby and R. Uberman, Influence of microcrystalline collagen on wound healing. I. Wound closure of normal excised and burn excised wounds of rats, rabbits, and pigs, *Proc. Soc. Exp. Biol. Med.* **140**(3):896–900.

8. S. K. Purna and M. Babu, Collagen based dressings: a review, *Burns* **26**:54–62 (2000).

9. J. B. Wright, D. L. Hansen and R. E. Burrell, The comparative efficacy of two antimicrobial barrier dressings: *in vitro* examination of two controlled release silver dressings, *Wounds* **10**(6):179–88 (1998).

10. J. B. Wright, K. Lam and R. E. Burrell, Wound management in an era of increasing bacterial antibiotic resistance: a role for topical silver treatment, *Am. J. Infect. Control* **26**(6):572–7 (1998).

27

New Generation Dressings

Aziz Nather and Chris Lee Choon Wei

Department of Orthopaedic Surgery
Yong Loo Lin School of Medicine
National University of Singapore, Singapore

Introduction

In the last decade a large variety of new generation wound dressings have appeared on the market for treating diabetic wounds. The trend includes the use of silver as an anti-microbial agent impregnated in the dressings as well as other anti-microbial agents such as iodine. Dressings are also now designed to support moist wound healing. For this, various materials have been used including alginate, hydrofibre, foams, soft silicone and Ringer's solution. Wound care product specialists from the private sector now play an important role in the healing of our diabetic wounds. The health care professionals or wound nurses treating the wounds must study the characteristics of the wounds to choose the appropriate dressing that best suits the individual needs of a particular wound. This chapter serves a very important purpose — namely to make health care professionals treating diabetic wounds to be aware of the availability of these new generation dressings that have been designed using the latest technology.

Use of the Silver Absorbent Dressing* in the Management of Surgical Amputations of the Foot in Diabetic Patients

Authors: N. Tagand, F. Ouliac and C. Salomon

Introduction

In diabetic patients infections take hold with increased frequency in established wounds of neuropathic and/or ischemic origin: perforating ulcer of the foot or distal ischemic necrosis. The development of secondary infection in the diabetic foot represents a particularly unfavourable turning point in the course of the condition, since it leads to a high number of foot amputations. Do we need to remind ourselves that infection is the cause of 30 to 40% of amputations in diabetics? Deep infections of the foot are dominated by the development of osteitis, quickly complicated by osteomyelitis, spreading the infection to the bone segment. The picture may be even more alarming if there is also extension to the fascias, requiring more extensive surgical debridement. The author reports her experience in the management of surgical diabetic foot amputations. The situations presented are stagnations in the healing process, which may have lasted for several months, following initially inappropriate treatment versus appropriate and early management. In our specialised department, management of this type of wound combines general measures (non-weight bearing on the wound, control of blood glucose levels, coordination of home care), with careful local wound care: debridement or cleaning of necrotic or fibrinous tissue, use of silver-containing dressings in the event of suspected significant bacterial colonisation before the onset of local inflammatory signs. It is in this latter indication that we use URGOCELL® Silver, a hydrocellular dressing combined with a silver lipido-colloid interface.

---

*Brand name: The antibacterial absorbent dressing is URGOCELL® Silver (Cellosorb® Ag) from Laboratoires URGO.

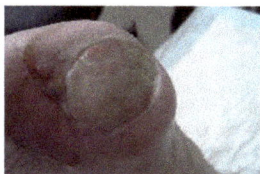

On admission (D0) on 22/08/2007: Fibrinous, foul-smelling wound covered with a greenish-whitecoating with peripheral oedema. Immediate offloading (Barouk shoe), local debridement and Silver absorbent dressing* given the clinical context.

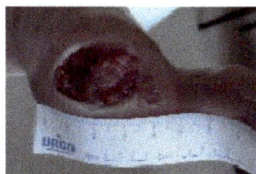

W1 (30/08/07): Total debridement of the wound and disappearance of inflammatory signs of local infection. Bulky fleshy buds are filling the cavity.

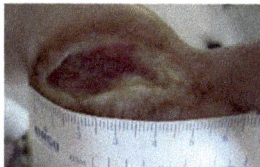

Appearance at W3 (15/09/07): Levelling of granulation tissue and peripheral epidermal mobilisation.

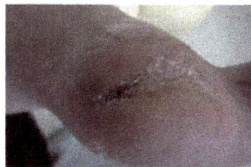

W8 (24/10/07): Definitive healing.

Patient No. 1: Sixty-three-year-old diabetic male patient, admitted to the department two months after amputation of the left big toe due to non-improvement of his wound.

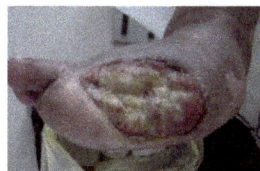

1st consultation (D0) on 29/03/2007:The wound measures 8 cm x 4 cm, covered with adherent fibrinous deposits requiring mechanical debridement (bistoury and dissecting tweezers). Prescription of Silver absorbent dressing* to be repeated daily at home then every two days depending on the course of the exudate.

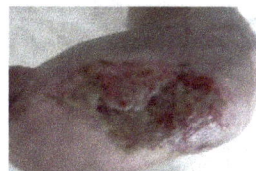

W4 (26/04/2007): Gradual debridement of the wound and satisfactory granulation. Start of peripheral epidermal margination.

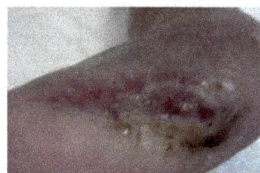

W10 (07/06/2007): Levelling of granulation and epidermal progression. The wound surface area has been reduced by half in comparison with the initial surface area.

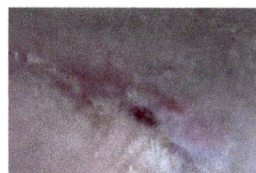

W15 (12/07/2007): Close-up on definitive healing.

Patient No. 2: Big toe post amputation wound in a 69-year-old male diabetic patient on dialysis managed as part of a wound consultation at the request of the Infectious Department.

---

*Brand name: The antibacterial absorbent dressing is URGOCELL® Silver (Cellosorb® Ag) from Laboratoires URGO.

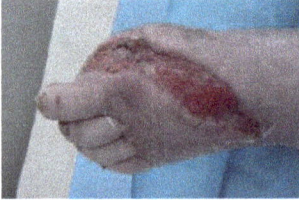

D0: The patient leaves on 28/08/2007 with a Silver absorbent dressing* and offloading of the foot using a Baroukshoe. The wound is deep, atonic and exuding.

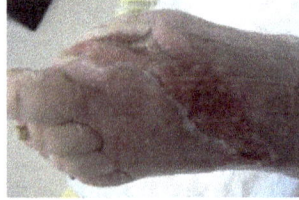

W1: Consultation of 03/09/2007: The wound measures 16.7 cm^2 and remains highly exuding with a fibrinous coating in places. Good-quality granulation and epidermal migration.

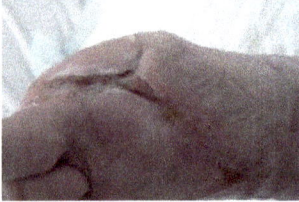

W6: Consultation of 08/10/2007: Total epithelialisation of the front of the foot. The zone at the amputation point only measures 2.8 cm^2. Hypertrophic granulation prevents the margins from meeting and will be treated with nitrate. Treatment will be continued with an absorbent dressing**(Cellosorb® Lite).

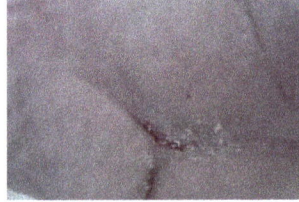

W10: 06/11/2007: Close-up of the previous zone. Almost definitive healing.

Patient No. 3: Sixty-seven-year-old female, insulin-dependent patient. Amputation of the big toe following perforating ulcer of the foot, complicated at home. Extensive excision due to the spread of cellulites to the front of the foot.

Conclusion

The cases reported in this poster illustrate the course of amputation wounds, initially complicated due to a superficial infectious component and which were persisting for several months. The use of antibacterial silver dressing* led to a resumption of the healing process with local improvement and the disappearance of fibrin and inflammatory signs until complete epithelialisation. In the event of early use of silver absorbent dressing* wound closure is observed within less than 2 months.

*Brand name: The antibacterial absorbent dressing is URGOCELL® Silver (Cellosorb® Ag) from Laboratoires URGO.

**Brand name: The absorbent dressing is Cellosorb® Lite from Laboratoires URGO, available only in France.

We gratefully acknowledge the support of Laboratoires URGO for the production of this poster 04/2008.

UrgoTul SSD, Contact Layer with Silver Sulphadiazine
Urgo Medical

UrgoTul SSD is a 2-in-1 contact layer based on the combination of Silver Sulphadiazine with the Technology Lipido-Colloid. It combines an efficient release of silver ions and a safe antibacterial activity strictly in contact with the wound bed. A sufficient amount of silver is essential to fight against bacteria and rebalance the bacterial burden. Yet, an adequate amount of silver is needed to prevent the penetration of silver ions into human tissues and the risk of a systemic reaction of the human body.

Action

UrgoTul SSD offers a patented technology — TLC-AG — that releases active, ionic silver within a lipidocolloid gel formed by Carboxymethyl cellulose in contact with the wound's exudates for a safe antibacterial action.

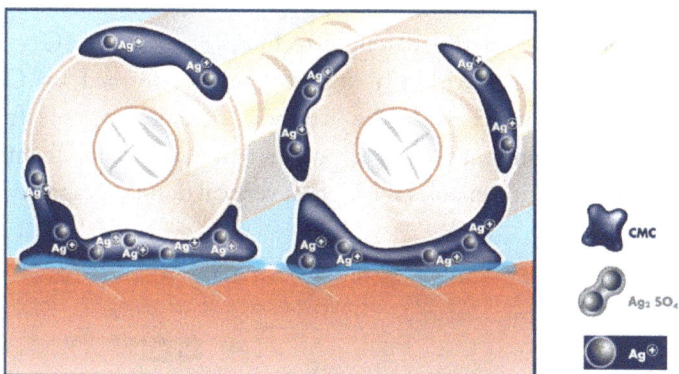

Ag+ ions are released strictly at the surface of the TLC interface

Benefits

UrgoTul SSD has proven its clinical efficacy against main common wound pathogens, including MRSA, *Pseudomonas aeruginosa* and *Candida albican.*[1]

UrgoTul is significantly less cytotoxic on fibroblasts, one of the main cells involved in repairing the wound dermis, than its competitors.[2]

Indication

UrgoTul SSD is indicated in all acute and chronic low exuding infected wounds (traumatic, post-operative wounds, burns, ulcers) or wounds at risk of infection.

UrgoCell Silver, Absorbent Foam Dressing with Silver

Urgo Medical

UrgoCell Silver is a 3-in-1 absorbent foam dressing based on the combination of Silver Sulphate with the Technology Lipido-Colloid. It combines an efficient and safe release of silver ions strictly in contact with the wound bed and an optimal drainage capacity of wound's exudates. An adequate amount of silver is essential to fight safely against bacteria. Besides, the wound's exudates need to be managed properly in order to prepare the wound bed for granulation stage and further healing.

Action

UrgoCell Silver offers a patented technology — TLC-AG — that releases active, ionic silver within a lipidocolloid gel formed by Carboxymethyl cellulose in contact with the wound's exudates for a safe antibacterial action. The combination of a polyurethane absorbent foam and a semi-permeable backing enables the highest vertical drainage capacity in the market place.

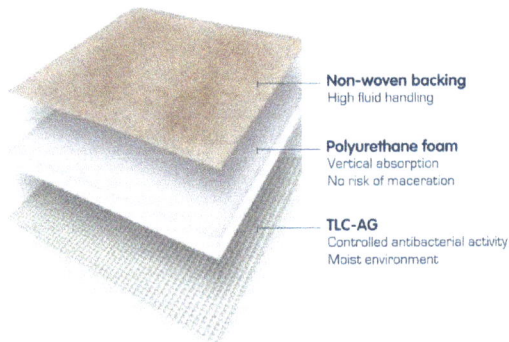

Non-woven backing
High fluid handling

Polyurethane foam
Vertical absorption
No risk of maceration

TLC-AG
Controlled antibacterial activity
Moist environment

Benefits

UrgoCell Silver has proven its clinical efficacy against main common wound pathogens, including MRSA, pseudomonas aeruginosa and candida albican.[1]

After 4 weeks of treatment using UrgoCell Silver on critically colonized venous leg ulcers, UrgoCell Silver has showed excellent results in reducing the signs of colonization and the wound surface area as a consequence.[3]

Indication

UrgoCell Silver is indicated in all acute and chronic exuding infected wounds (traumatic, post-operative wounds, leg ulcers, pressure ulcers, diabetic foot ulcers).

UrgoStart and UrgoStart Contact, The First Treatment to Accelerate Wound Healing by 2

Urgo Medical

UrgoStart is a new generation of dressing based on the combination of Nano Oligo Saccharide Factor (NOSF) particles with the Technology Lipido-Colloid. It contains NOSF, a Matrix Metallo Proteases (MMPs) inhibitor, which will restore the wound equilibrium of chronic wounds. Often stuck in the inflammatory phase, all chronic wounds present an excess of MMPs that keep degrading the newly formed tissues and prevent a normal healing process to take place.

Action

UrgoStart offers a patented technology — TLC-NOSF — that releases active NOSF within a lipidocolloid gel formed by Carboxymethyl cellulose to preferentially bind and inactive excess MMPs. Besides, thanks to the Technology LipidoColloid (TLC), UrgoStart improves fibroblasts proliferation for an enhanced healing.

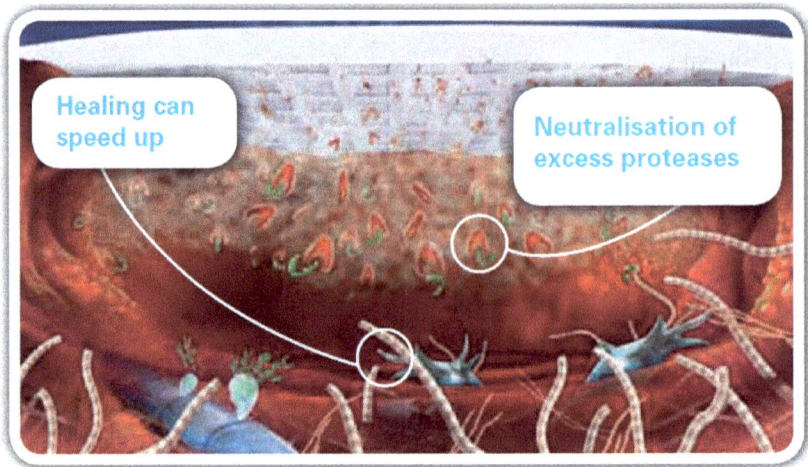

Benefit

By restoring the chronic wound equilibrium, UrgoStart shows a significant superiority in accelerating wound healing by 2 versus a neutral absorbent foam dressing. And, for the 1st time in the wound care arena, a dressing's efficacy has been proven in a double-blind randomized controlled trial.[4]

As a consequence, UrgoStart helps to reduce the cost of treatment for both hospitals and patients bringing back a smile to anxious and depressed patients.

Indications

UrgoStart range is split into two main products: UrgoStart and UrgoStart Contact.

UrgoStart is an absorbent foam dressing indicated in all exuding chronic wounds (pressure ulcers, leg ulcers, long standing acute wounds) as a first intention treatment.

UrgoStart Contact is a Contact Layer indicated in all low exuding chronic wounds such as diabetic foot ulcers.

UrgoClean, Hydro-Desloughing Dressing

Urgo Medical

UrgoClean is a new generation of Hydro-Desloughing dressing based on the Technology Lipido-Colloid. It combines resistant hydro-desloughing fibers for an optimal absorption of exudates and slough and soft-adherent lipidocolloid technology to maintain a moist wound environment favorable to healing. In order to accompany the wound bed preparation of sloughy and highly exuding wounds, UrgoClean simplifies the debridement stage for the medical staff and make it painless for the patients.

Action

In contact with the wound's exudates, UrgoClean's resistant hydro-desloughing fibers will gel, absorb exudates and trap sloughy residues to be removed in one piece upon dressing removal.

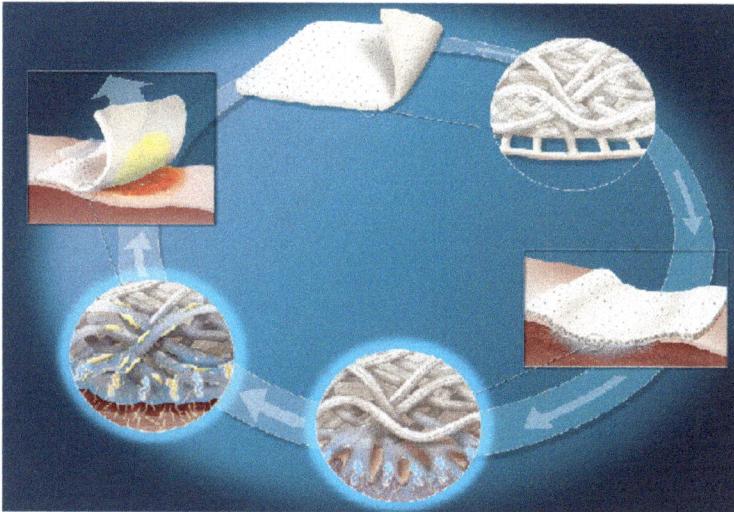

Benefits

UrgoClean offers an effective debridement that can easily be performed by the medical staff. After 6 weeks of treatment with UrgoClean, an average reduction of slough by 75% has been observed on leg ulcers.[4]

Thanks to the Technology LipidoColloid, UrgoClean does not adhere to the wound for a painless removal.

Indications

UrgoClean is indicated for all acute and chronic sloughy and/or highly exuding wounds.

References

1. *In vitro* studies of the antimicobial efficacy of the TLC-AG interface. Data on file.
2. A. Burd, A comparative study of teh cytotoxicity of silver-based dressings in monolayer cell, tissue explant and animal models, *Wound Repair Regen.* **15**:94–104 (2007).
3. I. Lazareth, Evaluation of a new silver absorbent dresssing in patients with critically venous leg ulcers, *J. Wound Care* **16**(3):129–32 (2007).
4. S. Measure, Management of chronic wound at sloughy stage with a new hydro-desloughing dressing: result of a clinical study. Data on file. Urgo (2011).

ConvaTec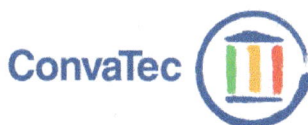

AQUACEL
Hydrofiber™ Wound Dressing

Introduction

AQUACEL® Hydrofiber® Dressing is a soft, highly conformable and absorbent dressing composed of hydrocolloid fibers using advanced technology unique to ConvaTec.

AQUACEL® Hydrofiber® rapidly absorbs exudate **up to 25 times its own weight directly into its fibers by vertical wicking action, minimizing risk of maceration**. It has higher retention capacity than any leading alginate dressing or gauze, even under compression.

Action

It creates a soft and soothing gel upon immediate contact with exudate and maintains a moist environment that supports the body's healing process and aids in the removal of unnecessary material from the wound (autolytic debridement) without damaging the newly formed tissue.

It also sequesters bacteria by preventing the release of bacteria into the wound. This helps to minimize cross-contamination during dressing changes.

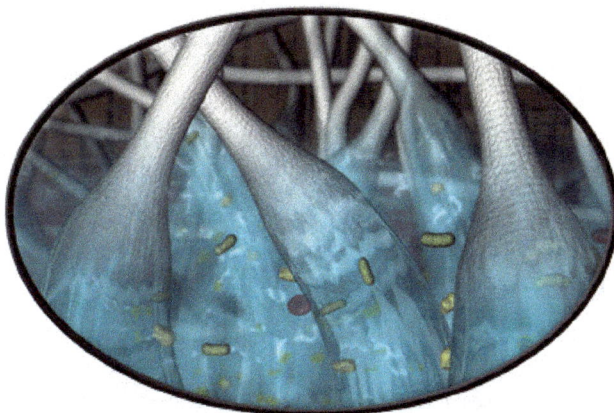

Indication and Benefits

AQUACEL® Hydrofiber® is ideal for many types of exuding wounds. Indications include chronic and acute wounds, pressure ulcers, venous and arterial leg ulcers, diabetic ulcers, post operative wounds and partial thickness burns.

It is virtually pain-free and easier to remove than gauze or alginate dressings and has a longer wear time. **It may be left in place for up to 7 days.**

Product Presentation

AQUACEL® Hydrofiber® Dressing is available in the following sizes:

Description	Pack Size	Product Code
5 × 5 cm	10	177901
10 × 10 cm	10	177902
15 × 15 cm	5	177903
2 × 45 cm rope with Strengthening Fiber	5	403770

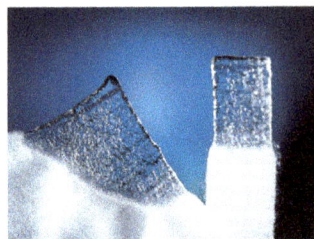

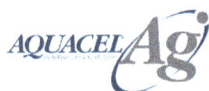

AQUACEL Ag

Introduction

AQUACEL® Ag Hydrofiber® Dressing is a soft, highly conformable antimicrobial dressing composed of hydrocolloid fibers impregnated with ionic silver.

The silver in the dressing kills bacteria present, reducing the number of bacteria and aids in creating an antimicrobial environment.

Action

AQUACEL® Ag releases active, ionic silver in a controlled manner as wound exudate is absorbed into the dressing to provide an optimum level of silver for **broad-spectrum antimicrobial action, including MRSA, VRE and bacteria in biofilms** that are physically less susceptible to antimicrobial agents.

AQUACEL® Ag absorbs high amounts of exudate and creates a soft, cohesive gel that intimately conforms to the wound surface, while maintaining a moist environment and aiding in the removal of non-viable tissue from the wound (autolytic debridement).

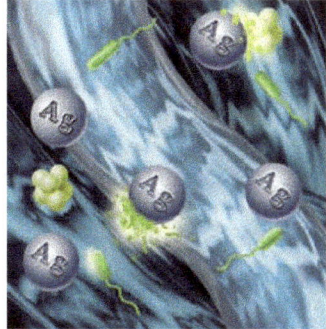

Main Benefits

Wound infections may be reduced by providing a moist wound healing environment and controlling wound bacteria to support the body's healing process.

AQUACEL® Ag also contains all the benefits of Hydrofiber® which include bacteria sequestration, vertical wicking effect to help reduce maceration and non-trauma to newly granulating tissue upon removal.

Indication

AQUACEL® Ag is ideal for many types of wounds. Indications include chronic and acute wounds, pressure ulcers, venous and arterial leg ulcers, diabetic ulcers, post-operative wounds, partial thickness burns and infected wounds.

It is significantly less painful and easier to remove than gauze or alginate dressings and has a longer wear time. **It may be left in place for up to 7 days.**

Product Presentation

AQUACEL® Ag is available in the following sizes:

Description	Pack Size	Product Code
5 × 5 cm	10	403706
10 × 10 cm	10	403708
15 × 15 cm	5	403710
20 × 30 cm	5	403711
2 × 45 cm rope with Strengthening Fiber	5	403771

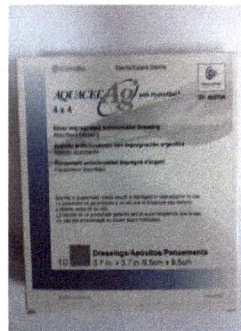

CarboFlex™
Odor Control Dressing

Introduction

CarboFLEX® Odor Control Dressing is a non-adherent dressing that effectively manages malodorous acute and chronic wounds through an innovative, multi-layered dressing design.

Action

It consists of a highly absorbent wound contact layer (containing Alginate and Hydrofiber®) which forms a gel to maintain a moist environment that supports the body's healing process and aids in autolytic debridement, without damaging newly formed tissue.

Main Benefits

In addition to the high absorbent action, the main benefit of CarboFLEX® is the **double-knit activated charcoal central pad to effectively absorb odor** and a smooth water resistant film to keep the dressing dry.

Product Presentation:

CarboFLEX® Odor Control Dressing is available in the following size:

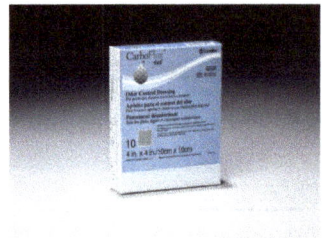

Description	Pack Size	Product Code
10 cm × 10 cm	10	403202

DuoDerm® Hydroactive® Gel

Introduction and Benefits

DuoDERM® Hydroactive® Gel is a clear hydrocolloid containing gel. It releases moisture into dry wounds and absorbs more than double its weight in exudate.

It creates a moist wound healing environment which facilitates **autolytic debridement and allows for non-traumatic removal of the secondary dressing** without damaging newly formed tissue.

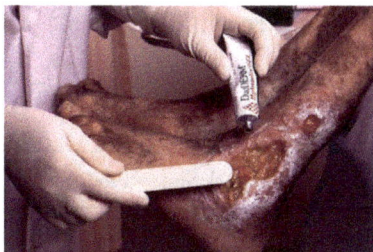

Indication

DuoDERM® Hydroactive® Gel is indicated for use in chronic and acute wounds including dry and sloughy wounds, or in cavity wounds as a filler to reduce dead space.

Product Presentation

DuoDERM® Hydroactive® Gel is available in the following sizes:

Description	Pack Size	Product Code
15 gm tube	10	187990
30 gm tube	3	187987

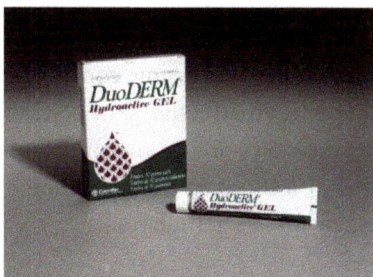

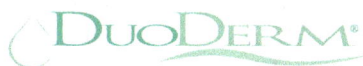

DUODERM® Hydroactive® Paste

Introduction and Benefits

DuoDERM® Hydroactive® Paste has a higher concentration of hydrocolloid than DuoDERM® Hydroactive® Gel, effective for **removal of necrotic tissue and adherent slough.**

It interacts with wound exudate to form a moist wound environment supportive of the healing process by aiding autolytic debridement and allowing the non-traumatic removal of the dressing without damaging the newly formed tissue.

Indication

DuoDERM® Hydroactive® Paste is indicated for the management of lightly exuding dermal ulcers, including full-thickness wounds, such as leg ulcers, pressure ulcers and diabetic ulcers.

Product Presentation

DuoDERM® Hydroactive® Paste is available in the following size:

Description	Pack Size	Product Code
30 gm tube	1	187930

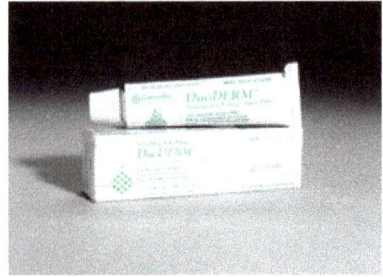

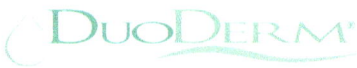 **CGF Dressing**

Introduction and Actions

DuoDERM® CGF (Controlled Gel Formula) Dressing is a self-adhesive Hydrocolloid Dressing consisting of a flexible, water-resistant foam outer layer and an adhesive skin contact layer that contains polymers to enhance the dressing's ability to contain wound exudate. It forms a cohesive gel to provide a moist wound environment which facilitates autolytic debridement and promotes granulation.

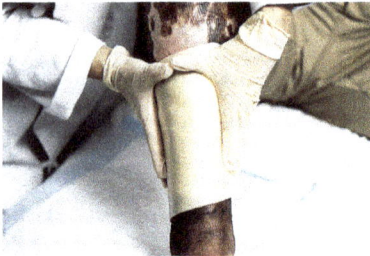

DuoDERM® CGF Dressing **stimulates angiogenesis** by providing a total occlusive environment which also acts as an **effective barrier against bacterial, viral and other external contaminants**, including HIV-1 and HBV.

Indication

DuoDERM® CGF is indicated for use on lightly to moderately exuding wounds, including pressure ulcers, leg ulcers, diabetic ulcers, post-operative wounds, open surgical wounds, traumatic wounds, lacerations, donor sites, first and second degree burns.

Product Presentation

DuoDERM® CGF is available in the following sizes:

Description	Pack Size	Product Code
10 × 10 cm	5	187660
20 × 20 cm	5	187662
10 × 13 cm w/Border	5	187973

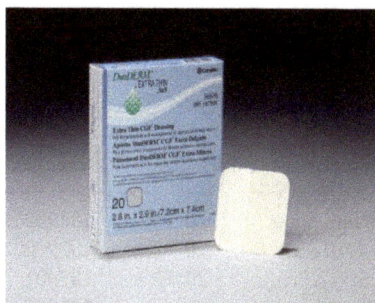

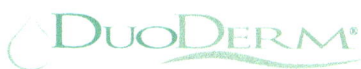

DuoDerm® Extra Thin CGF Dressing

Introduction and Actions

DuoDERM® Extra Thin CGF (Controlled Gel Formula) Dressing is a self-adhesive Hydrocolloid Dressing consisting of a flexible, water-resistant film outer layer and an adhesive skin contact layer that contains polymers to enhance the dressing's ability to contain wound exudate. It forms a cohesive gel to provide a moist wound environment which facilitates autolytic debridement and promotes granulation.

DuoDERM® CGF Dressing **stimulates angiogenesis** by providing a total occlusive environment which also acts as an **effective barrier against bacterial, viral and other external contaminants**, including HIV-1 and HBV.

Indication

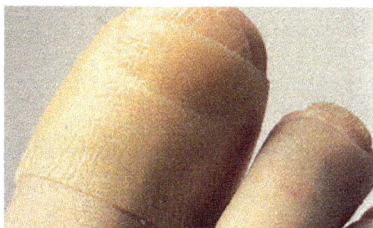

DuoDERM® Extra Thin CGF is indicated for use on minimally exuding wounds, over sutured sites or **difficult-to-dress anatomical areas** and also on intact skin to protect and prevent skin breakdown.

Product Presentation

DuoDERM® Extra Thin CGF is available in the following sizes:

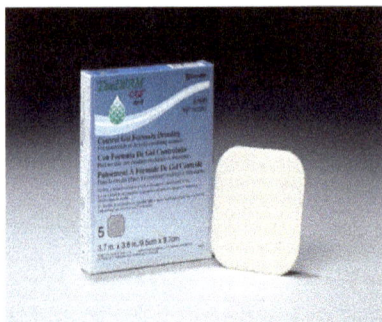

Description	Pack Size	Product Code
40 mm Spots	20	187932
5 × 10 cm	20	187900
7.5 × 7.5 cm	20	187901
10 × 10 cm	10	187955
5 × 20 cm	10	187961

KALTOSTAT® Calcium-Sodium Alginate Wound Dressing

Introduction and Action

KALTOSTAT® is a highly absorbent calcium- Sodium alginate dressing derived from naturally occurring brown seaweed. **It absorbs up to 17 times its own weight** and forms a firm, web-like gel via an ion-exchange mechanism where sodium ions in exudate are exchanged for calcium ions in the KALTOSTAT® dressing.

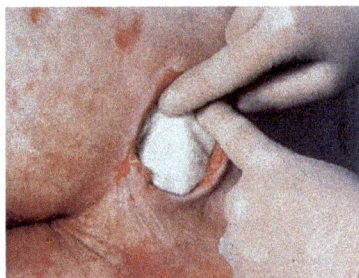

The gel forms a moist wound environment that is supportive of the healing process by aiding autolytic debridement. In addition, the dressing may be easily removed in one piece without damaging the newly formed tissue. KALTOSTAT® also has **haemostatic properties** and may be used to control minor bleeding.

Indication

KALTOSTAT® is indicated for use on moderately to heavily exuding wounds, including pressure ulcers, leg ulcers, diabetic ulcers, post-operative wounds, open surgical wounds, sinuses, traumatic wounds, lacerations and donor sites.

Product Presentation

KALTOSTAT® is available in the following sizes:

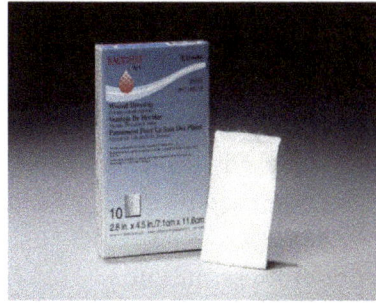

Description	Pack Size	Product Code
5 cm × 5 cm	10	168210
7.5 cm × 12 cm	10	168212
10 cm × 20 cm	10	168214
15 cm × 25 cm	10	168215
2 gm rope	5	168117

Versiva® XC® Gelling Foam Dressing

Introduction and Action

Versiva® XC® Gelling Foam Dressing is an interactive, semi-occlusive dressing containing Hydrofiber® Technology which maintains an optimal moist wound environment that kick-starts wound healing. Versiva® XC® dressing combines the gelling action of Hydrofiber® Technology with the simplicity of foam to provide a unique Gelling Foam dressing to redefine patient care.

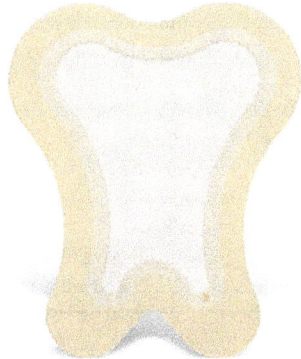

Benefits

- Retain exudate within the wound area, preventing its spread onto healthy periwound skin.
- Control exudate levels while still maintaining a moist wound healing environment.
- Remove harmful bacteria and enzymes from the wound bed, trapping them in the exudate and aiding the wound's healing process.
- Minimise patients' pain and discomfort when dressings are in place and at dressing change.

Indication

Versiva® XC® Gelling Foam Dressing is indicated for use on leg ulcers (venous leg ulcers, arterial ulcers and leg ulcers of mixed etiology), pressure ulcers (partial & full thickness), diabetic ulcers, skin tears, surgical wounds (left to heal by secondary intention, donor sites, dermatological excisions), second degree burns and traumatic wounds.

Product Presentation

Versiva® XC® Gelling Foam Dressing is available in the following sizes:

Description	Pack Size	Product Code
7.5 × 7.5 cm non-adhesive	10	410606
11 × 11 cm non-adhesive	10	410607
15 × 15 cm non-adhesive	5	410608
20 × 20 cm non-adhesive	5	410614
10 × 10 cm adhesive	10	410609
14 × 14 cm adhesive	10	410610
19 × 19 cm adhesive	5	410615
22 × 22 cm adhesive	5	410611
18.5 × 20.5 cm adhesive Heel	5	410612
21 × 21 cm adhesive Sacral	5	410613

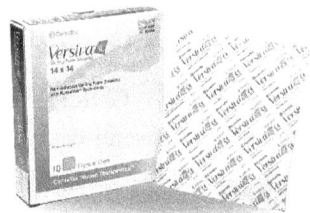

The VAC Therapy System

1. Integrated Therapy System with Innovative Technology Features

Since 1995, over 3 million patients worldwide have been treated successfully with V.A.C.® Therapy. The V.A.C.® Therapy system (V.A.C.® Therapy) is used in a wide variety of wound types including Acute Wounds, Traumatic Wounds, Sub-Acute Wounds, Dehisced Wounds, Chronic Wounds, Ulcers (Diabetic, Venous Stasis and Pressure Ulcers), Burns, Flaps and Grafts.[1-9]

The integrated system (see Figs. 1 and 3) consists of the following 3 major components which play a critical role in the clinical outcomes reported in the literature:

The 3rd Generation units (InfoV.A.C.® and ActiV.A.C.®) have the following functionality that promotes therapeutic outcomes for all the indicated wound types:

✓ **V.A.C.® Therapy Dressings:** V.A.C.® GranuFoam™ has an open reticulated pore foam structure that has been proven to stimulate wound healing faster than gauze under negative pressure[10]

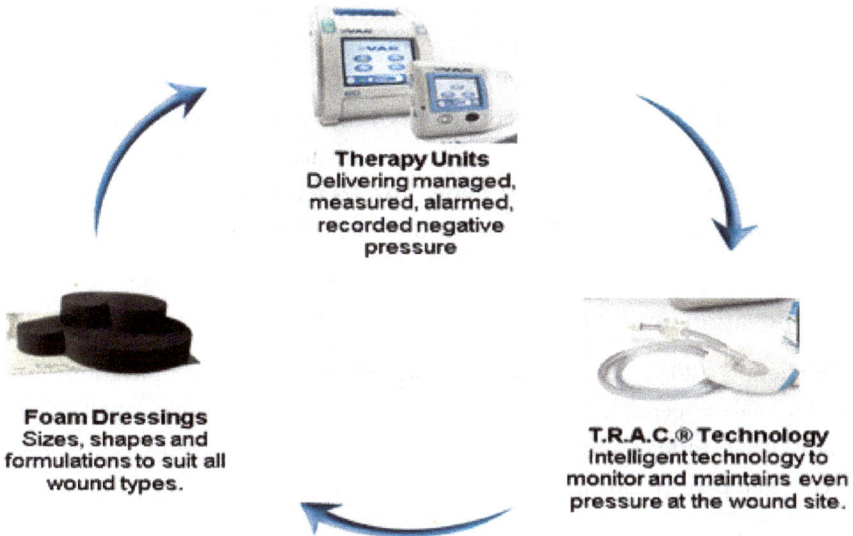

Therapy Units
Delivering managed, measured, alarmed, recorded negative pressure

Foam Dressings
Sizes, shapes and formulations to suit all wound types.

T.R.A.C.® Technology
Intelligent technology to monitor and maintains even pressure at the wound site.

Figure 1.   The integrated V.A.C.® therapy system

V.A.C. – VIA – ULTA   Prevena – Incision management system

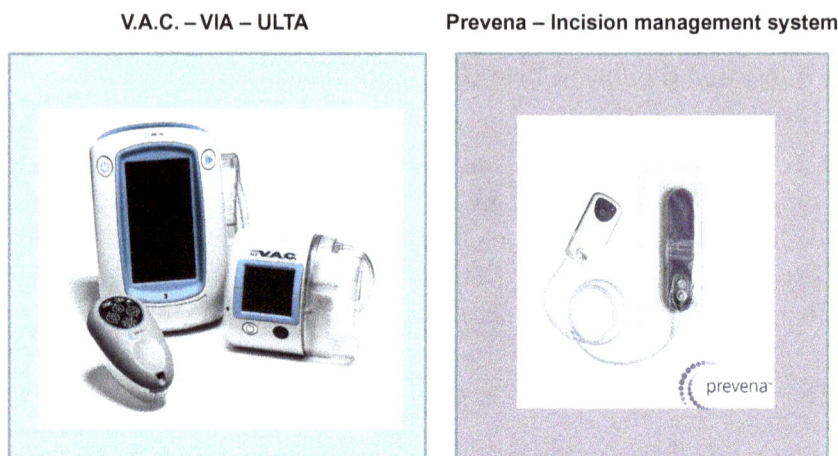

Figure 2.   Product innovation at KCI

✓ **Settings Guide** offers appropriate therapy settings for different wound types providing better clinical outcomes and improved safety.

✓ **Measurement Tool** enables clinicians to upload and displayed images directly on the therapy unit which provides improved and simplified documentation and feedback on the wound healing process. Wound size and volume are automatically calculated, reducing clinician-to-clinician variance in wound measurement. More timely patient care decisions are aided by improved wound information.

✓ **Detailed Therapy and Patient History** which allows clinicians to monitor and track therapy settings, durations and alarms. A record of wound treatment and therapy progression provides feedback and information to ensure quick therapy adjustments for best therapy results.

2. Innovation on the Horizon

ABThera™ (2010) is specifically designed to address complications for abdominal surgery (open abdomen, trauma etc.) ABThera™ will avoid additional theatre requirements, improve outcomes, reduce complications and step down patients quickly from high cost intensive care settings.

Prevena™ (Fig. 2) is the first and only negative pressure product designed for incision management to prevent surgical infection by holding wound edges together and creating an environment that promotes wound healing (reducing oedema, increasing perfusion, removing exudates and infectious material and reducing microbial colonisation)

V.A.C. Via™ (2010) is the first single patient use disposable NPWT device that provides 7 days of V.A.C. Therapy with options for continuous therapy or dynamic pressure control, ideal for transitioning patients, and is designed for moderate to low severity wounds. Improvement in patient's compliance through technology leads to better clinical outcomes.

V.A.C. Ulta™ (2011) KCI's premier therapy system to provide either NPWT only installation or combination therapy. This product will make a substantial difference to treating infected prosthesis for hip and knee replacements successfully and thereby significantly reducing cost (theatre and hospital stay)

3. Efficacy of the Therapy — Therapeutic Outcomes

The V.A.C.® Therapy System is an active, integrated wound healing system, designed to promote wound healing at the cellular level by way of its unique functions and mechanisms of action (MOAs)[10-12] including:

- Promoting wound healing by secondary or tertiary (delayed primary) intention by preparing the wound bed for closure[3,6,13-29]

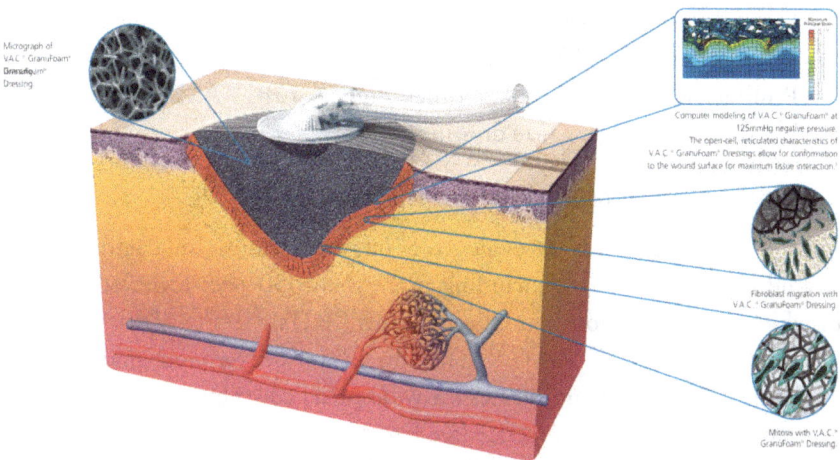

Figure 3. V.A.C.® therapy mechanism of action in action

- Reducing oedema[6,8,15,16,30−33]
- Promoting granulation tissue formation[3,9,12,13,15,17,34]
- Promoting perfusion[8,13,15,35−39]
- Removing exudates and infectious material[8,13,15]

The V.A.C.® Therapy System addresses these key factors especially in the inflammatory and proliferative phases of wound healing. The clinical and cost effective outcomes demonstrated in V.A.C.® Therapy's extensive body of evidence are a direct result of the system's unique functions and mechanisms of action as supported by scientific research.

— **V.A.C.® Therapy induces the formation of new blood vessels**[12] New blood vessels are critical to transport nutrition to the wound and improve effective wound healing

— **V.A.C.® Therapy has been proven to increase tissue growth**[13] by 103% in comparison to wounds without negative pressure

— **V.A.C.® GranuFoam™ induces stimulation** and division of new fibroblasts[10] which leads to rapid formation of granulation tissue. Fibroblast cells help to create collagen which is a key component of new tissue formation

— V.A.C.® GranuFoam™ demonstrates **3 × greater fibroblast migration** when compared with gauze[10]

— In cells exposed to V.A.C.® Therapy with V.A.C.® GranuFoam™ Dressings, the **mitochondria were very prominent**, indicating **increased metabolic activity** [(10)] when compared to gauze under suction[40]

— **Proliferation rates were 1.4 times higher** with V.A.C.® GranuFoam Dressings than with gauze dressings[10]

4. Evidence Based Medicine

V.A.C.® Therapy's body of evidence is one of the most substantial in the wound care industry[41,42] including more than 550 peer-reviewed articles, of which 18 are Randomized Clinical Trials (RCTs).[3,4,7,9,17,18,22,26,34,43−48] The incorporation of V.A.C.® Therapy in various wound management guidelines[49−56] also demonstrates the widespread contributions of this active system to wound healing practice (see Fig. 4).

To date, 94% (all forms NPWT, 580 of 618 articles) and 97% (commercial NPWT products only, 580 of 596 articles) of all published NPWT literature[57]

Wound Indication	No. of References	Highest Level of EBM	No. of Patients	Assessment
Stage III and IV Pressure Ulcers	21	1a	>1000	Superior to conservative methods in inoperable cases
Skin Graft Fixation	31	1b	>1000	Method of Choice
Leg Ulcers	9	1b	146	Method of Choice
Diabetic Foot Syndrome	24	1b	352	Firmly Integrated in the Treatment Algorithm
Burns	10	1b	39	Promising method for hand burns
Soft Tissue Infection	52	2b	>1000	Suitable Method
Temporary Closure of Open Abdomen / Abdominal Wall Wounds	32	3b	270	Suitable Method
Orthopaedic, Traumatic and Infected Wounds	33	3b	283	Suitable Method or promising option
Sternal Wound Infection	48	4	770	Method of Choice
Vascular Infection/Vascular Prosthesis Infection	10	4	86	Method of Choice
Cost effectiveness Studies	7	4	>1000	Calculated in USA and Germany
Varied studies across multiple wound indications	50	1b	>500	Multiple assessments

Figure 4. Subjective overview classifying a portion of V.A.C.® therapy literature by wound indication

is V.A.C.® Therapy specific; thus evidence on other forms of NPWT is extremely limited and does not clearly identify scientific foundations, MOAs, clinical outcomes, or economic outcomes as equivalent to V.A.C.® Therapy. Because these devices use interface materials other than GranuFoam™ dressings and do not provide controlled, self adjusting pressure technology in the studied pressure ranges, it cannot be presumed that data from those products can be pooled and clinically evaluated with V.A.C.® Therapy, nor can their evidence be construed to represent the same outcomes as V.A.C.® Therapy.

5. Cost Effectiveness

Several studies demonstrate that V.A.C.® Therapy can result in fewer adverse events, which results in fewer hospitalizations, less emergent care incidents, reduced complications, fewer amputations, less dressing changes, decreased personnel commitments, shorter hospitalization, and reduced treatment times.[3,5,14,34,49,58,59]

- Early use of V.A.C.® Therapy is both clinically efficacious and cost effective. Compelling results show that V.A.C.® Therapy accelerates wound healing and therefore reduces the cost of treatment significantly. V.A.C.® Therapy reduces both direct treatment cost and nursing time expenses.[9,60]

- One study showed a 76% risk reduction for the number of surgical procedures, including debridement and additional amputations when patients were prescribed V.A.C.® Therapy over other standard care.[14]
- A recent diabetic foot ulcer randomised controlled trial demonstrated a significantly greater proportion of patients treated with V.A.C.® Therapy (43.2%) achieved complete wound closure compared to patients treated with advanced moist wound therapy (28.9%).[3]
- In a diabetic amputation study, the average direct cost per patient treated for eight weeks or longer was $27,270 in the V.A.C.® Therapy group, versus $36,096 in the advanced moist wound therapy group, resulting in a savings of almost $9,000.[14]
- V.A.C.® Therapy is supported by the following clinical evidence to demonstrate its ability to deliver fast and effective results:

  — **V.A.C.® Therapy prepares the wound bed over twice as fast** compared to advanced moist wound dressings. Time to wound bed preparation is shown to be reduced from 17 days to 7 days with V.A.C.® Therapy.[9]

  — **V.A.C.® Therapy significantly reduces time of wound healing** in the treatment of Diabetic Foot Ulcers compared to advanced moist wound dressings, AMWD (V.A.C.® Therapy = 96 days, AMWD >112 days).[34]

  — **V.A.C.® Therapy demonstrated a shorter mean time to heal** on full thickness wounds.[9]

  — **V.A.C.® Therapy is 71% more effective in reducing wound area.** Wound Area reduced by 4.32 cm^2 under V.A.C.® Therapy compared to only 2.53 cm^2 with control group.[34]

6. Quality of Life

V.A.C.® Therapy has proven to provide overall significant improvement in a patient perceived quality of life[9,61] (Fig. 5).

The V.A.C.® Freedom system and ActiV.A.C, KCI's portable V.A.C.® Therapy devices, offers increased patient mobility and allows healing to occur within the home setting.

A German patient review conducted by Augustin *et al.*[61] in response to a request from the Institute for Quality for Economics in Healthcare (IQWIG)

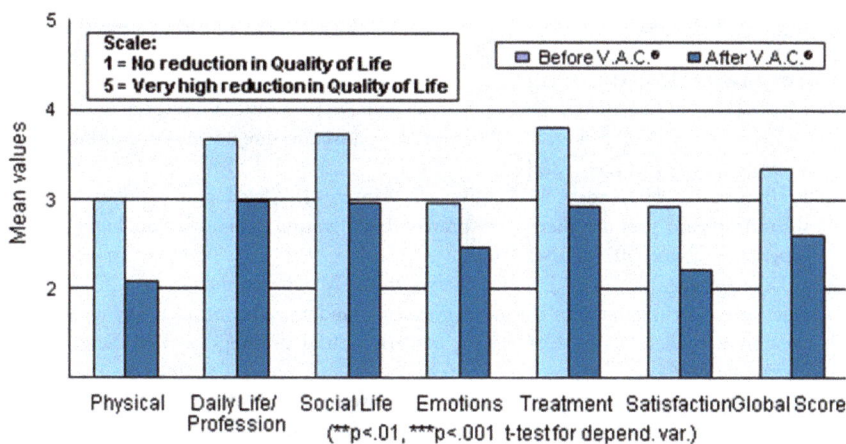

Figure 5. Quality of life before and after V.A.C.® therapy[60]

to evaluate medical devices from a patient's perspective, showed a significant positive improvement in quality of life from V.A.C.® Therapy in the following ways:

- Improved mobility
- Increased independence
- Faster return to social life and willing to mix with others
- Reduced pain and discomfort
- Reduced depression and feelings of fear

References

1. E. T. Powell, The role of negative pressure wound therapy with reticulated open cell foam in the treatment of war wounds, *J. Orthop. Trauma* **22**(10 Suppl):S138–41 (2008).
2. V.A.C. Therapy Clinical Guidelines: A Reference Source for Clinicians. 7–1–2007. Ref. Type: Pamphlet.
3. D. G. Armstrong and L. A. Lavery, Diabetic Foot Study Consortium. Negative pressure wound therapy after partial diabetic foot amputation: a multicentre, randomised controlled trial. *Lancet* **366**(9498):1704–10 (2005).
4. J. P. Stannard, J. T. Robinson, E. R. Anderson, G. McGwin, Jr., D. A. Volgas and J. E. Alonso, Negative pressure wound therapy to treat hematomas and surgical incisions following high-energy trauma, *J. Trauma* **60**(6):1301-6 (2006).
5. T. Schwien, J. Gilbert and C. Lang, Pressure ulcer prevalence and the role of negative pressure wound therapy in home health quality outcomes, *Ostomy Wound Manage.* **51**(9):47–60 (2005).

6. A. J. DeFranzo, L. C. Argenta, M. W. Marks, *et al.*, The use of vacuum-assisted closure therapy for the treatment of lower-extremity wounds with exposed bone, *Plast. Reconstr. Surg.* **108**(5):1184–91 (2001).

7. E. Moisidis, T. Heath, C. Boorer, K. Ho and A. K. Deva, A prospective, blinded, randomized, controlled clinical trial of topical negative pressure use in skin grafting, *Plast. Reconstr. Surg.* **114**(4):917–22 (2004).

8. L. P. Kamolz, H. Andel, W. Haslik, W. Winter, G. Meissl and M. Frey, Use of subatmospheric pressure therapy to prevent burn wound progression in human: first experiences, *Burns* **30**(3):253–8 (2004).

9. J. D. Vuerstaek, T. Vainas, J. Wuite, P. Nelemans, M. H. Neumann and J. C. Veraart, State-of-the-art treatment of chronic leg ulcers: a randomized controlled trial comparing vacuum-assisted closure (V.A.C.) with modern wound dressings, *J. Vasc. Surg.* **44**(5): 1029–38 (2006).

10. A. K. McNulty, M. Schmidt, T. Feeley and K. Kieswetter, Effects of negative pressure wound therapy on fibroblast viability, chemotactic signaling, and proliferation in a provisional wound (fibrin) matrix, *Wound Repair Regen.* **15**(6):838–46 (2007).

11. V. Saxena, C. W. Hwang, S. Huang, Q. Eichbaum, D. Ingber and D. P. Orgill, Vacuum-assisted closure: microdeformations of wounds and cell proliferation, *Plast. Reconstr. Surg.* **114**(5):1086–96 (2004).

12. A. K. Greene, M. Puder, R. Roy, *et al.*, Microdeformational wound therapy: effects on angiogenesis and matrix metalloproteinases in chronic wounds of 3 debilitated patients, *Ann. Plast. Surg.* **56**(4):418–22 (2006).

13. M. J. Morykwas, L. C. Argenta, E. I. Shelton-Brown and W. McGuirt, Vacuum-assisted closure: a new method for wound control and treatment. Animal studies and basic foundation, *Ann. Plast. Surg.* **38**(6):553–62 (1997).

14. J. C. Page, B. Newswander, D. C. Schwenke, M. Hansen and J. Ferguson, Retrospective analysis of negative pressure wound therapy in open foot wounds with significant soft tissue defects, *Adv. Skin Wound Care* **17**(7):354–64 (2004).

15. L. C. Argenta and M. J. Morykwas, Vacuum-assisted closure: a new method for wound control and treatment. Clinical experience, *Ann. Plast. Surg.* **38**(6):563–76 (1997).

16. M. J. Morykwas, L. R. David, A. M. Schneider, *et al.*, Use of subatmospheric pressure to prevent progression of partial-thickness burns in a swine model, *J. Burn Care Rehabil.* **20**(1 Pt 1):15–21 (1999).

17. S. K. McCallon, C. A. Knight, J. P. Valiulus, M. W. Cunningham, J. M. McCulloch and L. P. Farinas, Vacuum-assisted closure versus saline-moistened gauze in the healing of postoperative diabetic foot wounds, *Ostomy Wound Manage.* **46**(8):28–34 (2000).

18. M. T. Eginton, K. R. Brown, G. R. Seabrook, J. B. Towne and R. A. Cambria, A prospective randomized evaluation of negative-pressure wound dressings for diabetic foot wounds, *Ann. Vasc. Surg.* **17**(6):645–9 (2003).

19. N. Smith, The benefits of VAC therapy in the management of pressure ulcers, *Br J Nurs* **13**(22):1359–65 (2004).

20. T. E. Philbeck, W. J. Schroeder and K. T. Whittington, Vacuum-assisted closure therapy for diabetic foot ulcers: clinical and cost analyses, *Home Health Care Consult.* **8**(3):27–34 (2001).

21. D. G. Genecov, A. M. Schneider, M. J. Morykwas, D. Parker, W. L. White and L. C. Argenta, A controlled subatmospheric pressure dressing increases the rate of skin graft donor site reepithelialization, *Ann. Plast. Surg.* **40**(3):219–25 (1998).

22. M. G. Jeschke, C. Rose, P. Angele, B. Fuchtmeier, M. N. Nerlich and U. Bolder, Development of new reconstructive techniques: use of Integra in combination with fibrin glue and negative-pressuretherapy for reconstruction of acute and chronic wounds, *Plast. Reconstr. Surg.* 113(2):525–30 (2004).

23. S. N. Carson, K. Overall, S. Lee-Jahshan and E. Travis, Vacuum-assisted closure used for healing chronic wounds and skin grafts in the lower extremities, *Ostomy Wound Manage.* 50(3):52–8 (2004).

24. J. P. Agarwal, M. Ogilvie, L. C. Wu, *et al.*, Vacuum-assisted closure for sternal wounds: a first-line therapeutic management approach, *Plast. Reconstr. Surg.* 116(4):1035–40 (2005).

25. K. N. Cowan, L. Teague, S. C. Sue and J. L. Mahoney, Vacuum-assisted wound closure of deep sternal infections in high-risk patients after cardiac surgery, *Ann. Thorac. Surg.* 80(6):2205–12 (2005).

26. D. H. Song, L. C. Wu, R. F. Lohman, L. J. Gottlieb and M. Franczyk, Vacuum assisted closure for the treatment of sternal wounds: the bridge between debridement and definitive closure, *Plast. Reconstr. Surg.* 111(1):92–7 (2003).

27. P. R. Miller, J. W. Meredith, J. C. Johnson and M. C. Chang, Prospective evaluation of vacuum-assisted fascial closure after open abdomen: planned ventral hernia rate is substantially reduced, *Ann. Surg.* 239(5):608–14 (2004).

28. J. Bickels, Y. Kollender, J. C. Wittig, N. Cohen, I. Meller and M. M. Malawer, Vacuum-assisted wound closure after resection of musculoskeletal tumors, *Clin. Orthop. Relat. Res.* 441:346–50 (2005).

29. B. M. Parrett, E. Matros, J. J. Pribaz and D. P. Orgill, Lower extremity trauma: trends in the management of soft-tissue reconstruction of open tibia-fibula fractures, *Plast. Reconstr. Surg.* 117(4):1315–22 (2006).

30. P. Stone, J. Prigozen, M. Hofeldt, S. Hass, J. DeLuca and S. Flaherty, Bolster versus negative pressure wound therapy for securing split-thickness skin grafts in trauma patients, *Wounds* 16(7):219–23 (2004).

31. M. Kaplan, Negative pressure wound therapy in the management of abdominal compartment syndrome, *Ostomy Wound Manage.* 50(11A Suppl):20S–5S (2004).

32. K. Bookout, S. McCord and K. McLane, Case studies of an infant, a toddler, and an adolescent treated with a negative pressure wound treatment system, *J. Wound Ostomy Continence Nurs.* 31(4):184–92 (2004).

33. M. J. Morykwas, H. Howell, A. J. Bleyer, J. A. Molnar and L. C. Argenta, The effect of externally applied subatmospheric pressure on serum myoglobin levels after a prolonged crush/ischemia injury, *J. Trauma* 53(3):537–40 (2002).

34. P. A. Blume, J. Walters, W. Payne, J. Ayala and J. Lantis, Comparison of negative pressure wound therapy using vacuum-assisted closure with advanced moist wound therapy in the treatment of diabetic foot ulcers: a multicenter randomized controlled trial, *Diabetes Care* 31(4):631–6 (2008).

35. J. A. Molnar, J. L. Simpson, D. M. Voignier, M. J. Morykwas and L. C. Argenta, Management of an acute thermal injury with subatmospheric pressure, *J. Burns Wounds* 4(5):83–92 (2005).

36. Meeting, Topical Negative Pressure (TN) Therapy, Museum of London (4–6 December 2003). 12-4-2003. Ref Type: Abstract.

37. L. A. Scherer, S. Shiver, M. Chang, J. W. Meredith and J. T. Owings, The vacuum assisted closure device: a method of securing skin grafts and improving graft survival, *Arch. Surg.* 137(8):930–4 (2002).

38. B. T. Andrews, R. B. Smith, K. E. Chang, J. Scharpf, D. P. Goldstein and G. F. Funk, Management of the radial forearm free flap donor site with the vacuum-assisted closure (VAC) system, *Laryngoscope* **116**(10):1918–22 (2006).
39. M. S. Timmers, C. S. Le, P. Banwell and G. N. Jukema, The effects of varying degrees of pressure delivered by negative-pressure wound therapy on skin perfusion, *Ann. Plast. Surg.* **55**(6):665–71 (2005).
40. R. Wilkes, Y. Zhao, K. Kieswetter and B. Haridas, Effects of dressing type on 3D tissue microdeformations during negative pressure wound therapy: a computational study, *J. Biomech. Eng.* **131**(3):031012-1-031012-12 (2009).
41. G. Chaby, P. Senet, M. Vaneau, *et al.*, Dressings for acute and chronic wounds: a systematic review, *Arch. Dermatol.* **143**(10):1297–304 (2007).
42. C. Willy, H. U. Voelker and M. Englehardt, Literature on the subject of vacuum therapy: review and update 2006, *Eur. J. Trauma Emerg. Surg.* **33**(1):33–9 (2007).
43. M. B. Wanner, F. Schwarzl, B. Strub, G. A. Zaech and G. Pierer, Vacuum-assisted wound closure for cheaper and more comfortable healing of pressure sores: a prospective study, *Scand. J. Plast. Reconstr. Surg. Hand Surg.* **37**(1):28–33 (2003).
44. E. Joseph, C. A. Hamori, S. Bergman, E. Roaf, N. F. Swann and G. W. Anastasi, A prospective, randomized trial of vacuum-assisted closure versus standard therapy of chronic nonhealing wounds, *Wounds* **12**(3):60–7 (2000).
45. C. N. Ford, E. R. Reinhard, D. Yeh, *et al.*, Interim analysis of a prospective, randomized trial of vacuum-assisted closure versus the healthpoint system in the management of pressure ulcers, *Ann. Plast. Surg.* **49**(1):55–61 (2002).
46. A. Braakenburg, M. C. Obdeijn, R. Feitz, I. A. van Rooij, A. J. van Griethuysen and J. H. Klinkenbijl, The clinical efficacy and cost effectiveness of the vacuum-assisted closure technique in the management of acute and chronic wounds: a randomized controlled trial, *Plast. Reconstr. Surg.* **118**(2):390–400 (2006).
47. T. Wild, S. Stremitzer, A. Budzanowski, T. Hoelzenbein, C. Ludwig and G. Ohrenberger, Definition of efficiency in vacuum therapy — a randomised controlled trial comparing with V.A.C.™, *Int. Wound J.* **5**(5):641–7 (2008).
48. C. M. Moues, M. C. Vos, G. J. Van Den Bemd, T. Stijnen and S. E. Hovius, Bacterial load in relation to vacuum-assisted closure wound therapy: a prospective randomized trial, *Wound Repair Regen.* **12**(1):11–7 (2004).
49. M. Kaplan, P. Banwell, D. P. Orgill, *et al.*, Guidelines for the management of the open abdomen, *Wounds* **17**(Suppl1):S1–S24 (2005).
50. M. Baharestani, J. De Leon, S. Mendez-Eastman, *et al.*, Consensus Statement: A practical guide for managing pressure ulcers with negative pressure wound therapy utilizing vacuum-assisted closure- understanding the treatment algorithm, *Adv. Skin Wound Care* **21**(Suppl 1):1–20 (2008).
51. J. Stannard, Complex orthopaedic wounds: prevention and treatment with negative pressure wound therapy, *Adv. Skin Wound Care* **17**(1):1–10 (2004).
52. D. P. Orgill, W. G. Austen, C. E. Butler, *et al.*, Guidelines for treatment of complex chest wounds with negative pressure wound therapy, *Wounds* **16**(SupplB):1–23 (2004).
53. S. Gupta, M. Baharestani, S. Baranoski, *et al.*, Guidelines for managing pressure ulcers with negative pressure wound therapy, *Adv. Skin Wound Care* **17**(Suppl2):1–16 (2004).
54. K. Harding, Vacuum assisted closure: recommendations for use. A consensus document. Principles of Best Practice, 1-10. 6-4-2008. MEP Ltd. 6-13-2008. Ref Type: Journal (Full).

55. Various Authors, Position Document: Topical negative pressure in wound management, EWMA, pp. 1–17 (1 May 2007).

56. G. Andros, D. G. Armstrong, C. Attinger, *et al.*, Consensus statement on negative pressure wound therapy (V.A.C.® Therapy) for the management of diabetic foot wounds, *Wounds* 52(6-Suppl):1–32 (2006).

57. KCI. Data on file. Count of literature published between Jan 1, 1996–Jan 12, 2009. 2-4-2009. Ref Type: Unpublished Work.

58. R. G. Frykberg and D. V. Williams, Negative-pressure wound therapy and diabetic foot amputations: a retrospective study of payer claims data, *J. Am. Podiatr. Med. Assoc.* 97(5):351–9 (2007).

59. J. A. Niezgoda, The economic value of negative pressure wound therapy, *Ostomy Wound Manage.* 51(2A Suppl):44S–7S (2005).

60. J. Apelqvist, D. G. Armstrong, L. A. Lavery and A. J. Boulton, Resource utilization and economic costs of care based on a randomized trial of vacuum-assisted closure therapy in the treatment of diabetic foot wounds, *Am. J. Surg.* 195(6):782–8 (2008).

61. M. Augustin and I. Zschocke, Nutzenbewertung der ambulanten und stationaren VAC-therapie aus patientensicht, *MMW Fortschritte der Medizin.* 148:25–32 (2006).

Avance Negative Pressure Wound Therapy (NPWT) with Safetac Technology

Mölnlycke Health Care

Introduction

NPWT is a proven and effective wound treatment strategy. Yet to date, NPWT systems have not prioritised minimising pain and skin trauma. This has meant use of aggressive fixation film adhesives to maintain an airtight seal, which can be very painful at removal as they strip and irritate the skin. Some adhesive films may also cause painful blistering.[1] The WUWHS recommends to always assess pain and select a dressing that is atraumatic to the wound and surrounding skin.[2]

Safetac Technology

Safetac is a patented adhesive technology that minimises pain to patients and trauma to wounds. Safetac technology is available exclusively on Mölnlycke Health Care range of dressings including dressings for Avance NPWT. Safetac technology's soft silicone moulds to the skin's uneven surface pores, while other adherents simply stick to the top of the skin's surface. This moulding action is the secret to why Safetac technology is so effective at minimising pain and preventing maceration

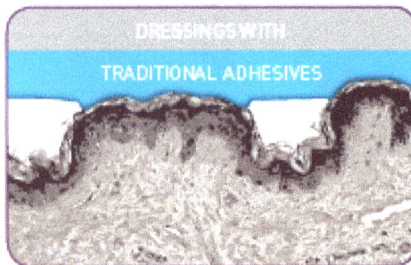

Traditional adhesives are less flexible and only adhere to the top of the skin pores and therefore need to stick harder to stay in place.

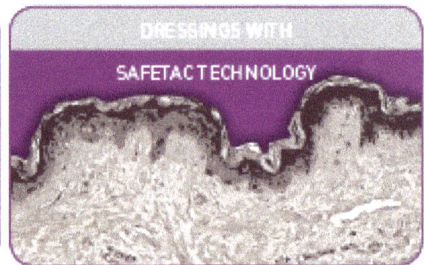

Safetac soft silicone adhesive conforms to the skin's pores, sealing the wound.

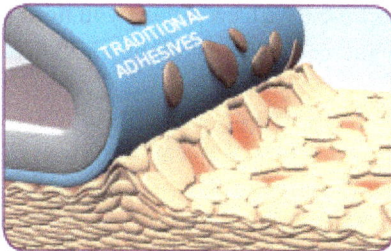

On removal, aggressive traditional adhesives strip epidermal cells, causing wound trauma and pain.

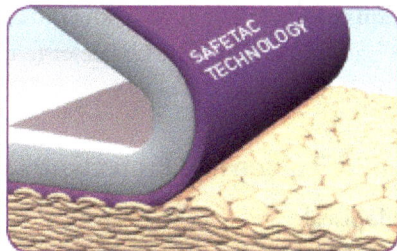

No epidermal cells are removed (no skin-stripping) with a dressing with Safetac technology[5].

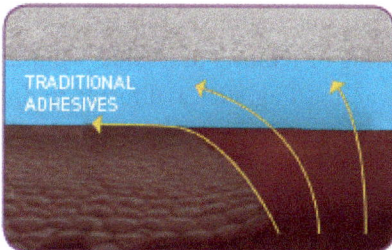

Traditional adhesives can't form a complete seal around the wound, which could lead to exudate spread.

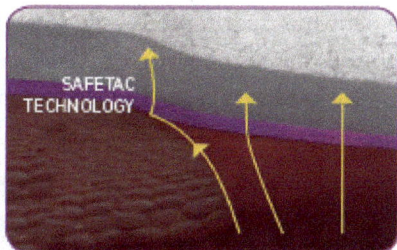

Safetac technology seals the wound margins, effectively minimising the risk of maceration.

Avance NPWT

Avance is a unique NPWT system that helps prevent unnecessary pain and skin trauma. Avance Film with Safetac and Mepiseal® sealant with Safetac help protect the periwound area against maceration,[3] prevent skin stripping at dressing changes,[4] and help prevent the formation of painful blisters.[5]

• **Easy to use.** Avance is lightweight and portable, and comes with a docking station for easy recharging. The same pump is used in hospital and at home.

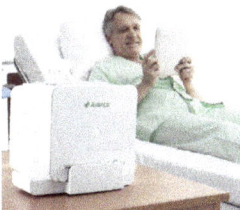

Pump with Docking Station

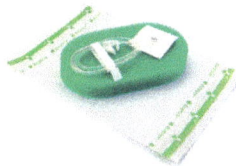

Foam Dressing Kit

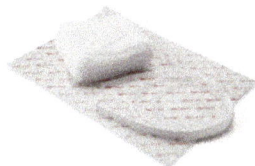

Gauze Dressing Kit

• **Convenience.** The Avance kit comes complete with everything you need for less painful NPWT. The choice of foam and gauze gives you the flexibility to treat all wounds.

Gentle Fixation and Protection

• **Mepiseal**

Mepiseal is a self-curing sealant with Safetac®, applied quickly and accurately from an intuitive, single-use applicator. It adheres effectively, yet gently comes off with no skin stripping or pain.[6] It also helps prevent exudate spreading to the periwound area, protecting skin against maceration and irritation. With Mepiseal there is no wasted time for cutting or removal of residues[6] and it is perfect wherever you need added fixation and sealing, such as difficult-to-dress wound areas

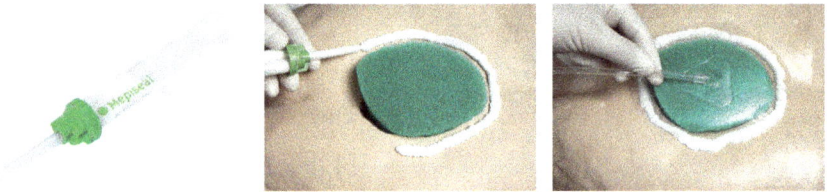

Avance® Film — Proven Less Skin Stripping[4,7,8]

Avance Film with Safetac was compared with two NPWT film dressings (B, C) and a hydrocolloid dressing (A), for their potential to strip skin and cause skin reactions. The dressings were applied to a dyed skin test area on 22 volunteers, and removed five times over 14 days. Colour changes and Transepidermal Water Loss (TEWL) were measured, and a visual assessment made, at each dressing change. Skin treated with Avance Film with Safetac showed the least change in colour and TEWL, and fewer skin reactions.

Mean value: **Erythema** - day 14

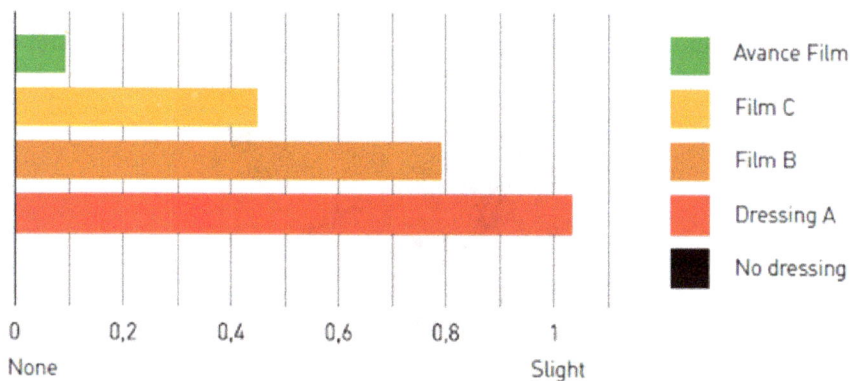

🟩	Avance Film
🟨	Film C
🟧	Film B
🟥	Dressing A
⬛	No dressing

0   0,2   0,4   0,6   0,8   1

None   Slight

Change in **skin colour** - day 14

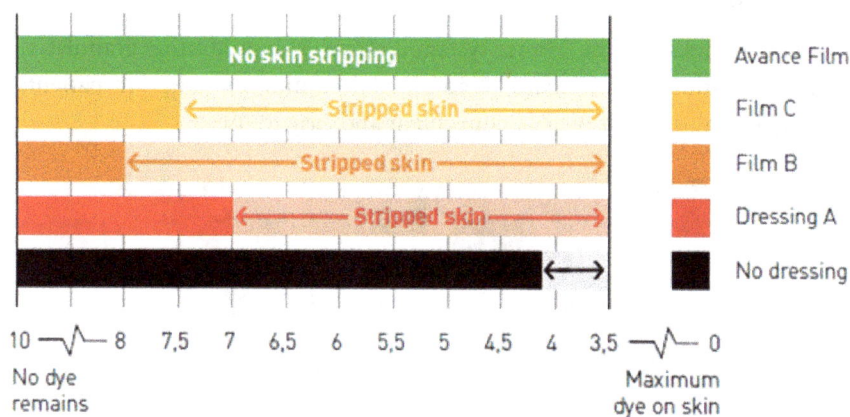

No skin stripping

Stripped skin

Stripped skin

Stripped skin

🟩	Avance Film
🟨	Film C
🟧	Film B
🟥	Dressing A
⬛	No dressing

10 —√— 8   7,5   7   6,5   6   5,5   5   4,5   4   3,5 —√— 0

No dye   Maximum
remains   dye on skin

- **Proven less pain with Mepitel**[9–11]

Several studies have shown that Mepitel as a contact layer between the foam and the wound bed reduces tissue ingrowth into the foam and thereby minimises pain

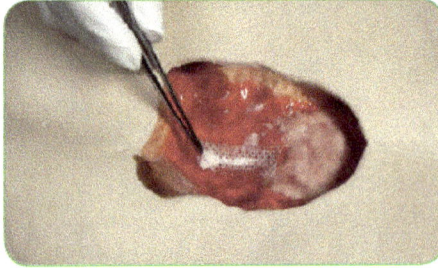

Mepitel on woundbed prior to foam application

Proven Effective and Easy to Use[12,13]

Clinical studies show the Avance system is effective in promoting granulation tissue formation and exudate removal, and minimizes pain for patients. Participants also found Avance convenient and easy to use.

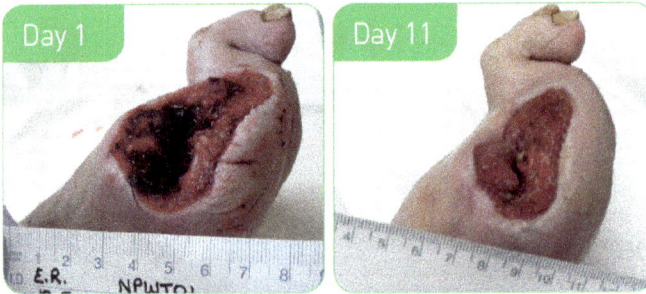

Treatment with Avance in a diabetes-related post amputation wound

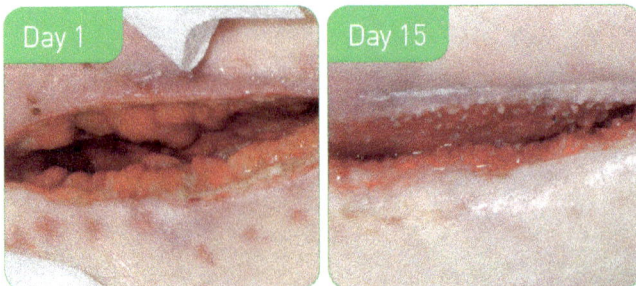

Treatment with Avance on a surgical wound dehiscence

Avance kits include a green foam for wound packing. In a recent study comparing foams and gauze, Avance green foam was proven better at contrasting against blood and exudates than black foam — making it easier to monitor healing progress.[14]

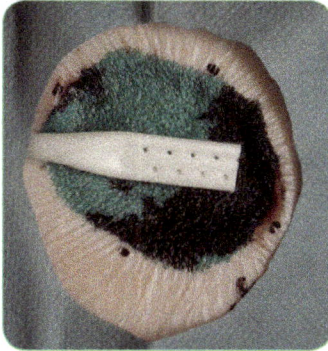 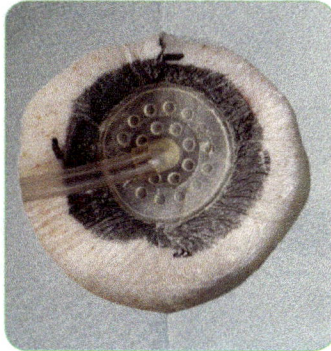

Green Foam　　　　　　　　Black Foam

With Avance Negative Pressure Wound Therapy system, patients use the same NPWT system at home as they did in hospital. Avance is simple to learn and operate for both patients and caregivers, which can help speed up the discharge process. Less pain and optimized sealing promotes better patient compliance, an important consideration in successful healing.

References

1. R. D. Howell, *et al.*, Blister formation with negative pressure dressings after total knee arthroplasty, *Curr. Orthop. Pract.* **22**(2):176 (March/April 2011).
2. Principles of Best Practice, Minimising pain at wound dressing related procedures: a consensus document, *Wounds Int.* (MEP Ltd, London, 2004).
3. S. Meaume, *et al.*, A study to compare a new self adherent soft silicone dressing with a self adherent polymer dressing in stage II pressure ulcers, *Ostomy Wound Manage.* **49**(9):44–51 (2003).
4. P. J. Dykes, *et al.*, Effect of adhesive dressings on the stratum corneum of the skin, *J. Wound Care* **10**(2):7–10 (2001).
5. T. Pukki, *et al.*, Assessing Mepilex® Border in post-operative wound care, *Wounds UK* **6**(1):30–40 (2010).
6. T. Brindle, *et al.*, Use of a novel injectable silicone dressing to improve outcomes with NPWT for complex wounds: a VCU experience. Poster presented at SAWC, Florida, USA (April 2010).
7. R. Zillmer, *et al.*, Biophysical effects of repetitive removal of adhesive dressings on periulcer skin, *J. Wound Care* **15**(5):187–91 (2006).
8. Data on file.

9. A. Dunbar, *et al.*, Silicone net dressing as an adjunct with negative pressure wound therapy, *Ostomy Wound Manage.* **51**(11A Suppl):21–2 (2005).

10. S. G. Terrazas, Adjuvant dressing for negative pressure wound therapy in burns, *Ostomy Wound Manage.* **52**(1):16,18 (2006).

11. M. Malmsjö, *et al.*, Green foam, black foam or gauze for NWPT: effects on granulation tissue formation, *J. Wound Care* **20**(6):294–9 (2011).

12. G. Stansby, *et al.*, Clinical experience with a new NPWT system in the treatment of diabetic foot ulcers and post-amputation wounds, *J. Wound Care* **19**(11):496, 498–502 (2010).

13. P. Chadwick, *et al.*, Avance® negative pressure wound therapy system: a clinical focus, *Wounds UK* **6**(4):114–22 (2010).

14. M. Malmsjö, *et al.*, Green foam, black foam or gauze for NWPT: effects on granulation tissue formation, *J. Wound Care* **20**(6):294–9 (2011).

※ We are **smith&nephew**

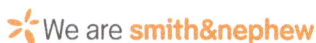

Smith & Nephew has been providing wound care solutions for over 150 years. As a market leader in advanced wound management we provide healthcare professionals with cost — effective solutions and services that help patients with chronic wounds heal quickly, with fewer complications, and get back to their normal life faster.

Wound Bed Preparation — The Path to Healing

Wound Bed Preparation (WBP) is a systematic approach to achieving rapid wound healing. In chronic wounds there are several barriers to healing, such as presence of bacterial overgrowth, necrotic or sloughy tissue, and an imbalance in moisture levels within the wound. Preparing the wound bed by selecting the treatment according to wound characteristics helps foster an ideal environment to advance healing.

The goals of WBP are to:

- Achieve a well-vascularized wound bed by removing necrotic tissue and slough
- Decrease the bacterial burden, reducing inflammation or infection
- Manage the exudate levels to avoid maceration, desiccation and create a moist wound environment

Debridement

INTRASITE° GEL is an excellent example of an advance wound care product which facilitates autolytic debridement by re-hydrating hard necrotic tissue. This amorphous hydrogel dressing also loosens and absorbs slough and exudate. Notably, during the later stages of wound closure, it provides an optimum moist wound environment.[1] This makes INTRASITE° Gel ideal for every stage in the wound management process and of particular importance in wound bed preparation.

Product indication

INTRASITE° Gel is used in shallow and deep open wounds.

Reference

1. J, Gates and G. A. Holloway, A comparison of wound environment, *Ostomy Wound Manage.* **38**(8):34–37 (1994).

VERSAJET◇ The innovative VERSAJET defines "hydrosurgery" as the use of specialized waterjet-powered surgical tools designed to establish new standards for patient care and procedural efficiency in wound debridement and other surgical applications.

The VERSAJET Hydrosurgery System enables surgeons to simultaneously hold, cut and remove damaged tissue and contaminants precisely-without the collateral trauma associated with current surgical modalities. Debridement of traumatic wounds, chronic wounds and other soft tissue lesions is achieved in a single step, with a single instrument, and single-handedly, while sparing healthy tissue and permitting the healing process to progress naturally (Figs. 1 to 3).

VERSAJET◇ II Hydrosurgery System enhances preservation of viable tissue during surgical debridement and reduces time to closure, while streamlining excision through procedural efficiency that delivers consistent clinical and economic value.

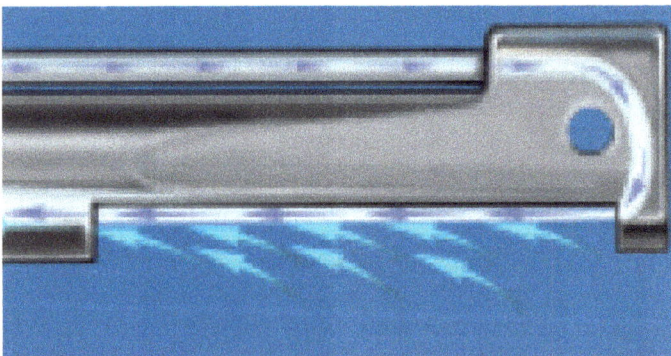

Figure 1.   Show venturi effect — a high velocity stream of sterile saline jets across the operating window and into an evacuation collector, creating a localized vacuum to hold and cut targeted tissue while aspirating debris from the site

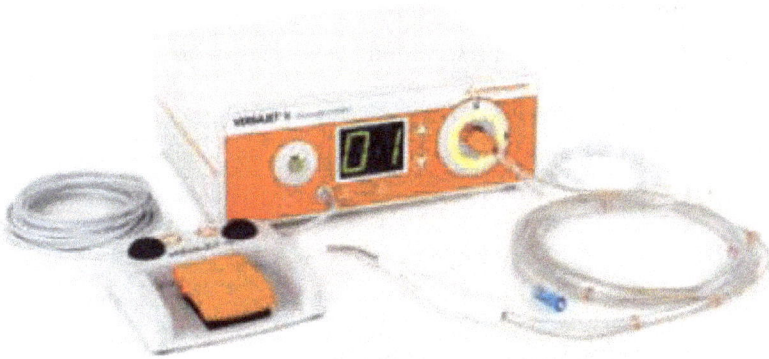

Figure 2. Versajet II hydrosurgery system

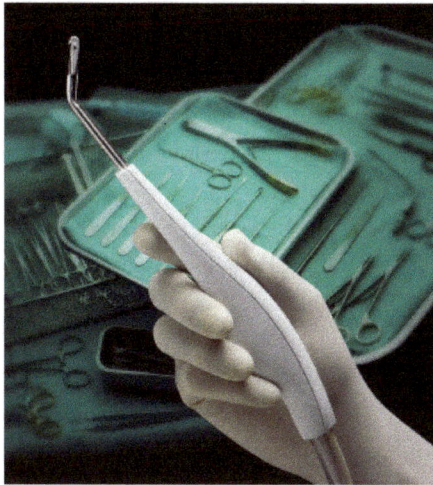

Figure 3. Versajet handset

Product indication

The VERSAJET II Hydrosurgery System is intended for wound debridement (acute, chronic wounds and burns), soft tissue debridement and cleansing of the surgical site in applications that, in the physician's judgment, require sharp debridement and pulsed lavage irrigation.

Clinical Examples:

Achieving maximum tissue preservation

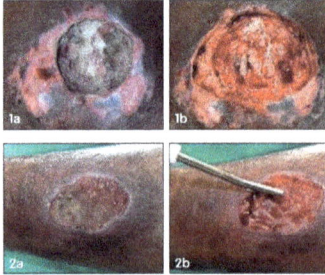

Tissue loss
Centripetal debridement:
Stage IV sacral decubitus
ulcer before (1a) and after (1b)
conventional surgical excision

Tissue preservation
Centrifugal debridement:
Chronic lower extremity ulcer
before (2a) and after (2b)
precise VERSAJET excision

Source: Adapted from Abernathie and Granick (2009)[4]

Managing Bacterial Burden, Inflammation and Infection

IODOFLEX°/IODOSORB° consist of Cadexomer matrix with Iodine, remove barriers to healing by its dual action antimicrobial and desloughing properties. The broad spectrum antimicrobial action is provided by the sustained release of iodine and the desloughing action is provided by the unique cadexomer matrix.

By effectively removing the barriers of bacteria, slough, debris and excess exudate, IODOFLEX°/IODOSORB° have been shown to create an effective wound healing environment and are effective for the management of chronic exuding wounds.

James *et al.* (2008) indicated that 60% of chronic wounds contain biofilms[1]; IODOFLEX°/IODOSORB° has been shown to not only prevent the formation of biofilms but also to substantially eradicate mature biofilms *(in-vitro)*[2,3] specifically on mature *Pseudomonas aeruginosa* PAO1 biofilm.

IODOFLEX°	IODOSORB° Power	IODOSORB° Ointment

Comparison between cadexomer iodine and povidone iodine	
Cadexomer iodine • Iodine is contained within the Cadexomer particles, physically bound • Cadexomer iodine is a reservoir which holds the iodine until it is required • Iodine levels below 1% are maintained with a lower concentration at the wound surface	Povidone iodine • Iodine is complexed to the PVP-1-chemically bound • PVP-1 is dissolved & becomes part of the wound fluid • PVP-1 is a kind of iodine, not just a reservoir. It is "fully" ready to act, which may potentially cause cytotoxic effects and have a short active life

Product indication

IODOSORB°/IODOFLEX° is a cadexomer matrix with iodine formulation indicated for the treatment and healing of chronic ulcers. It provides a broad spectrum antimicrobial action through the sustained release of iodine for up to 72 hours. It acts to:

- Debride and deslough the wound bed
- Reduce bacterial load/prevent and eradicate biofilm
- Absorb exudate and create a moist wound environment

References

1. G. A. James, *et al.*, Biofilms in chronic wounds, *Wound Repair Regen.* 16(1):37–44 (2008).
2. P. L. Phillips, *et al.*, Effects of antimicrobial agents on an (*in-vitro*) biofilm model of skin wounds, 1:299–304 (2010).
3. Smith and Nephew Research Centre Work Report #WRP-TSG015-07-001.
4. B. Abernathie and M. S. Granick, Centrifugal debridement: tissue sparing surgical treatment of chronic wounds, *J. Wound Technol.* 5:10–1 (2009).

ACTICOAT°, ACTICOAT° Flex, ACTICOAT° absorbent

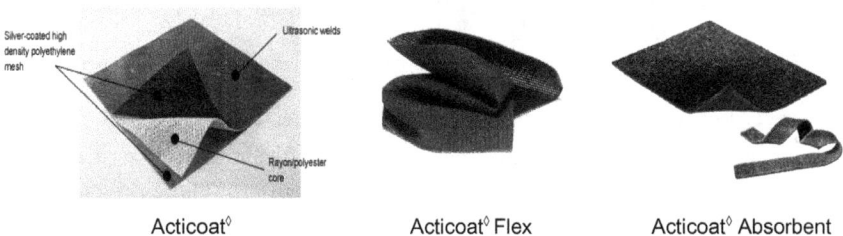

Silver-coated high density polyethylene mesh

Ultrasonic welds

Rayon/polyester core

Acticoat°   Acticoat° Flex   Acticoat° Absorbent

Product description

ACTICOAT° with SILCRYST Nanocrystals is a silver antimicrobial barrier dressing that releases the antimicrobial power of silver within the dressing and also to the wound bed, without inhibiting wound healing. It is a 3 layered dressing constructed of a silver-coated mesh applied to either side of rayon/poly ester core.

ACTICOAT° Absorbent with SILCRYST Nanocrystals combines all the antimicrobal benefits of ACTICOAT° with a highly absorbent alginate to provide a moist wound environment, high absorbency and the antimicrobial power of silver within the dressing and also to the wound bed.

ACTICOAT◇ Flex dressing consists of a flexible, low adherent polyester layer coated with nanocrystalline silver. ACTICOAT◇ Flex is a highly conformable dressing that follows the body contours to maintain contact with the wound surface. The dressing is low adherent, which helps to minimize wound trauma at dressing changes. Nanocrystalline silver provides an effective barrier to microbial contamination.

ACTICOAT◇ dressings, with SILCRYST silver, actively takle a broad spectrum of bacteria (*in vitro*)[1−7] and have proven to kill bacteria, including MRSA, in as little as 30 minutes (*in vitro*).[8]

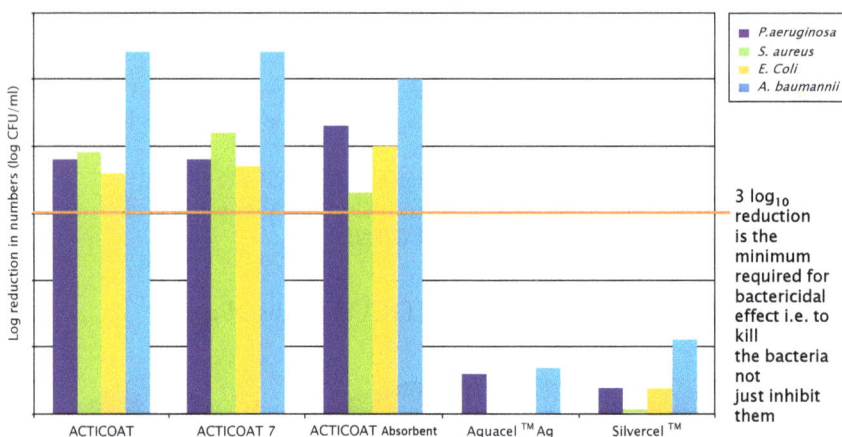

Figure 1. Log reduction in bacterial numbers generated by a range of silver containing wound management dressings after a 30 minute contact time[7]

Product indication

ACTICOAT◇ indicated as an antimicrobial barrier layer over partial and full thickness wounds such as pressure ulcers, leg ulcers, diabetic foot ulcers, burns and recipient graft sites.

ACTICOAT◇ Flex 3 indicated as an antimicrobial barrier dressing over partial and full thickness wounds such as burns, recipient graft sites, pressure ulcers, venous ulcers, diabetic ulcers. ACTICOAT◇ Flex 3 may be used to complement Negative Pressure Wound Therapy (NPWT) protocols for up to 3 days.

ACTICOAT◇ absorbent indicated as an antimicrobial absorbent dressing over full and partial thickness wounds such as pressure ulcers, venous ulcers, diabetic ulcers, burns, donor and recipient graft sites and cavity wounds

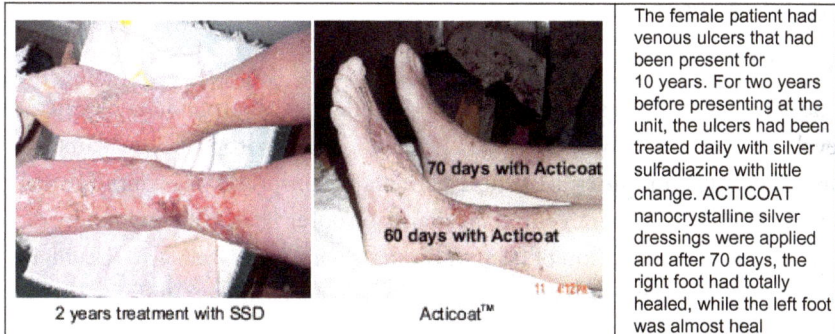

| | | The female patient had venous ulcers that had been present for 10 years. For two years before presenting at the unit, the ulcers had been treated daily with silver sulfadiazine with little change. ACTICOAT nanocrystalline silver dressings were applied and after 70 days, the right foot had totally healed, while the left foot was almost heal |

2 years treatment with SSD   Acticoat™

70 days with Acticoat
60 days with Acticoat

When to use ACTICOAT◊ vs IODOSORB◊

ACTICOAT range	IODOSORB range
• Low to high levels of exudate evident (choose appropriate option) • Wounds range from small to large surface areas • Three to seven day wear time required • Iodine not suited or well tolerated • Prevent biofilm formation	• De-sloughing required • Smaller wounds being treated (not suited to larger surface area wounds) • Moderate exudate levels evident • Up to three day wear time required • High risk wounds i.e. diabetic wounds are being treated • Eradicate biofilm and/or prevent biofilm formation

References

1. Smith & Nephew Data on file report 0810016.
2. Smith & Nephew Data on file report 0810017.
3. Smith & Nephew Data on file report 0810012.
4. Smith & Nephew Data on file report 0810013.
5. J. Wright, *et al.*, Wound management in an era of increasing bacterial antibiotic resistance: a role for topical silver treatment, *Am. J. Infect. Control* **26**(6):572–7 (1998).
6. J. Wright, *et al.*, Efficacy of topical silver against fungal burn wound pathogens, *Am. J. Infect. Control* **27**(4):344–50 (1999).
7. Westaim (Sherritt) Report Reference 93/001 Broad Spectrum Efficacy.
8. Smith & Nephew Data on file report 0507005.

Exudate Management

ALLEVYN◊

The ALLEVYN◊ dressing range provides effective management of exudate levels in chronic wounds.[1,2] ALLEVYN◊ is a hydrophilic polyurethane dressing with a unique triple-action technology comprised of a wound contact layer, a highly absorbent central layer and an outer layer which is waterproof and aids in the prevention of bacterial contamination. ALLEVYN◊ is a highly useful dressing that can be used for low to heavy exuding wounds.

Wound model studies show that, based on an exudation rate of a typical highly exuding wound, ALLEVYN◊ can be left in place for approximately four days without exudate leakage.[3] While being highly absorbent, ALLEVYN◊ also maintains a moist wound environment at the wound surface which may assist in the prevention of eschar or non-viable tissue. In addition, the ALLEVYN◊ dressings are easy to use, require less frequent dressing changes and are soft and conformable for patient comfort.

Since chronic wounds vary in size, severity and location, ALLEVYN◊ dressings are available to accommodate these differences. ALLEVYN◊ Ag is the new range added recently to our existing ALLEVYN◊ range of products.

References

1. S. Thomas, Foam dressings: a guide to the properties and uses of the main foam dressings available in the UK, *J. Wound Care* **2**(3):153–6 (1993).

2. M. J. Callam, Lothian and Forth Valley leg ulcer healing trial. Part 2: Knitted viscose primary dressing versus a hydrocellular dressing in the treatment of chronic leg ulceration, *Phlebology* 7:142–5 (1992).
3. J. W. L. Davis, *et al.*, A guide to the rate of non-renal water loss from patients with burns, *Br. J. Plast. Surg.* 27:325–9 (1974).

Negative Pressure Wound Therapy

RENASYS◇ GO offers clinicians a seamless Negative Pressure Wound Therapy (NPWT) package. Portable, compact and lightweight, patients on RENASYS◇ GO can start their therapy in hospital and proceed home with the therapy seamlessly.

Smith & Nephew is the first NPWT company to offer the choice of foam or gauze wound interface, giving clinicians the flexibility to tailor treatment to meet the individual needs of the patient, wound or care setting.

Published research[1,2] has shown that both foam and gauze fillers are equally effective at delivering negative pressure, wound contraction and stimulation of blood flow at wound edge.

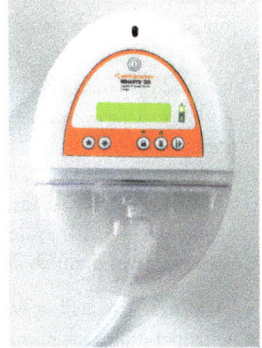

Measurement of Delivery of Negative Pressure to Wound Bed Through Foam or Gauze

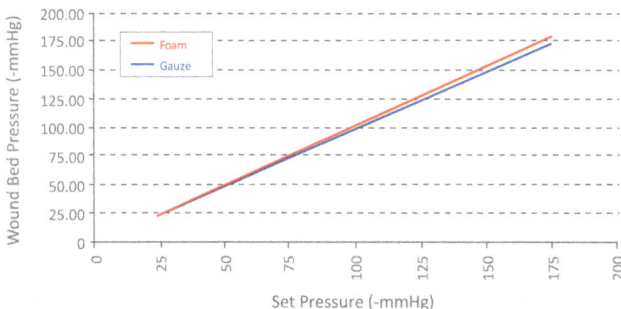

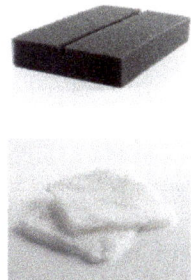

Studies are now emerging showing that the amount and character of granulation tissue formed may differ between the two dressings. The use of foam as a wound interface in NPWT produces thick, hypertrophic granulation tissue.[3–5] Gauze under NPWT results in less thick but dense granulation tissue.[3] The table below summarizes key characteristics of the two interfaces.

Gauze	Foam
Produce less thick but dense and more robust granulation tissue.[6]	Produce thick, hypertrophic but less robust granulation tissue.[6] Risk of in-growth of tissue into foam dressing.
Quick and easy to apply. Conformable to complex surfaces, tunneling and undermining.[9]	Easy to apply to deep, regular shaped wound. Requires cutting to size and shape of wound.
Gauze fillers are impregnated with the antimicrobial polyhexamethylene biguanide (PHMB) as standard.[7]	Routine open cell foam does not contain an antimicrobial, but silver impregnated foam is available.[8]
Comes with two drain choice:	Suction applied via a port fixed to the upper surface of the adhesive film.
• Flat drains for shallow wounds. • Channel drains for narrow wounds or tunnelling.[7]	

Comparison Between Foam and Gauze Filler for Wounds with Undermining Wound Bed

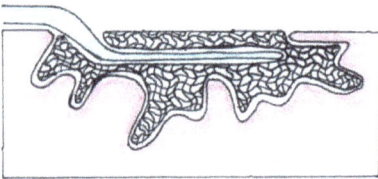

Gauze packed within a typical, irregular wound shape

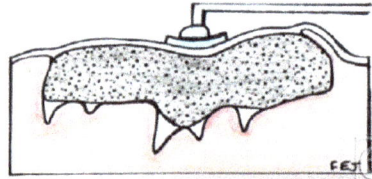

Foam under pressure in an irregular wound shape

Source: Lt Colonel Steve Jeffrey[9]

References

1. M. Malmsjo, R. Ingemansson, R. Martin, *et al.*, Negative pressure wound therapy using gauze or polyurethane open cell foam: similar early effects on pressure transduction and tissue contraction in an experimental porcine wound model, *Wound Repair Regen*. 17(2):200–5 (2009).
2. M. Malmsjo, R., Ingemansson, R., Martin and E. Huddleston, Similar physical properties of gauze and polyurethane foam in delivery of Negative Pressure Wound Therapy. Poster.

3. O. Borgquist, R. Ingemansson and M. Malmsjö, Micro- and macromechanical effects on the wound bed by negative pressure wound therapy using gauze and foam, *Ann. Plast. Surg.* **64**(6):789–93 (2010).

4. O. Borgquist, L. Gustafsson, R. Ingemansson, *et al.*, Tissue ingrowth into foam but not into gauze during negative pressure wound therapy. *Wounds* **21**(11):302–9 (2009).

5. M. Fraccalvieri, Negative pressure wound therapy using the gauze and the foam: immuno-histological and ultrasonography morphological analysis of the granulation tissue and the scar tissue. Preliminary report of a clinical study presented at the 3rd Congress CORTE 4–6 March 2010. Available from: http://www.corteitalia.org/ (accessed April).

6. M. Malmsjö and O. Borgquist, NPWT settings and dressing choices made easy, *Wounds Int.* **1**(3). Available from http://www.woundsinternational.com.

7. P. E. Campbell, G. S. Smith and J. M. Smith, Retrospective clinical evaluation of gauze based negative pressure wound therapy, *Int. Wound J.* **5**:280–6 (2008).

8. R. Gerry, S. Kwei, L. Bayer and K. H. Breuing, Silverimpregnated vacuum-assisted closure in the treatment of recalcitrant venous stasis ulcers, *Ann. Plast. Surg.* **59**(1):58–62 (2007).

9. S. Jeffrey, Advanced wound therapies in the management of severe military lower limb trauma: a new perspective, *Epalsty* **9**:e28 (2009).

Systagenix

PROMOGRAN® Protease Modulating Matrix

Introduction

PROMOGRAN® is sterile, freeze-dried composite of 55% Collagen and 45% Oxidised Regenerated Cellulose (ORC).

PROMOGRAN® is designed to promote an optimal healing environment.[1]

With PROMOGRAN®, stalled wounds close:

- Faster[1,2]
- Cost effectively[1,3,4]

In the presence of exudate the PROMOGRAN® matrix transforms into a soft and conformable, biodegradable gel: this allows contact with all areas of the wound.

How PROMOGRAN® Works?

Collagen/ORC has been proven to reduce levels of proteases such as MMPs and Elastase. This may restore the balance of the wound microenvironment, promoting granulation tissue and helping the wound close.[5]

PROMOGRAN® HAS ABILITY TO REDUCE WOUND SURFACE AREA

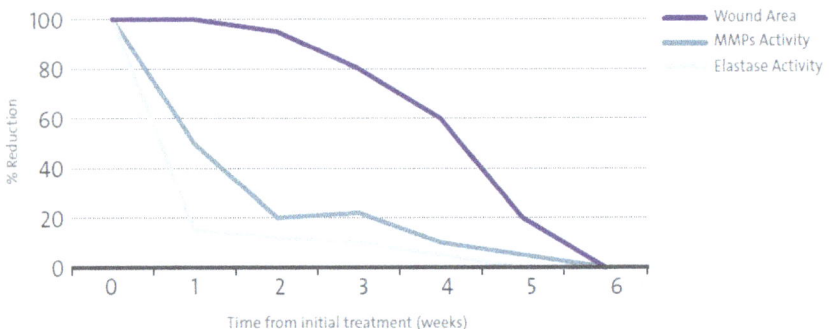

1) PROMOGRAN® binds and inactivates excess <u>PROTEASES</u> (once inactivated those proteases remain inactivated)
2) PROMOGRAN® binds and protects endogeneous <u>GROWTH FACTORS</u> (and afterwards those Growth Factors are released completely functional into the wound)

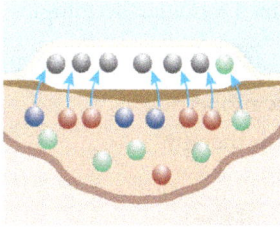

Deactivated
Protease MMPs
Protease Elastase
Growth factors and Cell proliferation

By reducing both MMP and Elastase activity the wound surface area has been shown to decrease in size. Collagen alone has been shown to be less effective at reducing protease activity than collagen/ORC.

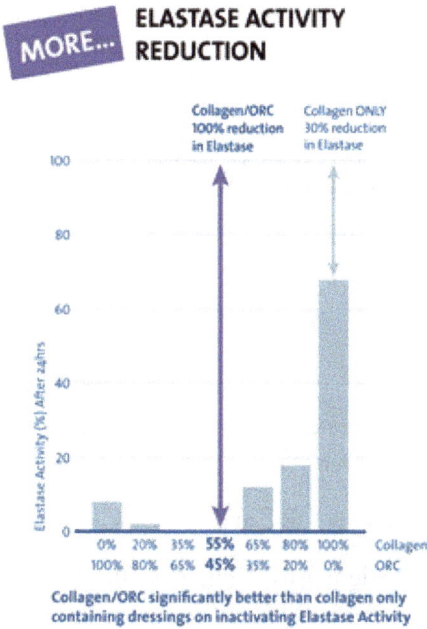

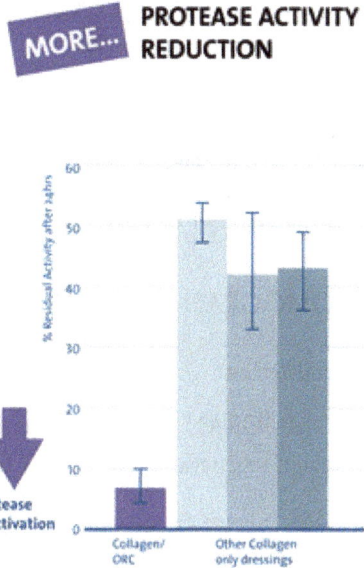

ELASTASE ACTIVITY REDUCTION

MORE...

PROTEASE ACTIVITY REDUCTION

MORE...

Collagen/ORC 100% reduction in Elastase — Collagen ONLY 30% reduction in Elastase

Collagen/ORC significantly better than collagen only containing dressings on inactivating Elastase Activity

Protease Inactivation

Indications:

PROMOGRAN® is indicated for the management of all wounds healing by secondary intent which are clear of necrotic tissue, including: Diabetic ulcers, venous ulcers, pressure ulcers, ulcers caused by mixed vascular aetiologies, traumatic and surgical wounds.

- PROMOGRAN® has demonstrated haemostatic properties
- PROMOGRAN® can be used under compression therapy

References

1. J. L. Lazaro-Martinez, *et al.*, Randomized comparative trial of a collagen/oxidized regenerated cellulose dressing in the treatment of neuropathic diabetic foot ulcers, *Circ. Esp.* **82**(1):27–31 (2007).
2. A. Veves, *et al.*, A randomized, controlled trial of Collagen/ORC vs standard treatments in the management of diabetic foot ulcers, *Arch. Surg.* **137**:822–7 (2002).
3. R. Snyder, Sequential therapies and advanced wound care products as a standard practice in the home care setting. Home health abstract for SAWC, San Diego, April 2008 (presentation at the J&J satellite symposium).
4. O. Ghatenekar, M. Willis and U. Persson, Health Economics. 'Cost effectiveness of treating deep diabetic foot ulcers with collagen/ORC in four European countries', *J. Wound Care* **11**(2) (Feb 2002).
5. B. Cullen, R. Smith, E. McCulloch, D. Silcock and L. Morrison, Mechanism of action of Collagen/ORC, a protease modulating matrix for treatment of diabetic foot ulcers, *Wound Repair Regen.* **10**:16–25 (2002).

PROMOGRAN PRISMA®

Introduction

PROMOGRAN PRISMA® matrix is a freeze-dried composite of collagen, oxidized regenerated cellulose (ORC) and silver.

- Made from a matrix of 55% collagen, 44% ORC and 1% ORC/Silver

PROMOGRAN PRISMA® matrix is designed to '**kick start**' the healing process while providing protection from infection.[1,2]

   In the presence of exudate PROMOGRAN PRISMA® matrix transforms into a soft and conformable, biodegradable gel; this allows contact with all areas of the wound.

   With PROMOGRAN PRISMA® Stalled wounds close:

- Faster[3–5]
- Cost effectively[3,6]
- While providing protection from infection[2,7]

How PROMOGRAN PRISMA® Works?

PROMOGRAN PRISMA® binds and inactivates proteases such as MMPs and Elastase to help rebalance the wound microenvironment, while providing low level silver to help prevent infection.[1,2]

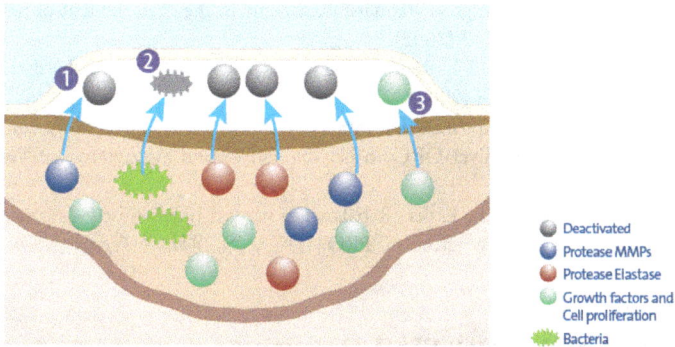

USING **PROMOGRAN PRISMA**®
HERE'S HOW IT WORKS

Legend:
- Deactivated
- Protease MMPs
- Protease Elastase
- Growth factors and Cell proliferation
- Bacteria

1 Collagen/ORC absorbs and inactivates Proteases [6-8]

2 Silver/ORC provides antimicrobial protection against bacteria and infection [6]

3 Protects growth factors [5]

Indications:

PROMOGRAN PRISMA® is indicated for is indicated for the management of all wounds healing by secondary intent which are clear of necrotic tissue, including: Diabetic ulcers, venous ulcers, pressure ulcers, ulcers caused by mixed vascular aetiologies, traumatic and surgical wounds.

- PROMOGRAN PRISMA® has demonstrated haemostatic properties and can be used under compression therapy.

References

1. B. Cullen, *et al.*, ORC/Collagen matrix containing silver controls bacterial bioburden while retaining dermal cell viability. Poster presented at EWMA Prague (May 2006).

2. S. Gregory, *et al.*, The ability of ORC/Collagen containing silver to reduce bioburden and retain dermal cell viability. Johnson & Johnson Wound Management, Gargrave, UK. Poster presented at ETRS Stuttgart (September 2005).
3. G. Nisi, *et al.*, Use of protease-modulating matrix in the treatment of pressure sores, *Chir. Ital.* **57**:465–8 (2005).
4. J. L. Lazaro-Martinez, *et al.*, Randomized comparative trial of a collagen/oxidized regenerated cellulose dressing in the treatment of neuropathic diabetic foot ulcers, *Circ. Esp.* **82**(1):27–31 (2007).
5. A. Veves, *et al.*, A randomized, controlled trial of PROMOGRAN® (a collagen/oxidised regenerated cellulose dressing) vs standard treatments in the management of diabetic foot ulcers, *Arch. Surg.* **137**:822–7 (2002).
6. B. Cullen, T. Domnelly and T. Rennison, Can excessive levels of silver be detrimental to healing?, SAWC, San Diego (2008).
7. B. Cullen, L. Nisbet, M. Gibson, S. Lanzara and P. Zamboni, A clinical study examining the effect of ORC/Collagen/Silver-ORC on healing and wound biochemistry, SAWC, Dallas (2009).
8. B. Cullen, L. Kemp and L. Essler, Rebalancing wound biochemistry improves healing: a clinical study examining effect of PROMOGRAN, *Wound Repair Regen.* **12**(2):A4 (2004).

SILVERCEL® NON-ADHERENT Dressing

Introduction

SILVERCEL® NON-ADHERENT Dressing is the next generation of Silver Antimicrobial Dressing with the unique features of a **Non-Adherent layer** to maximise protection of the wound bed particularly at dressing change.

The unique composition: a mixture of alginate, carboxymethylcellulose, and silver coated nylon fibres manages exudate effectively in infected or heavily colonised wounds. Whilst the unique EasyLIFT® film layer keeps the dressing simple and convenient to use, minimising pain and trauma at dressing change for your patients.

How SILVERCEL® NON-ADHERENT Works?

SILVERCEL® NON-ADHERENT is designed to absorb and retain high amounts of exudate, whilst allowing easy, intact and **atraumatic** pain free removal from the wound bed.[1]

The silver ions within the dressing protect the wound from bacterial contamination.[1]

SILVERCEL® NON-ADHERENT DESIGNED NOT TO STICK

- Maintains a sustained release of silver ions for up to 7 days *in vitro*.[1]
- Stays strong for intact removal, even when wet.[2]
- Optimally spaced perforations allow 'free flow' of exudate into the dressing, and also ensures the dressing stays intact.

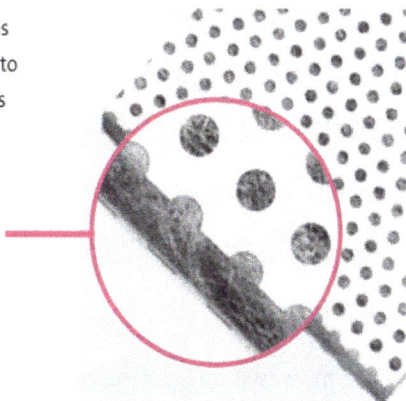

Optimally spaced perforations allow 'free flow' of exudate into the dressing, and also ensures the dressing stays intact.

Easy**LIFT**™ PRECISION FILM

- Conforms to the wound bed for complete coverage when moist, and is designed not to stick to the wound bed at dressing change.
- SILVERCEL® NON-ADHERENT has been proven to be 75% Less Adherent than the market leading silver dressing.[3]

Indications:

SILVERCEL® NON-ADHERENT Dressing is intended for use in the management of all moderate to heavily exuding, partial and full-thickness, chronic and acute wounds including: decubitus (pressure) ulcers, venous ulcers, diabetic ulcers, donor sites, traumatic, surgical wounds. As the product contains alginate it may assist in supporting the control of minor bleeding in supercial wounds. It is also suitable for use, under medical supervision, in the management of infected wounds, or wounds in which there is an increased risk of infection.

References

1. R. Clark, S.-A. Stephens, M. Del Bono, O. Abloye and S. Bayliff, The evaluation of absorbent silver containing dressings in vitro; Systagenix wound management. Poster Presentation CAWC Quebec City (October 2009).
2. R. Clark, M. Del Bono, S.-A. Stephens, O. Abioye and S. Bayliff, Simulated in use tests to evaluate a non-adherent antimicrobial silver alginate dressing. Presentation Quebec City (October 2009).
3. R. Clark, S.-A. Stephens and M. Del Bono, From lab to leg: the importance of correlating in-vitro and in-vivo test systems to clinical experience. Poster presented SAWC (2010).

TIELLE® Family: HYDROPOLYMER Dressing

Introduction

The TIELLE® Family has a unique design compared to ordinary foams:

- It contains LiquaLock® technology, which cleverly retains exudate while also letting moisture vapour pass through the dressing, helping to provide an optimal moist wound healing environment.
- Managing exudate better helps wounds heal faster and increases patient comfort. For instance, in a clinical evaluation of **6993 patients** TIELLE® dressings were proven to be clinically efficacious in all wound types studied, with 95% healing or improvement after 4 weeks of treatment, and to improve the patients' quality of life.[1]
- The TIELLE® Family comes in a wide range of sizes, shapes and absorbencies, allowing you to find a dressing that suits your patients' needs.

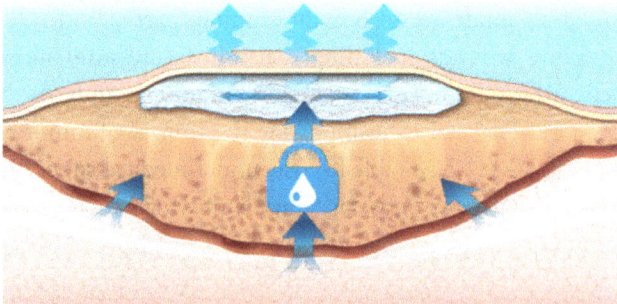

How TIELLE Family Works?

As exudate is absorbed by the dressing, it is designed to expand and conform to the contours of the wound bed, which helps minimise exudate build-up and the chance of maceration.

Under normal use, the **LiquaLock® technology** locks fluid into the cell walls, which means reduced potential for it to be released back into the wound.[2–4]

From September 2011 all TIELLE® Family variants are more absorbent, increasing by up to 41% in some variants — look for the Comfort Plus sticker on the pack.

The vapour-permeable backing allows moisture vapour to transfer through the back of the dressing, allowing for absorption of additional exudate.

Indications:

The TIELLE® range of dressings is indicated for the management of different types of wounds and exudate levels.

TIELLE® Family	LIQUA LOCK	Exudate level	Adhesive	Cut-able
TIELLE®	🔒	●●○	✔	—
TIELLE® Lite	🔒	●○○	✔	—
TIELLE® Sacrum	🔒	●●○	✔	—
TIELLE® Packing	🔒	●●●	—	✂
TIELLE® Plus	🔒	○●●	✔	—
TIELLE® Plus Sacrum	🔒	○●●	✔	—
TIELLE® Plus Heel	🔒	●●●	✔	—
TIELLE® Xtra	🔒	●●●	—	✂

References

1. C. Diehm and H. Lawall, Evaluation of TIELLE® hydropolymer dressings in the management of chronic exudating wounds in primary care, *Int. Wound J.* **2**(1):26–35 (2005).
2. A. Taylor, C. Lane, J. Walsh, S. Whittaker, K. Ballard and S. R. Young, A non-comparative multicentre clinical evaluation of a new hydropolymer adhesive dressing, *J. Wound Care* **8**(10):489–92 (1999).
3. K. Carter, Hydropolymer dressings in the management of wound exudate, *Br. J. Comm. Nursing* **8**(9)(Suppl):10–6 (2003).

4. S. Foster and P. Mistry, The evaluation of fluid retention in foam dressings, *Wounds UK* (2010).

INADINE®

Introduction

INADINE® is a non-adherent topical dressing with 10% povidone iodine equivalent to 1.0% available iodine, polyethylene glycol and purified water. It is a broad spectrum antimicrobial slow release iodine contact layer and has no reported cases of acquired resistance.[1]

INADINE® dressing is designed to protect the wound, even if infected.

Comparison of commonly used antimicrobials: microbial properties

	Gram +	Gram -	Fungi	Spores*	Viruses	Resist Resistance
Chlorhexidine	+++	++	+	0	+	+
Honey	+++	+++	+++	0	+	0
Iodine	+++	+++	+++	+++	++	0
Maggots	+++	++	ND	ND	ND	0
Silver	+++	+++	+	ND	+	+

0 no effect   ND no data   *Endospores

Source: Noreen Campbell RN BScN MA IIWCC LT(Vodder), Donna Campbell RN IIWCC, Foot & Leg Ulcer Clinic, Vancouver Island Health Authority, BC, Canada

How INADINE® Dressing Works?

The Povidone molecule provides an effective release of iodine. The polyethyleneglycol provides a water-soluble environment, which allows the Iodine to reach the bacteria in the wound.

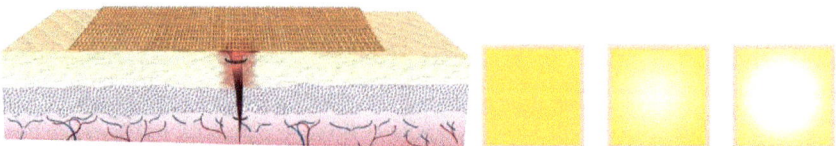

- The frequency of dressing changes depends primarily upon the condition of the wound.

- If large quantities of exudate are produced, daily changes will probably be required; but if the wound is relatively dry, the interval between changes may be extended.
- Fading of the colour of the dressing indicates the loss of antiseptic efficacy and this is when the INADINE® dressing should be changed.

References

1. A. R. McLure, *et al.*, *In-vitro* evaluation of povidone-iodine and chlorhexidine against methicillin-resistant *Staphylococcus aureus*, *J. Hosp. Infect.* 21(4):291–9 (1992).

28

Advances in Wound Management

Aziz Nather and Teo Zhen Ling

Department of Orthopaedic Surgery
Yong Loo Lin School of Medicine
National University of Singapore

Introduction

Wound healing depends on both intrinsic and extrinsic factors. The wound must have a good blood supply and be free from infection and significant biomechanical forces. Recently, there have been several advances in technology to enhance wound healing. These include the development of new generation antibiotics, new generation of dressings — silver dressings, negative pressure technique, mechanical techniques of debridement and maggot therapy.

Ultrasonic Debridement

Necrotic and nonviable tissue impairs wound healing. They also increase the risk of infection. Hence debridement is required to remove nonviable tissues, fibrin deposits and bacteria so that good wound healing can take place. Ultrasonic debridement,[1,2] a form of mechanical debridement, provides an alternative treatment to surgical debridement.

Basic Science

In ultrasonic debridement, low frequency ultrasound (25 to 42 kHz) and normal saline solution is delivered to the wound surface. The energy delivered causes the tissue molecules to oscillate. The effects of ultrasound on wound tissues are:

- *Cavitation* — Ultrasound creates microscopic bubbles in tissue fluids. These bubbles expand and contract according to changing pressure. At certain amplitudes of sound waves, the bubbles implode, forming tiny shock waves. Cavitation aids healing in two ways:
    - It destroys and clears away necrotic tissue:
      As necrotic tissue has less tensile strength than viable tissue, generated shock waves liquefy necrotic tissue, wound debris and biofilm. Viable tissue is left uninjured.
    - It has antibacterial properties:
      Ultrasound breaks up the biofilm in the wound, exposing bacteria to antibiotics. This improves the action of antibiotics on biofilm infections. In addition, ultrasound allows the saline solution to penetrate the tissue deeper. This provides a mechanical rinsing effect. Fibrin deposits and bacterial growth are flushed out of the wound.

- *Acoustic streaming* — Ultrasound pressure waves cause uni-directional movement of body fluids. Acoustic streaming aids healing in two ways:
    - It stimulates cellular activity: The movement of bodily fluids stimulates cellular activity, enhancing wound healing.
    - It has antibacterial properties: It facilitates the transport of antibiotics through the bacteria cell membrane.

In addition, the application of low-frequency ultrasound increases tissue temperature. Blood flow is thus increased, enhancing tissue perfusion. This leads to better wound healing.

The NUH Diabetic Foot Team employs the Ultrasonic Assisted Wound Therapy (UAWT) Unit from Sonoca[3] (Fig. 1). So far, 10 patients with diabetic foot ulcer have been treated with ultrasonic debridement from July 2010 to December 2011.

Case Study 1

A 55-year-old Malay female with Diabetes Mellitus was admitted with a right plantar foot abscess. Ankle Brachial Index (ABI) and Toe Brachial Index (TBI) were normal for both feet. Neuropathy was present with 5.07 Semmes

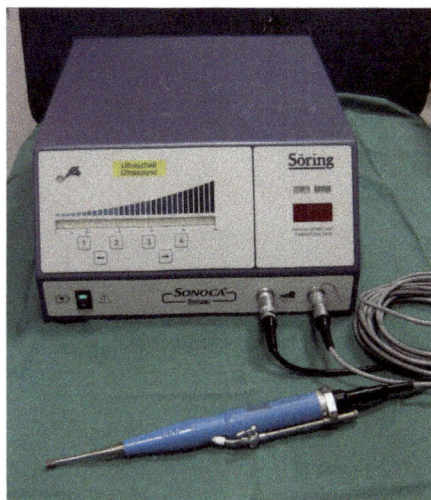

Figure 1. Ultrasonic assisted wound treatment (Sonoca)

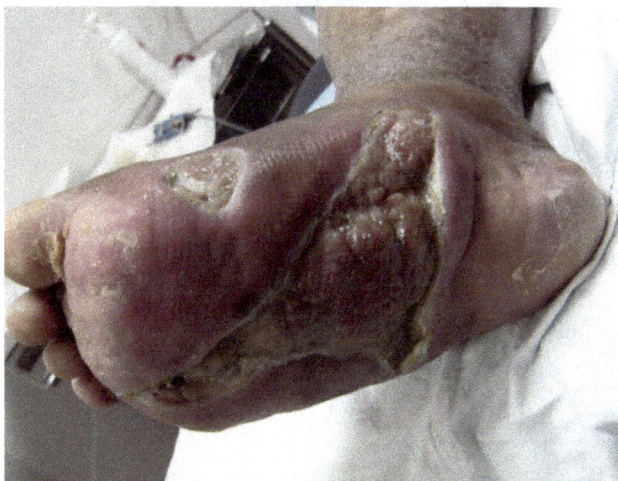

Figure 2. Ulcer with slough, after multiple surgical debridements

Weinstein Monofilament Test (3/10) and Vibration Perception Threshold (VPT) testing (40 V). She did not experience any pain in the foot. Wound cultures were positive for MRSA and Pseudomonas *aeruginosa*. She was treated with intravenous Vancomycin and oral Ciprofloxacin.

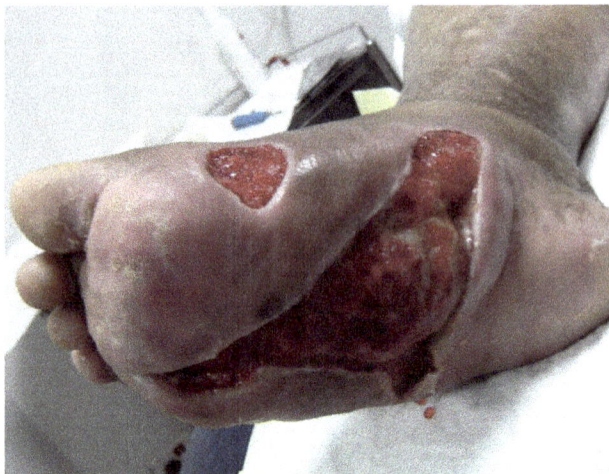

Figure 3. Ulcer after first ultrasonic debridement

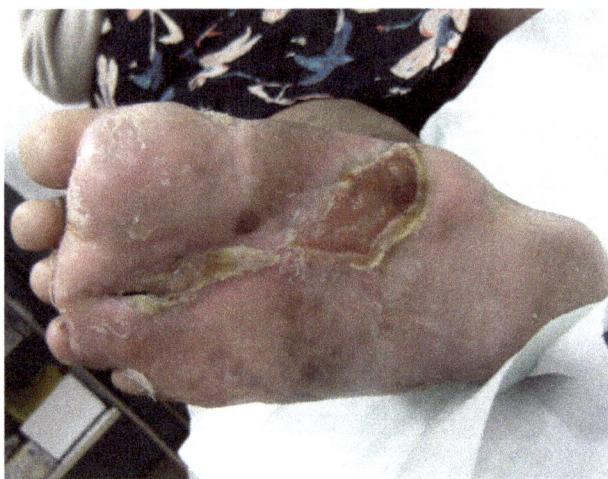

Figure 4. Ulcer healed after 3 months

Surgical debridement of the abscess was first done (Fig. 2). Subsequently, ultrasonic debridement was performed once per week (Fig. 3). Each treatment session was 12–17 minutes with an intensity of 40-50%. After each session, a Seasorb Ag dressing coupled with Mepilex foam dressing, was applied to the wound. 4 sessions of ultrasonic debridement was performed. 3 months post-surgical debridement, the ulcer healed completely (Fig. 4).

Case Study 2

A 68-year-old Malay female with Diabetes Mellitus was admitted with cellulitis of the left foot. ABI were 1.2 and TBI was 0.7. Neuropathy was present with an abnormal VPT reading (32V) and Monofilament test reading (7/10). The patient presented with erythema and a blister over the lateral aspect of the left foot. Wound cultures were positive for Pseudomonas *aeruginosa*. The wounds were treated with intravenous Ceftazidime and Cloxacillin.

During admission, the blister was surgically deroofed. The patient was later discharged with Seasorb Ag dressing. During follow-up, the wound was found to be filled with slough (Fig. 5). Ultrasonic Debridement was performed (Fig. 6) in the outpatient clinic — 2 sessions in total, one session per week. Each session lasted 7 minutes with an intensity of 25%. Dressings applied were supplemented with local Baneocin (antibiotic) powder. The wound responded well to the treatment (Fig. 7) and healed completely in 3 months.

From out limited experience with the use of Ultrasonic debridement (10 cases), the results have been encouraging. Immediately after each session, the wound is red and clean. The redness disappears after a few days. It is not until the next UAWT session that it looks red, raw and healthy again. Nonetheless, a proper randomized control study must be performed before one can conclude that it works well.

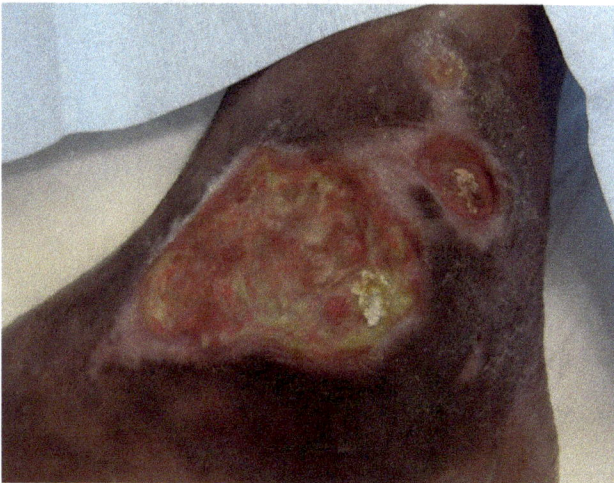

Figure 5.   Ulcer with sloughy wound floor

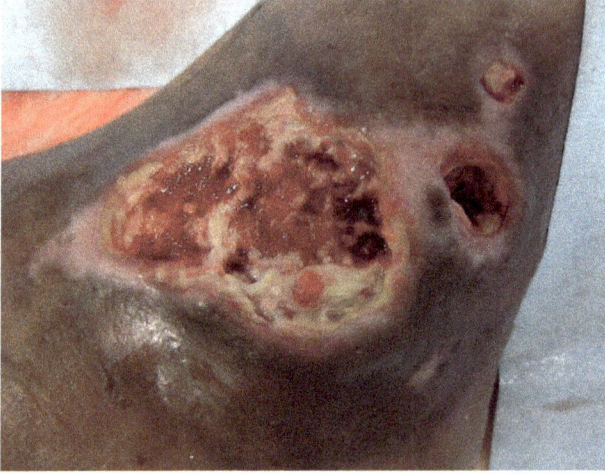

Figure 6. Ulcer after ultrasonic debridement

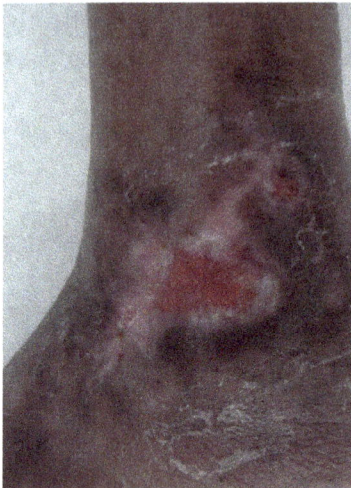

Figure 7. Ulcer almost healed after 1 month since ultrasonic debridement

Maggot Therapy

Maggot therapy[4] is another alternative to surgical debridement.

Basic Science

In maggot therapy, the larvae of *Lucilia cuprina* or *Lucilia sericata* are used to digest necrotic tissue, slough and pathogens in the wound. (Fig. 8) About

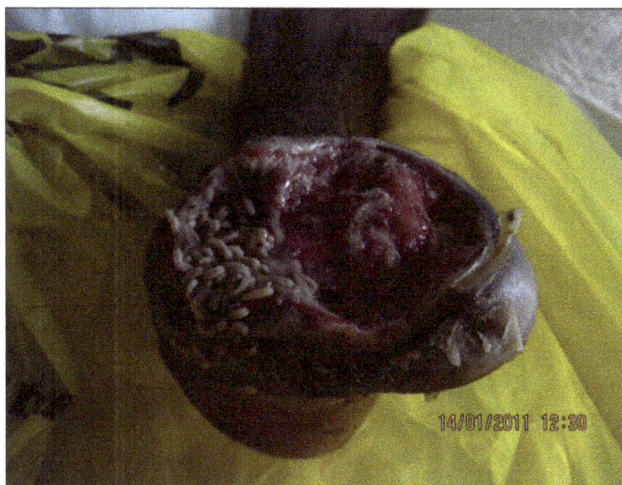

Figure 8. Sterile maggots left on a wound

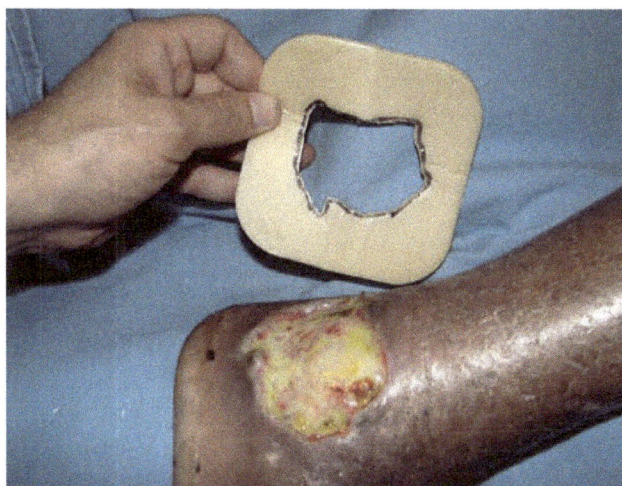

Figure 9. A cut ring of hydrocolloid dressing is placed around the wound

3 to 10 sterile maggots are applied to each square centimeter of the wound surface. They are left within a cage-like dressing[5] or a biobag® dressing for 24–48 hours.

The cage-like dressing is made by first cutting a ring of hydrocolloid dressing, such as Duoderm (Fig. 9). The hydrocolloid dressing is placed onto the skin surrounding the wound to protect the surrounding skin from maggot secretions. The maggots are added to the wound. A covering of porous dacron chiffon or a nylon stocking is then secured to the hydrocolloid ring with glue and tape. This cage-like dressing is then topped with a light gauze pad to absorb the necrotic drainage. The top layer of gauze is replaced every 4–6 hours.

Maggot Therapy enhances wound healing in the following ways:

- *It provides wound debridement* — The maggot secretions and excretions contain powerful enzymes that lyse necrotic tissue without injuring healthy, viable tissues. One such degrading enzyme is trypsin. The maggots then ingest the lysed necrotic tissue.
- *It removes pathogens* — Maggot secretions contain antimicrobial substances that are bactericidal and capable of destroying biofilms.
- *It stimulates granulation tissue formation* — Maggot secretions contain substances such as calcium carbonate, urea, allantoin and ammonia. These substances promote granulation tissue formation and cellular migration. The mechanical stimulation of the wound surface by movements of maggots can also stimulate tissue growth.

Maggot therapy is especially useful for ulcers overlying joint capsules, bones, tendons, vessels and nerves. These vital structures will not be debrided by the maggots.

Case Study:

A patient had a wound following 2nd, 3rd and 4th ray amputations. The wound extended over the dorsum and sole of the right foot (Fig. 10). It was subjected to maggot therapy. Figure 11 shows the ability of maggot therapy to remove slough, leaving behind good granulation tissue.

As shown by Sherman,[5] Maggot therapy is potentially a good alternative to surgical debridement. Once again, a good randomized control study must be performed to show evidence that it is effective.

A good advantage of maggot therapy is that it can be carried out without the need for general or local anesthesia. Patients with bad ulcers but are medically unfit to undergo general anesthesia required for surgical debridement can undergo maggot therapy instead.

A disadvantage of this treatment is that many patients are unable to psychologically accept the placement of maggots on their wounds.

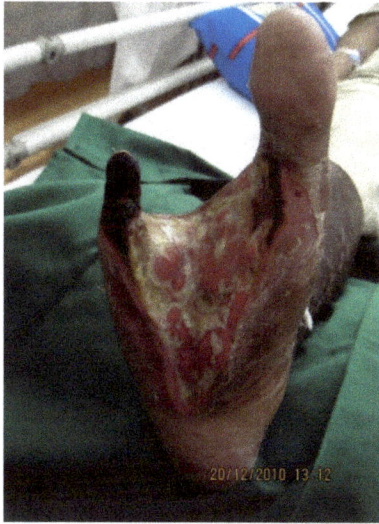

Figure 10. Wound before maggot therapy

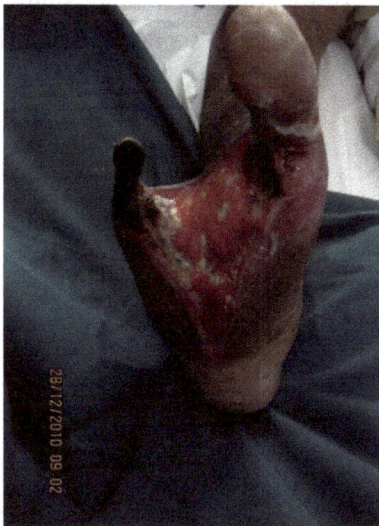

Figure 11. Day 3 after 1st application of maggot therapy

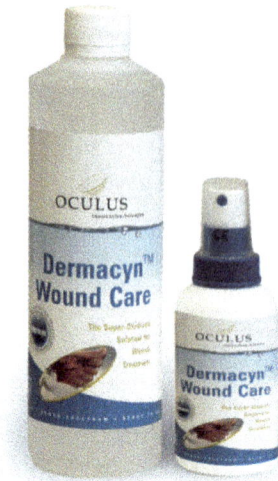

Figure 12.   Demacyn solution

Dermacyn

Dermacyn (Fig. 12) is a super-oxidised antiseptic solution. It can be used for the cleansing of wounds after debridement or during each change of dressing.

Basic Science

Dermacyn[6] is a neutral solution containing reactive species of chlorine and oxygen.

It can be applied directly onto the wound.

Dermacyn (Fig. 12) promotes wound healing in the following ways:

- It creates a moist wound environment.
- It irrigates and debrides the wound.
- It reduces the bacterial load. It degrades bacteria cell wall, causing an osmotic shock that kills bacteria.

Dermacyn may incur high costs if it is used for cleansing of all diabetic wounds. However, it could be used selectively for the cleansing of the following wounds:

- Wound after debridement for Necrotising Fasciitis.
- Infected Below Knee Amputation stump wound.
- Wound infected with *Pseudomonas aeruginosa*.

- Wound infected with Methicillin- Resistant *Staphylococcus Aureus* (MRSA).

Deramcyn can be an effective treatment for such infected diabetic wounds. However, surgical debridement must first be performed to remove all necrotic and infected tissue before Dermacyn can work effectively.

Negative Pressure Wound Therapy

Negative pressure wound therapy,[7] also known as Vacuum Assisted Closure (VAC) therapy, is commonly used in the management of surgical wounds.

Basic Science

VAC therapy accelerates wound healing in several ways:

- *It provides a semi-occlusive environment that keeps the wound moist and clean.* The moisture in the wound prevents desiccation. It also promotes migration and development of epithelial tissue.
- *It physically stimulates granulation tissue formation.* The direct mechanical stress applied on the wound creates a biochemical effect at the cellular level. Cell division, angiogenesis and granulation tissue formation is promoted.
- *It reduces wound exudate and decrease wound oedema.* VAC therapy removes wound exudate. It also reduces extracellular fluid and oedema. Excess fluid at the wound can inhibit the proliferation of keratinocytes, endothelial cells and fibroblasts — cells essential for wound healing. Proteases and cytokines in the wound fluid can cause continued inflammation of the wound. VAC therapy removes these.
- *It improves blood flow.* VAC therapy facilitates optimal blood flow in the wound. This improves the delivery of oxygen, nutrients and inflammatory mediators to the wound. Tissue perfusion is enhanced.
- *It alleviates infection by facilitating the removal of bacteria.*

Application of VAC Dressing

A sterile polyurethane foam (GranuFoam) dressing is trimmed to fit into the wound. (Figs. 13 to 15) The foam has a pore size of 400–600 μm to promote

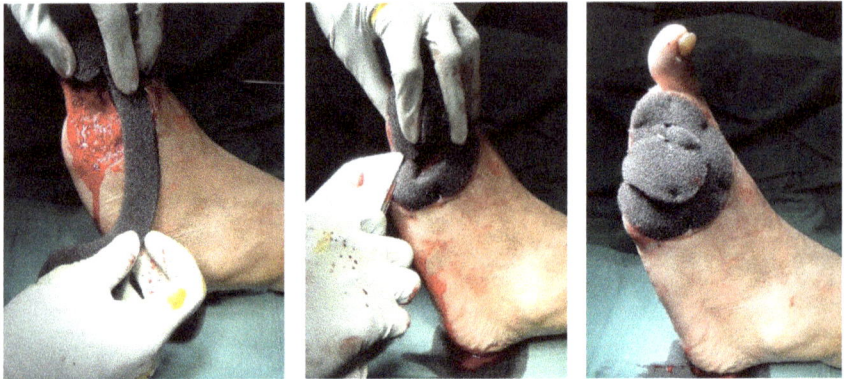

Figures 13 to 15. Step by step application of foam to the wound

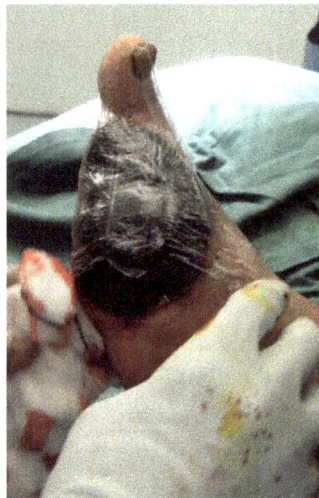

Figure 16. Application of adhesive tape over foam and surrounding skin

in-growth of granulation tissue. Adhesive tape is used to cover the foam and surrounding skin (Fig. 16). A non-collapsible tube connected to an electronic vacuum pump (Fig. 17) is embedded in the foam (Fig. 18).

Alternatively, a Bridge VAC dressing can be applied. In a Bridge VAC dressing, the GranuFoam dressing is placed over the wound and secured with adhesive drape. The bridge foam is then applied to allow placement of the suction pad away from the wound (Fig. 19). By allowing placement of the

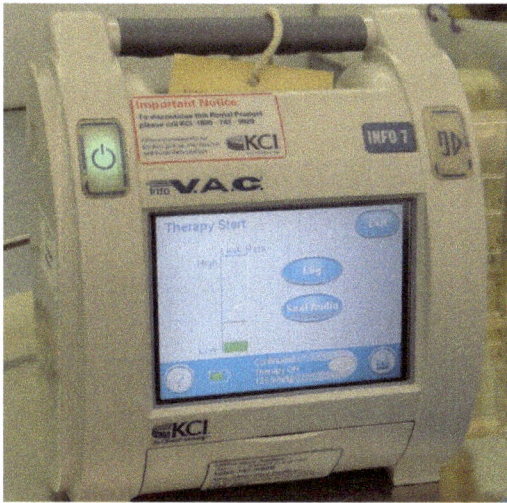

Figure 17. Electronic vacuum pump

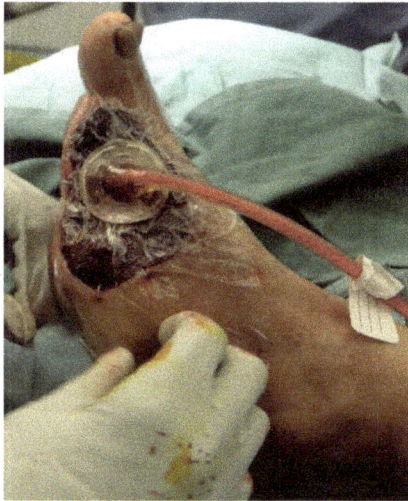

Figure 18. Completed VAC dressing with the non-collapsible tube

suction pad outside the foot area, patients can wear protective shoes and walk with crutches.

After the application of either forms of VAC dressing, negative pressure is then applied continuously or intermittently. At an optimal pressure of

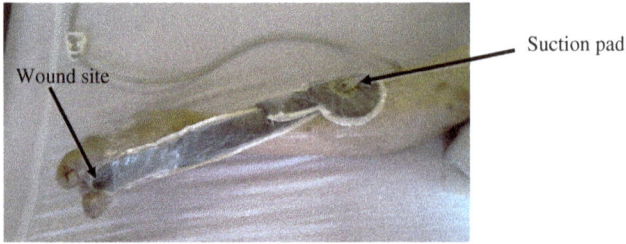

Figure 19. Bridge VAC dressing

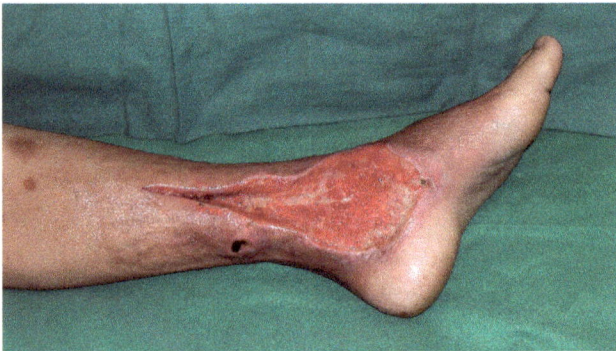

Figure 20. Ankle wound after initial surgical debridement. The medial malleolus was exposed in the wound

125 mmHg, an alternating pressure cycle of 5 minutes turned on followed by 2 minutes turned off is carried out. Cyclical application of pressure is used to alter cell structures.

Case Study 1

A 60-year-old female developed necrotising fasciitis of the left ankle after minor trauma. Surgical debridement was performed. The large ulcer resulting from this aggressive wound debridement was treated with VAC therapy. Figures 20 to 23 show the progress of wound healing in the ulcer treated with VAC therapy. The ulcer eventually showed good healing. The healthy granulation bed allowed a skin graft to be applied successfully (Fig. 23).

In a study of 11 consecutive patients with diabetic foot problems treated by the NUH Diabetic Foot team, the author found that VAC Therapy facilitates

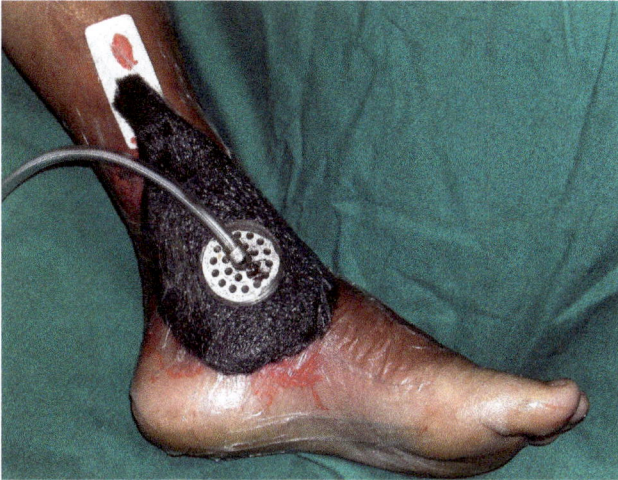

Figure 21. VAC therapy was applied for 2 weeks

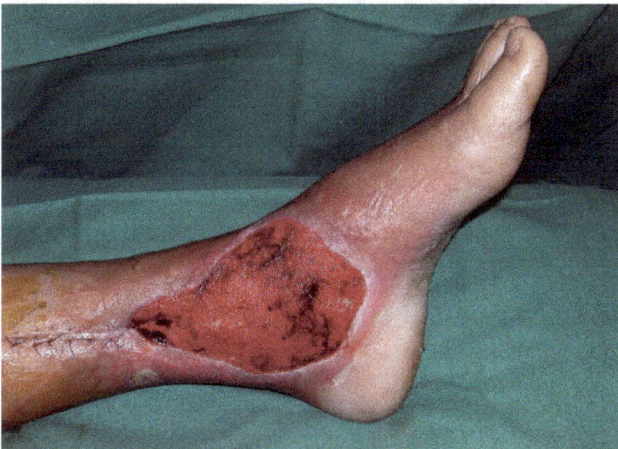

Figure 22. Significant healthy stable granulation tissue developed after 2 weeks

healing in all cases[8]. The study was conducted from January 2008 to February 2009. The number of VAC dressings required ranged from 5 to 18. (1 exceptional case required 37 dressings). The average length of treatment was 23.3 days. 9 wounds were closed with Split Skin Grafting and 2 by secondary closure.

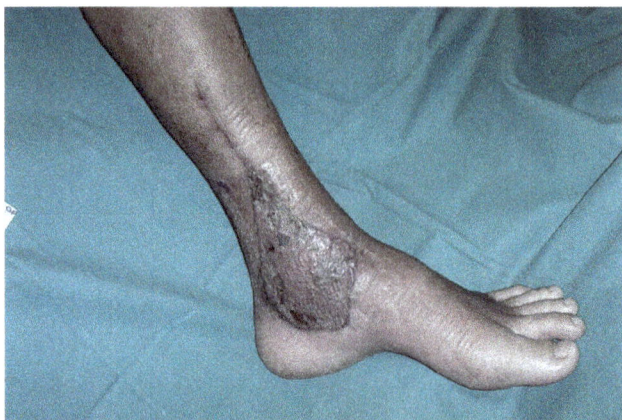

Figure 23. Final outcome after skin grating at 2 months post injury

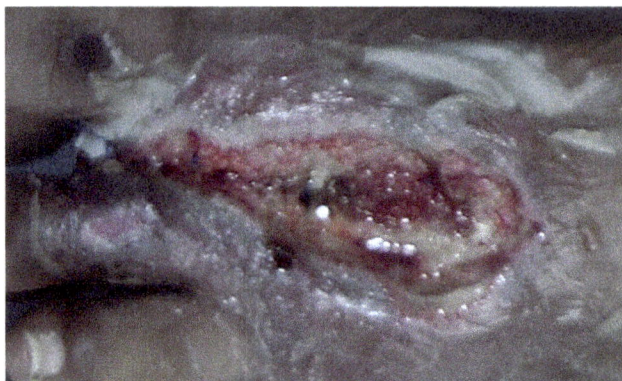

Figure 24. 2nd toe Ray Amputation wound on Day 1

Case Study 2

A 58-year-old Malay female presented with wet gangrene of the left 2nd toe. ABI was 1.0 and TBI was 0.9. Both dorsalis pedis and posterior tibial pulses were palpable. A 2nd ray amputation was performed. A Bridge VAC dressing was applied over the 2nd ray amputation wound in the operating theatre. Bridge VAC dressing was used, to allow this patient to put on footwear

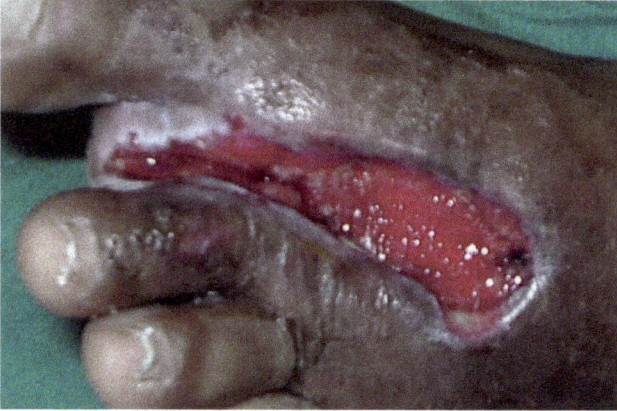

Figure 25. 2nd toe ray amputation wound on Day 22

readily. From Day 1 (Fig. 24) to Day 22 (Fig. 25) of Bridge VAC dressing application:

- *Wound Area* decreased by 12.5 cm^2 (41.7%)
  - Initial Area (Day 1): 30.0 cm^2
  - Final Area (Day 22): 17.5 cm^2
- *Granulation tissue* first appeared on Day 4 till sufficient granulation was observed on Day 22

A total of 8 Bridge VAC dressings were used and a Split Skin Graft was eventually performed after 22 days.

In a study of 5 consecutive cases of diabetic patients with foot ulcers, treated by the NUH Diabetic Foot team, Bridge VAC dressing was found to be effective in all cases.[9] The study was conducted from May 2011 to October 2011. The number of dressings required ranged from 8 to 10. The average length of treatment was 33 days. 4 wounds healed by Split Skin Graft and 1 wound healed by secondary closure.

Anodyne Therapy

Anodyne therapy, also known as Monochromatic Infrared Energy (MIRE) therapy, is another modality available for the treatment of diabetic foot ulcers.

Basic Science

Nitric oxide has several functions that are important for wound healing. Red blood cells store large amounts of nitric oxide in the form of nitrosothiols. Diabetic patients have elevated levels of glycosylated haemoglobin (HbA1C) which bind avidly to nitric oxide. As a result, there is a general lack of bioavailable nitric oxide in diabetic patients. This can contribute to the poor blood supply in the foot. Hence foot ulcers in diabetic patients often take a long time to heal.

MIRE enables more nitric oxide to be released from haemoglobin into the blood stream in diabetic patients. MIRE therapy (at a wavelength of 890 nm) has been found to stimulate local increase in nitric oxide concentration in the bloodstream from haemoglobin in red blood cells. This causes vasodilation of blood vessels and thus improves the microcirculation. Anodyne Therapy is therefore useful in the healing of diabetic foot ulcers that show poor healing.

Nitric oxide that is released into the bloodstream has several functions:[10]

- *It increases blood flow*
  - It causes vasodilation of blood vessels, increasing blood flow (Figs. 26 and 27).
  - Nitric oxide is a mediator of angiogenesis.

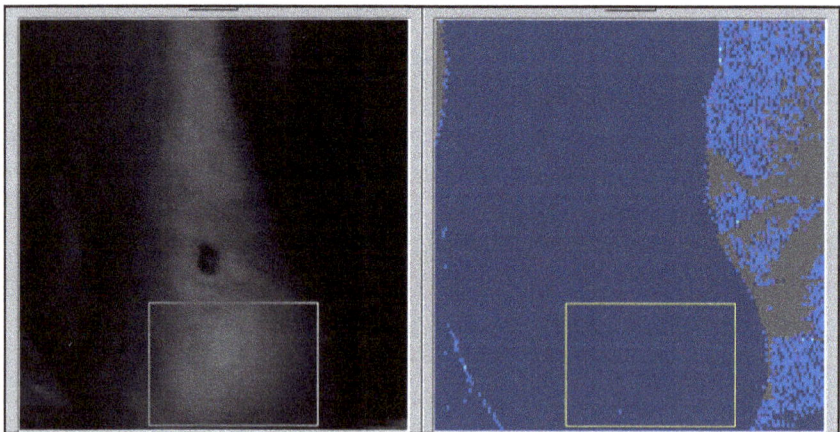

Figure 26. Scan and Laser Doppler Imaging of foot before MIRE irradiation

Source: http://www.anodynetherapy.in/increases-in-circulation

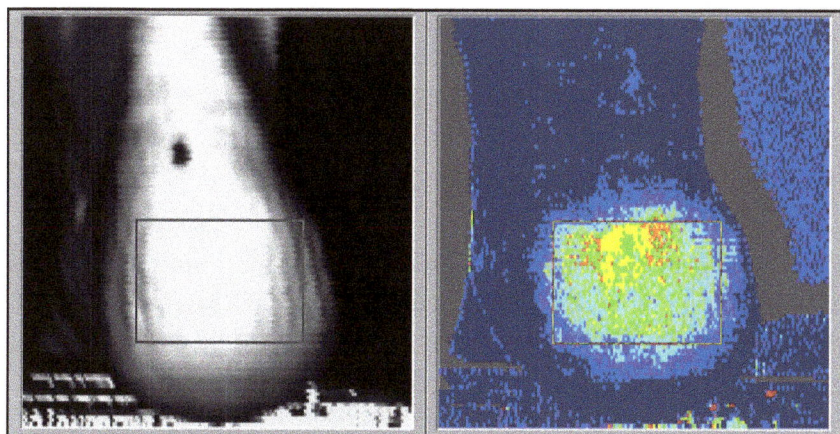

Figure 27. Scan and laser doppler imaging of the same foot after 20 minutes of MIRE irradiation showing an increase in perfusion by 32 times

Source: http://www.anodynetherapy.in/increases-in-circulation.

- *It improves neural function and pain relief*
  - **Direct**
    — Nitric oxide is a signal molecule that affects cGMP (cyclic guanosine monophosphate), thus allowing phosphorylation of ion channels especially potassium channels. This is necessary for the normal transmission of nerve signals.
    — Normal neural function then allows opioids (morphine) to act, relieving pain.
  - **Indirect**
    — It increases blood flow, allowing sufficient oxygen and glucose to be transported to the nerve cells.
    — The increased blood circulation restores normal membrane potential, reducing oedema. This reduces the pressure on the nerves caused by local oedema. Hence pain is reduced.
- *It promotes wound healing*
  - It stimulates cell division and maturation for tissue growth.
  - It acts as a signal molecule for collagen synthesis.
  - It is required for collagen fibril alignment. This reduces scar tissue and maximizes the tensile strength of healed tissue.

- o It has anti-inflammatory properties: It shortens the inflammatory stage of wound healing.
- o It strengthens immune response: Nitric oxide increases the concentration and activity of T-lymphocytes. In addition, nitric oxide mediated vasodilation aids in the delivery of antibiotics and white blood cells to the wound.

The Optimum treatment protocol for Anodyne therapy[11] consists of 3 sessions per week. Each session lasts for 30–40 minutes and has a bar setting of 6 to 8 professional units. The placement of therapy pads depends on the site of the wound.

Flexible therapy pads, each with 60 superluminous gallium-aluminum-arsenide diodes, are wrapped around each lower extremity (Fig. 28).

Case Study

A 68-year-old Malay man was admitted for a gangrenous left 5th toe. He had Diabetes Mellitus for 4 years. A ray amputation of his left 5th toe was performed. Anodyne therapy was started about a month later.

The surgical ulcer was Wagner's Grade 2 in depth. It measured 5×3.5 cm in size (Fig. 29). The wound decreased progressively in size (Figs. 30 and 31).

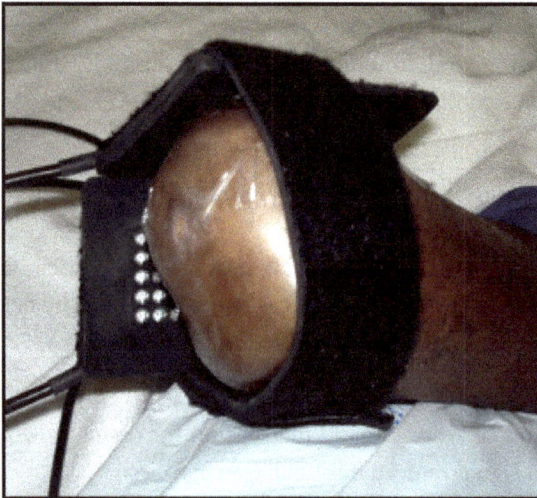

Figure 28. Application of 2 anodyne flexible therapy pads on a lower leg stump

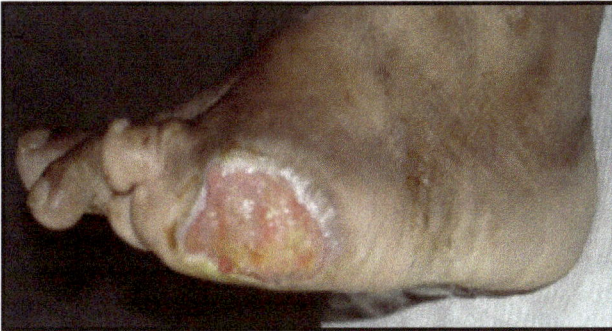

Figure 29. Surgical ulcer on day 1 of anodyne therapy

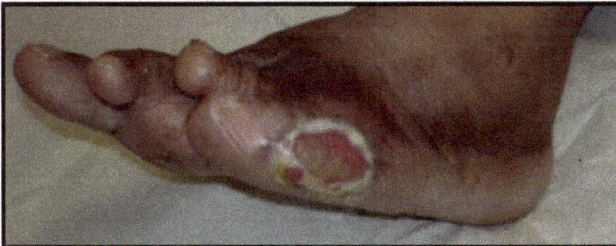

Figure 30. Surgical ulcer on day 24 of anodyne therapy

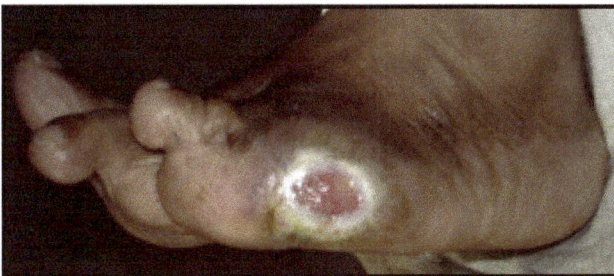

Figure 31. Surgical ulcer on day 40 of anodyne therapy

45 days later, the wound had shrunk by more than 50%, measuring 3 × 2 cm. (Fig. 32). Anodyne Therapy was stopped and daily duoderm gel dressing was continued. After a further 21 days, the ulcer healed completely.

In a study of 4 consecutive cases of diabetic patients with foot ulcers, treated by the NUH Diabetic Foot team, Anodyne therapy produced good

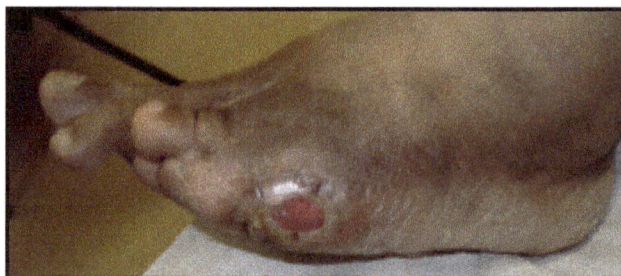

Figure 32.   Surgical ulcer on day 45 of anodyne therapy

healing in all 4 ulcers.[12] The study was conducted from September 2005 to February 2006. Anodyne therapy can be used to augment wound healing in patients where the wound shows poor healing or anergy. A disadvantage of Anodyne therapy is that it is labour intensive. It requires home visits by nurses/doctors 3 times per week. This is difficult to implement and limits the number of patients that can be treated. A viable alternative is to provide patients with home therapy units and educate the patients on its use.

Hyperbaric Oxygen Therapy (HBOT)

Hyperbaric Oxygen therapy[13,14] is the inhalation of 100% oxygen at pressures higher than sea-level in a treatment chamber. The treatment may be carried out in a monoplace (Fig. 33) or multiplace chamber (Figs. 34 and 35). HBOT was previously used to treat decompression sickness, carbon monoxide poisoning and even complement the effects of radiation in cancer treatment. It was first used to assist wound healing in 1965.

Basic Science

During HBOT treatment, a patient inhales pure oxygen through a mask or hood (Fig. 36). The oxygen is delivered at 2–3 times and up to 6 times that of atmospheric pressure for monoplace and multiplace chambers respectively. The treatment of non-healing wounds typically requires 20 to 30 HBOT sessions.

Henry's law states that the amount of gas dissolved in a liquid is proportional to the partial pressure of the gas exerted on the surface of the liquid. The increased atmospheric pressure in the HBOT chamber allows more

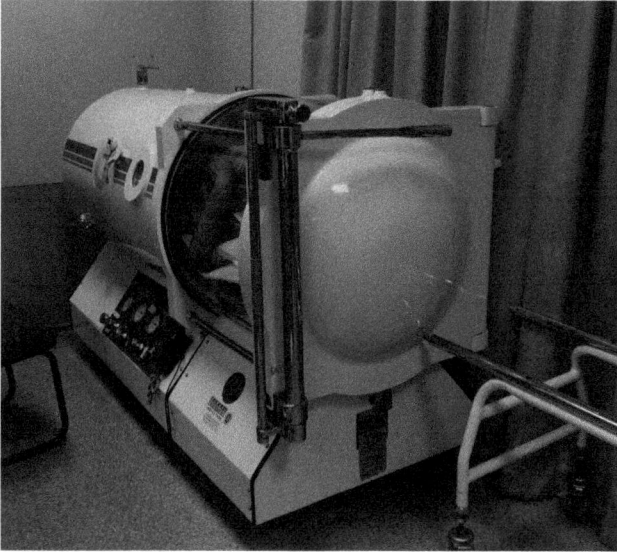

Figure 33. Diagonal view of a monoplace hyperbaric oxygen chamber at Tan Tock Seng Hospital (TTSH)

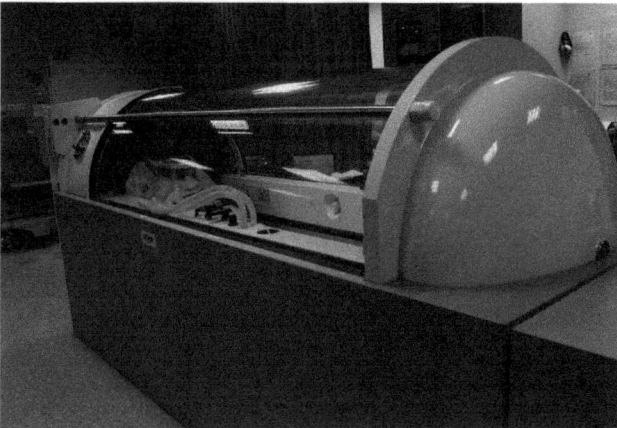

Figure 34. Diagonal view of a 3-person multiplace hyperbaric oxygen chamber at Tan Tock Seng Hospital (TTSH)

oxygen to be dissolved into the blood plasma than at surface pressure. This increased amount of oxygen dissolved in the blood plasma increases the amount of oxygen in a patient's blood. As the oxygen is in the blood plasma, it can reach areas where the red blood cells may not be able to pass, increasing tissue

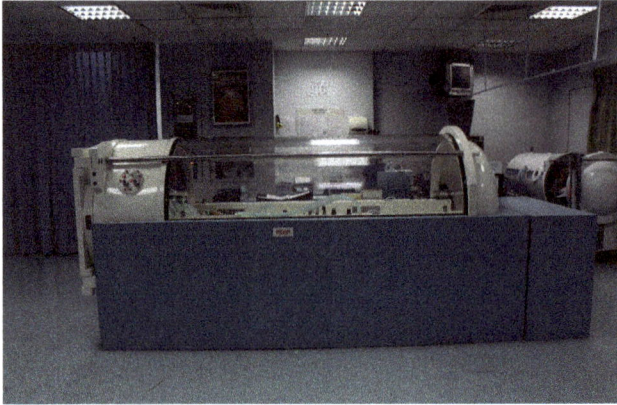

Figure 35.   Side view of a 3-person multiplace hyperbaric oxygen chamber at Tan Tock Seng Hospital (TTSH)

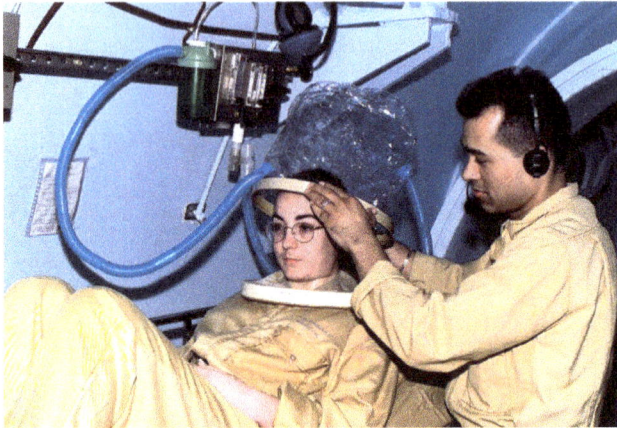

Figure 36.   Patient putting on a hood for hyperbaric oxygen therapy

Source: http://www.worldwidewounds.com

perfusion. It can also provide tissue oxygenation in the setting of impaired haemoglobin concentration or function.

In addition, based on Boyle's Law that volume is inversely proportional to pressure, the increased pressure reduces the size of oxygen bubbles. The smaller oxygen bubbles are able to pass through the circulation or at least travel into a smaller vessel.

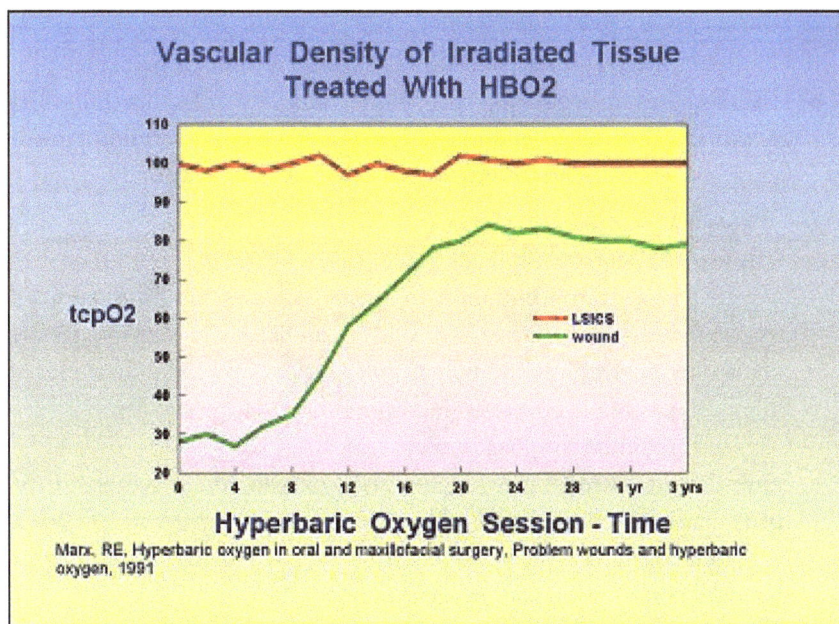

Figure 37. Increase tcpO2 readings with HBOT

Source: www.worldwidewounds.com

The effect of increasing blood oxygen concentration by HBOT can be observed using Transcutaneous oximetry (TcpO2). TcpO2 measures the amount of oxygen that reaches the skin through the blood circulation. The increase in blood oxygen concentration results in an increased amount of oxygen at the skin level, increasing TcpO2 values (Fig. 37).

HBOT has the following effects on wound healing:

- *It supports hypoxic tissue.*
  It restores aerobic metabolism to ischaemic tissue.
- *It reduces oedema through the vasoconstrictive effects of oxygen.*
  The increase in blood oxygen concentration causes vasoconstriction which reduces oedema. Reduction of oedema reduces the intercapillary diffusion distance and thus increases the rate of entry of oxygen into the tissues. It is to be noted that even with vasoconstriction, there is enough extra oxygen carried by the blood. Hence there is a net increase in tissue oxygen delivery.

- *It promotes tissue growth and repair.*
  - o Fibroblasts are stimulated to synthesise collagen through peroxides.
  - o HBOT causes up-regulation of cytokines and growth factors (fibroblast growth factor, vascular endothelial growth factor, transforming growth factor and platelet-derived growth factor) required for wound healing.
- *It helps to combat infection.*
  - o Activation of neutrophils.
    Increased oxygen concentration in tissue increases the production of oxygen radicals and superoxides. Oxygen radicals and superoxides are required by neutrophils and polymorphonuclear cells to kill bacteria.
  - o Enhancement of phagocytosis, increasing macrophage activity.
    Oxygen is required for phagocytosis.
  - o Inhibition of bacterial growth: Increased oxygen concentration in the tissue causes the production of large amounts of oxygen free radicals. These kill bacteria. Anaerobic bacteria are particularly susceptible to increased concentrations of oxygen.
  - o Inhibition of the release of bacterial endotoxins that cause tissue injury and death.
  - o Improves antibiotic effects.

Indications for HBOT

HBOT is especially useful for the healing of ischaemic wounds. The therapy increases the concentration of oxygen delivered to the wound.

HBOT is also beneficial to patients who underwent distal amputations with only 1 distal pulse present. A patient with only 1 distal pulse may not have adequate vascularity for wound healing.

A patient who underwent angioplasty and has a borderline perfusion (TcPO2 < 30 mmHg) can also undergo HBOT. HBOT will allow additional increase of oxygenated blood flow to the wound.

Case Study

A 67-year-old Chinese lady with Type 2 Diabetes Mellitus for 7 years presented with bilateral infected wet gangrene of the toes (Fig. 38). There was a purulent discharge for one month. Both dorsalis pedis pulse and posterior tibial pulse were not palpable. In the left foot, ABI was 0.4 and TBI was 0.2. In the right foot, ABI was 0.8 and TBI was 0.55.

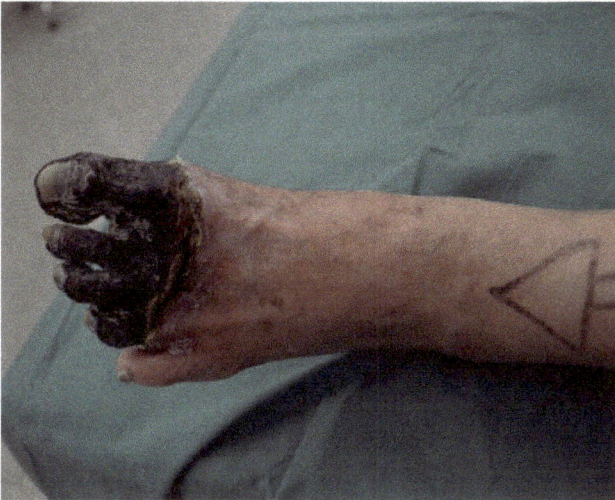

Figure 38. Infected wet gangrene of the left toes

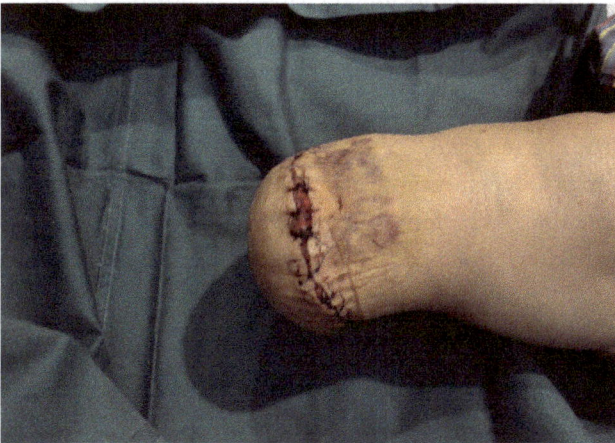

Figure 39. Right Below Knee Amputation stump on post operative day 18

A right Below Knee Amputation was done. As a bilateral BKA would lead to too high an energy expenditure for ambulation, a Pirogoff amputation was done on the left foot. Since vascularity was borderline, the patient underwent HBOT. She completed a course of 30 sessions. Both wounds have healed successfully (Figs. 39 and 40).

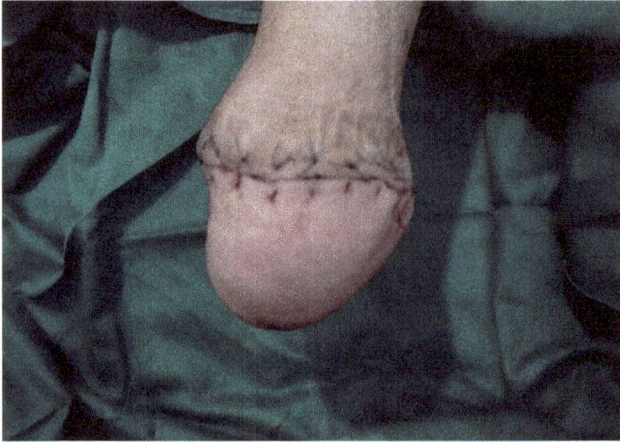

Figure 40. Left Pirogoff amputaiton stump on post operative day 13

Tissue Engineering

Currently, there are no well-documented research showing good results of using tissue engineering for diabetic foot wounds. Driver (Boston, USA) piloted a Multi-Centre study on intra-arterial injection of Mesenchymal Stem Cells (MSCs) to limb salvage cases to promote angiogenesis. The outcome of this study has yet to be reported.

However, tissue engineering[15] has huge potential in regenerative medicine. There is a potential to develop tissue engineered wound products which could promote the healing of diabetic wounds. Keratinocytes have been successfully cultured.

Basic Science

The tissue engineering triad (Fig. 41) consists of:

- Adult Mesenchymal Stem Cells
- Scaffolds
- Signalling Molecules (Cytokines)

Scaffolds

Scaffolds[16] provide the structural support for cell attachment and subsequent tissue development.

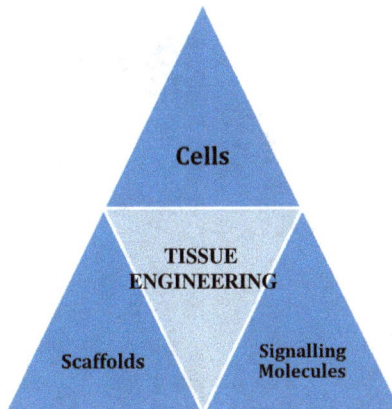

Figure 41. The tissue engineering triad

Several important properties of a scaffold:

- Architecture:
  - It should allow blood vessels, new cells and host cells to grow on it. It should facilitate integration with the host upon implantation.
  - The scaffold should be porous enough to allow efficient nutrient and metabolite transport without compromising its mechanical stability.
  - It should bioresorb and degrade at a rate matching the rate of new matrix production by developing tissue.
- Cytocompatibility and tissue compatibility:
  The biomaterials used to fabricate the scaffolds must be compatible with the cellular components of the engineered tissues and endogenous cells in host tissue. This is to allow the cells to attach, grow and differentiate on the scaffold.
- Bioactivity:
  Scaffolds may interact with the cellular components of the engineered tissues actively to facilitate and regulate their activities. The scaffold may serve as a delivery vehicle or reservoir for exogenous growth-stimulating signals such as growth factors to speed up regeneration.
- Mechanical property:
  The intrinsic mechanical properties of the biomaterials used for scaffolding or their post-processing properties should match that of the host tissue.

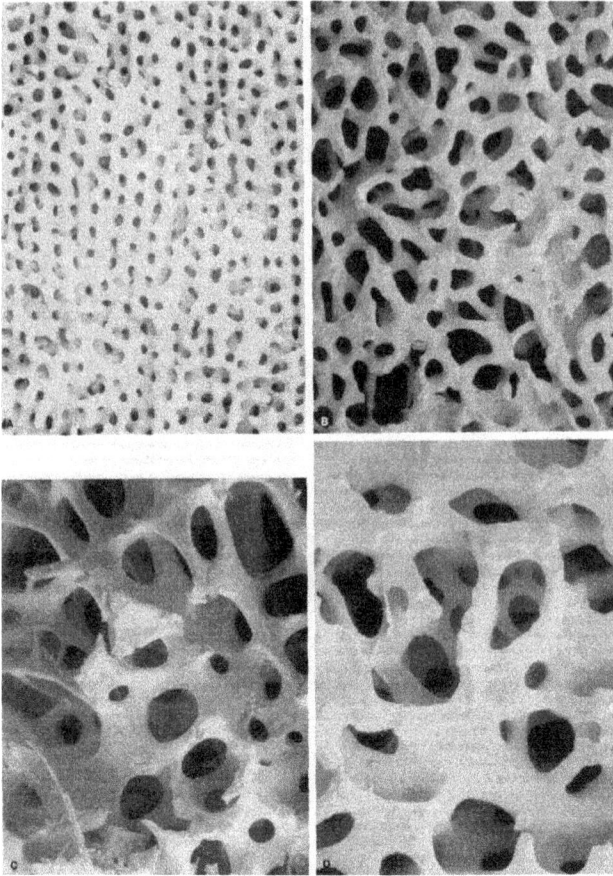

Figure 42. Coral ceramic scaffold

There are several types of scaffolds:

- Ceramics
  - Hydroxyapatite
  - Coral (Fig. 42)
- Allografts
  - Deep-Frozen (Fig. 43)
  - Freeze-Dried (Fig. 44)
  - Demineralised

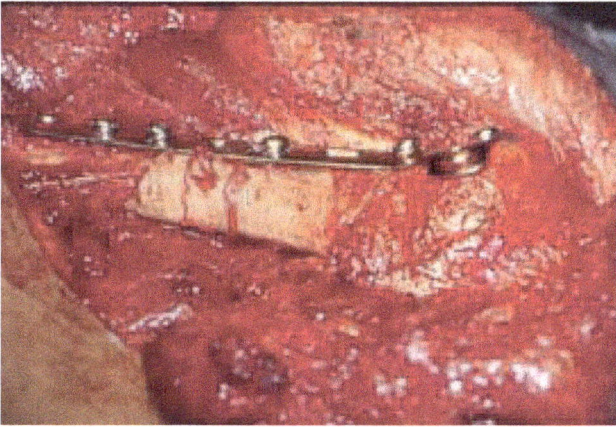

Figure 43. Deep-Frozen allograft

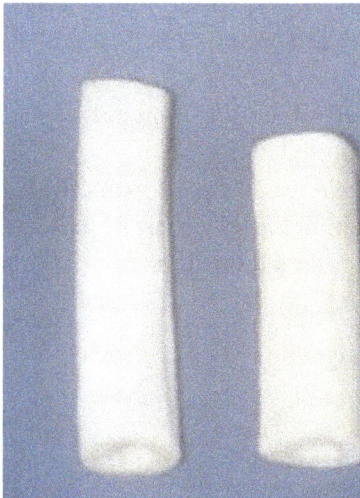

Figure 44. Freeze-Dried allograft

Adult Mesenchymal Cells

Adult Mesenchymal Stem cells (MSCs) are multipotent precursor cells. These cells give rise to multiple mesenchymal tissue types including bone, cartilage, tendon, muscle, fat and bone marrow. Donor sites of procurement include the bone marrow and adipose tissue.

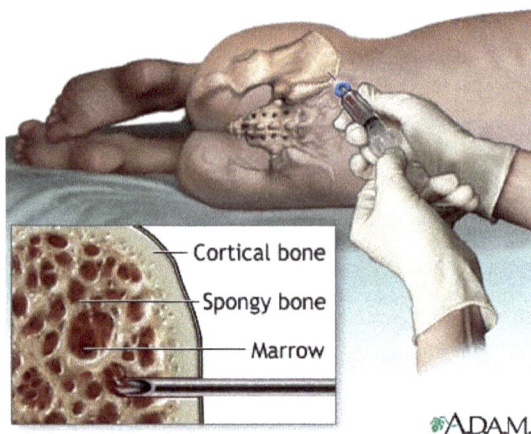

Figure 45.   Bone marrow aspiration from posterior iliac crest

The advantage of using adult MSCs is that it is largely free of bioethical controversy. MSCs are also more stable cells, resulting in lower risk of carcinogenesis.

In bone marrow aspiration, a small amount of bone marrow is taken from the bones, usually the posterior iliac crest (Fig. 45). The marrow aspirate is then subcultured to obtain mesenchymal stem cells.

Mesenchymal cells from the bone marrow possess multi-lineage potential to differentiate (Fig. 46) and mature into:

- Osteocyte (bone)
- Chondrocyte (cartilage)
- Myocyte (muscle)
- Tendocyte (tendon)
- Bone marrow stroma cells
- Adipocyte (fat/adipose tissue)
- Keratinocyte (skin epidermis)

The commitment and lineage progression to a particular pathway depends on the action of specific growth factors/cytokines.

Isolation of Mesenchymal Stem Cells[17]

The sample of bone marrow procured is mixed with 10 to 15 ml of Phosphate buffer solution (PBS). The cells are concentrated by centrifugation at 1500 rpm

Mesengenic process

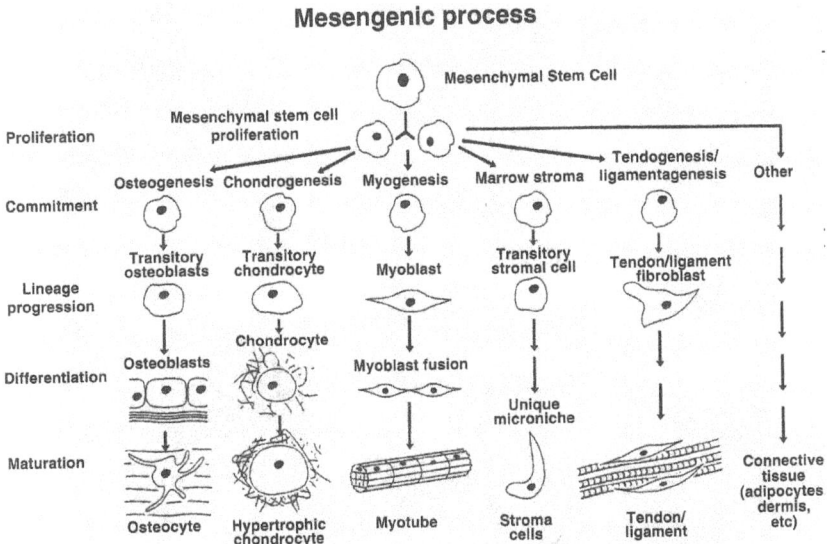

Figure 46. Diagram showing differentiation of human bone marrow MSCs into the main 6 groups of specialized cells

for 10 minutes at 20°C. The marrow separates into an upper serous layer and a lower density packed cellular layer. The supernatant is removed with a pipette. The pellet is resuspended in 10ml of PBS and centrifuged at 1500 rpm for 10 minutes to wash the cells. The supernatant is again removed, and the cells are suspended in 10 to 15 ml of complete medium. This is further centrifuged at 1500 rpm for 10 minutes. The supernatant is discarded. The pellet of cells is then reconstituted in 6 ml of complete medium and transferred to a T-75 culture flask (initial density of about 1×10^4 cells/cm^3).

Cell Culture

The T-75 culture flask is incubated at 37°C in a humidified 5% carbon dioxide environment, generated in a carbon dioxide incubator. On Day 5 of culture, non-adherent cells are removed along with the cultured medium. MSCs adhere to the glass or plastic approximately 5 days after isolation (unique characteristic of MSCs).

Adherent cells are mixed with 15ml of complete medium. The culture medium is changed every 3 days to ensure adequate cellular nutrition and removal of metabolic waste products. The cells are regularly inspected, using the inverted microscope, to look for confluence of cells.

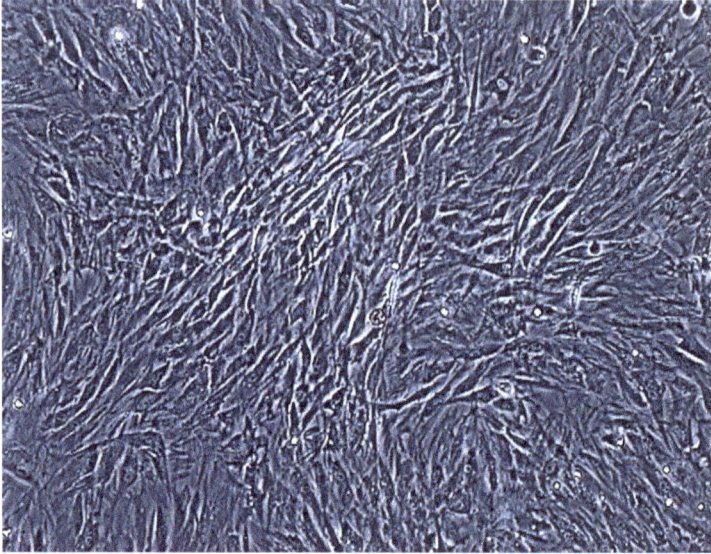

Figure 47.   About 80–90% confluence of cells achieved in primary culture

Passage of MSCs

Once 80–90% confluence of cells is achieved (Fig. 47), the cells are then passaged or sub-cultured. Usually, the Passage 2 cells are used for implantation.

Signal Molecules

Signalling molecules can be found in the Platelet-Rich Plasma (PRP). They are important in tissue engineering as they stimulate new tissue growth. The important signalling molecules are:

- *Growth Factors*
  Bone Morphogenetic Proteins (BMP), a subfamily of Transforming Growth Factor — Beta (TGF-β), are especially important.
- *Cytokines*
- *Chemokines*

Platelet-Rich Plasma (PRP) Gel

Platelet-Rich Plasma gel[18] aids in the natural healing process of wounds. It enhances the healing of allografts and bone grafts from the iliac crest (autografts). It is also suitable for exudative wounds such as diabetic ulcers, leg ulcers, pressure ulcers and surgical wounds.

Naturally, platelets are the principle source of growth factors in wounds. The autologous gel is thus a source of multiple autologous growth factors for bone grafts. It contains many proteins (growth factors, cytokines and chemokines) that stimulate tissue repair and regeneration. Key growth factors present in platelets and important for wound healing are:

- *Platelet Derived Growth Factor (PDGF)*
  PDGF stimulates cell replication and angiogenesis.
- *Transforming Growth Factor — Beta (TGF-β)*
  TGF-β, especially Bone Morphogenetic Proteins (BMPs), activate osteo-progenitor and mesenchymal cells. Activation of these cells induce bone matrix formation through osteogenesis. They also influence osteoblasts to lay down the collagen matrix, supporting capillary ingrowth.
- *Transforming Growth Factor — Alpha (TGF-α)*
- *Endothelial Growth Factor (EGF)*
- *Insulin-like Growth Factor (IGF)*
- *Platelet Derived Angiogenic Factor (PDAF)*

The highest concentrations of PDGF and TGF-β are found within blood platelets.

All these factors promote cell endothelial migration and the formation of granulation tissue thus allowing the wound healing to progress beyond the inflammatory phase.

Preparation of the PRP gel[19]

A 60 ml blood sample is first drawn from the patient (Fig. 48) using a 20-gauge needle in a syringe containing 6 ml of citrate-based anticoagulant (ACD-A). The syringe is then inverted 5 to 6 times to ensure that the ACD-A is adequately dispersed. Employing a sterile technique, the blood is then transferred to a plastic bag (Bag 1) of the collection set. Bag 1 is then loaded onto the platelet concentrate collection system. A second container of saline that is identical in weight to Bag 1 is used as a counter balance (Fig. 49). It is then centrifuged (Fig. 50) via the Platelet Concentrate Collection System (PCCS) to obtain the platelet rich layer.

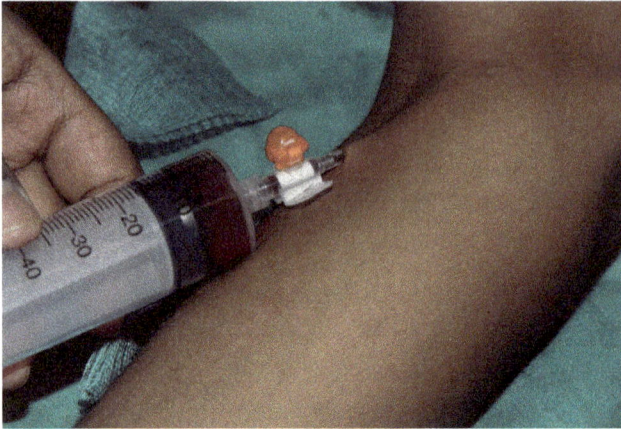

Figure 48.   Taking a whole blood sample

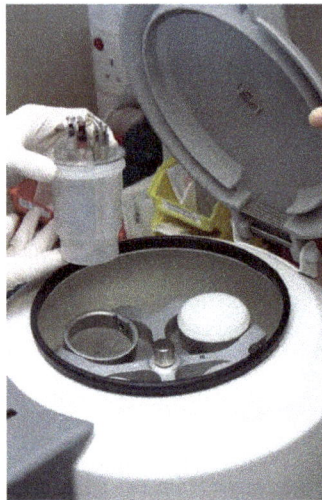

Figure 49.   Adding a counterbalance to Bag 1

The initial centrifugation is at 3000rpm for 3:45 minutes to separate the red blood cells from the plasma. The pellet formed comprises the red blood cells (about 40% of the original sample) and the supernatant is made up of platelets and plasma (Fig. 51). The PRP is pushed into Bag 2 using air and a manual 60 ml syringe, leaving the red blood cells in Bag 1 (Fig. 51).

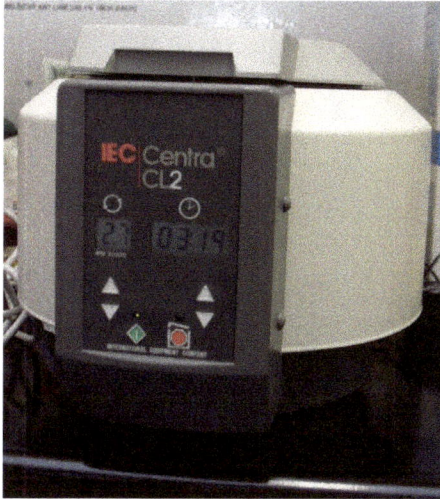

Figure 50. Outer view of the centrifuge

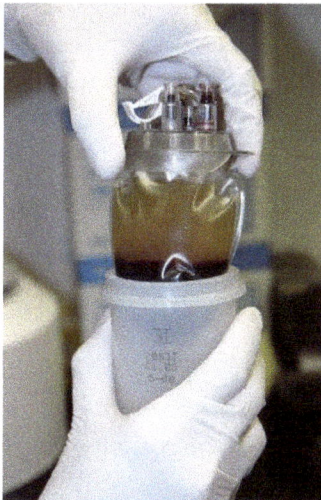

Figure 51. Soft spin showing the red blood cells below the supernatant (plasma and platelets)

The supernatant in bag 2 is then centrifuged at 3000 rpm for 13 minutes. The resultant supernatant is Platelet Poor Plasma (Fig. 52). The pellet consists of PRP. It is also called the "buffy" coat layer. The Platelet Poor Plasma (PPP) in the supernatant is allowed to enter Bag 1, leaving the PRP in Bag 2. The PRP obtained is about 15% of the original sample, about 5 to 7 ml.

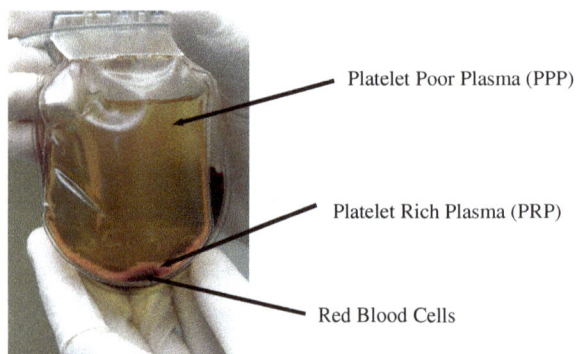

Figure 52. Hard spinning gives the layer of platelet concentrate and plasma (Platelet Rich Plasma). At this juncture, the "buffy" coat layer is rich in platelets

The final PRP sample is then mixed with 1 ml of 10% calcium chloride solution and 1000 units of topical human thrombin. This initiates the coagulation process and produces a gel-like material. The PRP gel can now be directly applied to the diabetic wound. The gel can be applied to the wound every twice a week for over 5 weeks.

So far, there has been no report of randomized control studies on the role of PRP gel in promoting the healing of diabetic wounds.

Traditional Chinese Medicine (TCM)

Traditional Chinese Medicine (TCM) is part of Asian Culture and thus widely practiced in Asia. It is used for diabetic wounds and has the potential to benefit wound healing.

The underlying principle of TCM is the Yin-Yang balance in the body. Orally administered chinese herbal prescriptions are thus highly individualized. The most commonly applied prescriptions[20] are:

- *Ulceration in the extremities with ulcer exudate:*
  Zeng ye (增液) decoction (Fig. 53) is used to nourish the yin.
  Si miao yong an (四妙勇安) decoction is used to activate the blood to clear heat and remove toxins.
- *Ulceration with severe gangrene:*
  Di huang yin zi (地 • 飲子) (Fig. 54) decoction is applied to improve wounds with gangrene, nourish yin and assist yang.

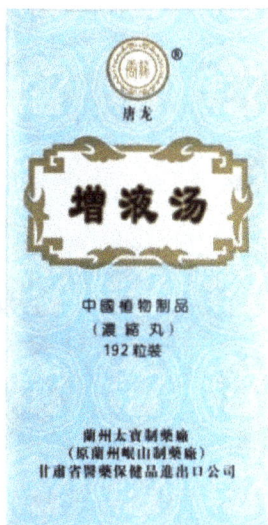

Figure 53. *Zeng ye* (增液) decoction

Source: www.chinesemedicinepractice.co.za

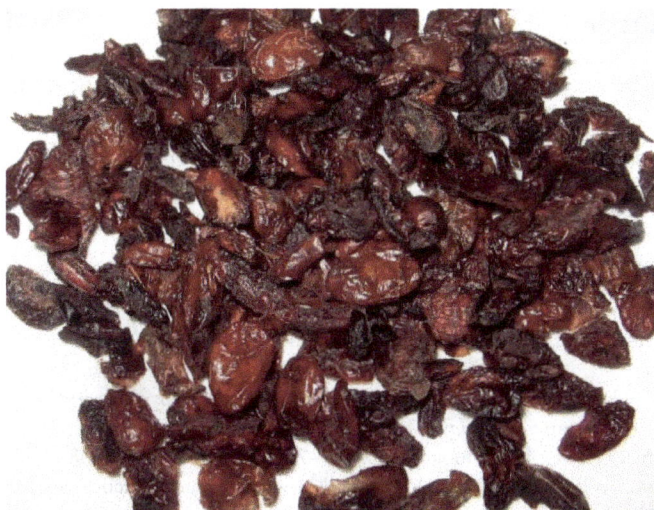

Figure 54. *Di huang yin zi* (地・飲子)

Source: www.wenyaotang.net

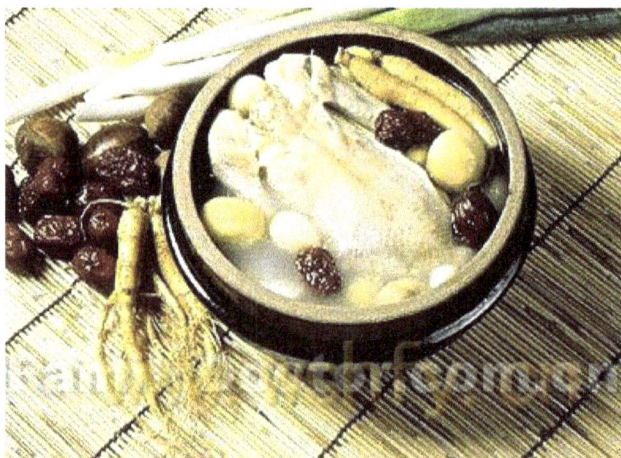

Figure 55. *Er-Xian* (二仙) decoction

Source: www.wshfy.cn

Er-Xian (二仙) decoction (Fig. 55) is used to promote local blood circulation and remove toxin.

- *Si miao yong an* (四妙勇安) decoction activates blood to clear the heat and remove toxin.

Professor P. C. Leung showed that the 2-Herb Formula is as good as the 3-Herb Formula (see Chapter 20)

The use of TCM in managing diabetic foot problems holds great potential. Good documented research is required to evaluate its healing potential.

References

1. W. J. Ennis, W. Valdes, M. Gainer and P. Maneses, Evaluation of clinical effectiveness of MIST ultrasound therapy for the healing of chronic wounds, *Wound Care* **19**(8):437–46 (2006).
2. W. A. Conlan and D. Weir, Ultrasound assisted wound therapy: an exceptional adjunct to wound bed preparation, *Todays Wound Clinic* (2009).
3. A. Nather, Diabetic Foot Problems. pp. 459–73 (World Scientific, 2008).
4. Mexican Association for Wound Care and Healing, Clinical Practice Guideline for the Treament of Acute and Chronic Wounds with Maggot Debridement Therapy (2010).
5. R. A. Sherman, Maggot therapy for treating diabetic foot ulcers unresponsive to conventional therapy. *Diabetes Care* **B26B**(2):446–51 (February 2003).
6. A. A. Gutiérrez, The science behind stable, super-oxidized water, *Wounds* **18**(Suppl.):7–10 (January 2006).

7. Centre for Evidence-based Purchasing, Evidence Review: Vacuum Assisted Closure Therapy, *CEP 08017* (June 2008) nhscep.useconnect.co.uk/ShowDocument.ashx?id=46&i=true

8. A. Nather, S. B. Chionh, A. Y. Han, P. P. Chan and A. Nambiar, Effectiveness of vacuum-assisted closure (VAC) therapy in the healing of chronic diabetic foot ulcers, *Ann. Acad. Med. Singapore* **39**(5):353–8 (May 2010).

9. A. Nather, Y. H. Ng, K. L. Wong and J. A. Sakharam, Effectiveness of bridge V. A. C. dressings in the treatment of diabetic foot ulcers, *Diabet. Foot Ankle* **2**:5893 (March 2011).

10. T. Burke, *Nitric Oxide and Its Role in Health and Diabetes*, www.diabetesincontrol.com (2002).

11. Anodyne Therapy Professional System, Model 480: Important Safety information and instructions.

12. A. Nather, Y. E. Sim, L. L. J. Chew and S. H. Neo, Anodyne therapy for recalcitrant diabetic foot ulcers: a report of four cases, *J. Orthop. Surg.* **15**(3):361–4 (2007).

13. J. Wright, Hyperbaric oxygen therapy for wound healing, *World Wide Wounds* (May 2001).

14. E. Latham, M. A. Hare and M. Neumeister, Hyperbaric oxygen therapy, *Medscape Reference*: Article 1464149 (May 2010).

15. Y. Ikada, Challenges in tissue engineering, *J. R. Soc. Interface* **3**(10):589–601 (October 2006).

16. B. P. Chan and K. W. Leong, Scaffolding in tissue engineering: general approaches and tissue-specific considerations, *Eur. Spine J.* **17**(Suppl 4):467–79 (December 2008).

17. A. Nather, S. Das De and C. W. Lee, Culturing mesenchymal stem cells from bone marrow. In: *Bone Grafts and Bone Substitutes: Basic Science and Clinical Applications* (World Scientific, 2005), pp. 321–33.

18. D. Man, H. Plosker and J. E. Winland-Brown, The use of autologous platelet-rich plasma (platelet gel) and autologous platelet-poor plasma (fibrin glue) in cosmetic surgery, *Plast. Reconst. Surg.* **107**(1):229–37 (2001).

19. S. Das De, R. Manohara and A. Nather, Platelet-rich plasma in orthopaedic surgery: basic science and clinical applications. In: *Bone Grafts and Bone Substitues: Basic Science and Clinical Applications* (World Scientific, 2005), pp. 387–403.

20. Y. Huang, M. Jiang, C. Zhang, Y. Guo and A. Lu, Managing diabetic foot ulcers using Chinese medicine, *Ostomy Wound Manage.* (2011).

29

Wound Products for Diabetic Foot Problems

Geoff Sussman

Faculty of Medical and Health Science
Faculty of Medicine
University of Auckland
Monash University

Introduction

The management of the diabetic limb wound is multifaceted with the application of wound products being only one aspect of patient treatment. Wound products should have the following features according to Turner:[1]

1. Removal of excess exudates and toxic components
2. Maintenance of high humidity at wound dressing interface
3. Gaseous exchange
4. Thermal insulation
5. Protection from secondary infection
6. Free from particulate or toxic contamination
7. Allow removal without trauma at dressing changes[2]

The role of a dressing is to be an adjunct to total patient management and to act on the wound environment to remove impediments to healing and to enhance the ability of tissue to heal.

Wound Management Principles

- Cleanse with minimal trauma
- Removal of slough/necrosis
- Adequate absorption of exudate
- Prevention/reduction of contamination/infection
- Protect damaged/healing tissue[3,4]

Consider:

- Cost/Who and How often?/Ease of use/Skin and Keep it simple

Definition of Wound Management

Wound management and product selection is only a part of the total patient management of the diabetic. The important considerations include : Disease control and management, off-loading, infection prevention, vascularization, cleansing, debridement and finally dressings.

What is wound management? I define it as: The provision of the appropriate environment for healing by both direct and indirect methods together with the prevention of skin breakdown. The prevention aspect is the most important one in the diabetic patient. The more that can be done to educate diabetic patients in the care of their feet and the regular consultations with a podiatrist will have a significant impact on reducing wounds and as a result lessen the potential for digit or limb amputation.

Major Issues

Infection Prevention and Treatment

The most critical issue with the diabetic patient is that of infection due to the high risk in the diabetic. Every effort must be made to limit the risk and to ensure the patient understands the basic rules of foot care. If a skin break occurs, swift and aggressive management is essential, given that 86% of all diabetic foot amputations first presented as a minor wound. If a wound is identified as being infected, post culture and sensitivity, the antibiotic shown to be the one that will destroy the bacteria causing the infection should be administered. In addition, a topical antiseptic, but not a topical antibiotic, to reduce the bacterial load in the wound, should be used.

The major issue with the use of most dressings in the management of the diabetic wound is the lack of published evidence. In making the decision to use a particular dressing the wound specific factors must be considered and most important it is essential to have a clear understanding of the properties of a dressing and how it best addresses the wound issues.

For many years the products used were of the 'passive' or the 'plug and conceal' concept including gauze, lint, non-stick dressings and tulle dressings. They fulfill very few of the properties of an ideal dressing, and have very limited use (if any) as primary dressings. Some are useful as secondary dressings. It is clear that there are a number of negative aspects in the use of gauze. Interactive dressings help to control the micro- environment by combining with the exudate to form either a hydrophilic.gel, or by means of semipermeable membranes, control the flow of exudate from the wound into the dressing. They may also stimulate activity in the healing cascade and speed up the healing process. Interactive dressings may also react with the cytokine and MMP levels in a chronic wound to re-balance the wound in line with the principles of Wound Bed Preparation.[2−4]

Wound Cleansing and Care of the Skin

Most soaps and detergents are alkaline and induce an increase in cutaneous pH, which affects the physiologic protective "acid mantle" of the skin by decreasing the fat content. DO NOT USE SOAP. Instead, use a pH balanced surfactant wash is best. The 'acid mantle' of the Stratum Corneum seems to be important for both permeability barrier formation and skin antimicrobial defense. Changes in the pH are reported to play a role in the cause of skin diseases like irritant contact dermatitis, Atopic Dermatitis, Acne Vulgaris and fungal infections, leading to an increased colonization of the skin with coagulase-negative staphylococci.[4]

Skin Moisture

The use of a good emollient is important as dry skin is more vulnerable to damage. The emollient should provide a barrier function as well as providing moisture. Simple water based creams such as Sorbolene cream are of little value. In particular, the diabetic should take care of their heel skin. The use of a specific foot balm will be helpful.

Wound Dressings

There are a number of dressing products available for use on diabetic wounds. They include Film Dressings, Hydrocolloid Dressings, Foam Dressings, Alginate Dressings, Hydroactive (Foam-like) Dressings, and Hydrogels (Amorphous and Sheet).

Non-Absorbing Dressings (for nil to low exudate)

Film dressings

Film dressings (including island dressings) consist of a thin, poly-urethane membrane coated with a layer of acrylic adhesive. Their physical properties include being gas and water vapour permeable, impermeable to microorganisms, and being transparent and flexible. They allow easy wound assessment and are conformable offering considerable patient comfort. They provide a moist environment and encourage autolysis. However, they do not have the ability to absorb exudate. They are particularly useful in superficial, clean wounds and in the prevention of breakdown and pre-ulcers in pressure wounds. They should *not* be used in infected wounds. There are no absolute contradictions for their use. However some local irritation has been observed to the adhesive. Examples include Opsite™ and Tegaderm. If there is a small amount of exudate in the wound, an Island film that includes a non-stick pad is best, e.g. Opsite post op™ and Tegaderm with pad.[2-6]

Absorbing Dressings (for low exudate)

Hydrocolloids

Hydrocolloids are a combination of polymers held in a fine suspension and an adhesive. When placed on a wound the polymers combine with the exudate and form a soft, moist gel-like mass. They also encourage autolysis to aid in the removal of slough from a wound. Hydrocolloids have a polyurethane film or foam backing, and are occlusive. Hydrocolloid products are used in low to moderately exudating wounds-including ulcers, and granulating wounds-and act as a secondary dressing. They may also be used in conjunction with a hydrocolloid paste or powder. The paste or powder is used in a deeper ulcer or cavity. They convert to the same hydrophilic gel and are covered with the normal hydrocolloid wafer.

Hydrocolloids also are available in thin forms. These dressings are permeable, and are also very light and comfortable. They are used over sutured wounds and incision sites, as a protective dressing and on lightly exudating wounds, since they have the ability to cope with some exudation. Because of their occlusive nature producing an anoxic environment, which may lead to increase in (anaerobic) infection and pain they are contraindicated on foot ulcers in patients with diabetes and/or PAD. In addition exudate control is often not adequate using this dressing, e.g. Duoderm®/Comfeel™, Replicare Ultra™ and Hydrocoll®.[2-7]

Absorbing Dressings (for medium to high exudate)

Poly-urethane foams

These products meet many of the standard requirements for an ideal dressing, in that they allow the passage of exudate through the non-adherent surface to be absorbed in the main body of the product, while maintaining a moist environment and being insulating. They may be composed of a soft, open cell hydrophobic foam, the contact layer having been heat treated to produce a non-adherent hydrophilic layer. Some foams have a soft hydrophilic foam bonded to a semi permeable polyurethane film and covered with a three dimensional plastic net. These products are highly absorbent of exudate, and maintain a moist environment without maceration of surrounding tissue. Their uses are mainly in moderate to heavily exudating wounds including ulcers, donor sites and minor burns. They act as a secondary dressing-particularly as a covering with the use of amorphous hydrogels. They come in a variety of sizes including shaped cavity devices which may be inserted into pressure wounds or dehisced surgical wounds, e.g. Lyofoam™, Allevyn™, Lyofoam Extra™ and PermaFoam®. A new presentation of Foam dressings are the Soft Silicone Foam Dressings This is a new style of dressing composed of a multiple layer foam dressing. The surface of the foam has a soft silicone surface adhesive for non-traumatic removal, e.g. Mepilex,a thin version called Mepilex Lite and a waterproof version Mepilex border. The other brand is Allevyn gentle which also is presented as a waterproof form Allevyn gentle border.

A simple method to apply a foam dressing to a digit is to cut the foam in the shape of the letter L. Apply the length of the L around the digit, hold with tape and then flip the foot of the L across the wound foam, hold with tape and forming a sock-like dressing.[2-6]

Hydroactives (foam-like) dressings

Hydroactive dressings are composed of absorbent polymers that absorb exudate into their structure and expand, while maintaining a moist environment. They aid autolysis without maceration of the surrounding tissue. They are used on moderate to heavily exudating wounds-including ulcers, and granulating wounds. Some of these dressings are confused for foam dressings in that they may appear to be similar. However, whilst the foams absorb by siphon and hold exudates in the air spaces, the hydroactive dressings absorb exudates into the polymer structure and expand in shape. They are available in many forms including thin, non-adhesive, cavity and island forms, e.g. Cutinova Hydro™, Biatane™ and Tielle™.[2−6]

Alginates

Alginates are the calcium or sodium/calcium salts of alginate acid, obtained from seaweed. When applied to a wound, the sodium ions present in the wound exchange with the calcium in the alginate to form sodium alginate, a hydrophilic gel. This gel has the ability to absorb exudate into itself while maintaining a moist environment at the interface between the dressing and the wound. The physical properties include the ability to absorb exudate forming a gel, and produce a moist environment without maceration of the surrounding tissue. In addition, a number of these products also have haemostatic properties.

They are used on donor sites, bleeding sites, exudating leg ulcers and cavities. They come in a number of different forms, including sheets, packing rope and in combination with charcoal for exudating malodorous wounds, e.g. Kaltostat®, Algisite M™, Sorbsan™ and Comfeel Seasorb™. In addition there are fibre dressings called hydrofibres composed of sodium carboxymethylcellulose. These dressings absorb exudates and form a firm gel. They differ from alginates in that they do not wick laterally. Therefore, they may be place not only in the wound but around it and will protect the peri-skin from maceration, e.g. Aquacel™ and Versiva®.[2−6]

Moisture Donating Dressings (for dry or sloughy wounds)

Hydrogels

Hydrogels are a group of complex organic polymers having a high water content from 30 to 90 percent. They have the properties of both rehydrating dry tissue, and absorbing certain amounts of fluid into themselves. They are provided as either amorphous gels- used to help re-hydrate sloughy wounds and necrotic tissue to aid in the autolytic debridement of wounds. They are also used in the management of burns — including sunburn, scalds and other partial thickness burns. Amorphous hydrogels have also been used in the management of chicken pox and shingles. It is applied liberally to the eruptions four to five times a day. They provide a moist environment and relieve the discomfort of the lesion, and also reduce the probability of scarring.

Hydrogels are also available in sheet form consisting of a cross-linked polymer hydrogel and water held in a backing. These products are particularly useful in the management of superficial burns. It also aids the removal of necrotic tissue in pressure wounds. In general, most modern wound dressings have a place in the management of Diabetic wounds, e.g. IntraSite gel™, Comfeel Purilon Gel™, Solosite™, DuoDERM Gel®, Solugel™ and Hydrogel Sheet, e.g. Aquaclear™ and Nu-gel™.

Flaminal® hydrogels are based upon gelled alginate and not on other polymers Flaminal® hydrogels use the enzymes glucose oxidase and lactoperoxidase to control the bioburden in a similar way to honey. Flaminal® contains lactoperoxidase which is an enzyme extracted from milk and acts as an important natural antimicrobial. It has been shown to be bacteriostatic against Gram-positive organisms. It exhibits pH-dependent bactericidal action against Gram-negative organisms in the presence of hydrogen peroxide and thiocyanate.[2–6]

In general, the use of moist wound healing is appropriate for neuropathic wounds. However, it is considered inappropriate in ischaemic wounds. Such wounds have poor perfusion and should remain dry to prevent bacterial invasion.

Antiseptic dressings

These dressings play a role in the reduction of the bioburden in many wounds, particularly in patients with diabetes. They are used in conjunction with systemic antibiotics in infected wounds and in the early management of minor trauma wounds in the diabetic to prevent infection. There are, however, some antiseptics known to be toxic to healing dermal cells, e.g. Hydrogen peroxide, acetic acid and povidone iodine.

New antiseptics

Prontosan® range is a ready to use solution containing Polyhexanide and Betaine for cleansing and moistening of wounds. PHMB was recognised as possessing superior antimicrobial effect to other cationic biocides. As with the biguanides, PHMB was shown to bind rapidly to the envelope of both Gram-positive and Gram-negative bacteria, and in doing so, displaces the otherwise stabilising presence of Ca^{2+}. This binding is to the cytoplasmic membrane itself, and also to lipopolysaccharide and peptidoglycan components of the cells wall.

Betaine is a surface active solution that penetrates difficult coatings and removes debris, bacteria powerfully yet gently. Both ingredients are known to be extremely safe when used on skin and mucous membranes. Effective wound irrigation is highly important as it prepares the wound bed by removing debris, bacteria and coatings from the wound. This allows full inspection of the wound so the correct treatments can be applied.

The two main antiseptic product groups used are Iodine and Silver.

Inadine

Inadine, consists of a knitted viscose fabric impregnated with a polyethylene glycol (PEG) base containing 10% povidone-iodine, equivalent to 1.0% available iodine. In the presence of wound fluid, the povidone-iodine, a potent antimicrobial agent with a broad spectrum of activity, is readily released from the PEG base. The dressing, which is designed as a low adherent wound contact material, is orange in colour. Unlike paraffin or lanolin used in manufacture of some medicated paraffin gauze type products, the PEG base used in the production of Inadine is water-soluble and easily removed from the skin or wound surface.

Cadexomer iodine dressings (Iodosorb/Iodoflex)

This product is a cross-linked polymer containing Iodine. When it absorbs exudate from the wound it forms gel with exudate. It releases iodine as gel forms at 0.1% (not cytotoxic) over 72 hours. The product helps in slough removal. There is evidence that Iodine may stimulate growth factors and macrophage function. In addition, it reduces the pH of the wound, enhancing antimicrobial effect. Because it is pro-inflammatory it 'kick 'starts chronic wound healing. Due to its antibacterial effect, it has also been shown to reduce malodour in a wound. The known contraindications are in patients with Iodine/shellfish sensitivities (Hashimoto's thyroiditis, Graves disease). It is recommended that the weekly maximum dose must not exceed 150 grams. In use, it should be reapplied every third day. It is also essential to remove all product residue before reapplication. It is important to warn patients that some pain may be experienced when it is first applied.

There are a number of published studies confirming the impact of this product on improved wound healing with low toxicity. It is useful in diabetic wounds as it will stimulate an inflammatory response, often lacking in the diabetic, remove bacteria, odour and slough and stimulate healing.[3,4,6,8,9]

Silver-containing dressings

Silver has been used for many years and it has proven antimicrobial activity. It is broad spectrum — inactivates almost all known bacteria including MRSA and VRE. No documented cases of bacterial resistance have been reported. Chemically, metallic silver is relatively inert but its interaction with moisture on the skin surface and with wound fluids leads to the release of silver ions and its biocidal properties. Silver ion is a highly reactive moiety and avidly binds to tissue proteins, causing structural changes in bacterial cell walls and intracellular and nuclear membranes. The anti-microbial properties of silver stem from the chemical properties of its ionized form, Ag^+. This ion forms strong molecular bonds with other substances used by bacteria to respire, such as molecules containing sulfur, nitrogen, and oxygen. Once the Ag^+ ion complexes with these molecules, they are rendered unusable by the bacteria, depriving it of necessary compounds and eventually leading to the bacteria's death. Silver exerts its antimicrobial effects by interfering with the respiratory chain at the cytochromes. Silver ions also interfere with components of the microbial electron transport system and bind DA and inhibit DNA replication. Thus Silver ions attack multiple microbial cells sites compared with antibiotics that mostly attack only one.[10,11]

Silver has been used in particular in the treatment of burns as Silver Sulphadiazine Cream. This cream has also been applied to some wound. The difficulty is the fact that the cream is formulated to be applied to intact skin. When applied to a wound it encourages the development of muscilagenous slough. Contemporary silver dressings allow for continued release up to 7 days. The level of silver contained in the various dressings varies greatly. Their mode of action also varies. Some release the silver into the wound. Some partly release the silver and hold some in the dressing, while others keep the silver within the dressing. The choice of dressing will depend on the level of infection, the size, the depth and the amount of exudate, e.g. Acticoat®, Mepilex Ag® Biatain Ag®, Aquacel Ag™ and Atrauman Ag™.[4-6]

Silver dresssings may be composed of metallic silver or silver salts.

The ACTICOAT◇ family is a unique range of antimicrobial barrier dressings for use over partial, full thickness and acute wounds. Unique Patented Silver technology: SILCRYST Nanocrystalline Silver Antimicrobial protection provides an effective barrier to over 150 wound pathogens. It is available as a polyethylene mesh enclosing a single layer of rayon (as a three or seven day form), as an alginate, a foam, a post op dressing, or as a single layer of flexible One–way stretch knitted polyester (also available in three or seven day form).

Allevyn Foam Dressing ALLEVYN Ag contains silver sulphadiazine (SSD) particles embedded within the structure of its foam layer It releases silver over 7 days.

ALGISITE Ag

An absorbent type 1 calcium alginate dressing non-woven dressing of silver impregnated calcium alginate fibre ALGISITE Ag forms a gel on contact with fluids. This creates a moist wound healing environment, to assist faster ealing. ALGISITE Ag provides an antimicrobial barrier.

SeaSorb®-Ag alginate dressing with silver is a unique mix of high G (guluronic acid) and highly absorbent carboxymethylcellulose (CMC) with the addition of an ionic silver complex, which releases silver ions in the presence of wound exudate. As exudate is absorbed, the dressing forms a soft, cohesive gel that intimately conforms to the wound surface.

Physiotulle — Ag is a non-adherent, moist wound healing contact layer with silver sulphadiazine that maintains a moist wound healing environment.

The hydrocolloid particles and petrolatum contained in Physiotulle — Ag swell to form a cohesive gel. This helps maintain an ideal moist wound healing environment and ensures atraumatic dressing changes.

BIATAIN Ag is a Soft and flexible foam-like,dressings prepared with hydro-activated silver, which is released into the wound during wear. It is available as surface sheets and as packing sheets.

Mepilex Ag combines the unique features of Safetac technology with the bacteria reducing power of silver. Mepilex Ag goes to work quickly, inactivating wound pathogens within 30 minutes and for up to 7 days. At dressing removal, Mepilex Ag does not stick to the wound or strip surrounding skin, minimising patient pain and wound trauma.[12]

AQUACEL® Ag dressing incorporating unique Hydrofiber® Technology with 1.2% (w/w) silver combines the favourable gelling characteristics of Hydrofiber® Technology with the broad-spectrum antimicrobial properties of ionic silver (Ag$^+$). It is available in surface sheet and reinforced ribbon for cavity packing.

Atrauman Ag is an ointment impregnated silver containing wound contact layer. It prevents secondary dressings from sticking to wounds, provides skin care for the wound edges and is antibacterially effective when bacteria come into direct contact with the dressing.

Silvercel is an antimicrobial Alginate dressing. It is a sterile, non-woven pad composed of high tensile strength alginate, carboxymethylcellulose (CMC) and silver-coated fibers. It contains elemental silver (8%) as a sustained release formulation.

There are some specific studies of the use of silver products in the management of diabetic wounds. It is important that many more clinical studies be undertaken in order to clearly demonstrate the mechanism of action of silver in clinical wound management and its antibacterial, anti-inflammatory and wound-healing properties.

Other Treatment of Diabetic Wounds

David G. Armstrong, Lawrence A. Lavery, for the Diabetic Foot Study Consortium
Negative pressure wound therapy after partial diabetic foot amputation: a multicentre, randomised controlled trial demonstrated NPWT delivered by the VAC Therapy System seems to be a safe and effective treatment for complex diabetic foot wounds, and could lead to a higher proportion of healed wounds, faster healing rates, and potentially fewer re-amputations than standard care.

Growth Factors and Other Pharmacological Treatments

There continues to be considerable research in the area of growth factors. It is now clearly understood that growth factors play an important role in would healing. Although at this stage, it is not clear as to their precise role, Growth Factors may be divided into two groups: Tissue-generated Growth Factors and Haematopoietic Growth Factors.

Tissue generated growth factors include platelet-derived growth factors, macrophage growth factors, fibroblast growth factors, transforming growth factors alpha and beta, vascular endothelial growth factors, insulin-like growth factors and epidermal growth factors.

Haematopoitic Growth Factors include GCSF and GMCSF. They have been used in the treatment of Necrobiosis Lipoidica Diabeticorum.

Commercially there are a few Topical Growth Factors available. The most widely used is Becaplermin (Regranex®). This product contains Platelet Derived Growth Factors and is used in the treatment of diabetic foot ulcers. The results of the pooled integrated analyses are consistent with those reported from the 4 pre-approval studies showing that Regranex Gel 0.01% significantly increases the incidence of complete healing and reduces the time to complete closure of diabetic neuropathic ulcers. These results reinforce the position that Regranex Gel 0.01% is a useful adjunct for the treatment of diabetic foot ulcers.

There have been some limited studies with the topical or systemic use of drugs to improve diabetic wound healing. These include Phenytoin, Doxycycline, L-arginine and other NO stimulators. More research is needed to confirm the usefulness of these products to improve diabetic wound healing.

References

1. T. D. Turner, Surgical dressings and their evolution. In: D. J. Leaper, K. G. Harding and T. D. Tumer (eds.), *Proceedings of 1st European Conference on Advances* (Macmillan Magazines, London, 1992), pp. 181–7.
2. S. Thomas, *Wound Management and Dressings* (Pharmaceutical Press, London, 1990).
3. G. Sussman, Wound dressings: removing the confusion, *Aust. J. Podiatr. Med.* 32(4):145–8 (1998).
4. G. Sussman, Management of the wound environment with dressings and topical agents. In: C. Sussman and B. Bates-Jensen (eds.), *Wound Care: A Collaborative Practice Manual for Health Professional*, 4th Edition (Lippincott Williams & Wilkins, Philadelphia, 2001), pp. 502–21.
5. S. Thomas, *Surgical Dressings and Wound Management* (Medetec Publications Cardiff, 2010).
6. C. Weller and G. Sussman, Wound dressing update, *J. Pharm. Pract. Res.* 36(4):318–24, (2006).
7. J. Apelqvist, *et al.*, Topical treatment of necrotic foot ulcers in diabetic patients: a comparative trial of DuoDerm and MeZinc, *Br. J. Dermatol.* 123:787–92 (1990).

8. J. Sundberg and R. A. Meller, Retrospective review of the use of Cadexomer Iodine in the treatment of chronic wounds, *Wounds* 9(3):68–86 (1997).

9. K. Moore, A. Thomas and K. Harding, Iodine release from the wound dressing Iodosorb modulates the secreation of cytokines by human macrophages responding to bacterioal lipopolysaccardide, *Int. J. Biochem. Cell Biol.* 29(1):163–71 (1997).

10. A. B. Lansdown, Silver 1: its antibacterial properties and mechanism of action, *J. Wound Care* 11(4):125–30 (2002).

11. A. B. Lansdown, Silver 2: toxicity in mammals and how its products aid wound repair, *J. Wound Care* 11(5):173–7 (2002).

12. J. W. K. Tong, Case reports on the use of antimicrobial (silver impregnated) soft silicone foam dressing on infected diabetic foot ulcers, *Int. Wound J.* 6:275–84 (2009).

Section 8

Footwear

30

Diabetic Footwear

Aziz Nather and Gurpal Singh

Department of Orthopaedic Surgery
Yong Loo Lin School of Medicine
National University of Singapore

Introduction

Diabetic footwear has long been used in the primary prevention of diabetic foot problems as well as in the treatment and secondary prevention of re-ulceration in patients who have already developed foot ulcers. Repeated emphasis on footcare and proper selection of footwear are two important strategies.[1] Basic foot care includes the proper trimming of toenails, avoidance of foot trauma and not walking barefoot (even at home).

In the prescription of therapeutic diabetic footwear, based on International Diabetes Federation (IDF) Guidelines (2005),[2] IDF Guidelines (2007),[3] National Institute for Health and Clinical Excellence (NICE) Guidelines[4] and Foster *et al.* (1999)[5] the following guidelines should be included:

(1) Wearing well-cushioned walking shoes or athletic shoes. Extra-wide shoes with extra depth may be required if there are foot deformities such as hammer toes or bunions. If problems are severe, custom-made shoes are required.

(2) Avoidance of shoes with high heels or pointed toes. They can create pressure, which might contribute to bone and joint disorders as well as diabetic ulcers.

(3) Avoidance of open-toed shoes or sandals with a strap between the first two toes.

(4) Presence of well-cushioned, tailor made insoles
Proper fitting of shoes. A large number of ulcers are attributed to ill-fitting shoes. Shoe size is often estimated by the salesperson by looking at the foot, or with reference to the size of the shoe currently being used by the patient. There is diversity in size measurement systems — European, United Kingdom and United States systems (Fig. 1). Also, these sizing systems reflect only the length of the shoe and do not take into account the width and depth.

(5) Footwear should be light, preferably less than 700 grams per pair.

(6) Stockings or socks should always be worn with shoes to avoid blisters. Soft cotton socks should be used to reduce shear stress (Fig. 2)

(7) Shoes should be purchased in the afternoon because feet swell a little during the day

(8) The heel of the shoe (Fig. 3) should be under 5 cm high to avoid weight being thrown forward onto the metatarsal heads.

(9) Shoes should be fastened with adjustable lace, strap or Velcro high on the foot

(10) The toe box (Fig. 3) should be sufficiently long, broad and deep to accommodate the toes without pressing on them, with a clear space between the apices of the toes and the toe box so that the toes are not too cramped to function.

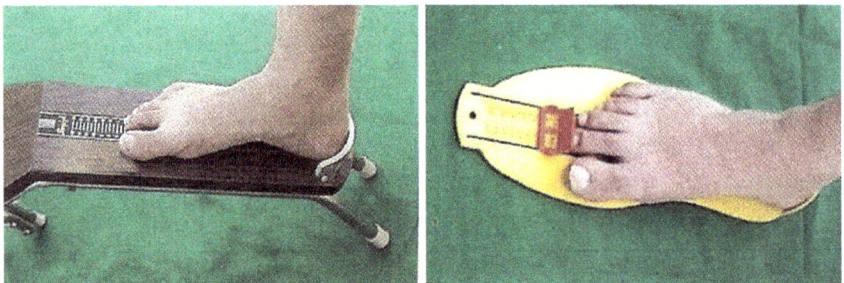

Figure 1. Measurement of foot

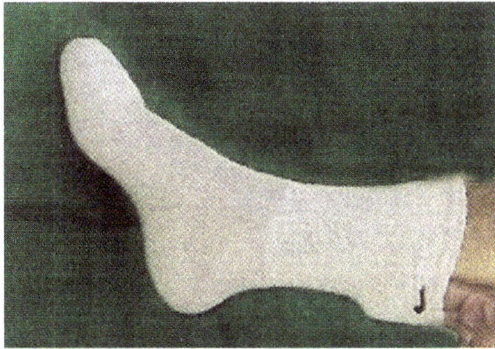

Figure 2. Soft cotton socks without tight elastic

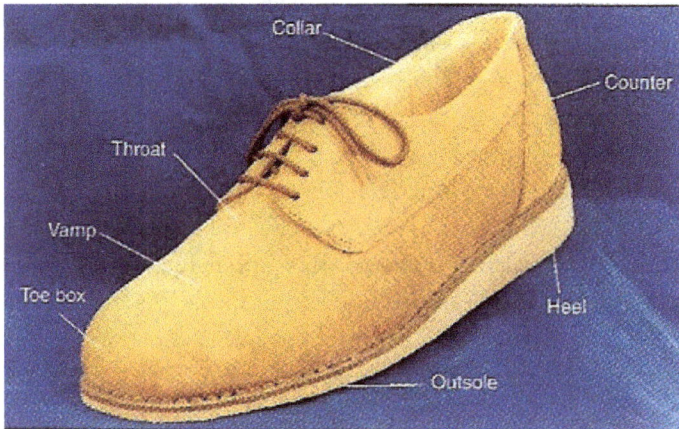

Figure 3. Nomenclature for parts of a shoe

Foot Pressure Measurements

There is evidence to demonstrate that the prescription of diabetic footwear leads to a reduction in new foot ulceration and as a result, a reduction in lower extremity amputation rates. Studies using pedobarography with in-shoe pressure sensing devices show that diabetic footwear is effective to reduce plantar foot pressure (See Fig. 10 in Chapter 6: Biomechanics of the Foot). Lobmann *et al.* (2001)[6] concluded that early insole support is successful in reducing plantar pressure but a repeat adjustment must be done every 6 months to prevent foot pressure increment. A study by Viswanathan *et al.*

(2004)[7] showed that there were lower foot pressures in diabetic patients who were using diabetic footwear compared with patients who were using routine non-custom made footwear. Foot (plantar) pressures were measured using the RS scan in shoe pressure measurement system and the peak pressure was taken to be from the metatarsal heads. Sarnow *et al.* (1994)[8] published similar findings on foot pressure differences between patients who routinely use therapeutic diabetic footwear versus those who do not. Chantelau *et al.* (1990)[9] described that incidence of diabetic foot lesions in patients who regularly used diabetic footwear was 45% lower than in those who did not regularly use diabetic footwear. With regards to preventing re-ulceration in diabetic patients with existing foot ulcers, the evidence is more controversial. Maciejewski *et al.* (2004)[10] conducted a review of several studies and reported statistically significant protective effects from therapeutic footwear in this group of patients. There was a large variation in the incidence of re-ulceration and footwear design and patient compliance issues may be confounding the results (annual re-ulceration varied from 8.4–59.3%). Also, diabetic footwear with the intention to prevent re-ulceration seems to be more effective in patients with existing severe foot deformities.

Reduction of peak pressures is an effective tool for managing the diabetic foot. Non-diabetic footwear does not reduce foot pressures and thus predisposes to foot ulceration and compromises healing of foot ulcers. Viswanathan *et al.* (2004)[11] suggests three possible materials for production of diabetic shoes — polyurethane, ethylene vinyl acetate (EVA) and microcellular rubber (MCR) and cork. Majority of the patients prefer wearing 10 mm MCR for insoles with rubber outer-sole.

Fitting of Shoes

Ill-fitting of shoes remains a significant problem, especially in the elderly. These patients have difficulty in getting access to shops or centres where their feet can be measured and correct sizes fitted. Ill-fitting shoes are a risk for falls and a significant cause of ulceration.[12] Amongst diabetics, up to 37% wear ill-fitting shoes that result in diabetic foot ulcerations in 20% of patients. Even in non-diabetic patients, 24% wore shoes that were of the wrong size. Older patients tend to wear shoes which are too big. Of patients assessed, 65% wore shoes which were too long and wide for the foot. Only 6% wore shoes which were too small. Movement of the foot in an oversized shoe causes friction and leads to ulceration.[13] Morbach *et al.* (2004)[14] concluded that despite having more access to special diabetic footwear, shoe-related injuries are the major cause of diabetic foot related problems. Ill-fitting footwear is associated with most of these problems and two thirds of diabetics wear shoes of incorrect size.[15] Footwear fitting does play an important part in achieving better outcomes in protection of the diabetic foot.

Compliance of Footwear

Another important issue to consider is patient compliance to diabetic footwear. For diabetic footwear to be effective, it needs to be worn for more than 60% of the time. Most patients fall short of this level.[16]

Aesthetic considerations need to be taken into account. Weight of the shoes and cost are two very important factors directly correlating with patient compliance.

More choices in styles and perhaps involvement of patients in footwear design and selection would be helpful. Cost and cosmetic appearance were quoted as the reasons for non-compliance by a series of patients interviewed at Manchester Diabetes Centre, UK by Knowles and Boulton. Most diabetic footwear were perceived as 'ugly' by patients and this led to poor compliance.[17] Diabetic footwear perceived as being ugly or cosmetically unattractive is a major contributory factor to non-compliance. Jannink *et al.* (2004)[18] concluded from an epidemiological survey that 70% of patients with given orthopaedic shoes are not using them.

Pendsey Recommendations for Footwear

An important basic principle in the design of diabetic footwear is pressure offloading.[1,2] Pendsey[19] recommended the following guidelines for selecting footwear, based on the IWGDF Risk Stratification Tool:

(i) Risk Category 0 — No history of foot problems and no neuropathy.[20,21] These patients can wear shoes available over the counter (Fig. 4).
(ii) Risk Category 1 — Loss of protective sensations without any deformities. These patients should wear soft cushioned sports shoes or preventative footwear (Figs. 5a to 5c).

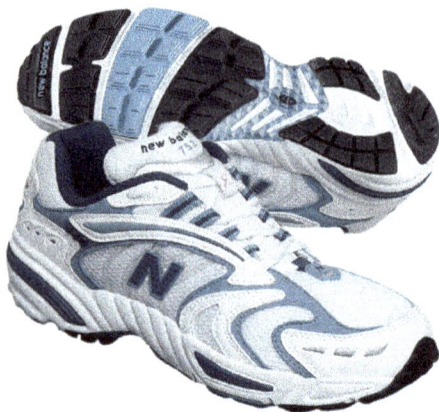

Figure 4.   Sports shoe

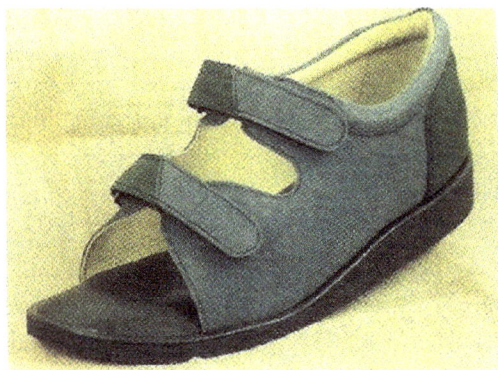

Figure 5a.   Preventive sandal with velcro straps

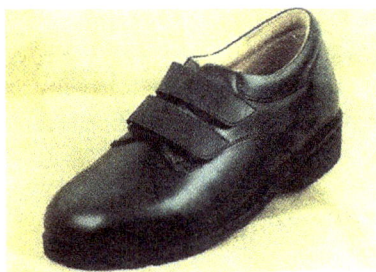

Figure 5b.   Preventive shoe with velcro straps

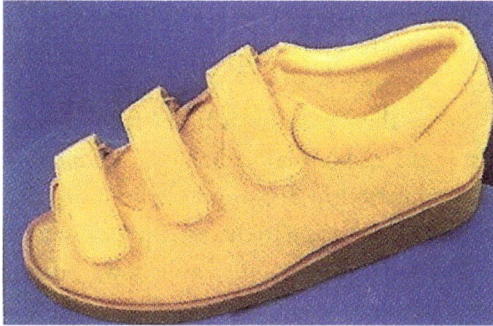

Figure 5c. Preventive sandal with velcro straps

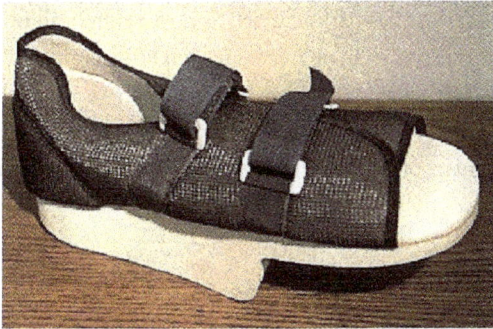

Figure 6. Healing sandal

(iii) Risk Category 2 — Loss of protective sensations and presence of foot deformities. These patients need shoes with extra depth, width, high toe box and soft insoles. Custom-made footwear can be used for this risk category.

(iv) Risk Category 3 — History of previous ulcer or partial foot amputation. Foot wear as detailed in category 2 above may be used but the majority of these patients require custom-made footwear (Fig. 6).

Finally, footwear needs can vary in different cultures. There is a marked difference in footwear habits in developed countries compared with under-developed countries.[13] In underdeveloped countries, people tend to wear sandals and slippers and some do not wear shoes at all due to poverty or religious reasons. In Asian countries, people tend not to wear shoes in the house. This is often due to the belief that the home environment is safe.[22]

This causes difficulties in the prevention and management of diabetic foot problems. Patients tend to be just as active at home as when they go out.

The lower socio-economic group of patients prefers wearing only sandals. Nather *et al.*[23,24] found that diabetics without foot problems presenting to the endocrinologist in the diabetic clinic had socio-economic status similar to that of the general population in Singapore. In contrast, diabetics who have developed foot problems presenting to the orthopaedic surgeon in the diabetic foot team clinic were found to be mainly in the lower socio-economic group with educational level of up to secondary school only and an average monthly household income of less than SGD$2000 (US$1333).

A large proportion of patients that are at risk of ulceration are in the elderly age group and tend to spend more time at home. Thus, there is an additional need to design footwear that can be worn at home, and will be accepted by the patient. Local adaptations may be necessary depending on our tropical climate and our local resources. Patients do not like to wear footwear because they are too hot and sweaty for our climate. They prefer to walk barefeet at home. This makes them susceptible to unnoticed trauma, especially in patients with sensory neuropathy.

Footwear Habits in Singapore

Nather *et al.*[25] conducted a footwear survey of 100 patients seen in the NUH Diabetic Foot Team from January to June 2005. The cohort included 60 patients with diabetic foot problems and 40 patients with diabetes but no foot complications. The latter came to the team for an annual foot screening examination.

A detailed questionnaire was employed including patient profile, type of footwear, fixation of footwear, ability to fit off-loading insoles and patient's preference for footwear. For the selection of footwear preference, patients were shown a chart with photographs of 6 types of footwear (Fig. 7) and were asked to indicate their preference.

Results showed that 54% did not wear footwear at home whilst 38% wore slippers. All patients used footwear outdoors, with 49% of them wearing shoes, 26% wearing slippers and 25% wearing sandals. Leather footwear was used outdoors by 51%. Majority of outdoor footwear did not have fixation and removable insoles. Only 11 patients used socks indoors. 51 patients used socks outdoors.

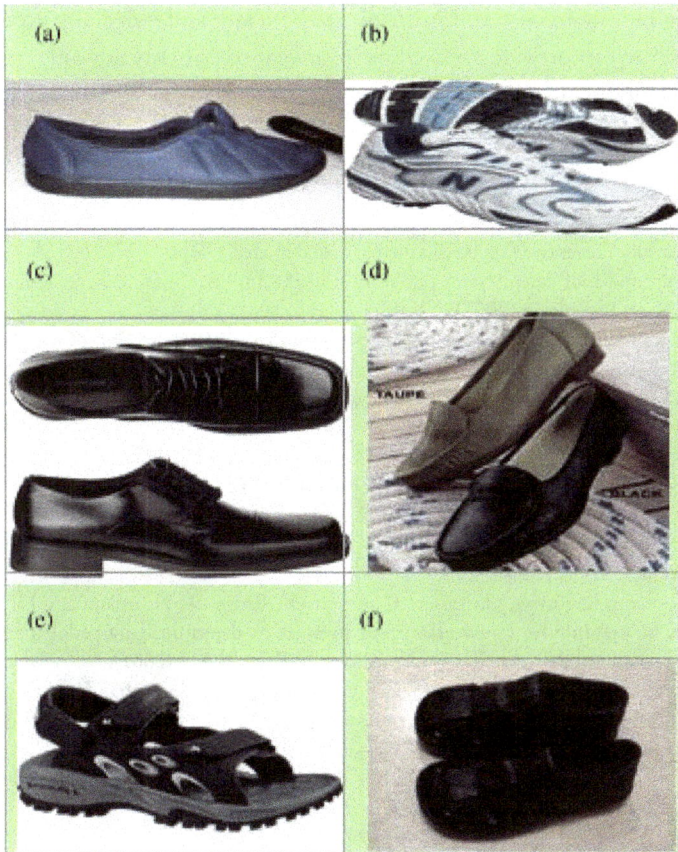

Figure 7. Six types of footwear for patient to indicate preference

Conclusion

Wearing the correct diabetic footwear is a very important aspect of PREVENTION. All patients diagnosed with diabetes must pay particular attention to using preventive footwear. Those who have already developed foot complication should be given therapeutic footwear to prevent re-ulceration. Major problems with footwear include ill-fitting shoes, especially seen in the elderly, and compliance to footwear. Shoes must not only be affordable but must also be aesthetically and culturally acceptable.

There is a need to develop a diabetic footwear centre in NUH, to design fashion and manufacture preventive and therapeutic footwear. The footwear must also be low in cost and must be aesthetically and culturally acceptable. Such a centre can provide appropriate footwear to patients not only in NUH, but to all patients in Singapore.

References

1. J. A. Mayfield, G. S. Reiber, L. J. Sanders, D. Janisse and L. M. Pogach, American Diabetes Association, Preventive foot care in people with diabetes, *Diabetes Care* 26: S78–79 (2003).
2. Diabetes and foot care, A joint publication of the International Diabetes Federation — Chapter on Prevention (2005).
3. International working group on the diabetic foot/consultative section of the IDF 2007, Practical Guidelines on the Management and Prevention of the Diabetic Foot — based on the International Consensus on the Diabetic Foot, prepared by the International working Group on the Diabetic Foot.
4. NICE (National Institute for health and Clinical Excellence) Clinical Guidelines for Type 2 Diabetes. http://www.nice.org.uk/page.aspx?o=38551.
5. M. E. Edmonds and Alethea VM Foster, Managing stage 1: The normal foot. In:*Managing The Diabetic Foot*, eds. M. E. Edmonds and A. V. M. Foster (Blackwell Science, United Kingdom, 2000), pp. 25–34.
6. R. Lobmann, R. Kayser, G. Kasten, U. Kasten, K. Kluge, W. Neumann and H. Lehnert, Effects of preventative footwear on foot pressure as determined by pedobarography in diabetic patients: a prospective study, *Diabet. Med.* 18:314–9 (2001).
7. V. Viswanathan, M. Sivagami, R. Seena, C. Snehalatha, A. Ramachandran and A. Veves, Increased forefoot to rearfoot plantar pressure ratio in South Indian patients with diabetic foot ulceration, *Diabet. Med.* 21(4):396–7 (2004).
8. M. R. Sarnow, A. Veves, J. M. Giurini, B. I. Rosenblum, J. S. Chrzan and G. M. Habershaw, In-shoe foot pressure measurements in diabetic patients with at-risk feet and in healthy subjects, *Diabetes Care* 17(9):1002–6 (1994).
9. E. Chantelau, T. Kushner and M. Spraul, How effective is cushioned therapeutic footwear in protecting diabetic feet? A clinical study, *Diabet. Med.* 7(4):355–9 (1990).
10. M. L. Maciejewski, G. E. Reiber, D. G. Smith, C. Wallace, S. Hayes and E. J. Boyko, Effective of diabetic therapeutic footwear in preventing reulceration, *Diabetes Care* 27(7):1774–1782 (2004).
11. V. Viswanathan, S. Madhavan, S. Gnanasundaram, G. Gopalakrishna, B. N. Das, S. Rajasekar and A. Ramachandran, Effectiveness of different types of footwear insoles for the diabetic neuropathic foot: a follow-up study, *Diabetes Care* 27(2):474–7 (2004).
12. G. E. Reiber, D. G. Smith, C. Wallace, K. Sullivan, S. Hayes, C. Vath, M. L. Maciejewski, O. Yu, P. J. Heagerty and J. Lemaster, Effect of therapeutic footwear on foot reulceration in patients with diabetes: a randomized controlled trial, *JAMA* 287(19):2552–8 (2002).
13. S. L. Burns, G. P. Leese and M. E. T. McMurdo, Older people and ill fitting shoes, *Postgrad. Med. J.* 78:344–6 (2002).
14. S. Morbach, J. K. Lutale, V. Viswanathan, J. Mollenberg, H. R. Ochs, S. Rajashekar, A. Ramachandran and Z. G. Abbas, Regional differences in risk factors and clinical presentation of diabetic foot lesions, *Diabet. Med.* 21:91–5 (2004).

15. S. J. Harrison, L. Cochrane, R. J. Abboud and G. P. Leese, Do patients with diabetes wear shoes of the correct size?, *Int. J. Clin. Pract.* **61**(11):1900–4 (2007).

16. D. J. Macfarlane and J. L. Jensen, Factors in diabetic footwear compliance, *J. Am. Podiatr. Med. Assoc.* **93**(6):485–91 (2003).

17. E. A. Knowles and A. J. Boulton, Do people with diabetes wear their prescribed footwear?, *Diabet. Med.* **13**(12):1064–8 (1996).

18. M. J. Jannink, J. de Vries, R. E. Stewart, J. W. Groothoff and G. J. Lankhorst, Questionnaire for usability evaluation of orthopaedic shoes: construction and reliability in patients with degenerative disorders of the foot, *J. Rehabil. Med.* **36**(6):242–8 (2004).

19. S. Pendsey, Preventative footwear, In: *Diabetic Foot — A Clinical Atlas* (Martin Dunitz, London, 2004), pp. 171–5.

20. D. J. Janisse and E. J. Janisse, Pedorthic and orthotic management of the diabetic foot, *Foot Ankle Clinic* **11**(4):717–4 (2006).

21. H. B. Leung and W. C. Wong, Footwear — Hong Kong experience. In: *Diabetic Foot Problems*, ed. A. Nather (World Scientific, New Jersey, London, Singapore, 2008).

22. D. G. Armstrong, L. A. Lavery and L. B. Harkless: Treatment based classification system for assessment and care of diabetic feet, *JAPMA* **86**:311 (1996).

23. A. Nather, S. B. Chionh, K. L. Wong, S. Q. O. Koh, Y. H. Chan, X. Li and A. Nambiar, Socioeconomic profile of diabetic patients with and without foot problems, *Diabet. Foot Ankle* **1**:5523 (October 2010).

24. A. Nather, S. B. Chionh, Y. H. Chan, X. Y. Li, L. Yan and P. H. Wu, Socio-economic factors of diabetics with and without foot problems. In: *Diabetic Foot Problems*, ed. A. Nather (World Scientific, Singapore, 2008).

25. A. Nather, T. Tsao, K. Stone and Z. Aziz, Footwear habits in patients with diabetic foot problems. In: *Diabetic Foot Problems*, ed. A Nather (World Scientific, Singapore, 2008).

31

What is in the Market at the Moment? A Look at the Industry

Adam Jorgensen

Principal Podiatrist
Camden Medical Centre
Singapore

What is in the Market at the Moment

Firstly, most diabetic footwear originate from Europe and the United States of America (USA), both with temperate climates and with different cultural footwear habits compared to regions such as South East Asia and Asia both with tropical climates.

Worldwide centres of shoe manufacture include China, Indonesia, Vietnam, USA, Spain, Portugal and countries in Eastern Europe.

Current Prominent Brands Include

- Apex Ambulator shoes (US)
- Darco Gentlestep (USA product manufactured in China)
- PW Minor (USA)

Corresponding author: Dr. Adam Jorgensen, Principal Podiatrist, The Foot Practice, Unit 10-04A Camden Medical Centre, 1 Orchard Boulevard, Singapore 248649, Tel: (+65) 6836-4515, Fax: (+65) 6836-4516, E-mail: adamj@thefootpractice.com

- Acor (USA)
- Klaveness (Norway)
- Mollitor, Podartis (Italy)
- Fits all (Portugal)
- Nimco (The Netherlands)
- Bata (Czech Republic).

Types of Shoes

There are currently 3 main categories of shoes. These are:

- Healing sandals/Post op shoes
- Standard street shoes
- Walking shoes

Healing Sandals/Post Op Shoes

One of the best known is the Darco Post Op Shoe. This is made up of a simple rigid rubber sole with soft fabric upper and velcro straps. It is designed primarily to allow temporary post-operative ambulation. It allows for accommodation of bulky bandaging. It has been adapted as diabetic footwear as the extra depth allows for orthoses and the rigid sole aids in reducing forefoot pressures (Fig. 1). It is unisex, aesthetically ugly, breaks down quickly and can be unsafe

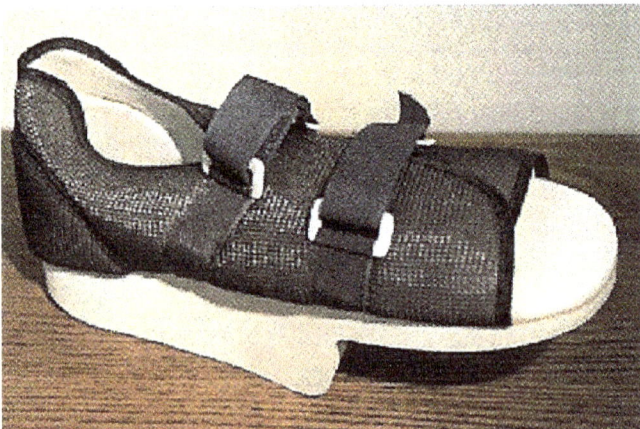

Figure 1.   Healing sandal

for those with poor balance when worn as a pair. It remains relatively cheap at approximately \$20–\$30 for 1 pair. Darco also carries Orthowedge post-op shoes with rear foot or forefoot wedging to offload these areas as required.

Standard Street Shoes

Currently majority of diabetic footwear is of this variety. The standard men's shoes has brogue appearance with complete covering, laces or velcro. They will have a soft, smooth lining with removable insoles to increase the depth or to allow for custom orthotic insertion. Newer innovations have been the use of Lycra, an expandable material to accommodate deformities more readily. Sandals have only recently appeared on the market with brands such as Apex, Klaveness and Podartis.

Rocker soles have also begun to appear in the market. These are believed to be more effective in offloading the forefoot while still allowing for reasonable ambulation.

Walking/Exercise

Exercise is an important aspect of diabetes/health management. Patients are encouraged to walk for exercise. Shoes companies have slowly discovered the demand for sports shoes in the market and are now developing these models without having to significantly redesign their footwear (Fig. 2).

Asics is developing a health exercise shoe, primarily with deeper toe box and seamless inner lining. New Balance shoes (costing SGD200–SGD250 a pair) and Brooks shoes are also good sports shoes or Health Walking Shoes.

Singapore Shoe Market

In Singapore only a very small number of DM Shoes/Orthopaedic Shoes are available in the general market. Running shoes have been the shoe of choice for recommendation. These shoes have cushioned sole, so, completely covered upper, lace or Velcro strapping, and are readily available and reasonably priced. However, our elderly women are usually resistant to wearing them as they are not compatible with the Cheongsam, Kebaya or the Saree. Products which are available currently in Singapore include the Darco Healing Sandal/Post Op Shoes, Darco Gentlestep, Apex Ambulator shoes.

Orthotic Capable Brands have existed for the past 3 years and include Kumfs, X-Sensible, Naot, Mephisto, Birkenstock (with a cost range of SGD200–SGD300) and Ecco-Primo Sandals (\$150–\$200).

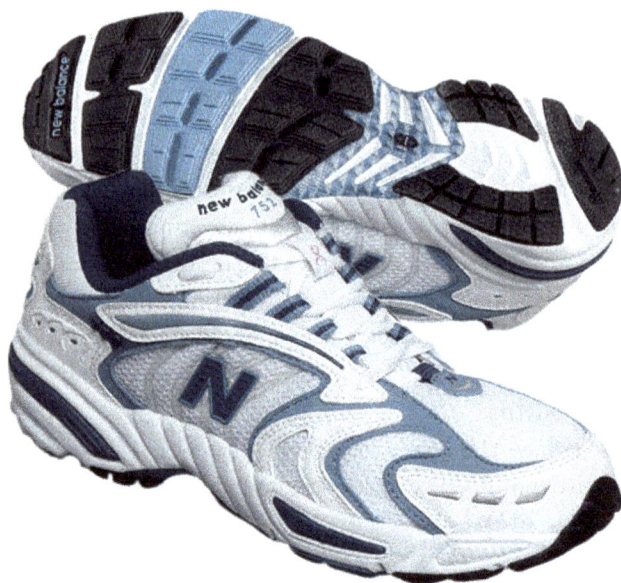

Figure 2. Sports shoe

Exercise Shoes

New Balance did bring in diabetic friendly models but these have since been withdrawn because of poor sales.

Conclusion

There is a demand for Diabetic Footwear for Diabetics belonging to Pendsey Risk Stratification Groups 1 and 2. Currently, most of this demand is taken up by wearing exercise shoes from the open shoe market. There is very little specialised footwear catering to the needs of such diabetics. Whilst Darco is available, they are cosmetically and culturally unacceptable. The majority do not want to wear such footwear and use sandals instead even for outdoor use. There is a great demand for designing, fashioning and fabrication of special shoes (for outdoor use), special sandals (for indoor use) and therapeutic sandals that is acceptable in technical design and fashion and culturally acceptable by our local population.

Section 9

A Patient's Guide

32

Caring for Your Diabetes

Teo Zhen Ling, Chin Yu Xuan and Aziz Nather

Department of Orthopaedic Surgery
Yong Loo Lin School of Medicine
National University of Singapore

Introduction

Currently, there is no cure for diabetes. However, if a patient takes good care of his diabetes, he can prevent the development of complications. There are 3 important aspects in the care of diabetes:

1) Treatment
2) Monitoring and
3) Healthy lifestyle

Treatment

Proper medication is the first step in controlling diabetes. There are many different insulin regimes prescribed according to the patients' needs. These regimes mimic the normal insulin requirement of the body in the fasting state and after a meal.

Take the medication as prescribed by endocrinologist.

For Type 1 Diabetes:

- Insulin injections

Insulin is usually given as an injection (Fig. 1), using a syringe and needle or pen injector, into the layer of fat under the skin (Fig. 2). Avoid injecting at the

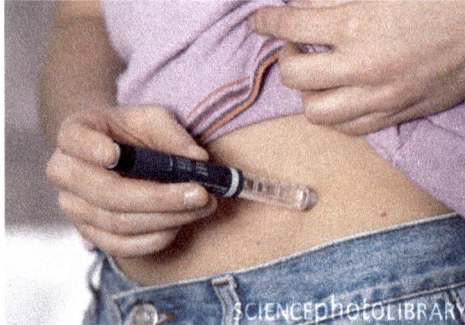

Figure 1. Injection at the abdomen

Source: *www.sciencephoto.com.*

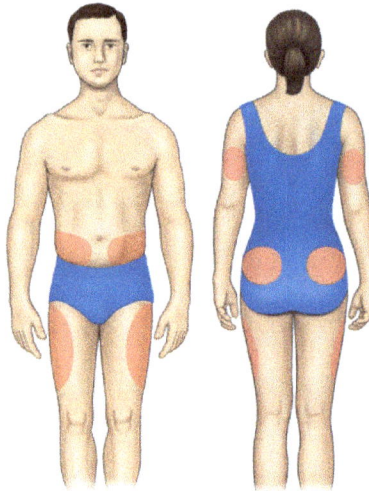

Figure 2. Injection sites are shaded

Source: *www.uptodate.com.*

same spot each time as this may lead to a loss or accumulation of fatty tissue, causing a lump or dent in the skin.

- 3 times a day, before meal

For Type 2 Diabetes:

- Oral tablets

Oral tablets contain hypoglycaemic agents such as

➢ Insulin secretagogues stimulate the pancreas to release insulin.
➢ Biguanides reduce glucose production from the liver, delaying glucose absorption from the intestines and increasing the usage of glucose by cells in the body.
➢ Alphaglucosidase inhibitors slow down the digestion and absorption of glucose in the intestines.
➢ Thiazolidinediones make tissues more sensitive to insulin.

• 3 times a day, before meal

Monitoring

Regular monitoring of one's diabetes is important to prevent diabetic complications. As a patient with diabetes, you should undergo the following:

1. Hypocount self-monitoring
2. HbA1C test
3. Annual foot examination
4. Annual eye examination
5. Foot care: Monitoring your feet daily

Hypocount self-monitoring

You can test you own blood glucose level at home by using a glucometer (Figs. 3 and 4). Monitoring your own blood glucose levels allows you to learn how your body reacts to daily events. This allows you to control your diabetes.

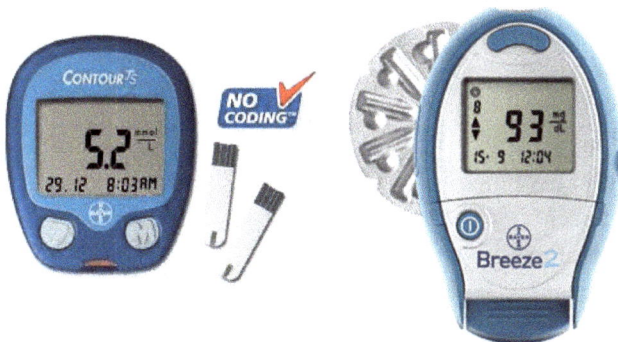

Figure 3. Two types of glucometer

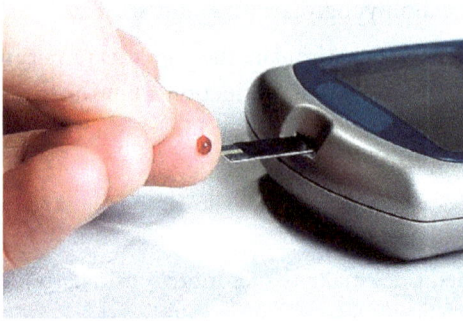

Figure 4. Testing for hypocount

How often should I test my blood glucose levels?

Diabetes type	Frequency of self-monitoring of blood glucose
Type 1 (insulin treated i.e. injection)	3–4 times daily (even at 2 am if needed)
Type 2 (insulin treated i.e. injection)	2–3 times per day, 2–3 days a week
Type 2 (non-insulin treated i.e. no injection)	Frequent enough to achieve glucose targets

Detailed recommended timings for blood glucose testing (Fig. 5)

- Before breakfast
- 1–2 hours after breakfast
- Before lunch
- 1–2 hours after lunch
- Before dinner
- 1–2 hours after dinner
- Before bedtime

Postprandial Blood Glucose (PPBG) is the rapid rise in blood-glucose levels after a meal

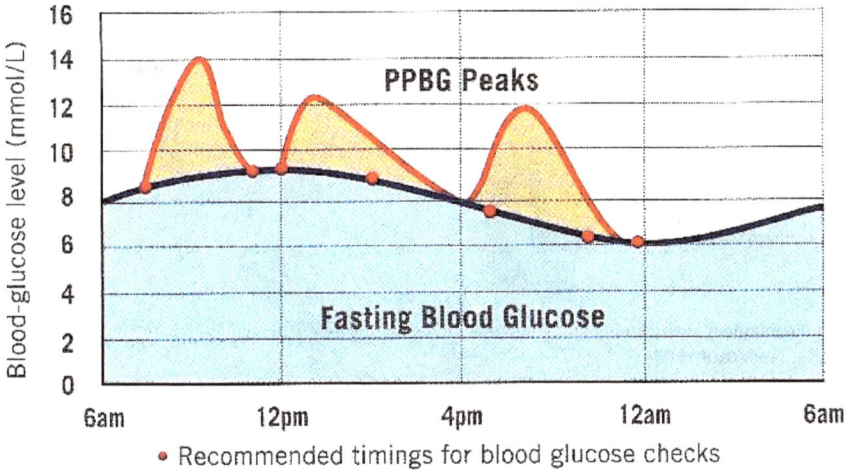

Figure 5. Graph showing the recommended timings for blood glucose checks

What is the normal blood glucose level?

Time	Normal (non-diabetic levels)	Good (target goal for diabetics)	Acceptable	Poor
	Glucometer reading (mmol/L)			
Before meal	4.0–6.0	6.1–8.0	8.1–10.0	>10.0
After meal	5.0–7.0	7.1–10.0	10.1–13.0	>13.0

Hypoglycaemia

Hypoclycaemia is when blood sugar levels are too low (<3.9 mmol/L).

Symptoms:

How it feels like

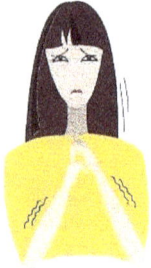

**Trembling Hands/
Nervousness**

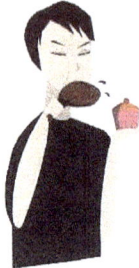

Hunger

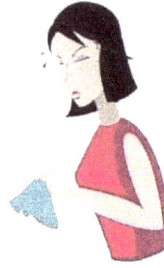

Sweating

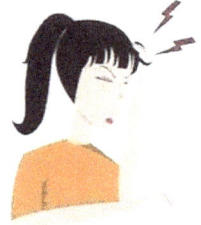

**Dizziness/
Headache**

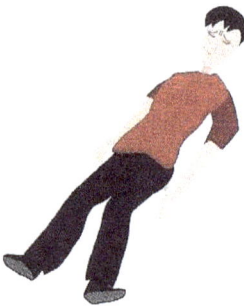

Coma

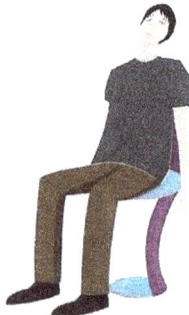

Tiredness

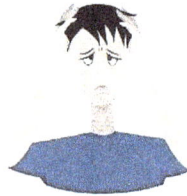

Moody/Confused

What you should do:

- Check your blood sugar level (low if it is <3.9 mmol/L)
- Take your meal or snack immediately if it is already planned for within the next 30 minutes; otherwise
- Take some sugar (15 g) = 120 ml of regular Coke or 3 glucose tabs
- Check your blood sugar level again in 15 minutes

Hyperglycaemia

Hyperglycaemia is when blood sugar levels are too high (>14 mmol/L).

Symptoms:

Fatique &
Weakness

Weight
Loss

Frequent
Urination

Constant
Thirst

Blurred
Vision

Nausea &
Vomiting

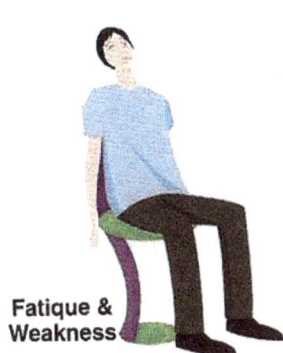

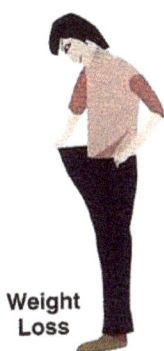

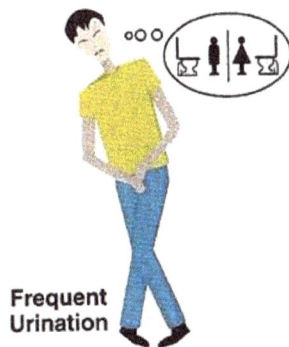

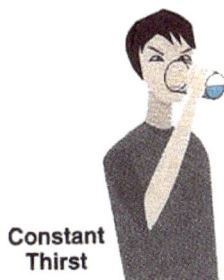

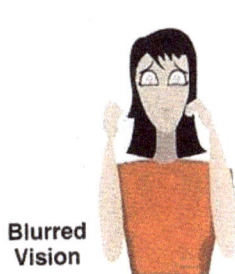

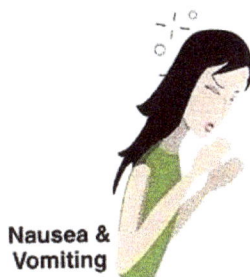

What you should do:

- Check if you are unwell
- Ensure that you have taken your medication
- Check your blood sugar level (2–4 hourly) until it is less than 14 mmol/L
- Check urine ketones
- Call your doctor or nurse if:

  ➢ Blood sugar levels are 14 mmol/L or greater for more than 6 hours
  ➢ Urine ketones are present for more than 6 hours
  ➢ Unable to take fluids or food for 4 hours
  ➢ Severe abdominal pain
  ➢ Still feeling unwell

HbA1C test

HbA1c (glycated haemoglobin) measures how much glucose is attached to your haemoglobin. It reflects an average blood glucose level over a period of 2 to 3 months.

How often should I test for blood glucose levels?

For good diabetes control: Check your HbA1C levels twice a year
For poor diabetes control: Check your HbA1C level 4 times a year

What is a good HbA1C reading?

	Ideal (non-diabetic levels)	Optimal (target goal for majority of patients)	Suboptimal	Unacceptable
HbA1C (%)	4.5–6.4	6.5–7.0	7.1–8.0	>8.0

Annual eye examination

Visit the hospital/polyclinic for an eye examination every year (Fig. 6).

Annual foot examination

Visit the hospital/polyclinic for foot examination every year (Fig. 7).

Foot care: monitoring your feet daily

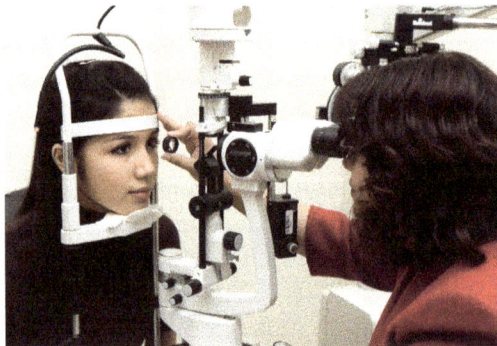

Figure 6. Patient undergoing eye examination

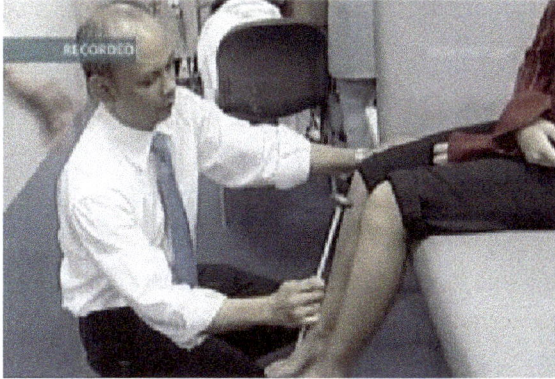

Figure 7.   Patient undergoing foot examination

If you have diabetes, you are at risk of developing a diabetic foot complication. Poorly controlled diabetes can decrease the blood supply to your legs and feet and damage nerves. This can cause

- Poor healing of any injuries or sores on your feet.
- Numbness of your feet. You will not feel pain and thus not know if your feet were injured.

Therefore it is very important to control your blood sugar levels and take proper care of your feet. Clean and check your feet daily!

Cleaning your feet

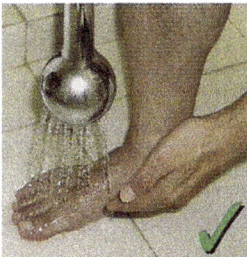

Wash your feet daily with mild soap and warm water

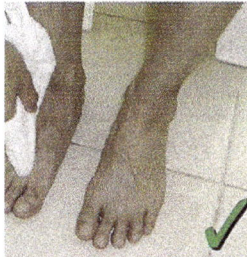

Dry feet well, especially between the toes

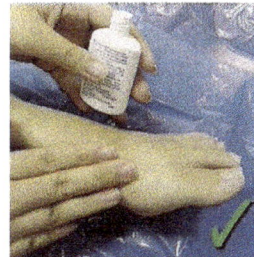

Apply moisturiser everyday to prevent your skin from cracking

Checking your feet

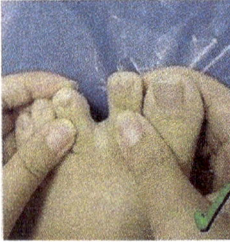

Check your feet everyday:

- Between your toes
- Around the heel
- Sole of foot

 Look for cuts, swelling, redness, blisters or pus (discharge)

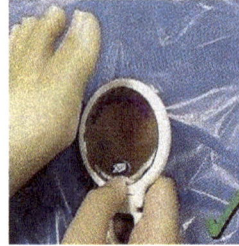

Ask someone to help or use a mirror if you have difficulty checking the soles of your feet

Healthy lifestyle

Leading a healthy lifestyle is essential in diabetes control and the prevention of diabetic complications. A healthy lifestyle consists of

- Maintaining a healthy weight
- Healthy diet
- Exercise

Maintaining a healthy weight

Excess body fat prevents insulin from working properly. It also raises your blood pressure, putting additional strain on your heart, leading to poor blood circulation.

 Keep check of your weight by calculating your Body Mass Index (BMI) regularly.

$$\text{CALCULATE YOUR BMI} = \frac{\text{WEIGHT (kg)}}{\text{HEIGHT} \times \text{HEIGHT (Metre)}}$$

BMI (kg/m^2) for adults	Health risk
27.5 and above	High risk
23–27.4	Moderate risk
18.5–22.9	Low risk (Healthy range)
Below 18.5	Risk of nutritional deficiency disease and osteoporosis

Healthy diet

Being on an oral diabetic medication or insulin, you have to take extra care to make sure that your food intake is balanced with exercise to better manage your blood glucose levels. When you make wise food choices, you can improve your overall health and can prevent further complications such as ischaemic heart disease and hypertension.

Use the Healthy Diet Pyramid (Fig. 8) to help you achieve a healthy diet:

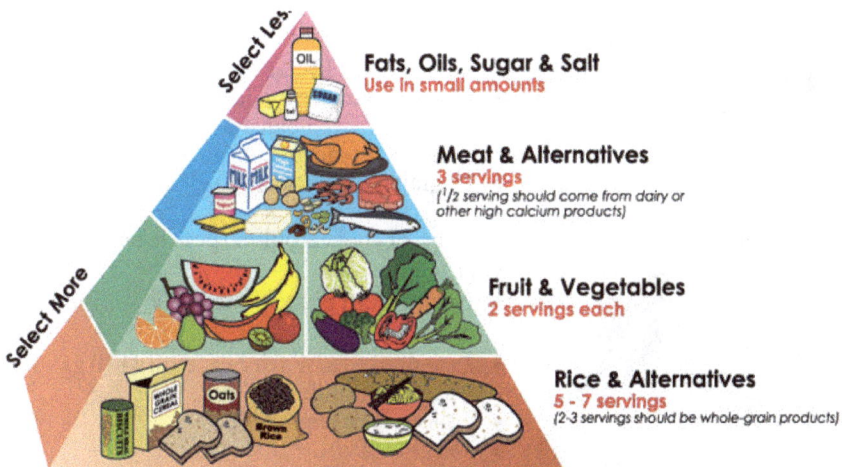

Figure 8. Healthy diet pyramid
Source: *Health Promotion Board, Singapore*

Examples of one serving size for each food group:

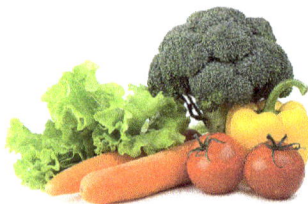

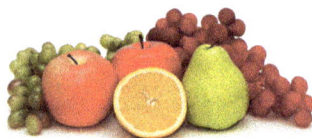

Food group	Example of one serving size
Rice & Alternatives	• 1 bowl of rice (100 g) • 1 bowl of noodles, beehoon or spaghetti (100 g) • 2/3 bowl of uncooked oatmeal (50 g) • 1 thosai (60 g) • 1 large potato (180 g) • 1 cup of plain cornflakes (40 g) • 2 bowls of rice porridge • 2 slices of bread (60 g) • 4 plain crackers (40 g)
Vegetables	• 150 g raw leafy vegetables • 100 g raw non-leafy vegetables • 1 mug of cooked leafy vegetables (100 g) • 1 mug of cooked non-leafy vegetables (100 g)
Fruit	• 1 small apple, orange, pear or mango (130 g) • 1 wedge of papaya, pineapple or watermelon (130 g) • 1 cup of pure fruit juice (250 ml) • 1 medium-sized banana • 1 cup of dried fruit (40 g) • 10 grapes or longans (50 g)
Meat & Alternatives	• 1 cup of cooked pulses (peas, beans, lentils) (120 g) • 1 palm-sized piece of meat, fish or poultry (90 g) • 2 small blocks of soft beancurd (170 g) • 2 glasses of milk (500 ml) • 2 slices of cheese (40 g) • 3 eggs (150 g) • 5 medium-sized prawns (90 g)

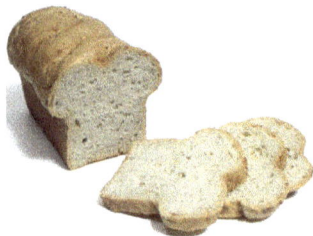

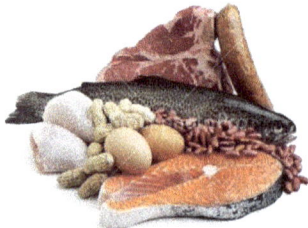

Carbohydrate counting

Carbohydrates are essential in your diet as they provide your body with energy. However, blood sugar is affected most by carbohydrates. Therefore in addition to the normal healthy diet, you need to focus on Carbohydrate Counting to ensure that your blood sugar level is effectively managed.

Carbohydrate Counting can make eating flexible, more enjoyable and give you better control over your blood sugar level. In Carbohydrate Counting, you need to count the amount of carbohydrates in your meals and snacks to tally up a daily total.

Find your carbohydrate allowance based on the recommended daily energy needs given by your dietician or doctor:

Recommended caloric intake	1200 calories	1500 calories	1800 calories	2000 calories
Amount of carbohydrates that is 50% of total calories	150 g/10 CHO exchanges	188 g/12 CHO exchanges	225 g/15 CHO exchanges	250 g/16 CHO exchanges
Amount of carbohydrates that is 60% of total calories	180 g/12 CHO exchanges	225 g/15 CHO exchanges	270 g/18 CHO exchanges	300 g/20 CHO exchanges

Note: 15 g of carbohydrates = 1 CHO exchange

For example:

You are advised to eat 1800 calories per day.
The amount of carbohydrates allowed per day
= 50% − 60% of your total calories (1800)
= 900 − 1080 calories
= 225 − 270 grams of carbohydrates*

*1 gram of carbohydrates = 4 calories

Spread your carbohydrate intake over meals and snacks:

For example:

Meal	Carbohydrates consumed
Breakfast	50 g/3 CHO exchanges
Lunch	75 g/5 CHO exchanges
Snack	25 g/1.5 CHO exchanges
Dinner	75 g/5 CHO exchanges
Snack	25 g/1.5 CHO exchanges
Total	250 g/16 CHO exchanges

Use the food chart to select the food items for each meal:

Ensure that the amount of carbohydrates is within recommended levels.

For example:

Meal	Food item	Carbohydrates consumed
Breakfast	1 piece of roti prata, plain	15 g
	1 baked red bean bun	16 g
	1 glass of soyabean drink, with sugar	19 g
Total	50 g	

Food chart

		Per serving	
Food item	Serving size	Energy (kcal)	Carbohydrates (g)
Breakfast			
3-in1 cereal	1 pack	89	13
Bread, white	1 slice	83.7	15

(Continued)

Food item	Serving size	Per serving	
		Energy (kcal)	Carbohydrates (g)
Bun, kaya	1 piece	213	34
Bun, pizza	1 piece	224	27
Bun, red bean, baked	1 piece	102	16
Bun, tuna	1 piece	205	23
Chapati, plain	1 piece	187	28
Chee cheong fun, plain with sauce	1 roll	133	26
Curry puff, chicken	1 piece	246	20

Food item	Serving size	Energy (kcal)	Carbohydrates (g)
Fried beehoon, plain	1 plate	250	46
Fried beehoon, vegetarian	1 plate	404	72
Lontong with sayur lodeh	1 plate	466	43
Lor mai kai	1 piece	322	55
Nasi lemak	1 packet	494	80
Pau, char siew	1 piece	363	45
Pau, lotus paste	1 piece	170	29
Porridge, century egg	1 bowl	364	38
Porridge, chicken	1 bowl	181	21
Porridge, duck	1 bowl	586	53
Porridge, fish	1 bowl	211	32
Porridge, fried peanuts and ikan bilis	1 bowl	344	37

(*Continued*)

(*Continued*)

Food item	Serving size	Per serving	
		Energy (kcal)	Carbohydrates (g)
Porridge, peanut and pork	1 bowl	211	19
Porridge, sweet potato	1 bowl	168	35
Rice dumpling, in lotus leaf	1 piece	315	52
Roti prata, plain	1 piece	96	15

Food item	Serving size	Energy (kcal)	Carbohydrates (g)
Roti prata with egg	1 piece	288	28

Lunch/Dinner

Ban mian, fish head, soup	1 bowl	832	82
Ban mian, soup	1 bowl	475	48
Beansprouts with salted fish, stir-fried	1 portion	89	2
Beef ball kway teow, soup	1 bowl	381	65
Beef hor fun	1 plate	697	95
Beef noodle, dry	1 bowl	395	72
Beef noodle, soup	1 bowl	303	47
Beehoon, fish head soup	1 bowl	666	83
Beehoon, fish slice soup	1 bowl	349	48
Beehoon, seafood soup	1 bowl	297	35
Beehoon with cuttlefish and kangkong	1 plate	382	61

(*Continued*)

Food item	Serving size	Per serving	
		Energy (kcal)	Carbohydrates (g)
Bittergourd with egg, fried	1 plate	400	8
Bread, focaccia, with sun-dried tomato	1 piece	245	23
Broccoli, stir-fried	1 portion	98	4
Char kway teow	1 plate	744	76

Food item	Serving size	Energy (kcal)	Carbohydrates (g)
Char Siew rice	1 plate	605	91
Cha Soba	1 portion	170	28
Chicken rice	1 plate	607	75

Food item	Serving size	Energy (kcal)	Carbohydrates (g)
Claypot rice	1 plate	899	93
Duck noodle, dry	1 bowl	500	67
Duck rice	1 plate	673	99
Ee mee with mixed seafood	1 plate	1007	78
Egg fuyong	1 plate	660	6
Egg sambal	1 plate	67	3
Egg with minced pork, steamed	1 portion	177	2

(Continued)

(*Continued*)

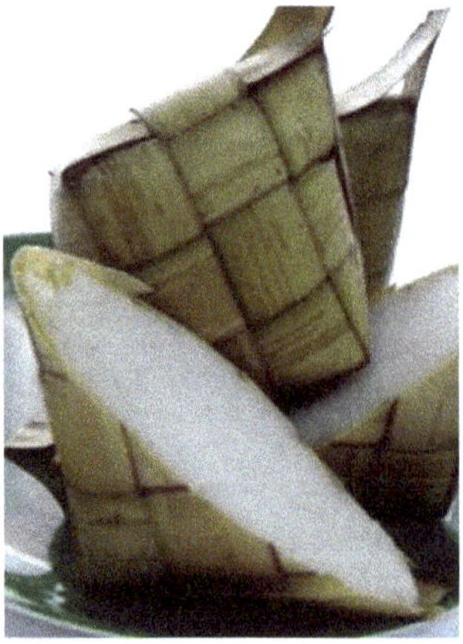

Food item	Serving size	Energy (kcal)	Carbohydrates (g)
Egg with tofu, steamed	1 portion	128	1
Egg, steamed, Japanese style	1 portion	116	3
Fishball noodle, dry	1 bowl	370	55
French beans, cooked with sambal chilli	1 portion	186	6
Fried Hokkien prawn mee	1 plate	522	69
Fried hor fun	1 plate	748	91
Fried rice	1 plate	508	66
Fried rice wrapped in omelette, Malay style	1 plate	805	80
Garlic bread	1 loaf	653	81
Ipoh hor fun	1 plate	453	66
Ketupat	1 whole	88	20
Kway chap with meat, intestine and taupok	1 portion	650	70
Laksa lemak	1 bowl	591	58

(*Continued*)

Food item	Serving size	Per serving	
		Energy (kcal)	Carbohydrates (g)
Laksa yong tau foo	1 bowl	634	51
Lo han chai	1 portion	157	6
Longbeans with tempeh, stir-fried	1 plate	869	9
Lor mee	1 bowl	383	55
Macaroni, chicken, soup	1 bowl	199	31
Mee goreng	1 plate	500	61
Mee hoon kway, soup	1 bowl	584	71
Mee rebus	1 plate	571	82
Mee siam	1 plate	694	92

Food item	Serving size	Energy (kcal)	Carbohydrates (g)
Mee soto	1 plate	433	60
Mee sua with kidney soup	1 bowl	277	38
Mui fun	1 plate	720	112
Murtabak, sardine	1 plate	787	69
Mushroom, mixed, braised	1 portion	39	0
Naan bread	1 piece	357	57
Nasi briyani	1 plate	619	109
Nasi goreng	1 plate	742	103
Noodles, meepok, minced pork and black mushroom, dry	1 bowl	511	57
Noodles, meepok, minced pork and black mushroom, soup	1 bowl	383	50
Ladyfingers with shrimp paste, fried	1 plate	149	8

(*Continued*)

(*Continued*)

Food item	Serving size	Per serving	
		Energy (kcal)	Carbohydrates (g)
Omelette, oyster	1 plate	645	32
Omelette, onion	1 plate	448	10
Penang fried kway teow	1 plate	510	59
Penang laksa	1 plate	377	71
Pineapple rice, Thai style	1 plate	815	119
Potato and cauliflower masala	1 portion	127	10
Prawn noodle, dry	1 bowl	461	65
Prawn noodle, soup	1 bowl	294	49
Rojak, Chinese style	1 plate	559	65

Food item	Serving size	Energy (kcal)	Carbohydrates (g)
Satay beehoon	1 plate	763	75
Shrimp dumpling noodle, dry	1 bowl	503	53
Shrimp dumpling noodle, soup	1 bowl	399	56
Soup, miso	1 bowl	13	0
Spinach, fried	1 portion	189	1
Sweet potato porridge	1 bowl	168	35
Tauhu telur	1 whole	811	21
Taukwa, pan fried	1 piece	103	0
Taupok, stewed	1 piece	89	2
Tempeh, deep fried	1 piece	128	1
Tofu, hong siew	1 plate	563	1
Tofu, hotplate	1 plate	782	4
Tofu, mapo	1 portion	226	1

(*Continued*)

Food item	Serving size	Per serving	
		Energy (kcal)	Carbohydrates (g)
Tofu, with minced pork, steamed	1 wedge	118	2
Udon, prawn tempura, soup	1 bowl	573	64
Unagi don, eel rice, Japanese style	1 bowl	626	91
Wanton noodle, dry	1 bowl	411	55
Wanton noodle, soup	1 bowl	290	41
Yam rice	1 bowl	435	88
You tiao, stuffed with squid paste, deep fried	1 piece	244	19

Snacks

Food item	Serving size	Energy (kcal)	Carbohydrates (g)
Apple	1 small one	77	21
Bak kwa, pork, lean	1 piece	370	47
Banana	1 medium one	105	27
Banana fritter	1 piece	197	36
Cake, banana	1 piece	146	16
Cake, butter	1 piece	180	19
Cake, cheese	1 piece	174	11
Cake, pandan chiffon	1 piece	135	15

Food item	Serving size	Energy (kcal)	Carbohydrates (g)
Chicken floss	1 portion	427	35
Cream cracker, plain	1 piece	40	5
Cream cracker, wholemeal	1 piece	39	4
Digestive biscuit	1 piece	49	7
Doughnut, sugared	1 piece (42 g)	164	19
Durian (Thai)	5 small seeds	267	48

(*Continued*)

(Continued)

Food item	Serving size	Per serving Energy (kcal)	Carbohydrates (g)
Egg tart, plain	1 piece	178	18

Grass jelly (chin chow)	1 bowl	55	14
Muffin, banana	1 whole	277	31
Muffin, blueberry	1 whole	248	30
Muffin, chocolate	1 whole	217	25
Papadum	1 piece	30	2
Pie, chicken	1 whole	456	37
Pineapple tart	1 piece	82	11
Popiah	1 roll	188	14

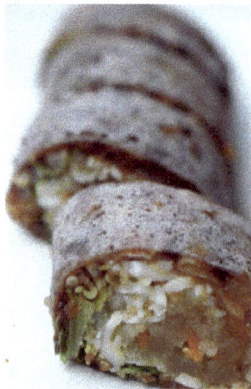

(Continued)

Food item	Serving size	Per serving	
		Energy (kcal)	Carbohydrates (g)
Prunes	3 pieces	69	18
Raisins	14g	42	11
Spring roll (chun juan)	1 piece	139	8
Tau huay, with syrup	1 bowl	317	60
Desserts			
Bubor cha cha	1 bowl	536	52

Bubor terigu	1 bowl	329	70
Cheng tng, clear soup	1 bowl	218	53
Red bean soup, without coconut milk	1 bowl	381	80
Tang yuan, peanut filling	1 bowl	90	11
Tang yuan, red bean filling	1 bowl	68	10
Tiramisu	1 portion	345	35
Yam paste (Or ni)	1 bowl	1417	182
Beverages			
Bandung	1 packet	152	32
Barley water	1 glass	55	14
Bubble tea	1 cup	160	27
Bubble tea with milk	1 cup	232	24.4
Bubble tea with milk and pearls	1 cup	340	52.7

(Continued)

(*Continued*)

Food item	Serving size	Per serving Energy (kcal)	Carbohydrates (g)
Café mocha	1 cup	185	26
Cappucino	1 cup	76	10
Coffee with evaporated milk	1 cup	8	1.5
Coffee, black, unsweetened	1 cup	5	1
Coffee, with condensed milk	1 cup	113	15
Coffee, with sugar	1 cup	66	12

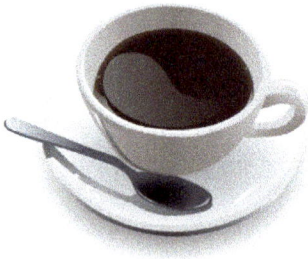

Cultured milk drink	1 bottle	89	21
Lassi, sweet	1 glass	78	8
Orange juice	1/2 cup	60	15
Pineapple juice	1/2 cup	60	15
Soyabean drink, with sugar	1 glass	138	19

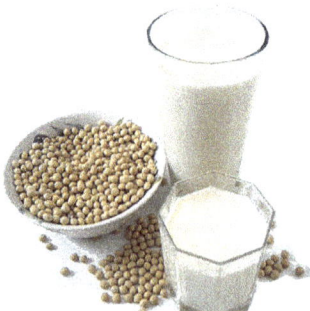

(*Continued*)

Food item	Serving size	Per serving	
		Energy (kcal)	Carbohydrates (g)
Soyabean drink, without sugar	1 glass	83	3
Tea with evaporated milk	1 cup	5	1.5
Tea, black, unsweetened	1 cup	2	1
Tea with sugar	1 cup	67	17

Sauces and Condiments

Food item	Serving size	Energy (kcal)	Carbohydrates (g)
Coconut milk, fresh, first squeeze	1 coconut	618	6
Commercial sweet & sour sauce	1 Tbsp	28.2	6.8
Gula meleka	1 whole piece	120	30
Gula merah (red sugar)	1 Tbsp	17	4
Oyster sauce	1 tsp	5	1
Sambal belacan	2 tsp	15	1
Sambal chilli	2 tsp	19	2
Satay sauce	1 portion	77	3

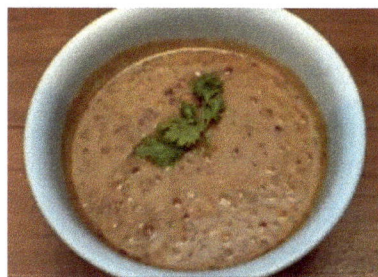

Food item	Serving size	Energy (kcal)	Carbohydrates (g)
Sauce, chee cheong fun	1 portion	241	45
Sauce, plum	1 portion	42	10
Sauce, wasabi	1 portion	5	1
Thai chilli sauce	1 Tbsp	40	9.9
White sugar	1 tsp	20	5
Yong tau foo, chilli sauce	1 portion	64	2
Yong tau foo, red sauce	1 portion	23	4

Source: Abbott Nutrition

Tips for eating out

- Know the ingredients in your food and portion size
- Keep portion sizes in check — eat the same portion that you would at home
- Make substitutions — ask for low-fat options if available
- Ask for condiments, sauces or dressings to be served on the side so that you can control how much you use
- Choose foods that are baked, broiled, poached, steamed or stir fried
- Try not to avoid whole food groups at a meal unless you are saving your carbohydrates for a small dessert
- Eat slowly
- Eat on time
- Compensate by reducing the amount of other carbohydrates in your meal

Exercise

Physical activity uses up blood glucose (lowers blood glucose levels) and burns body fat. This improves insulin action and helps to control body weight. Physical activity should be part of your daily routine. Regular exercise improves blood circulation, strengthens your heart, relieves stress and prevents the onset of diabetic complications.

Start an exercise routine that is safe and enjoyable:

- Engage in 30 minutes of physical activity a day on 5 or more days a week
- Exercise to achieve an energy expenditure of 1000–2000 kcal (roughly 5 hours of slow walking) per week

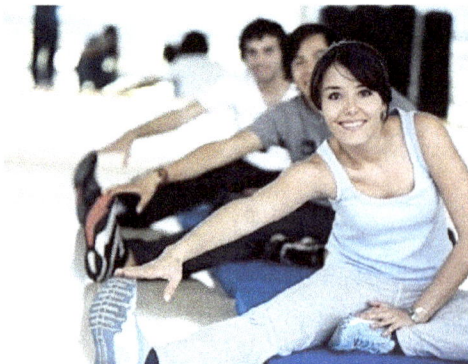

Tips for a safe exercise

- If you have any diabetic complications, consult your doctor before exercising
- Check your blood glucose before and after exercising to prevent hypoglycaemia. Test your blood glucose twice before you exercise, 30 minutes apart, to ensure that your blood glucose level is stable and not dropping.
- Avoid injecting insulin into exercising limbs
- When exercising in the evening, increase carbohydrate intake to minimize hypoglycaemia at night
- Always carry a fast-acting source of carbohydrate (e.g., glucose gel or tablets, soft drink, raisins) in case you experience hypoglycaemia
- Replace body fluids by drinking plenty of water
- Avoid exercising alone
- Always carry an identification tag
- Wear suitable and well-fitting shoes and socks
- Check your feet every day after each exercise session for redness, infected cuts or open sores

The greatest risk of exercise for patients with diabetes is exercise-induced hypoglycaemia.

Recommended dietary carbohydrate intake (g) before exercise

Intensity of exercise	Example	Blood glucose level before exercising (mmol/L)	Carbohydrate intake before exercising (g)
Brief, high-intensity	<30 min: Resistance training	6–10	No food required
Light	30 min: Walking or 60 min: Easy-pace aerobics	<6	15 g

(*Continued*)

(Continued)

Intensity of exercise	Example	Blood glucose level before exercising (mmol/L)	Carbohydrate intake before exercising (g)
Moderate	<45 min: Swimming, jogging	<6 6–10	30–45 g 15 g
Strenuous	>60 min: Triathlon, marathon, cycling	<6 mmol/L 6–10 mmol/L 10–14 mmol/L	45 g 30–45 g 15–30 g

In addition to a maintaining a healthy weight, a healthy diet and regular exercise, you can protect your health by ensuring that you:

- Do not smoke
  (Nicotine in cigarettes promote macrovascular and microvascular disease.)
- Do not consume alcohol
- Manage stress
- Treat any signs of sickness early

33

Care of Your Foot

Lynn Li Toh

Podiatrist
Department of Rehabilitation
National University Hospital

Introduction

Poor blood supply to the feet, as well as nerve damage, can result in foot complications in people with diabetes. Without the appropriate education and foot care, these foot complications may lead to amputations of the lower extremity.

To raise global awareness of the increasing health issues that diabetes poses, the International Diabetes Foundation (IDF), with the support of the World Health Organization (WHO) (Fig. 1), organizes the World Diabetes Day. This event is held annually on 14th November (Fig. 2).

With the number of amputations resulting from diabetes becoming unacceptable, the IDF, WHO and the International Working Group on the Diabetic Foot (IWGDF) collaborated to organize the World Diabetes Day. World Diabetes Day 2005 was themed "Put feet first: prevent amputations" (Fig. 3).

The campaign was an effort to reduce amputation rates by between 49% and 85% by raising awareness worldwide. This can be achieved by prevention and providing appropriate education for people with diabetes and healthcare professionals, so that they can better control diabetes (Fig. 4).

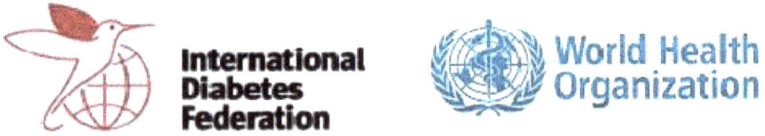

Figure 1.   International Diabetes Federation (IDF) and World Health Organization (WHO) are the organizers of World Diabetes Day

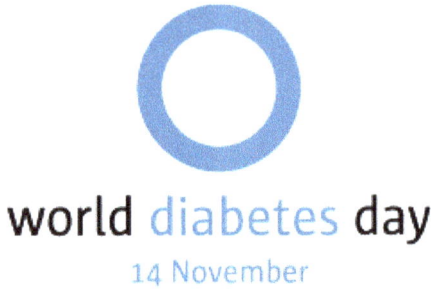

Figure 2.   World Diabetes Day is held annually on the 14th November to raise global awareness on Diabetes

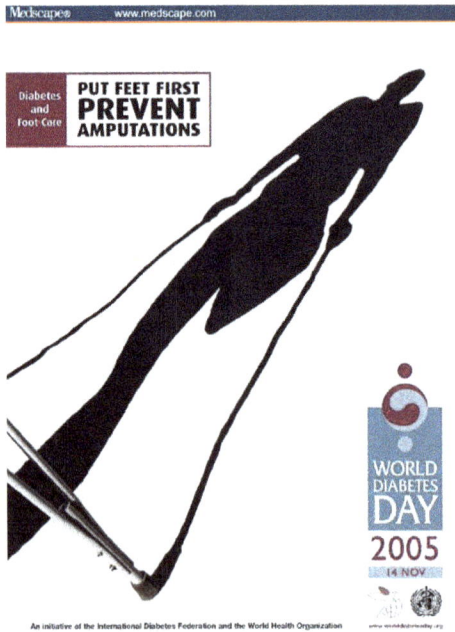

Figure 3.   World Diabetes Day 2005 themed "Put feet first: prevent amputations"

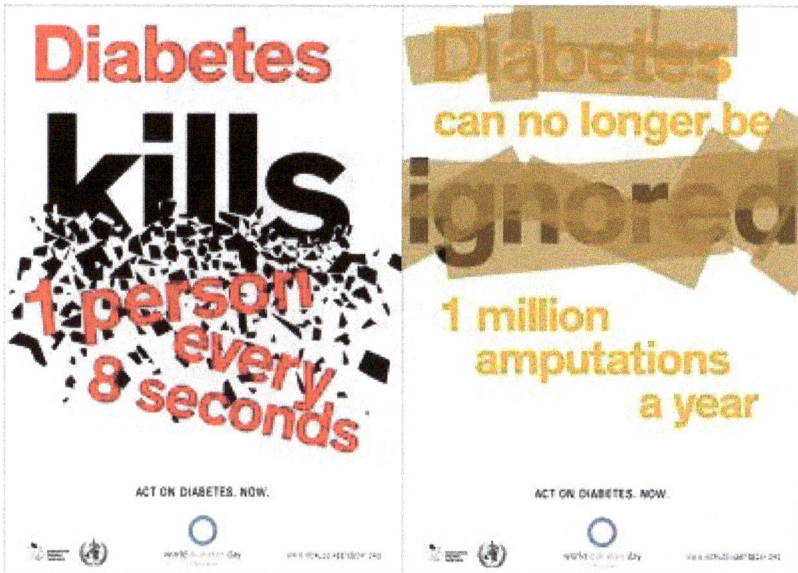

Figure 4. Posters used during World Diabetes Day

Approximately 85% of amputations are preceded by diabetic foot ulcers. Diabetic foot ulcers are mainly caused by:

- Poor blood supply to the feet (peripheral vascular disease)
- Nerve damage (peripheral neuropathy)
- Common foot deformities (bunions, hammer toes)
- Injuries (eg. stepping on a sharp stone)

With complications arising from diabetes, wound healing is impeded. There is a higher risk of infection as the body's ability to fight infection is weakened. If the infection is not detected early and becomes too serious, amputation may be inevitable. However, with proper foot care and good management of diabetes, foot ulcers can be prevented thus preventing amputations.

How to Take Care of Our Feet

There are 6 main aspects to diabetes foot care. These include:

- Foot hygiene
- Skin care

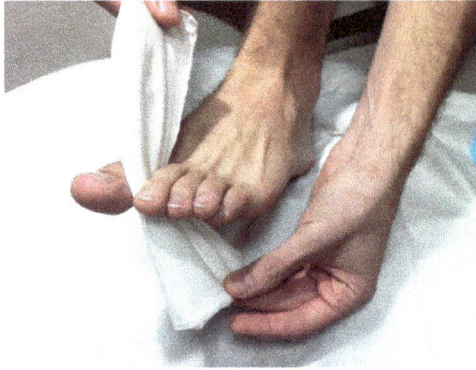

Figure 5. Dry between the toes to prevent maceration

- Nail care
- Inspection
- Footwear
- First aid

Hygiene

Basic foot hygiene is the first step in maintaining good foot care. Clean feet help to keep the skin healthy and prevent infection.

The following tips can help you maintain foot hygiene:

- Wash your feet with warm water and mild soap at least twice daily.
- Ensure that the spaces between your toes are also cleaned as these areas trap dirt easily.
- After cleaning, use a clean towel to dry the feet especially between the toes (Fig. 5). If the spaces between the toes are not properly dried, this can lead to skin maceration causing a break in the skin (Fig. 6). This becomes a portal of entry for fungal and bacterial infection.
- Avoid using any foot powder in between the toes as it tends to adhere to moist areas forming clumps. These hard clumps of powder can cause skin abrasions thus ulcerations.

Skin Care

The skin condition of patients with diabetes is usually dry and has a rough texture. It does not help if the skin is also constantly exposed to dry conditions

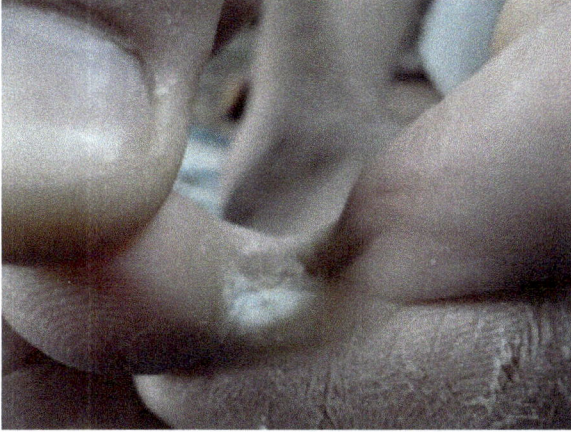

Figure 6.   Maceration between the toes is a common cause for fungal and bacterial infection

as contributed by the wide usage of air-conditioning in Singapore. Dry skin condition can lead to cracks in the skin exposing the skin to possible fungal and bacterial infections.

- Also with age, the skin loses its elasticity and becomes very thin and fragile. In the elderly, a small scratch on the skin can cause an ulcer. Therefore, it is important to maintain skin moisture for the skin to be smooth, elastic and resilient.
- Apply a good foot moisturizing cream to the feet daily. Foot balms and creams usually have ingredients such as urea and soft paraffin in them for better skin penetration as the skin at the sole of the foot is thicker than the rest of the skin of the body.
- With very dry feet, apply the foot cream at least three times daily.
- Apply all over the feet and legs EXCEPT the spaces between the toes as this can cause maceration.
- If you have trouble reaching your feet, enlist the help of a family member or friend to apply the cream. Alternatively, you can use a squirt bottle to squirt some cream on to your foot and use the other foot to rub the cream over the foot (Fig. 7). You can also put some cream on to a soft cloth tied to a long stick and use that to apply the cream.

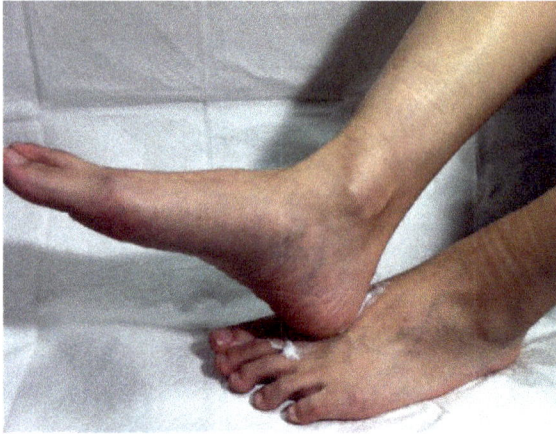

Figure 7. Use your other foot to help with applying cream if you are unable to reach

Nail care

Ingrown toenail is a common problem in patients with diabetes. It is often very painful and if there is a break in the skin, infection can become a problem. Poor eyesight and the inability to reach the feet especially in the elderly often leads to the skin being accidentally cut and can cause ulcer formation. Here are some suggestions for good toenail care:

- Trim toenails after shower as they are softer and easier to manage.
- Use nail clippers instead of scissors to prevent from cutting the skin.
- Trim toenails straight across and not too short to prevent ingrown toenails (Fig. 8).
- Do not cut down the corners of the nails. Use a nail file to gently file down any sharp corners.
- Do not dig into the corners of the nails as this can cause ingrown toenails (Fig. 9).
- If the toenail is thick and difficult to cut, file down the toenail first using a gentle nail file and try trimming again.
- If you are having problems seeing and/or reaching your feet, get a family member or friend to help trim your toenails. Alternatively, you can also visit a podiatrist for toenail care.

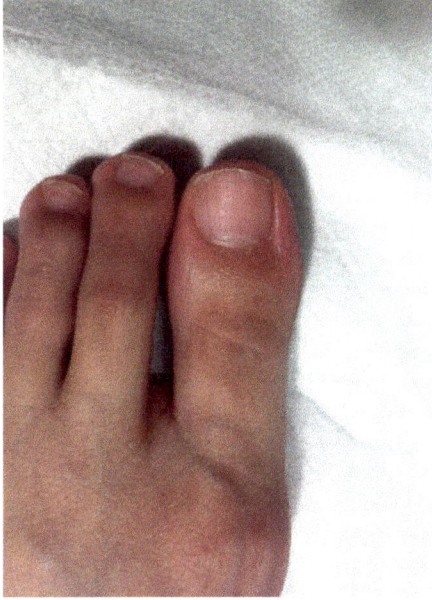

Figure 8. Trim toenails straight across and not down the corners

Inspection

If there is nerve damage due to diabetes (neuropathy), pain sensation is altered. Patients with diabetes who experience this do not realize when there is a cut on the foot or if they have stepped on a sharp object as they cannot feel the pain. They will only realize that there is a wound when they see blood stains on the floor or when there is an infection. Therefore, it is important to inspect the feet daily for early detection of problems.

- Inspect the feet every day.
- If you have vision problems, feel the feet for any abnormalities.
- If you are unable to reach the feet, use a mirror to aid you (Fig. 10).
- It is important to check the top of the foot, the sole, around the heels, between the toes (Fig. 11) and around the toenails.
- Look out for any cuts, blisters, abrasions, corns, calluses and changes in colour. See a doctor or podiatrist if there are any concerns.

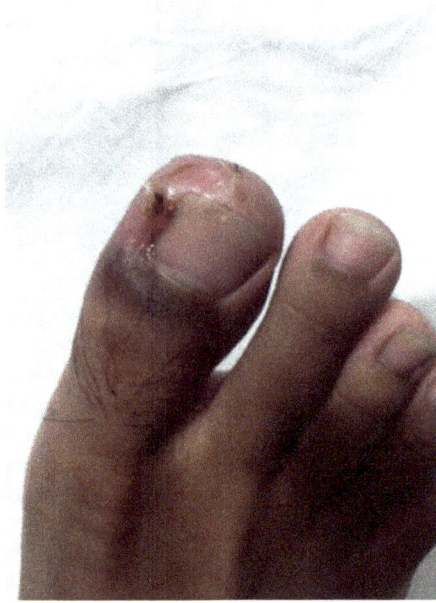

Figure 9. Infected ingrown toenail

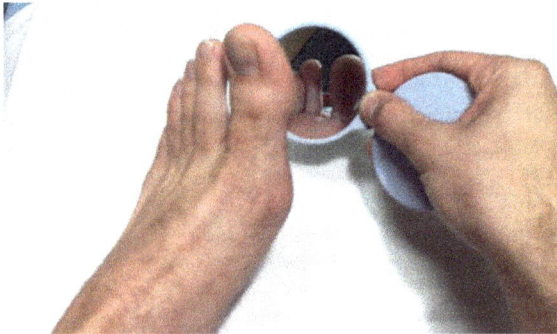

Figure 10. Use a mirror to look at the bottom of the foot

Footwear

In Singapore, patients prefer to wear slippers or sandals due to the hot humid weather. However, such footwear do not provide adequate protection for the feet.

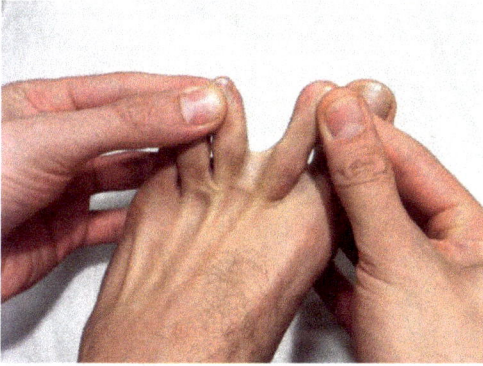

Figure 11. Check the spaces between the toes

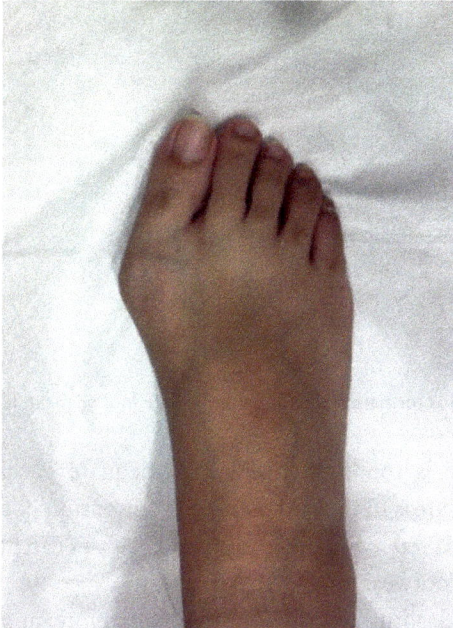

Figure 12. Bunion deformity requiring footwear with a wide toebox

It can also be difficult to find appropriate footwear to accommodate foot deformities such as bunions (Fig. 12) and hammertoes. Patients with severe foot deformities may need to consult an orthopedic shoemaker to have shoes to be custom made to accommodate the deformities.

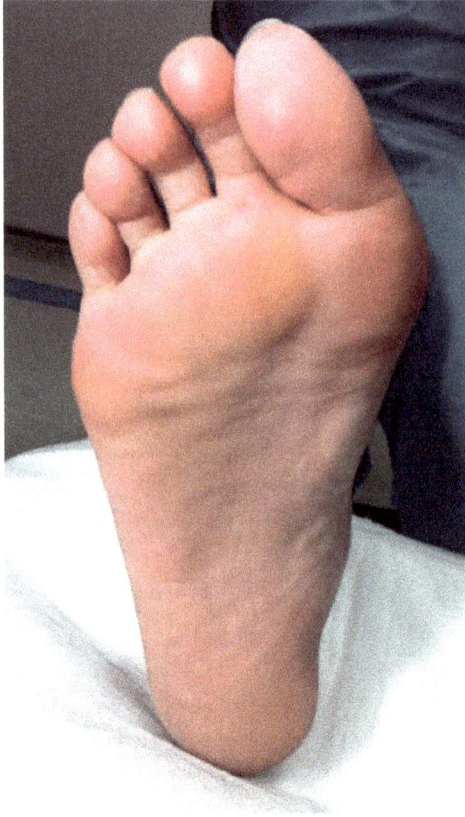

Figure 13. Callus formation due to inappropriate footwear can lead to ulceration

Footwear that is too tight or have inadequate cushioning can cause abnormal pressure areas in the foot leading to formation of corns and calluses. If the pressure is not removed, these corns and calluses can breakdown to form ulcers (Fig. 13). Footwear that is too large can cause the foot to move too much in the shoe, leading to skin abrasions. Therefore, appropriate footwear is important to protect the feet and to prevent foot complications.

- Wear footwear at all times. Wear covered shoes when outdoors and wear soft cushioned slippers when at home.
- Choose a good sport shoes with these components:
  - Soft lining
  - Good support

- Extra cushioning
- Extra depth and width
- Laces or Velcro straps to secure the shoe to the foot
- The space between the tip of the longest toe and the front of the shoe should be one thumb's width.
- The width of the shoe should be as wide as your foot.
- Wear cotton socks when wearing shoes as it gives extra protection to the feet and it is a good moisture absorber.
- Change socks regularly to maintain good hygiene.
- Check the insides of the shoes and shake them out before wearing to ensure that there are no foreign objects that can be harmful to the feet.
- Check the shoes for any wear and tear. Worn out shoes do not provide adequate protection for the feet.

First Aid

An open lesion creates a portal of entry for microorganisms leading to an infection. Also, with diabetes and its complications, the wound takes much longer to heal. It is important that any open lesion should be attended to immediately, to prevent from getting worse.

- Keep a well stocked first aid kit (Fig. 14). A first aid kit should have the following:
  - Cleaning solution
  - Gauze and cotton balls
  - Forceps
  - Antiseptic cream
  - Band-aid
- Clean the wound thoroughly with the cleaning solution.
- After the wound is cleaned and dried, apply the antiseptic cream.
- Cover the wound with a good band-aid.
- Look out for any clinical signs of infection such as redness, warmth, swelling, pus discharge, pain and loss of function. See a doctor or a podiatrist immediately if any of these signs appear.

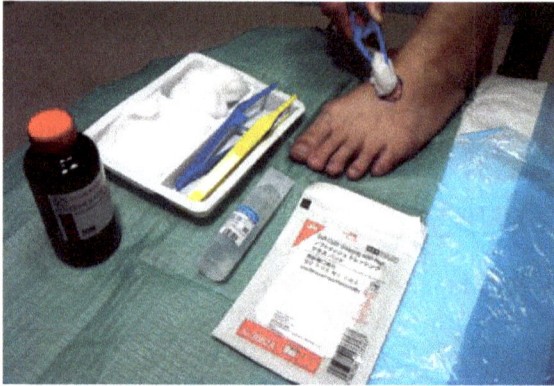

Figure 14. First aid kit

Summary

It is important to be aware about diabetes and its complications. It is good practice to have a foot screening done annually by the doctor, podiatrist or foot care nurse to detect any foot complication. Regular and proper foot care is a basic step in preventing a foot complication. In this way, major amputation can be avoided.

34

Choosing Your Own Footwear

Jun Morimoto

Podiatrist
Department of Rehabilitation
National University Hospital

1. Introduction

For patients with diabetes, poor footwear can lead to serious problems such as foot deformity, ulceration, infection and amputation in extreme cases. Therefore appropriate footwear plays a significant role in preventing foot complications. Often, patients with diabetes have to change their footwear to prevent foot complications. It is very important to encourage patients with diabetes to wear good footwear both indoors and outdoors.[1] Despite the proven effectiveness of appropriate diabetic footwear, patient compliance is a major issue. The most common reasons for non-compliance have been cited as aesthetics, comfort, durability, and cost.[2]

2. Why do people with diabetes need to wear good footwear?

Diabetes can cause loss of protective sensation (neuropathy) and poor circulation (peripheral vascular disease). In patients with neuropathy, even minor trauma can lead to development of chronic ulcers.[1] It can also cause changes in the shape of the foot. There may also be pressure areas that have high risk of developing callosities and ulcerations, if not protected by a good footwear or an insole. Poor circulation, in conjunction with poor footwear, can delay wound healing and predispose to infection. This may result in amputation if not treated properly.

Appropriate footwear will protect the diabetic foot from pressure, friction and trauma.[3] It will provide stability and comfort, reduce pain, and is also able to accommodate a therapeutic insole if necessary.

3. Assessment of each individual patient for suitable footwear

It is important to assess each individual for suitable footwear to improve compliance and efficacy of prevention and treatment of the foot complication present.

The assessment must include the following:

(1) **Presence of Complications** i.e. presence of neuropathy, deformity, ulcer or poor circulation.
(2) **Level of protection required** for each individual.
(3) **Employment** i.e. need for special shoes such as safety shoes, Wellington boots or smart shoes for offices.
(4) **Lifestyle and daily activities:** Elderly patients who stay at home most of the time have different needs from young active individuals.
(5) **Culture:** Some cultures do not include wearing covered shoes. In some countries, the hot climate results in people wearing slippers or sandals. In some cultures, walking barefoot indoors is the norm.

4. Features of good footwear

For all patients with diabetes, good footwear should have following features. (Fig. 1):

- Soft lining for protection and prevention from excessive friction and pressure
- Good supportive structure for stability.
- Good cushion for shock absorption and to reduce excessive stress on the feet.
- Extra depth and width to prevent pressure areas and to accommodate the foot deformity.
- Secure to ankle with lace or velcro strap to hold the foot in the shoe.

Figure 2 shows examples of good footwear.

5. Fitting of diabetic footwear

It is important to fit shoes correctly to prevent the development of abrasion and foot deformity from an ill-fitting footwear.

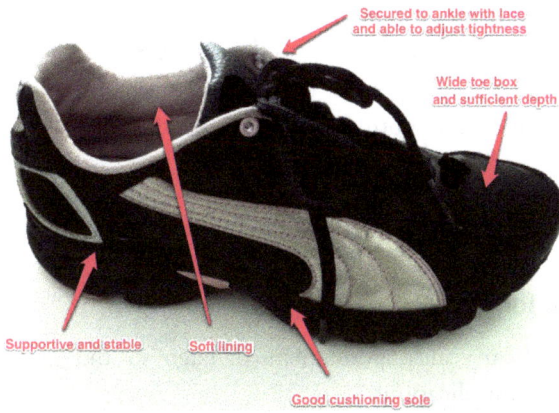

Secured to ankle with lace
and able to adjust tightness

Wide toe box
and sufficient depth

Supportive and stable

Soft lining

Good cushioning sole

Figure 1. Example of footwear suitable for patients with diabetes

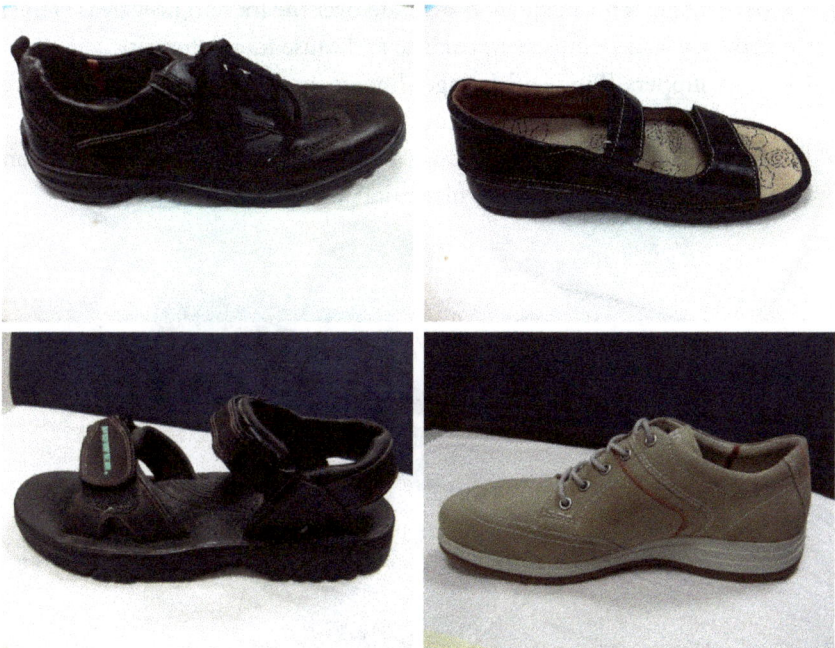

Figure 2. Examples of good footwear

- **Length:** Should have enough space for at least one finger to fit between longest toe and front of shoe.
- **Depth of toe box:** should be deep so that toes can wriggle freely.
- **Width:** Should be slightly wider than your feet when standing
- **Material:** Should be smooth inside and made of breathable material, such as leather.
- **Heel Height:** Should be less than 1 inch or 2.5 cm.

6. Avoid bad footwear

Ill-fitting shoes can cause permanent damage to the feet, resulting in deformities and complications.[4]

- **High-heeled shoes (Fig. 3):** Increases pressure on the forefoot area, may lead to ulceration. This type of shoes is very unstable to walk and risk of falls or soft tissue injury is high.
- **Slippers:** There is no adequate protection over the toe and heel areas. Thus, slippers may lead to muscle imbalance and cause foot deformity.
- **Massage slippers (Fig. 4):** Massage slippers increase unnecessary pressure and friction over the sole of foot and can cause skin breakdown.
- **Flip-flops (Fig. 5):** Flip Flops can cause increased pressure and friction between the toes and can cause ulceration.

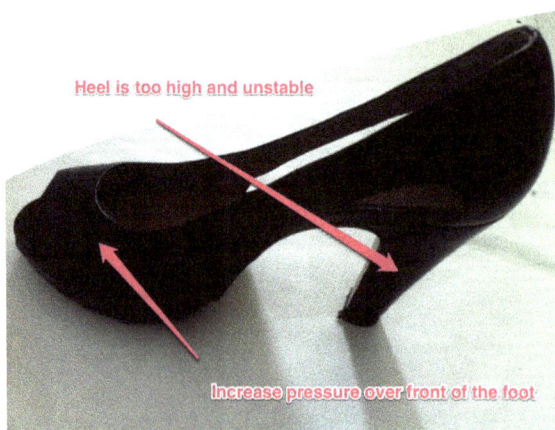

Figure 3. High-heeled shoe

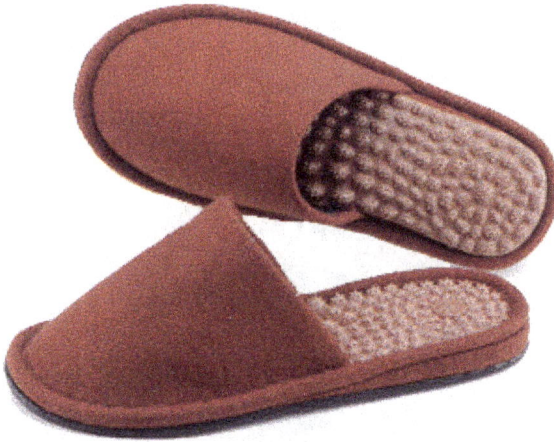

Figure 4. Massage slippers

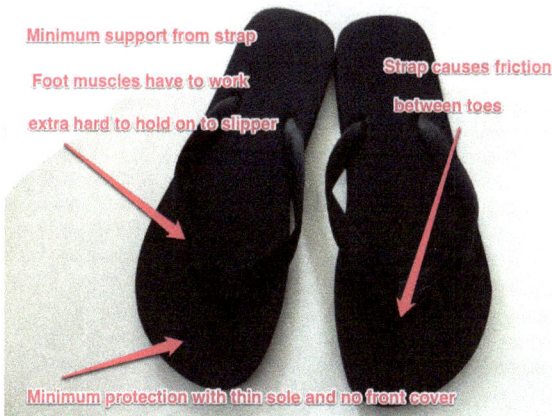

Minimum support from strap

Foot muscles have to work
extra hard to hold on to slipper

Strap causes friction
between toes

Minimum protection with thin sole and no front cover

Figure 5. Flip flops

- **Shoes with tight toe boxes (Fig. 6):** Such shoes cause overcrowding of toes and lead to skin breakdown between toes or over bony prominences.
- **Slip on shoes (Fig. 7):** These increases excessive movement inside shoes and cause friction.
- **Thin sole shoes:** These lack shock absorption and high impact goes through foot structures leading to repetitive trauma, fracture or skin breakdown.

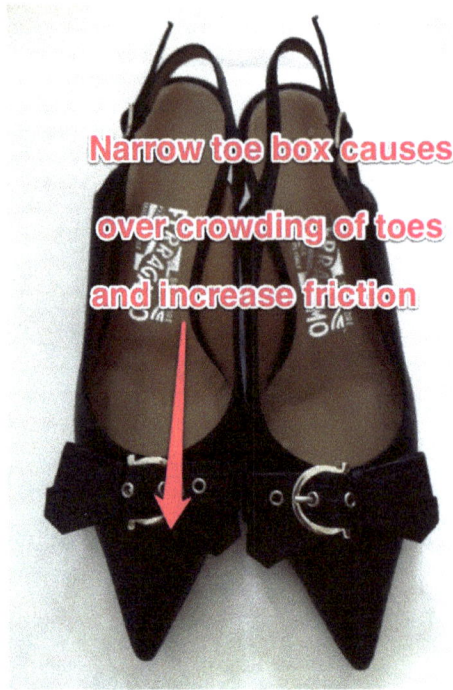

Figure 6. Shoes with tight toe box

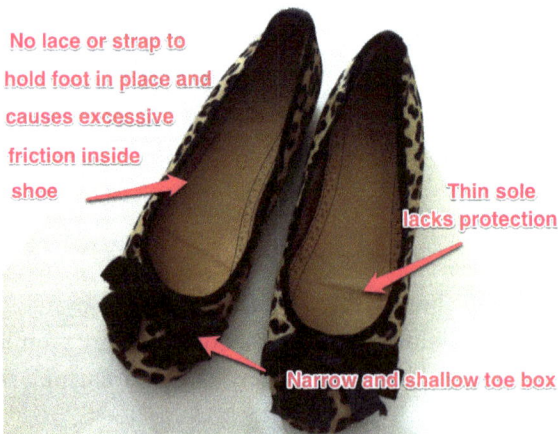

Figure 7. Slip-on shoes

Sharp nails or objects can pierce through a thin sole and cause injury without the patient knowing due to the presence of a neuropathy.

- **Oversized shoes:** Excessive movement inside shoes can cause more friction. It is harder for the foot to have a firm grip on the footwear. This may therefore cause muscle overuse injury.

7. Things to do before putting on shoes

- **Cotton socks should be worn:** This will help absorb excess moisture and prevent excess friction. Socks should be changed regularly to maintain good hygiene.
- **Check the shoes for excessive wear and tear inside and outside:** If the shoes are very old and worn out, replace them with new ones
- **Check inside the shoes for foreign bodies and shake them out before putting shoes on each time.**

8. Buying new shoes

- **Buy shoes in late afternoon:** Normal feet swell when people have been on their feet a lot.[4]
- **Avoid wearing a new pair of shoes for too long:** Check every hour for signs of blister, abrasion and redness.
- **Have at least 2 pairs of shoes:** Wear them alternatively so that there is always a pair of wearable shoes.

9. Special footwear

Some patients with diabetes have feet that cannot be accommodated in normal recommended footwear. Some patients require bulky dressing for treatment of an ulcer and are unable to fit into normal shoes. These patients require special footwear. There are a few different types of such footwear available.

Ready-made diabetic shoe with soft lining (Fig. 8)

Such shoes are usually very wide, and have a soft and seamless inside-lining. It is wide enough to accommodate a diabetic insole, if necessary.

Temporary surgical sandal and boot (Figs. 9 and 10)

These shoes come with adjustable velcro straps to hold the ankle and forefoot. They can accommodate heavy dressings. The attached insole can be modified

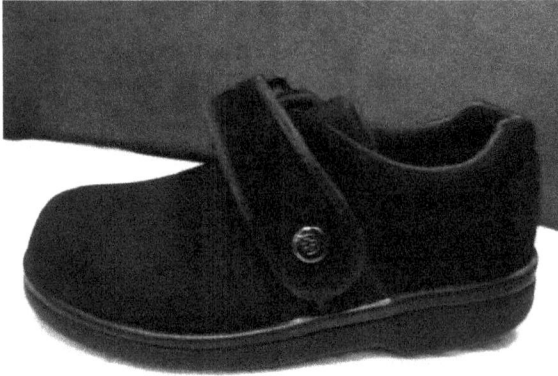

Figure 8. Ready-made diabetic shoe with soft lining

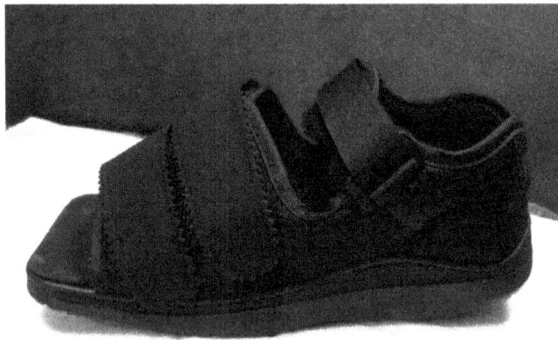

Figure 9. Temporary surgical sandal

to make an offloading insole by the podiatrist or orthotist.[5] The inner-lining of the shoes is soft and smooth. These shoes are therefore suitable for diabetic patients.

Forefoot wedge offloading shoe (Fig. 11)

This is special footwear to offload forefoot area when walking. It is useful when the patients have ulcers on forefoot areas. It should only be worn on one foot.

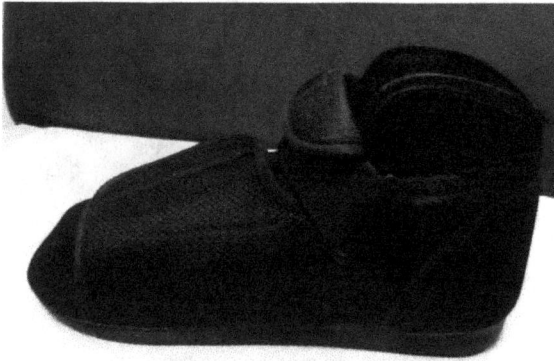

Figure 10. Temporary surgical boot

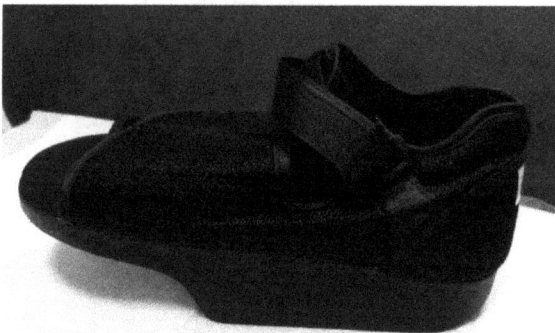

Figure 11. Forefoot wedge offloading shoe

Heel wedge shoe (Fig. 12)

This is another type of special footwear to offload the heel. It is useful for treatment of a heel ulcer. This should also be worn only on one side.

Pneumatic walker (Fig. 13)

This device is a removable cast boot with a flat bed insole that can be replaced with a customized insole. This device will immobilize foot movement and provide instant offloading.[6]

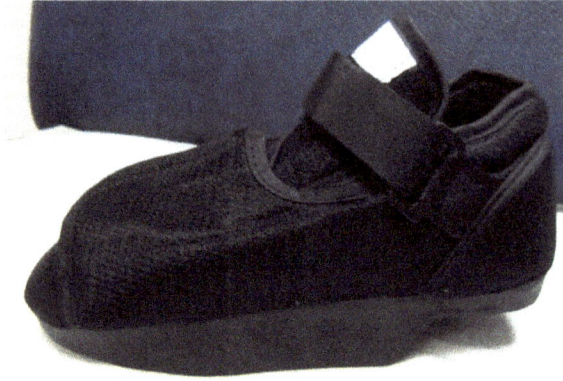

Figure 12.   Heel wedge shoe

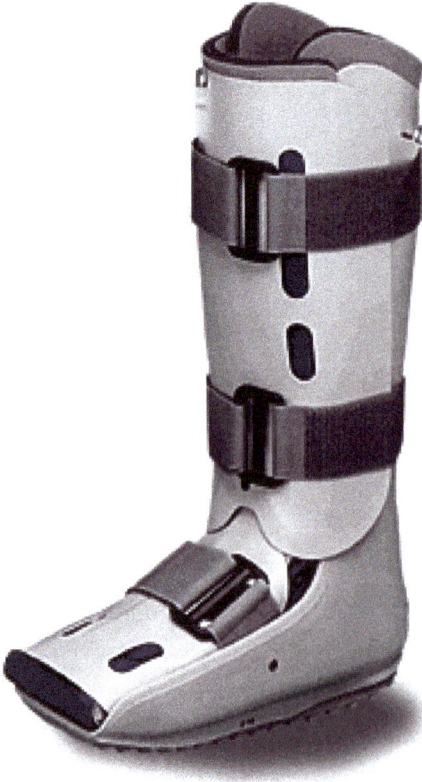

Figure 13.   Pneumatic walker

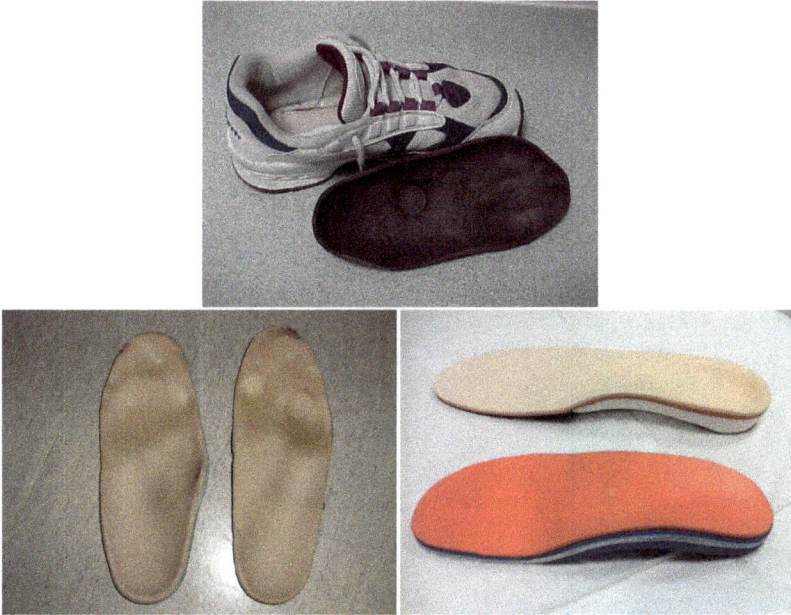

Figure 14. Therapeutic insoles

Therapeutic insole (Fig. 14)

Insoles accommodate pressure areas and redistribute areas of high pressure. They are usually worn inside shoes. However, it is also possible to wear them inside a surgical sandal/boot or a pneumatic walker to achieve ultimate wound healing.

10. Education and advice

After an assessment of the individual's shoe and habits, education must be provided if the footwear is inadequate.

Patients should be informed of:

- Reason why they have to change their footwear habits
- The styles and design parameters that are required
- Proper fitting of shoes
- Examples of shoes they could wear

Visual aids, sample of shoes or brochures will greatly help the patient to understand their exact needs and improve their compliance to wearing footwear.

References

1. J. Apelqvist, *et al.*, Practical guidelines on the management and prevention of diabetic foot, *Diabetes Metab. Res. Rev.* **24**(Suppl 1):S181–7 (2008).
2. D. J. Macfarlane, Factors in diabetic footwear compliance, *J. Am. Podiatr. Med. Assoc.* **93**:485–91 (2003).
3. M. J. Mueller, Therapeutic footwear helps protect the diabetic foot, *J. Am. Podiatr. Med. Assoc.* **87**:360–4 (1997).
4. M. E. Edmonds, *et al.*, *Diabetic Foot Care. Stage 1: The Normal Foot* (Blackwell Publishing, 2004), pp. 17–34.
5. M. E. Edmonds, *et al.*, *Diabetic Foot Care. Stage 2: The High-Risk Foot* (Blackwell Publishing, 2004), pp. 35–61.
6. M. E. Edmonds, *et al.*, *Diabetic Foot Care. Stage 3: The Ulcerated Foot* (Blackwell Publishing, 2004), pp. 62–101.

35

Footwear for Diabetic Foot

Harikrishna K. R. Nair

Head and Wound Care Consultant
Diabetic Foot Clinic
Kuala Lumpur Hospital, Malaysia

1. Introduction

The incidence of diabetes mellitus is rising in alarming proportions throughout the world but more so in the Asian population where obesity and other factors are becoming prevalent. Studies have shown that 25% of diabetics will develop foot complications. In addition, 85% of these amputations could be prevented.

Diabetic footcare is important for prevention of a below knee amputation (Fig. 1). It is an important part of Lower Extremities Amputation Prevention (LEAP).

There are 5 Ps of Prevention as shown below:

- Podiatric care
- Proper fitting shoes
- Pressure reduction
- Prophylactic surgery
- Preventive education

2. Socks

Why do diabetic patients need to wear socks?

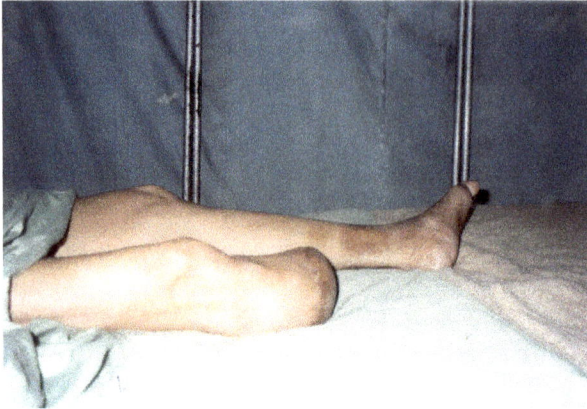

Figure 1. Below Knee Amputation

Socks add an additional layer of protection to the feet (Fig. 2a) and

- Reduce the risk of developing a blister
- Reduce the development of fungal infection
- Socks with extra padding reduce pressure to the soles of the foot

General tips:

- Do avoid tight socks that might affect your feet circulation
- Do change socks daily
- Do ensure the socks are clean (Fig. 2b)
- Do ensure that the socks fit properly (Fig. 2b)
- Do use cotton or wool socks that allow your feet to 'breathe'
- Do use socks without elastic tops (Fig. 2c) for those with reduced blood supply (Fig. 2d)

3. Footwear

Practical guidelines (the Do's in footwear selection):

- **Do** wear professionally fitted shoes (Fig. 3a) (length should be one thumb's width beyond the longest toe)
- **Do** wear comfortable shoes
- **Do** wear correct foot gear for the occasion

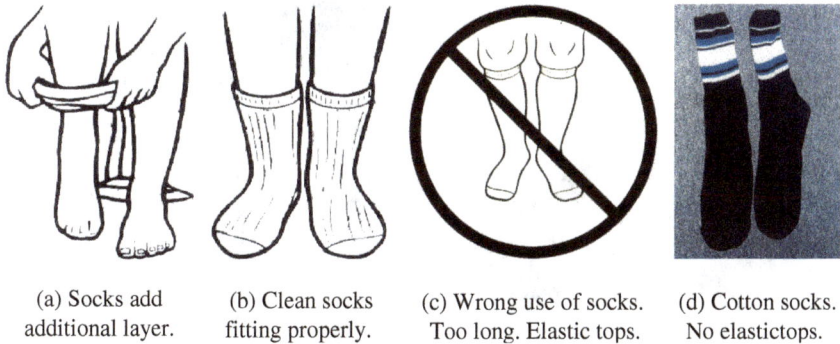

| (a) Socks add additional layer. | (b) Clean socks fitting properly. | (c) Wrong use of socks. Too long. Elastic tops. | (d) Cotton socks. No elastictops. |

Figure 2. Wearing socks

- **Do** wear shoes with a firm heel counter
- **Do** wear shoes with a heel height no greater than 2.5 cm because a broad heel gives greater stability
- **Do** wear closed shoes for protection. Sport shoes are ideal. However sandals are acceptable
- **Do** wear shoes with a broad rounded toe box (wide enough to accommodate the toe)
- **Do** wear shoes with a cushioning sole. Soles should be reasonably firm throughout and flex across the ball of the foot, rubber composition or EVA provides shock absorption)
- **Do** wear shoes with adjustable straps (laces, buckles or Velcro) for better ankle support and prevent foot fatigue. This well prevent the foot from sliding (Fig. 4)
- **Do** wear shoes from soft leather (especially the upper layer and the lining)
- **Do** wear shoes with no cutting/sharp edges at the inner lining of the shoes

Practical footwear guidelines — general hints:

- **Do** check inside the shoe for foreign objects, seams or torn linings before you put on the shoes (Fig. 5).
- **Do** try on new shoes gradually, i.e. 1 hour on the first day, 2 hours on the second day and so on until they are comfortable
- **Do** alternate between 2 pairs of shoes
- **Do** clean and wash the shoes regularly

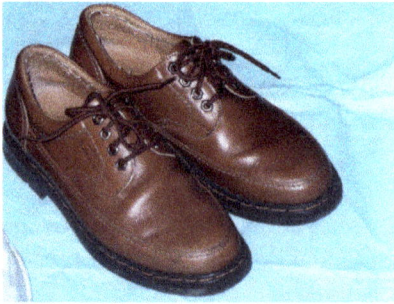

(a) Proper fitting shoes. Firm heel counter. Heel height <2.5cm. Rounded toe box.

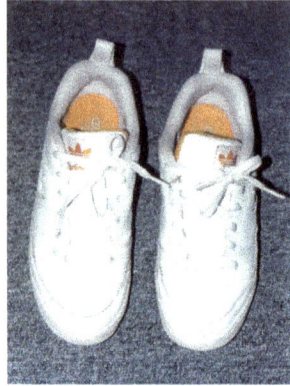

(b) Sports shoes – ideal.

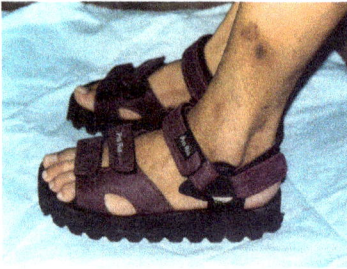

(c) Acceptable sandals with adjustable straps (Velcro) for better ankle support.

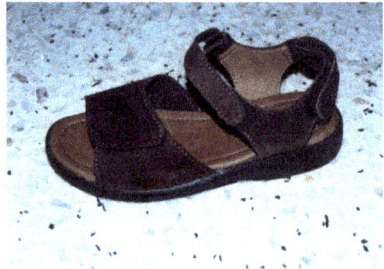

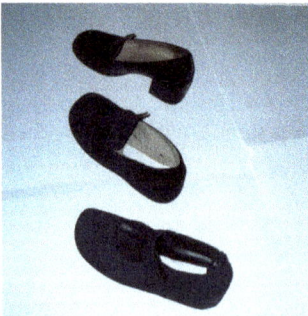

(d) Acceptable shoes.

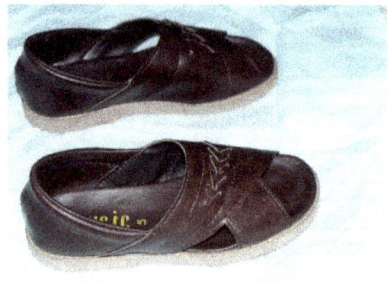

(e) Acceptable shoes with open toebox.

Figure 3. Proper footwear

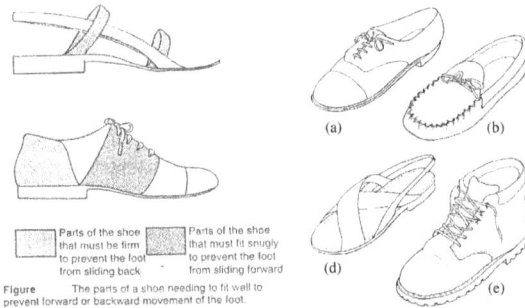

Figure | The parts of a shoe needing to fit well to prevent forward or backward movement of the foot.

Figure 4. Check inside the shoes

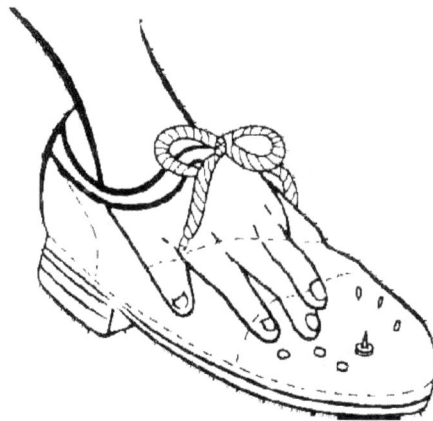

Figure 5. Proper fitting shoes to prevent sliding

- **Do** buy shoes in the afternoon as feet generally tend to swell towards the end of the day
- **Do** buy the shoes that fit the larger foot as often one foot is larger than the other
- **Don't** wear shoes that are too tight or too loose
- **Don't** wear shoes which needs to be stretched to provide a good fit
- **Don't** wear slippers or flip-flops (Fig. 6a)
- **Don't** wear shoes with pointy toes (Fig. 6b)
- **Don't** wear shoes with high heels (no stiletto or short, pointed heels) (Fig. 6c)
- **Don't** sacrifice comfort and protection for the sake of fashion

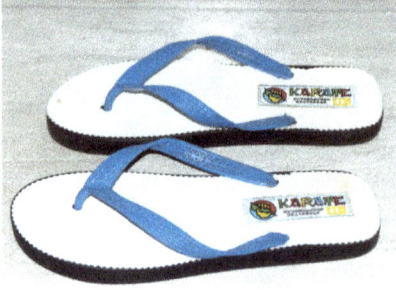

(a) Japanese slippers.

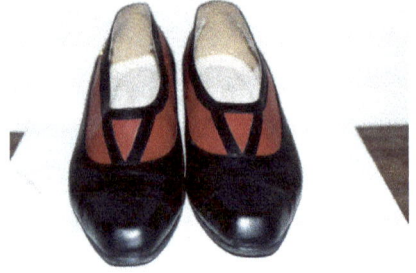

(b) Pointed shoes.

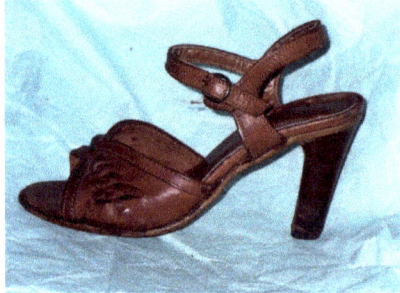

(c) Stilleto heels.

Figure 6.   Improper footwear

4. Conclusion

It is critical to wear proper diabetic footcare and footwear including customized insole and footwear for offloading the feet. This will prevent the formation of ulcers. It will also provide comfort to diabetics who tend to have neuropathic feet. Diabetic patients need to be counselled and given good footcare education. They must be taught how to look after their feet carefully including the proper usage of socks, the use of proper orthosis or insoles and good customized footwear to prevent the development of diabetic foot complications. The key to the management of diabetic foot is prevention — avoid the development of a diabetic foot complication. In this way, major amputation can be avoided.

36

Doing Your Own Dressings

Yuen Fun Alexis Lai* and Aziz Nather†

* Podiatrist
Department of Rehabilitation Medicine
National University Hospital
† Department of Orthopaedic Surgery
Yong Loo Lin School of Medicine
National University of Singapore

Introduction

In Singapore, upon discharge from the hospital ward, the daily dressings required are done by:

- Outpatient government polyclinics (majority)
- Patients' own general practitioner or family doctor (minority)
- Patients' own relative who is a staff nurse or assistant nurse (preferred choice, if available)
- Patients' own relative or domestic helper (maid)
- Patient himself (when there is no caregiver)

Wound Dressing in Government Polyclinics

There are problems encountered by patients sent to government polyclinics for regular wound dressings. Sometimes, nurses in polyclinics decide on their own choice of dressings. These could be dressings that the nurses usually apply. They may change the frequency of dressing to 3 or 2 times a week as they see fit, even though daily wound dressings are required and instructed. Also, one must not forget the inconvenience of bringing an elderly patient down to the polyclinics for such regular dressings. Bringing an elderly patient down by a car or taxi is costly and time-consuming.

Our Patients' Profile

Nather *et al.*[1] showed that the majority of patients with diabetic foot ulcers belong to the lower socio-economic group:

- Malays
- Education level of up to secondary school only
- Low average monthly household income of less than SGD2000

Many of our patients could not afford the costs to go to the polyclinics regularly for wound dressings.

Doing Your Own Dressings

Nather encourages his patients to do their own dressings. Having a caregiver to help patients do their own dressings at home offers the following advantages:

- Caregiver (maid or relative) can be trained in the ward 1 to 2 days before the patient's discharge by the ward nurses to be proficient in doing the dressing. This is better and more reliable than a dressing done by a nurse in a polyclinic who has never seen the wound before.
- Caregiver is committed. In contrast, in the polyclinic, the daily dressings may not be done by the same nurse on each visit. The nurse will not show the same level of commitment as the caregiver.
- Caregiver who sees the wound daily can monitor the progress of the wound better than the nurse in the polyclinic who sees the wound on an irregular basis.
- Another benefit is that the caregiver can be trained to do the dressings in the correct way as instructed, and will follow the wound dressing as prescribed.
- Caregiver can do the dressings more frequently without the added inconvenience and costs of frequent visits to the polyclinics.

What Patients Need for Doing Their Own Dressings

3 things are required:

1. Buy a simple basic dressing kit
2. Choose and buy the cleansing solution for cleaning the wound
3. Choose and buy the wound dressing selected for the wound

Dressing Set for Doing Their Own Dressings

The patient must purchase a single basic dressing set. It must contain the following items:

- Normal saline 0.9% vial x 1
- Dressing set (Figs. 1 and 2) comprises of:
  — Plastic drape
  — Paper towels
  — Waste bag
  — Cotton balls
  — Gauze
  — Forceps x 3
- Specific dressings as instructed by clinician (e.g. foam, alginate, Iodosorb powder)

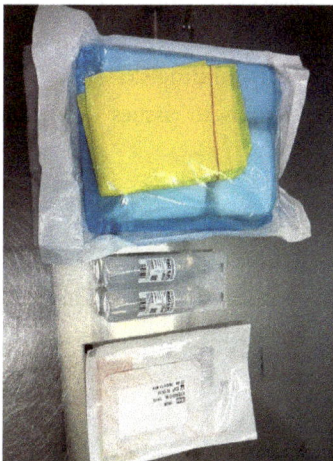

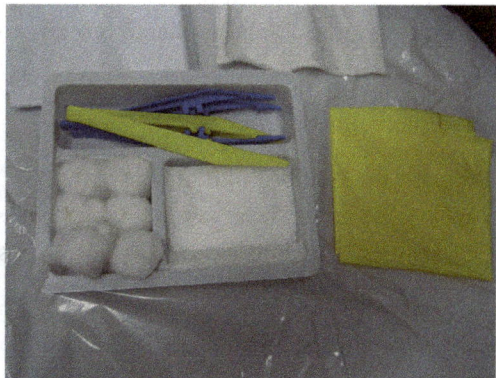

Figures 1 and 2. Dressing set and its items

Cleansing Solutions

The objectives of cleansing a wound include:

- To provide a moist environment through rehydration to the wound bed
- To remove foreign bodies from the wound
- To remove dressings that adhere to the wound
- To provide patient comfort

Cleansing solutions reduce the flora and bacterial contaminants in a wound.[2] Cleansing solutions used include normal saline, antiseptics, hypochlorite or tap water.[3]

Characteristics of a good cleansing solution are:

- It is non-toxic to wound tissue
- It is able to reduce microbacterial load
- It remains effective upon contact with the wound bed
- It is cost effective
- It is easily available
- It has a long shelf life[4]

Currently, normal saline solution is the preferred cleansing solution as compared to antiseptics and hypochlorite. Current studies suggest that antiseptic solutions have a shorter contact time with the wound surface. Hence they are not effective in removing infection.[3] They also cause detrimental effects on the cells in the wound and inactivate organic material in the wound. They also cause irritation to wound tissue and the surrounding skin.

Hypochlorite has been phased out due to its toxicity to tissues and mild wound cleaning properties.[2]

- Normal saline solution

Normal saline 0.9% solution is commonly used in the NUH wards as a cleansing solution. It is safe to use on most wounds as it is isotonic. It comes in vials or bottles. It can be purchased from the pharmacy and is inexpensive.

- Chlorhexidine/iodine/alcohol/hydrogen peroxide

These are commonly used as cleansing solutions for infected wounds. They reduce the growth and development of microorganisms in wounds. However, the use of antiseptic solutions impairs cell migration and blood circulation in the wound. They should be used less often as it can be toxic to the wound.

- Tap water

Tap water is an alternative solution for wound cleansing. However, there are concerns that tap water can increase the risk of infection. In addition, it is also not isotonic. In fact, it is a hypotonic solution.[4]

Wound Dressings

The functions of a good dressing include the following:

- Control microbial load
- Thermal insulation of wound
- Mechanical protection
- Conform to structure/size of wound
- Absorb exudate from wound
- Reduce the risk of infection

Choosing the appropriate wound dressing

The type of dressing to be chosen depends on the type of wound:

- Infected wound
- Ischaemic wound
- Infected and Ischaemic wound

Firstly, the wound must be assessed to accurately decide the type of wound being dealt with. The dressing used for an infected wound is different from that used for an ischaemic wound. It varies according to the phase of wound healing — acute phase versus chronic phase. In acute phase, with an exudative wound, an absorbent dressing must be used.[5]

Current dressings promote moist wound environment and rehydrate the wound. Interactive dressings promote migration of cells to enhance wound healing whereas passive dressings function to protect the wound.[6]

Types of Wound Dressings

Wound dressings can be classified into two groups:

(i) Passive Dressings:

Passive dressings include gauze, lint and non-stick dressings.

It is often used for superficial wounds or for wounds that are nearly completely healed.

(ii) Interactive Dressings:

Interactive dressings include film, hydrocolloid, alginate, hyrdoactive, foam and hydrogel dressings.

It reacts with the wound surface and environment to aid wound healing.

Wound Field Preparation

Before doing the dressing, the patient or caregiver must also decide on the type of wound field preparation that she intends to use.

There are 3 types of wound field preparation (Table 1):

- Sterile
- Aseptic
- Clean

The individuals or caregiver must be proficient in the use of aseptic principles to reduce the risk of infection. Sterile dressings and solutions must be used.[3]

Table 1. Types of wound field preparation

Sterile	Aseptic	Clean
• Eliminate microorganisms	• Minimise contamination by pathogens	• All fields are free of dirt and soiling
• Use of sterile gloves	• Reduce infection	• Clean dressing supplies
• Sterile fields and dressings	• Sterile gloves and gowns are not required	• Use of gloves
• Single usage of sterile solutions	• Dressing packs	
	• Hand washing before and after dressings	

It is difficult for the caregiver to achieve a sterile wound field preparation. However, at least an aseptic wound field preparation should be employed. For this purpose, sterile dressings and solutions must be used.[3]

Procedure for Doing Own Dressing

- Take a shower before changing your dressing. Do remember to use a plastic bag to cover the area with the wound so as to prevent water from seeping into your dressing
- If your wound feels painful, take your prescribed pain medication 30 minutes before the dressing change.
- Prepare all items required before opening the wound to reduce cross contamination through the touching of other objects.
- Wash your hands with soap and water, and dry your hands with a towel.
- Take off the dressing gently and discard in a plastic bag for disposal.
- Wash your hands after taking off the dressing.
- Open the dressing set (Fig. 3).
- Wear a pair of gloves.
- Open the container of the normal saline for its use (Fig. 4).
- When using chlorhexidine, clean the edge of the packet with alcohol wipe.
- Clean the wound as instructed by your health care professional (Figs. 5 to 8).

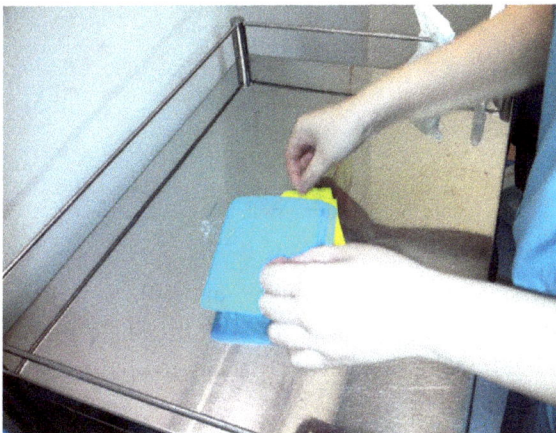

Figure 3. Opening the dressing set

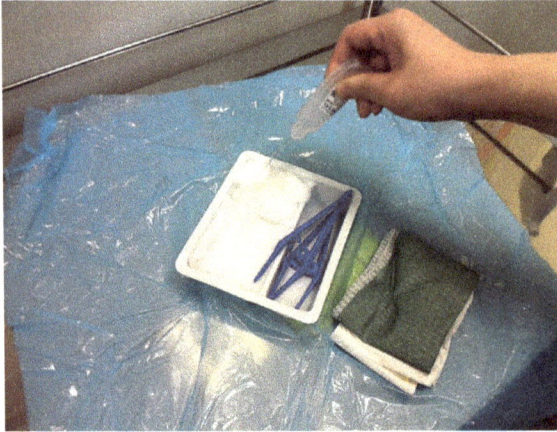

Figure 4.   Use of normal saline

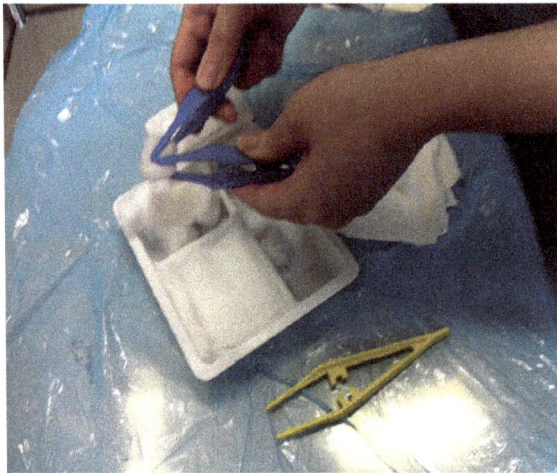

Figure 5.   Preparing swab of normal saline

- Apply the dressing to the wound (Figs. 9 and 10).
- Tape your dressing so that it will not fall off using a primapore dressing (Figs. 11 and 12). Do not wrap your dressing too tightly as it can cause the wound to deteriorate.
- Keep the dressing clean and dry until the next dressing change.
- If the wound exudates heavily, change the dressings more frequently.

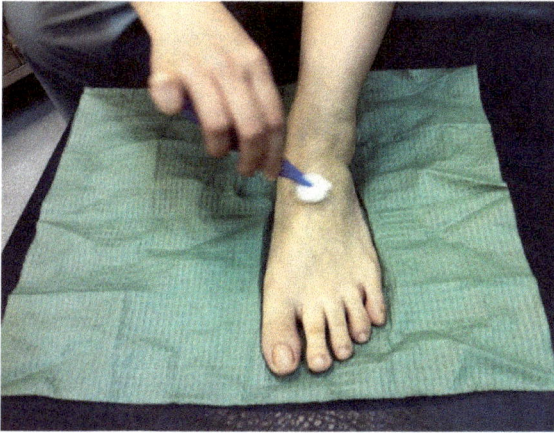

Figure 6. Cleaning with swab of normal saline

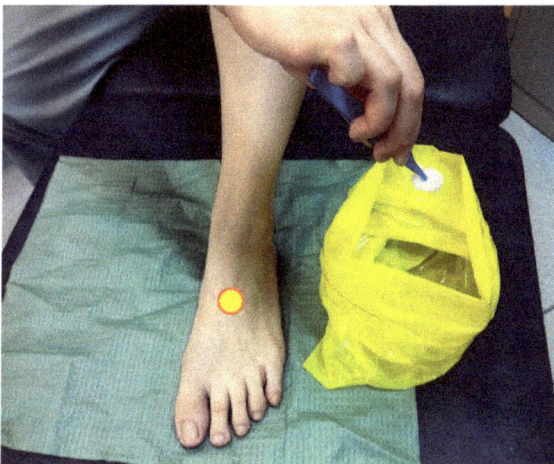

Figure 7. Discarding swab after use into biohazard bag

During daily wound care, look out for these indicators to identify wound infection:

- Fever
- The wound is painful and tender to touch
- Redness

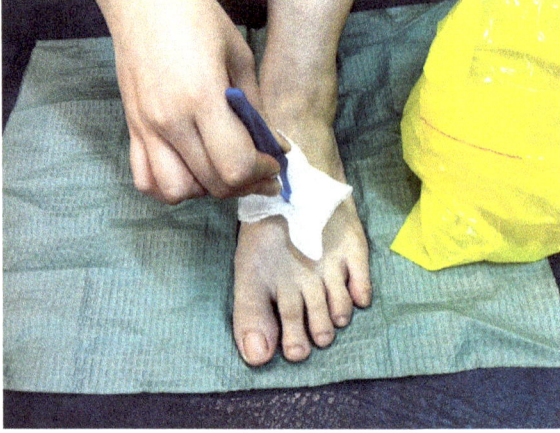

Figure 8. Drying the wound

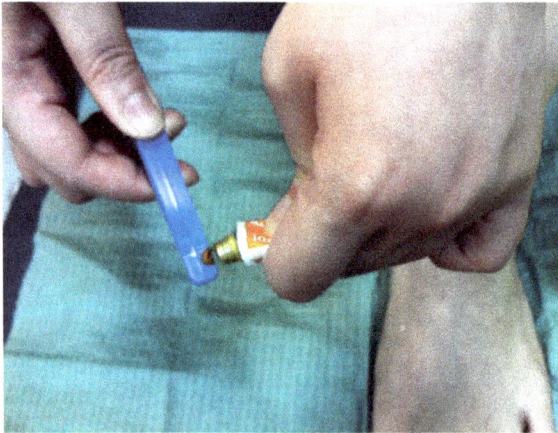

Figure 9. Squeezing dressing ointment onto spatula

- Wound exudation with pus (green or yellow discharge)
- Swelling
- Odour
- The wound bed has black or yellow tissue that was not previously there

If you experience any of the above, it is important to seek early treatment with your physician.

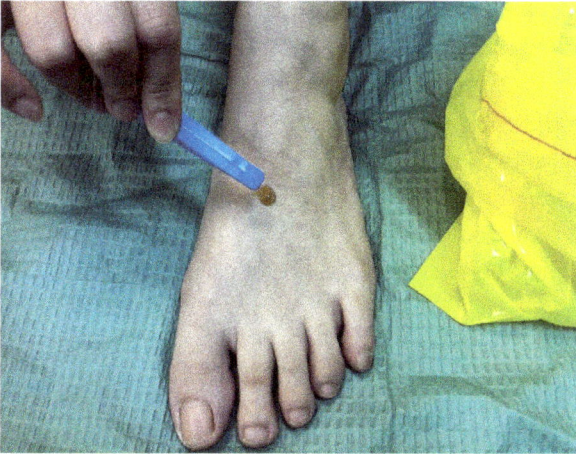

Figure 10.   Applying the dressing onto wound

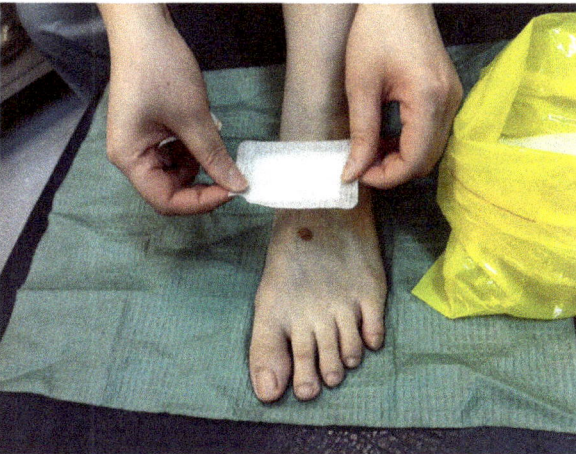

Figure 11.   Using a primapore dressing to cover wound

Dressing Different Types of Wounds

Patients should note that different types of wounds require different types of wound cleansing and dressing. Caregivers must be taught on how to dress the patients' wound in the appropriate way required.

Performing Cleansing for Different Types of Wounds:

1. *For shallow wounds (Fig. 13)*
   — Clean the centre of the wound in a circular fashion
   — Slowly work to the edges of the wound
   — Do not return to the same wound area after cleaning to minimise wound contamination
   — Dress the wound as recommended by clinicians

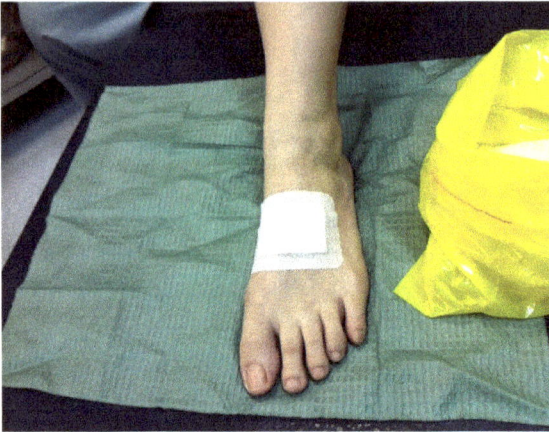

Figure 12.   The completed dressing

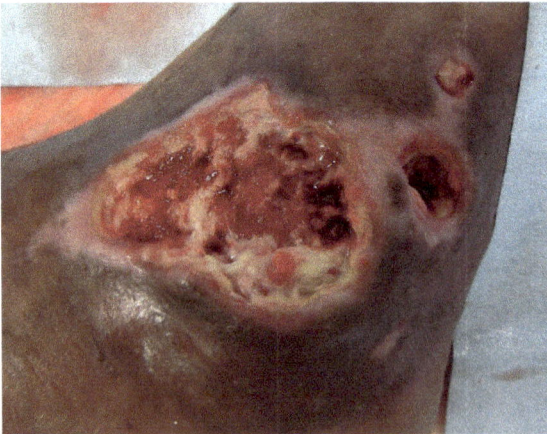

Figure 13.   Shallow wound

2. *For wounds with infection or inflammation (Fig. 14)*

   — Gently clean the wound
   — Reduce trauma to the wound by gently removing dressing without damaging viable tissue
   — Dress the wound as recommended by clinicians

3. *For a healthy granulating and epithelising wound (Fig. 15)*

   — Clean the wound gently to prevent further trauma to the wound surface
   — Avoid using an antiseptic solution on a healthy granulating wound as its toxicity can hinder healing
   — Wound dressing used must be non-adherent to minimise injury

4. *For an undermined wound*

   — Avoid irrigating normal saline into the wound as the wound could be deep
   — Fill the syringe with normal saline and use a basin to collect the fluid
   — Flush the wound using a syringe. Ensure that the tip of the syringe does not come into contact with the wound
   — Massage the wound gently to drain out the remaining fluid
   — Repeat two to three times

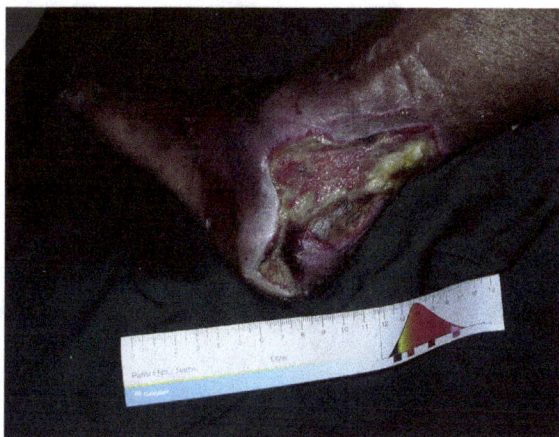

Figure 14. Infected wound showing swelling and inflammation

5. *For a necrotic wound with poor healing (Fig. 16)*

  — For a necrotic wound, use septanol to minimize infection and to keep the wound as dry as possible to prevent wet gangrene
  — The main aim should be to allow necrotic tissue to desiccate. Autolytic debridement should not happen

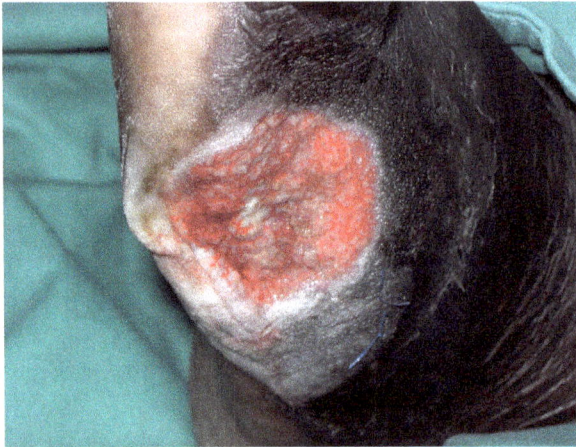

Figure 15.   Healthy, granulating wound

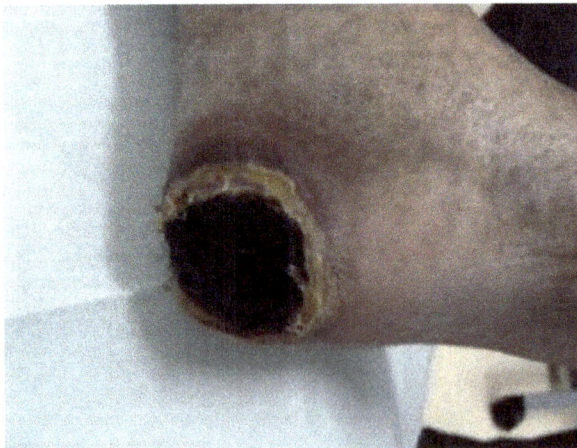

Figure 16.   Necrotic wound

— Leave the wound exposed to air if it is not exudative. If not, use a loose non-woven gauze to cover the wound. Ensure that the gauze is not occlusive or adherent to the necrotic tissue
— Dressing should not be too tight as it will affect the blood circulation to wound

Conclusion

The appropriate application of wound dressings plays an important role in reducing infections. Patients can be educated by their healthcare provider on how to apply their own dressings.

References

1. A. Nather, S. B. Chionh, K. L. Wong, S. Q. O. Koh, Y. H. Chan, X. Y. Li and A. Nambiar, Socioeconomic profile of diabetic patients with and without foot problems, *Diabet. Foot Ankle* 1:5523 (2010).
2. R. G. Smith, A critical discussion of the use of antiseptics in acute traumatic wounds, *J. Am. Podiatr. Med. Assoc.* **95**(2):148–53 (2005).
3. L. Parker, Applying the principles of infections control to wound care, *Br. J. Nurs.* **9**(7):394–400 (2000).
4. M. Flanagan, Wound cleansing. In: M. Morison, C. Moffat, J. Bridel-Nixon and S. Bale (eds.), *Nursing Management of Chronic Wounds* (Mosby, London, 1997), Chap. 5.
5. K. F. Cutting, Addressing the challenge of wound cleansing in the modern era, *Br. J. Nurs.* **19**(11):S24–9 (2010).
6. K. Ballard and H. Baxter, Developments in wound care for difficult to manage wounds, *Br. J. Nurs.* **9**(7):405–12 (2000).

37

Rehabilitating Your Below Knee Amputation

Lim Kean Seng Andrew and Aziz Nather

Department of Orthopaedic Surgery
Yong Loo Lin School of Medicine
National University of Singapore

This chapter covers the very important aspect of rehabilitation following Lower Limb Amputation (below knee amputation: commonest major amputation performed). The objectives include pain control, wound care and control, contracture prevention and joint range of motion, physical conditioning and psychological support and education. The NUH Rehab Programme for the Below Knee Amputee is described in detail. An important part of rehab includes discharge planning and ultimately preparation of the stump for fitting of prosthesis.

Introduction

The loss of a limb can result in major disability and psychological trauma to the affected individual. An integrated comprehensive approach by an interdisciplinary team following limb amputation is paramount for successful surgical and functional outcome.

Two main goals of the management of limbs in the post-amputation, pre-prosthetic stage are obtaining maximal functional independence and optimizing the residual limb for prosthesis fitting.[1] The rehabilitation of the below knee amputee is described in detail to illustrate the various important principles involved in the rehabilitation of all major lower limb amputations.

Areas of focus would include the following:

— Pain control
— Wound care and oedema control
— Contracture prevention and joint range of motion
— Physical conditioning
— Psychological support and education

Pain Control

Pain can be from various sources. It is important to distinguish phantom pain from that of the surgical wound. Phantom pain is characterised as intermittent burning, stabbing or shooting pain perceived in the amputated part of the limb which occurs at rest and not necessarily with manipulation of the stump. This usually subsides with time, generally within 6 months, however 10% of patients will experience chronic intractable phantom pain.[2] Pharmacological agents used for phantom pain are similar to those for neuropathic pain. These include amitriptyline, carbamazepine and gabapentin.[3]

Wound Care and Oedema Control

Soft tissue swelling of the residual limb delays wound healing and causes pain. For a start, a soft dressing with an over the top elastic bandage wrapped in a figure-of-eight technique (Fig. 1), compressive Tubigrip stockinet or elastic shrinker is used. This is easily applied and allows for frequent wound inspection.

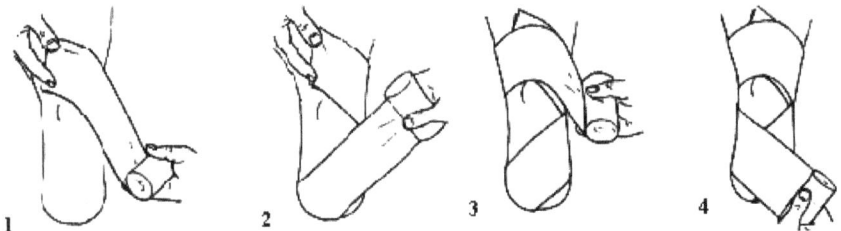

Figure 1. Bandaging technique for below-knee amputation

Contracture Prevention and Joint Range of Motion

As a result of the alteration of muscular balance and contraction of the wound after surgery, knee flexion contracture in transtibial amputees and hip contracture in a flexed, abducted and externally rotated position in transfemoral amputees occur.

A contracted joint affects the alignment of the limb when a prosthesis is applied and affects efficient ambulation. A knee flexion of more than 25 degrees and a hip abduction and flexion of more than 15 degrees in a below-knee amputee and above-knee amputee respectively will result in sub-optimal prosthesis use.[4]

Prevention of contractures include keeping the knee in an extended position at all times and the patient should sit with an extension board under the knee. The use of a pillow beneath the knee must be avoided.

A daily schedule for range of motion and stretching exercises with counteracting muscle group strengthening exercises help prevent joint contracture (refer to NUH Rehabilitation Programme).

Physical Conditioning

Amputees need to learn new techniques of bed mobility and transfers to adapt to the change in their body mechanics. A pivot manoeuvre or use of a transfer board allows easy transfer from a bed to a chair. Detachable armrests on wheelchairs are recommended to accommodate these transfer skills.

Ambulation using walking frames for short distances is a targeted goal upon discharge. The training of balance using parallel bars is commenced in the early post-operative period (refer to NUH Rehabilitation Programme). The use of proper footwear and care for the contralateral limb must be emphasized. Patients with a cardiac disease history may require close monitoring during therapy sessions.

Psychological Support and Education

The prevalence of clinical depression and adjustment disorders is high in the early post-operative phase. Counselling is essential to reduce a patient's anxiety level and is more effective if practised at the pre-operative stage. This should include discussion of the necessity for amputation, rehabilitation process, estimated time of prosthesis fitting and training with advice on projected functional outcome. Education on stump care and good glycaemic control is essential. Caregiver training may be required to assist with home management.

1. Start with bandage held in place on inside of thigh just above knee and unroll bandage such that laid diagonally down outer side of stump while maintaining about two-thirds of maximum stretch in bandage.
2. Bring bandage over inner end of stump and diagonally up outer side of stump.
3. Bring bandage under back of knee, continue over upper part of kneecap and down under back of knee.
4. Bring bandage diagonally down back of stump and around over end of stump. Continue up back of stump to starting point on inside of thigh and repeat sequence in a manner such that entire stump is covered when roll used up. It is important that tightest part of bandage be at end of stump.

(adapted from Malaysian Information Network on Disabilities)

NUH Rehabilitation Programme for the Below Knee Amputee

Day 1:

— Chest physiotherapy
— Straight leg raising (Fig. 2)
— Hip abduction
— Isoquads (isometric/static quadriceps exercises) (Fig. 3)
— Calf pumping (isometric gastrocnemius exercises)

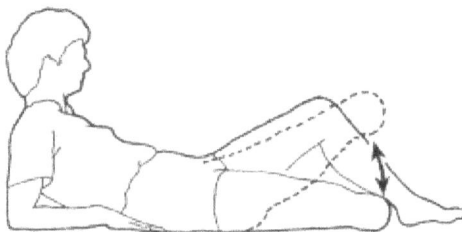

Figure 2.   Straight leg raising

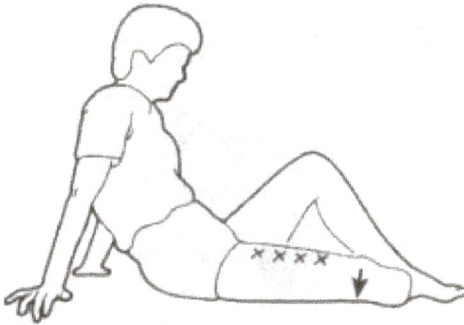

Figure 3. Isoquads

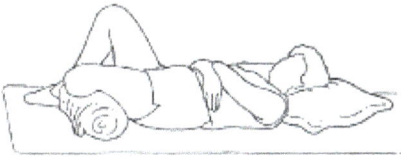

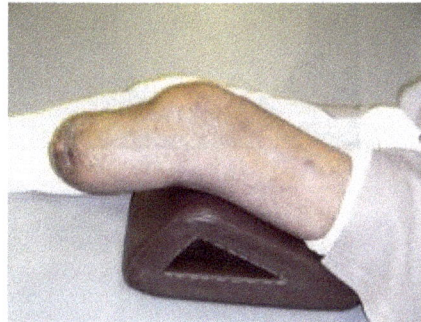

Figure 4. Stump exercises

Day 2:

— Thermoplastic splint fitting by occupational therapist
— Inner range quadriceps or stump exercises (0-30 degree knee flexion with roll of towel/support under thigh) (Fig. 4)
— Standing with walking frame
— Walking/balancing with walking frame

Day 3:

— Balancing across parallel bars at physiotherapy department orthopaedic gym
— Surgical drain removed and outer dressings lightened

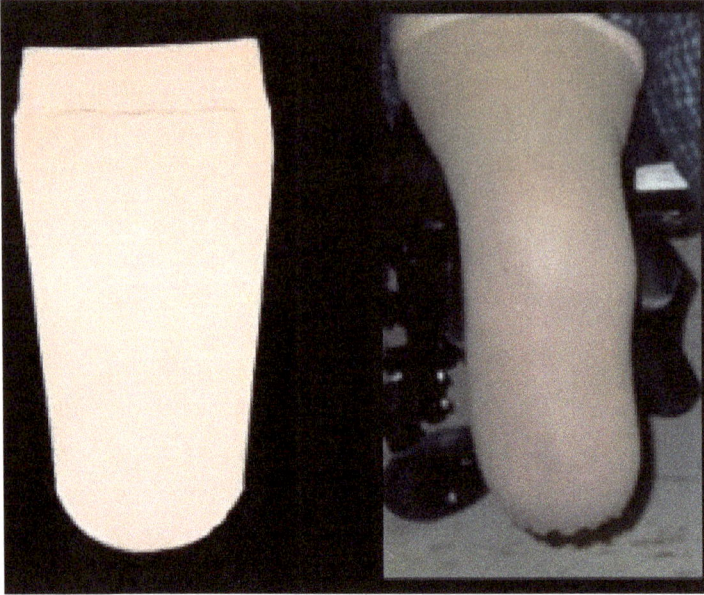

Figure 5.   Below knee elastic stump shrinker

Day 5:

— Wound inspection (done earlier if dressing becomes soaked, foul odour is smelt or if patient develops a fever)
— Primapore dressing
— Figure of 8 technique stump bandaging three times a day
— Tubigrip compressive stockinet or elastic shrinker (Fig. 5) may be applied for wound oedema
— Caregiver training on stump bandaging using 6 inches crepe bandage (on discharge patient must be prescribed 2 rolls of 6 inches crepe bandage)

Criteria for discharge home (target 1 week post-operative):

— Able to walk/balance with walking frame (Fig. 6)
— Able to achieve stump control
— Caregiver proficiency with stump bandaging

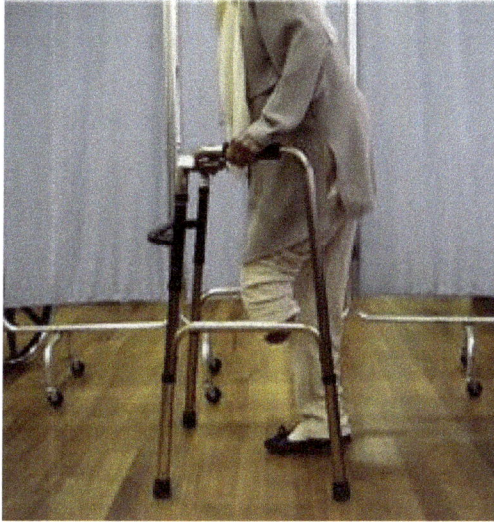

Figure 6. Walking frame ambulation

Plan for Discharge

— Planning must begin on day patient was admitted for the diabetic foot problem by Case-Manager and Nursing Officer in charge of ward
— Care-giver training must be provided from the first post-op day
— Lack of planning leads to unnecessary prolonged length of stay and increased hospitalisation cost

Follow-Up Clinic Appointments Required:

— Orthopaedic Clinic: Wound inspection and removal of sutures at 14th post-operative day or later (diabetics may take a longer time to heal — as long as 3 weeks or more)
— Diabetic Clinic: Diabetic control by endocrinologist, education on diabetes by nurse
— Podiatry: Education on footcare for other leg and advice on footwear +/− Cardiology, Renal, Ophthalmology Clinic

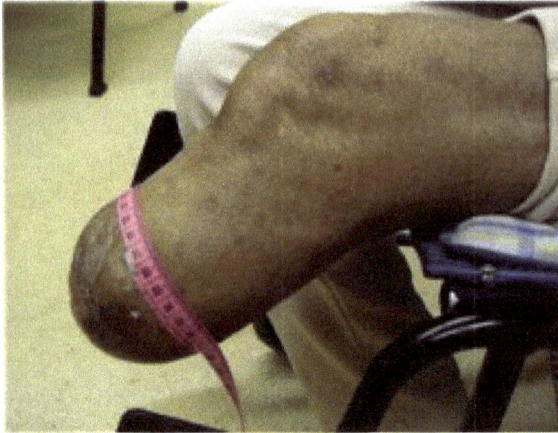

Figure 7.   Stump girth measurement

Preparation of Stump for Fitting of Prosthesis:

— Monthly serial measurement of stump girth during follow-up (Fig. 7)
— Maximal stump shrinkage usually achieved after about 3 to 4 months
— Prosthesis fitting at Artificial Limb Centre (In Singapore, there is a centralised prosthesis fitting centre for all hospitals in Tan Tock Seng Hospital.) (Fig. 8)
— Commencement of rehabilitation walking exercises
— Suitability of prosthesis checked after 2 weeks by Prosthetist (in Clinic at Tan Tock Seng Hospital) and Orthopaedic Surgeon in Diabetic Foot Clinic

Cost for Prosthesis

The majority of our amputees belong to the lower socio-economic group. Many may not be able to afford purchasing the below knee prosthesis. The cost of a prosthesis (subsidised by the Government is about SGD$900). Those that cannot afford to buy the prosthesis must be referred to the Medico-Social Worker for financial assistance.

It is very encouraging to note that recently the Ministry of Health has given priority to Diabetes Mellitus to be one of the ten chronic diseases where health costs can be obtained from the patient's own Central Provident Fund. This has been a great help to our patients many of whom are poor.

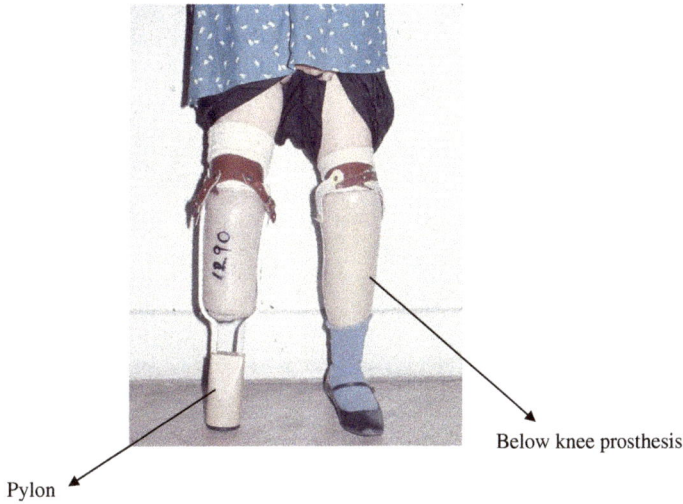

Below knee prosthesis

Pylon

Figure 8. Fitting of prosthesis

References

1. H. Jung, Comprehensive post-operative management after lower limb amputations: current concepts in rehabilitation, *SGH Proc.* **16**:58–62 (2007).
2. T. S. Jensen, *et al.*, Immediate and long-term phantom limb pain in amputee: incidence, clinical characteristics and relationship to pre-amputation limb pain, *Pain.* **21**:267–8 (1985).
3. M. Bone, P. Critchley and D. J. Buggy, Gabapentin in postamputation phantom limb pain: a randomized, double-blind, placebo-controlled, cross-over study, *Reg. Anesth. Pain Med.* **27**:481–6 (2002).
4. A. Moshirfar, *et al.*, Prosthetic options for below knee amputation after osteomyelitis and nonunion of the tibia, *Clin. Orthop.* **360**:110–21 (1999).

NUH Diabetic Foot Team

Aziz Nather

Chairman, Diabetic Foot Team
Department of Orthopaedic Surgery
Yong Loo Lin School of Medicine
National University of Singapore

Need for Diabetic Foot Service

In January of 2003, Professor K Satku first approached me to start a service for the diabetic foot. Professor K Satku was then the Chief of Orthopaedic Surgery in the National University Hospital (NUH) from 2002 to 2004. He is now the Director of Medical Services in the Ministry of Health (MOH).

At that time, I was 55, and my tenure with NUS was coming to an end. I was being reviewed for extension. During this critical period, Professor Satku set me a target to be met before considering renewing my contract. He asked me to set up a diabetic multi-disciplinary foot team, and set 3 parameters to assess the success of the diabetic service. The first was to reduce the average length of stay for diabetic foot problems by 10%, the second was to reduce the complication rates by 10%, and the final target was to reduce the below-knee amputation (BKA) rate by 10%. Should I be able to meet these targets within one year, Professor Satku assured me that he was more than willing to extend my contract.

He reiterated that it was not possible for me to succeed alone. Instead, a multi-disciplinary foot team had to be formed, involving an endocrinologist, an infectious disease (ID) specialist, a podiatrist and nurses.

In the past, care of diabetic feet faced enormous problems. There was a large clinical load — both inpatient and outpatient. Since all wounds had to be inspected daily, diabetic foot service would involve demanding and time-consuming ward rounds. A large majority of these patients were subsidized patients. In addition, surgery for these patients involved high risk, with mortality rates of about 20–50%, due to the multiple co-morbidities present.

I was initially disheartened upon hearing this. Having been specializing in spine surgery for the past 10 years, I had no experience in this field of work. However, after much careful consideration, I put my best efforts into assembling a diabetic foot team. I managed to persuade Dr Chionh Siok Bee, an endocrinologist, to join me on a team ward round once a week. We also managed to get an infectious disease specialist, Professor Paul Tambyah, and the principal podiatrist, Mr Adam Jorgensen to join the team round. We would also be assisted by a Case Manager, Ms Rose Low, who organized the patients that we needed to see during each team round.

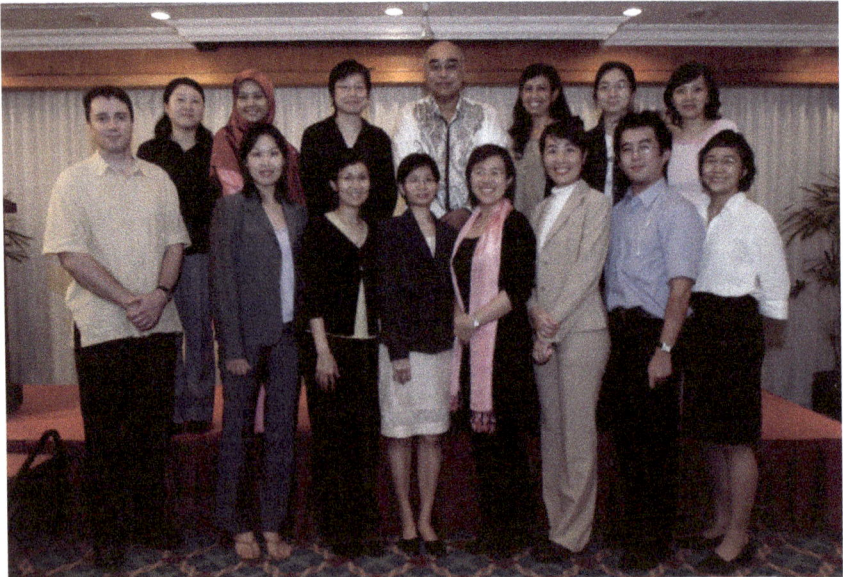

Pioneers of NUH Diabetic Foot Team (November 2004)

On careful review of literature, we found that the team approach had actually been very successful in reducing the major amputation rates from 40% to 23.5%, as reported by Faglio *et al.* in 1998. Furthermore, the formation of a "Specialized Foot Care Clinic" decreased the amputation rate dramatically from 9.9 per 1000 to 1.8 per 1000 over 5 years, as found by Driver *et al.* in 2005 in Boston.

The team approach works because it is patient-centered. In a team round, the management of patients is discussed by all specialists present. The surgeon decides whether surgery is required. The endocrinologist gives input on endocrine control, while the ID specialist advises on which antibiotics are to be used. The ward nurse directs the type of dressing to be applied. In this way, the best possible care is given to the patient in a holistic way. This team approach is not only highly cost effective, but also clinically efficient in managing diabetic foot problems.

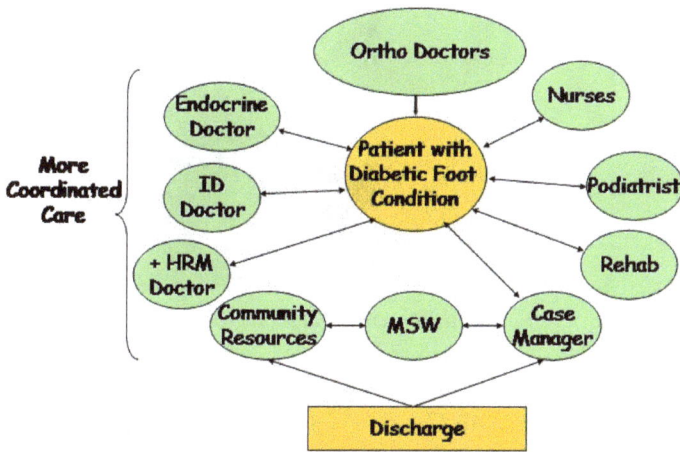

Patient-centred Team Approach

The team members simultaneously decided to design a clinical pathway. All patients admitted to NUH with diabetic foot problems were to be put on the pathway. In this pathway, detailed treatment plans were listed. For example, on the first day, professional input by various team members were to be provided. Investigations to be carried out were also outlined. Such guidelines must be adapted for all patients, day by day. The implementation of this clinical pathway was instrumental to the success of the team approach.

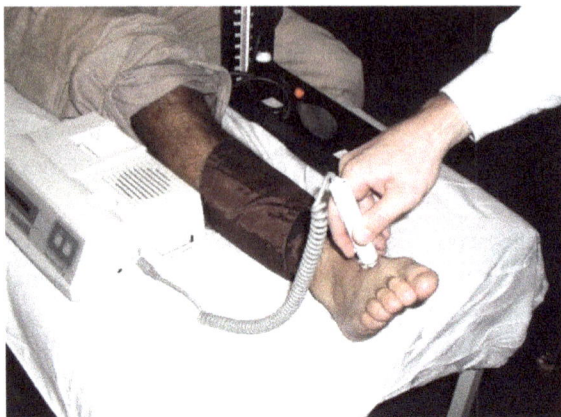

Doppler measurement of patient's foot

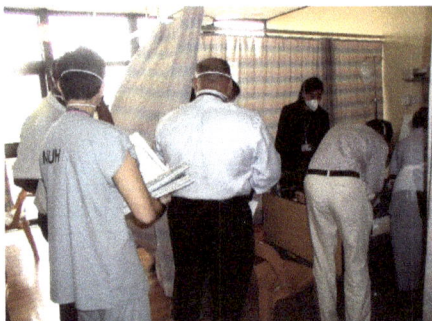

Team Round during SARS period (May 2003)

The NUH multi-disciplinary team for diabetic foot problems was launched in May 2003, with Dr. Nather as Chairperson and Dr Chionh Siok Bee as Co-Chairperson. At the same time, the Diabetic Foot Clinical Pathway was also launched.

In each diabetic team round on Tuesday mornings, cases were presented by the housemen and medical officers in Ward 54. In each teaching round, each session was awarded 1 point for Continuous Medical Education.

The Diabetic Foot Clinical Pathway was finalized and implemented in January 2004. The pathway was carefully explained to each new batch of

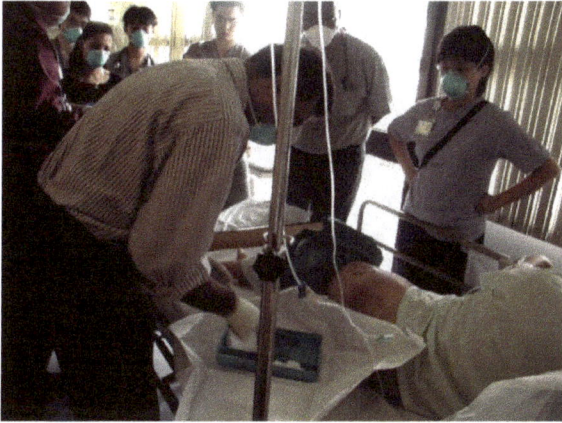

Dressing a patient's wound

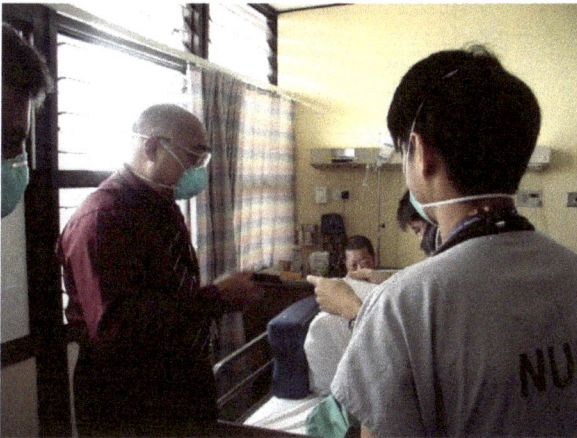

Discussing treatment plan with patient

housemen and medical officers by the Case Manager. Housemen were hence able to follow the pathway as case notes when they clerked the patients admitted to the hospital. In addition, the diabetic foot team also started a combined diabetic foot clinic on Wednesday mornings, led by the orthopaedic surgeon, together with a podiatrist and wound nurses.

Explaining Clinical Pathway to house officers and residents

After 1 year of work, results of our treatment were analysed. I presented the outcome of our Team Approach and Clinical Pathway during the keynote address given at the First National and Regional Conference on Diabetic Foot Problems in November 2004. This Conference included participation of consultants from Malaysia, Indonesia and Hong Kong. A total of 200 participants from 4 countries — Singapore, Malaysia, Indonesia and Hong Kong — attended the first conference.

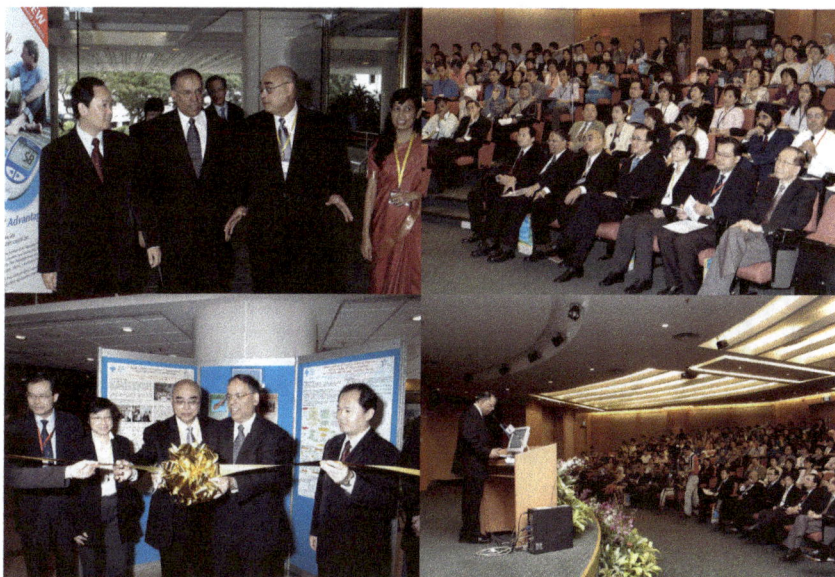

Opening Ceremony of First National and Regional Conference on Diabetic Foot Problems (20 Nov 2004)

The outcome of our team approach was successful. The average length of stay had decreased from 20.36 days before the team to 13.74 days after the team formation. The major amputation rate decreased from 31.15% in 2002 to 19.59% in 2004 — a significant reduction. Furthermore, the complication rate was reduced from 19.67% pre-team to 8.78% post-team. All 3 targets had been met. Our results showed that the multi-disciplinary team approach, combined with the clinical foot pathway, was indeed effective in providing good quality care for patients admitted with diabetic foot problems.

Research Projects with Junior College Students

Being an academic at heart, and being particularly fond of research, I couldn't help but notice that diabetic foot surgery was a field little explored. It provided great opportunities for research. We therefore embarked on several clinical research projects. Due to shortage of registrars and medical officers assigned to work with the Diabetic Foot Team, we piloted clinical research projects with the recruitment of research assistants from junior colleges. These were top students from the respective junior colleges who had completed their A levels and were eager to pursue medicine. They were employed from January to May full-time.

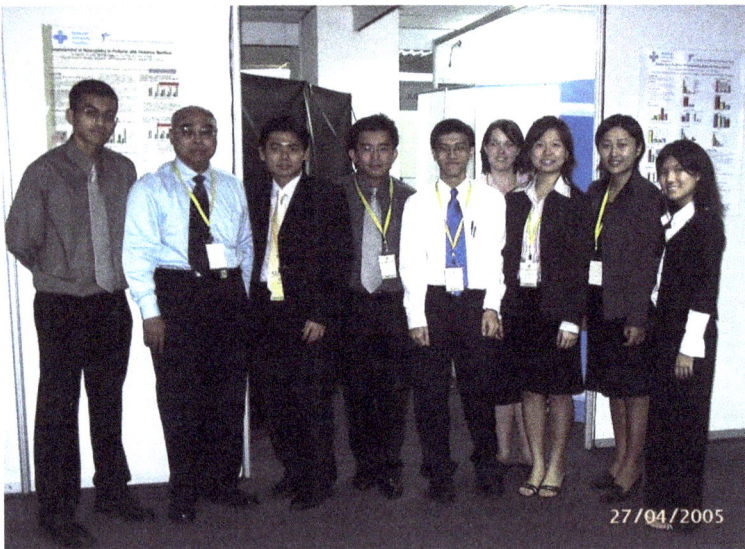

First Research Team MOA Conference in Miri, Sarawak

The first research team in 2005 included 3 students from Raffles Junior College (RJC) and 1 from Victoria Junior College (VJC). A total of 6 projects were completed, studying neuropathy in patients with diabetic foot problems, neuropathy in patients without diabetic foot problems, diabetic foot infections, diabetic footwear and diabetic vasculopathy. Of these, 2 were finally published in medical literature. The team presented a total of 9 papers at the 35th Malaysian Orthopaedic Association (MOA) meeting in Miri, Sarawak, in May 2005. This student research assistant pilot scheme was an outstanding success.

Their research includes the study of:

- Epidemology of Diabetic Foot Problems and Predictive Factors for Limb Loss
- Assessment of Sensory Neuropathy in Patients with Diabetic Foot Problems
- Assessment of Sensory Neuropathy in Patients without Diabetic Foot Problems
- Diabetic Foot Infections
- Diabetic Footwear
- Diabetic Vasculopathy

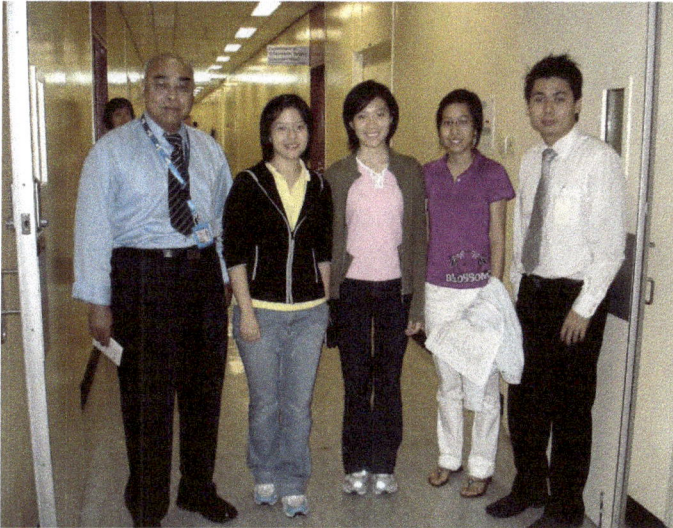

Second Research Team

Encouraged by the success of the first team, subsequent research teams were formed using JC students. The second research team in 2006 included 3 VJC students, who completed 3 research projects. Their work included the study of the use of anodyne therapy and the ultrasonic debrider. The team of 4 presented 5 papers at the 2nd APOA Trauma section meeting in Kuala Lumpur, Malaysia, in June 2006. These papers include

- Anodyne Therapy for Recalcitrant Diabetic Foot Ulcers: a report of four cases
- Detecting Neuropathy in Early Diabetics: CSB & Stanley's clinics

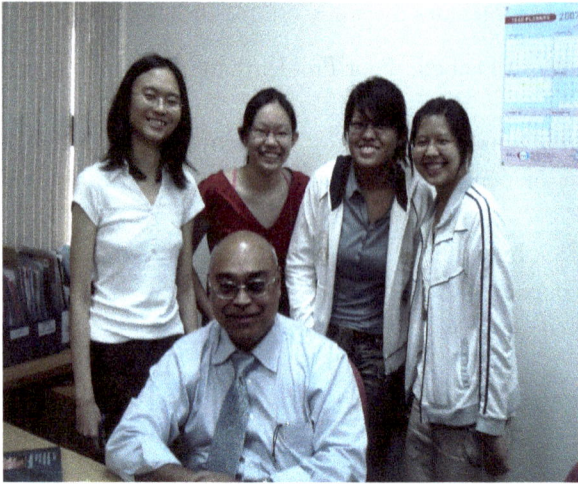

Third Research Team

The 3rd research team in 2007 included 4 RJC students. Their studies included a socio-economic survey on diabetics comparing one cohort with diabetic foot problems against a cohort without diabetic foot problems. The team of 4 presented 5 papers at the APOA 15th triennial congress in Seoul, Korea, in September 2007. This research team also assisted in writing most of the chapters in a book entitled Diabetic Foot Problems, published by World Scientific in 2008.

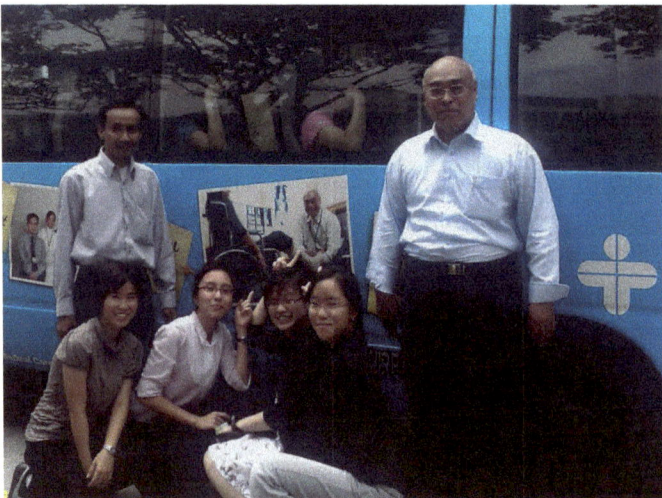

Fourth Research Team

The 4th research team consisted of 2 VJC students and 2 RJC students. More projects on diabetic foot were carried out, including a study on the role of Extracorporeal Shockwave Therapy (ESWT) in healing chronic diabetic ulcers. Research was funded by a grant obtained from Dornier Medtech. (This study was aborted after 6 months due to poor results.) The team also studied VAC dressings for diabetic wounds as well as the outcome of major and minor amputations for diabetic foot problems. This group also did the bulk of manuscript preparation for a book on tissue banking — Allograft Procurement, Processing and Transplantation — published in September 2010.

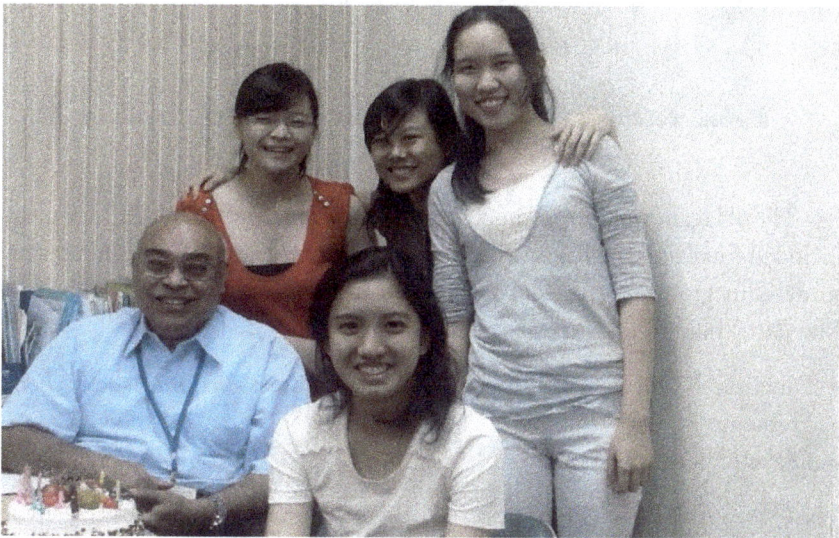

Fifth Research Team

The 5th research team in 2009 also comprised of 2 VJC and 2 RJC students. This group further wrote chapters for the book: Allograft Procurement, Processing and Transplantation. They also completed our clinical research projects on VAC dressings for diabetic wounds and on the outcome of below knee amputations. This team of 4 presented 4 papers at the 39th MOA Annual General Meeting (AGM)/ Annual Scientific Meeting (ASM) in May 2009 in Sabah, Malaysia.

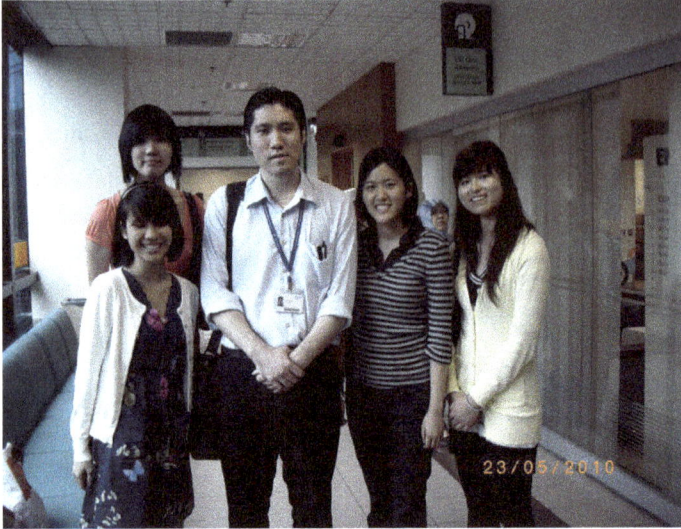

Sixth Research Team

The 6th team was formed in 2010 with 2 RJC and 2 VJC students. Projects included finalizing the below knee amputation study and the ray amputation study. This group of 4 presented 2 papers at the 40th MOA AGM/ ASM in May 2010 held in Johor Bahru, Malaysia:

- Functional Outcome Of Below Knee Amputees With Diabetic Foot Problems
- Diabetic Foot Infections

The 6th team also studied the effect of Bridge VAC Dressings, with the help of a grant by KCI. We studied 5 cases with Bridge VAC Dressings, from March to October 2010. This work was subsequently published in Diabetic Foot and Ankle.

I will never forget how one the students of this team, Jane, had lamented her fate as the group prepared for the conference. "What bad luck we have," she had remarked, "Of all the places we could go to, like Sabah or Sarawak, we only get to go to Johor Bahru, not even Kuala Lumpur!" What a remark! I laughed heartily and pointed out that we were fortunate not to be presenting in Singapore. Presenting in Johor Bahru meant that at least we got to travel out of the country. Indeed, all of us hope to travel for our research work, and travelling is a good motivation for all of us.

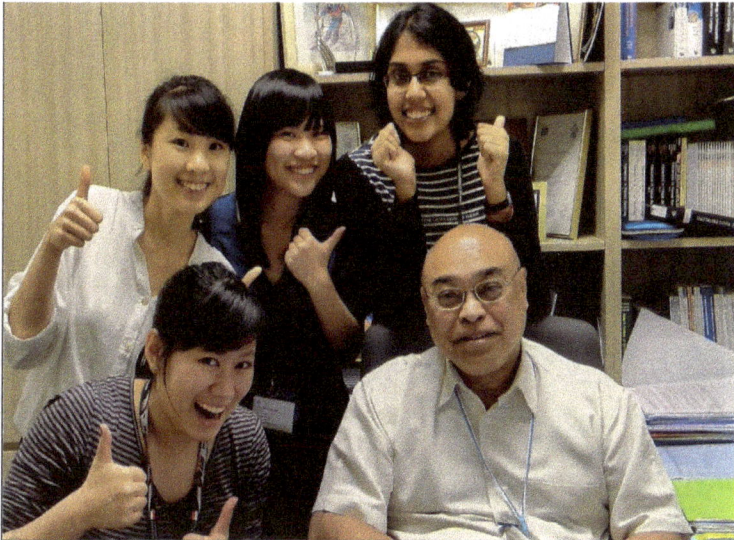

Seventh Research Team

The 7th research team was assembled in 2011, again with 2 RJC and 2 VJC students. The projects they embarked on included the study of the outcome of below knee amputations and ray amputations in the diabetic foot. They also started work on the MOH Grant — Predictive Factors for Below Knee Amputation in Patients with Diabetic Foot Problems. Their work was presented as 2 papers at the 41st MOA AGM/ASM in May 2011 at KLCC in Kuala Lumpur, Malaysia:

- Clinical Outcomes of Below-Knee Amputations in Diabetic Foot Patients
- Clinical Outcomes of Ray Amputations in Diabetic Foot Patients

This group was also responsible for doing the groundwork for 2 papers to be presented at the 6th International Symposium on the Diabetic Foot in May 2011, in Noordwijkerhout in The Netherlands. At last, after nearly 7 years full time in diabetic foot, I had reached the Mecca of Diabetic Foot Problems — the International Working Group on the Diabetic Foot (IWGDF) in the Netherlands. I was invited to participate in the Guidelines Experts Group Meeting as a corresponding member of the IWGDF. This was a great honour for Singapore. We participated in the foremost body formulating guidelines on the diabetic foot for the rest of the world.

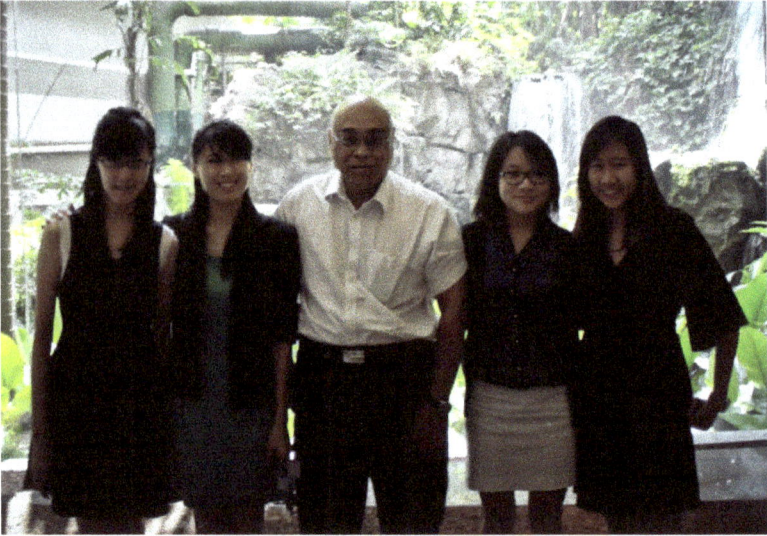

Eighth Research Team

The 8th research team was assembled in 2012 with 2 RJC students, 1 VJC student and 1 Hwa Chong Junior College (HCJC) student. The team carried out research projects mainly using funds from the MOH grant on Predictive Factors of the Diabetic Foot. The research projects were:

- Predictive Factors for Below Knee Amputations
- Socio-economic Factors in Patients with Diabetic Foot Problems
- The Role of the Oximeter in Indicating Tissue Perfusion in Diabetic Foot Problems
- The Oximeter as a Measure of Tissue Perfusion in the Foot (Control Study)

This group was also actively involved in the manuscript preparation of most chapters in the new book — The Diabetic Foot, published by World Scientific in September 2012. This book is targeted to first be launched in our 60th Anniversary Celebration in conjunction with the Singapore Orthopaedic Conference in October 2012. It is also targeted for a big launch in October 2013, at the 10th Asia Pacific Conference on Diabetic Limb Problems.

NUH Strategy

In summary, with 9 years of work full time on the diabetic foot from May 2003 to May 2012, the team approach and clinical pathway implemented have reduced the average length of stay, complication rate, and major amputation rate of patients coming to NUH with diabetic foot problems. The major amputation rate was reduced from 31% to 11% in 2007. However, we can reduce it further only if we can introduce more revascularization surgery, such as distal limb bypasses.

The quality service we provide for all patients with diabetic foot problems have certainly improved. We are now able to provide them with new generation silver dressings, VAC therapy, ultrasonic debridement, new generation antibiotics, and where needed, maggot therapy, to allow more feet to be saved.

However, in the long term, the key strategy for our NUH diabetic foot program is prevention. Prevention includes performing annual foot screening for all patients diagnosed with diabetes. Patients at risk of developing diabetic foot problems can then seek early intervention by podiatrists, vascular surgeons and orthopaedic surgeons. The use of preventive and therapeutic shoes for all patients with diabetes must also be encouraged.

All patients with diabetes must be treated carefully to reduce the onset of complications including diabetic foot problems. The principal aim is to reduce the HbA1c level to less than 7% to reduce the complication rate of diabetes. In particular, our diabetic foot program plans to screen all patients newly diagnosed with diabetes for risk factors to identify the foot at risk. By performing annual foot screenings, we can detect the formation of foot complications early. Attending to these foot complications at an early stage can help us reduce the incidence of major amputations. In addition, more attention must also be given to advising patients regarding proper footwear — preventive or therapeutic. The use of proper footwear specially designed for diabetic feet will reduce the development of foot complications.

Diabetes is given special attention on NUH Diabetes Day — a special day dedicated to the care of diabetes. It usually coincides with the World Diabetes Day. The theme for NUH Diabetes Day 2005 was the Care of the Foot. That year, our team put up posters on the care of the diabetic foot, and also provided free foot screening for all patients who had diabetes.

NUH Diabetes Day 2005

In 2006, the theme was Diabetes Care for Everyone. Forums were organized involving several specialties including the nephrologist, the ophthalmologist and the cardiologist for kidney, renal and heart screening. The NUH diabetic foot team also participated by providing free foot screening. From 2007 to 2008, the multi-disciplinary diabetic foot team continued being part of the celebrations on NUH Diabetes Day, providing free foot screening for all diabetic patients.

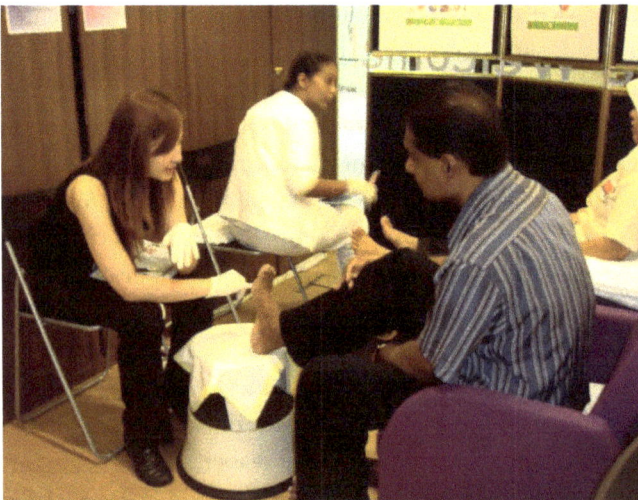

Screening a patient's foot

Such events earned the team much publicity among all doctors in the hospital, including key personnel such as the Chairman of the Medical Board, the President of the National University Healthcare System (NUHS), as well as the Chief Executive Officer of NUH. NUH Diabetes Day provides an avenue for professional education, helping other doctors to understand the seriousness of having a diabetic foot problem. Doctors will then refer all patients diagnosed with diabetes to attend annual foot screening.

NHG Strategy

The strategy of the National Healthcare Group (NHG) is to ensure that all hospitals in its group could provide foot screening for all patients diagnosed with diabetes. NHG is the western cluster of the 3 hospitals in Singapore: National University Hospital (NUH), Tan Tock Seng Hospital (TTSH) and Alexandra Hospital (AH). In May 2005, an NHG task force for the diabetic foot was set up, with 2 representatives from each hospital — Dr Nather and Dr Chionh Siok Bee represented NUH.

NHG encouraged patient education, and provided finance for us to print a public education guide in October 2005. Ms Torng Ay-Hwa from NUH produced a publication pamphlet for patient education in 4 languages — English, Mandarin, Malay and Tamil — for use in all 3 hospitals.

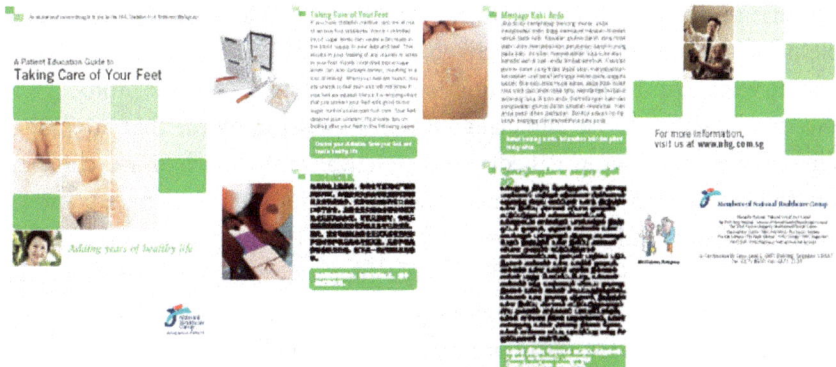

Patient Education Guide *"Taking Care of Your Feet"* in 4 Languages

Regional Training Course for Diabetic Foot Screening

NHG's key strategy was to provide annual foot screening services to all patients with diabetes in polyclinics in both the NHG and SingHealth clusters.

However, upon monitoring the attendance rate of patients with diabetes for foot screening, it was realized that there was only a 70% compliance rate. There was a difficulty in carrying out 100% annual foot screening in all 3 hospitals for all patients diagnosed with diabaetes. We faced the problem of shortage of podiatrists to conduct such screening. At that time, there were only 15 podiatrists in Singapore and none in Malaysia and Indonesia. Therefore, the taskforce felt that assistant nurses or staff nurses should be trained to do the tasks normally carried out by podiatrists — foot screening, education on foot care and education on footwear.

We implemented the NHG diabetes foot screening course to train nurse clinicians to perform foot screening. NHG provided a grant of $76500 in October 2005 for this purpose. The budget was used by each of the 5 hospitals to purchase one full set of equipment to perform foot screening, and also to cover costs for running a foot screening course. The nurse clinicians must be provided by the hospitals themselves, with 2 nurse clinicians each from NUH and TTSH, and 1 nurse clinician from AH. Dr Nather was the Project Director with Dr Tay Jam Chin, the vascular surgeon and endocrinologist from TTSH as Co-Director.

The task force designed a comprehensive curriculum for foot screening, to train nurse clinicians to perform foot screening, education on footcare and footwear, as well as education on diabetes care itself. A one-week hands-on Foundation Course on the use of the ABI and TBI Doppler ultrasound and the neurothesiometer, and on performing Semmes Weinstein Monofilament Testing with proper clinical examination was developed. A simple protocol was also developed for nurse clinicians for use in performing the foot screening. The course ended with a theory and practical exam. Each nurse clinician would be tested on the theory and practice of foot screening, by a board of examiners from the diabetic teams in NUH, TTSH and AH. Upon completing this course, nurse clinicians could practice foot screening, following a further attachment to a hospital for one month. The attachment includes sessions with an endocrinologist, orthopaedic surgeon or podiatrist.

The first NHG training course for foot screening was conducted in March 2006. There were 11 students including 2 occupational therapists from Universiti Kembangsaan Malaysia (UKM). This course was a great success.

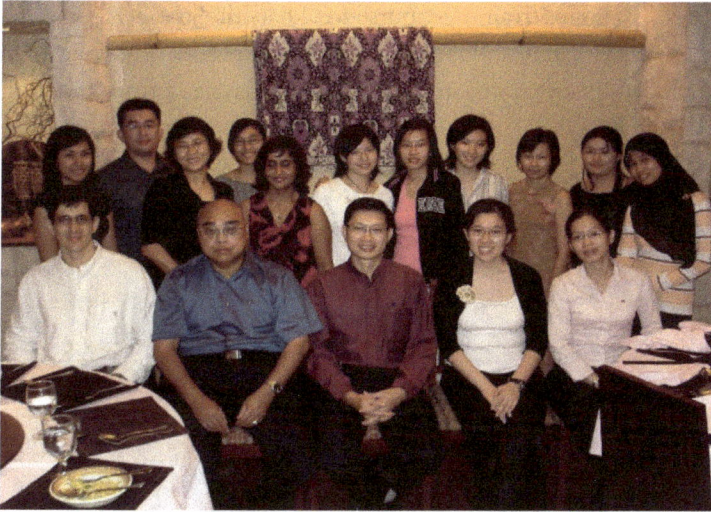

1ˢᵗ Regional Training Course for Diabetic Foot Screening (2006)

The 2ⁿᵈ Regional Training Course for Diabetic Foot Screening in March 2007 was subsequently organized by NUH on its own initiative. There were a total of 28 participants (all nurse clinicians) this year — 16 from Singapore, 10 from Malaysia, 1 from Indonesia and 1 from Hong Kong.

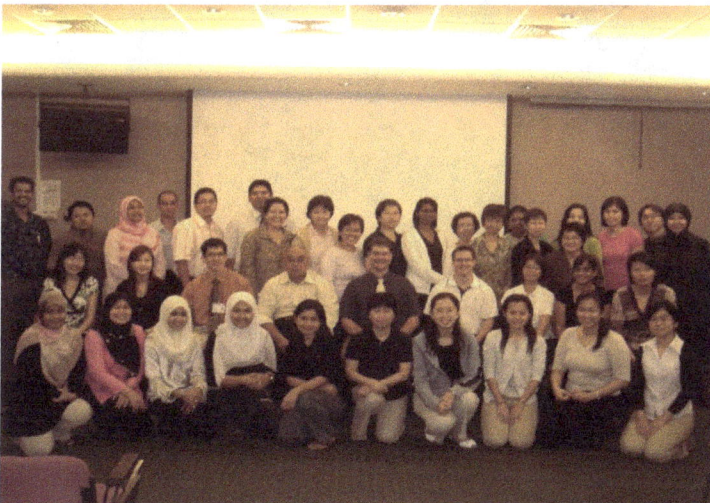

2ⁿᵈ Regional Training Course for Diabetic Foot Screening (2008)

The 3rd Regional Training Course for Diabetic Foot Screening followed in April 2008, with almost double the number of participants. The 43 participants included 29 from Singapore, 10 from Malaysia, 3 from Indonesia and 1 from Hong Kong.

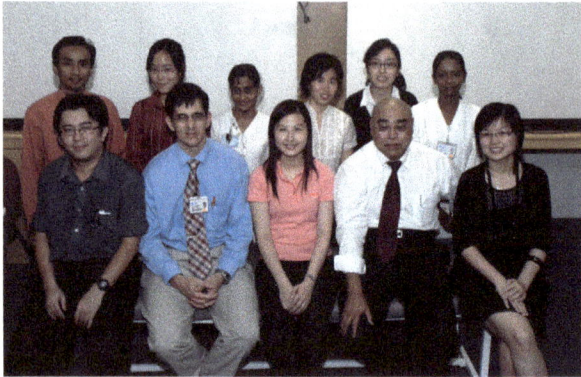

3rd Regional Training Course for Diabetic Foot Screening (2009)

The 4th regional training course continued in November 2010 with 20 participants — 12 from Singapore, 4 from Malaysia, 2 from Indonesia and 2 from Hong Kong.

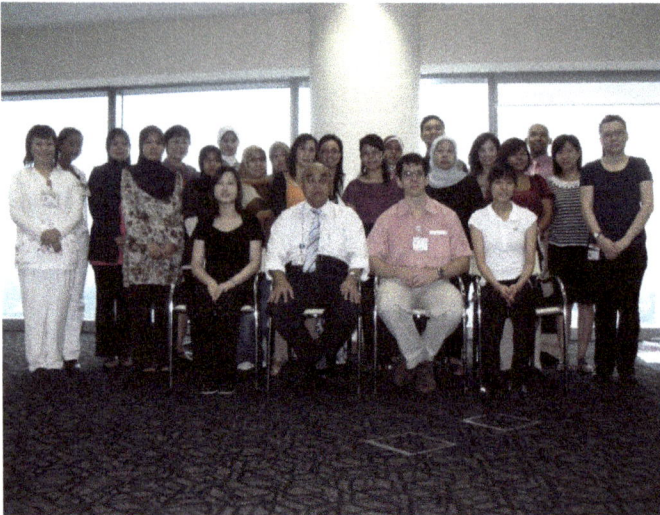

4th Regional Training Course for Diabetic Foot Screening (2010)

The 5th Regional Training Course for Diabetic Foot Screening was held from 21–25 November 2011. There were a total of 14 participants — 6 from Singapore, 7 from Malaysia and 1 from Indonesia.

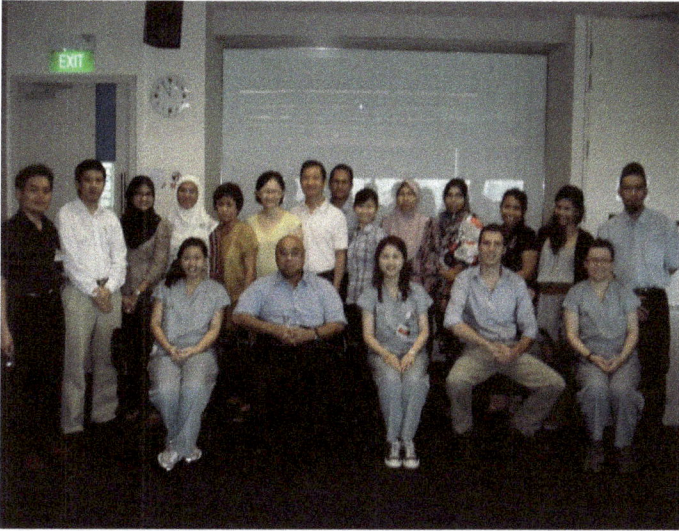

5th Regional Training Course for Diabetic Foot Screening (2011)

This year, the 6th regional training course will be held in November 2012.

As of December 2011, a total of 116 nurse clinicians had been trained by the NUH foot screening courses. This included 62 nurses in Singapore from polyclinics, as well as hospitals like the National University Hospital, Tan Tock Seng Hospital, Alexandra Hospital, Singapore General Hospital and Changi General Hospital. 31 nurse clinicians and 2 occupational therapists from Malaysia, 5 nurse clinicians and 2 orthopaedic surgeons from Indonesia, as well as 4 nurse clinicians from Hong Kong had also been trained.

The diabetic foot screening course, initiated by the NHG taskforce, proved to be an outstanding success. It not only trained nurse clinicans to start foot screening in several hospitals in Singapore, but also provided for foot screening in hospitals in Malaysia and Hong Kong.

The Regional Training Course for Diabetic Foot Screening also received publicity when it was covered in a news report by Channel News Asia on 21 April 2008. The news feature highlighted the aim to not only train nurses in Singapore, but also nurse clinicians in Malaysia, Indonesia and Hong Kong.

Dr Otman Siregar, from Medan, who travelled to Singapore to learn about the diabetic foot, emphasized the important role that NUH Diabetic Foot Team had played in helping to develop expertise to provide for diabetic foot screening in Indonesia.

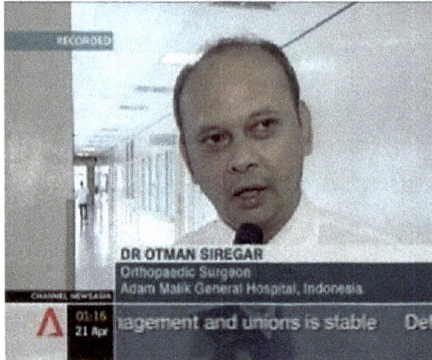

Interview with Dr Otman Siregar during News Feature by Channel News Asia

The equipment included an Ultrasonic Doppler costing about $4000, a Biothesiometer costing an estimated $2000, a monofilament test system, a tuning fork as well as a tendon tapper. The total price for each set of equipment was only about $5500. With only a small amount of about $6000, hospitals could start a good diabetic foot program by providing diabetic foot screening.

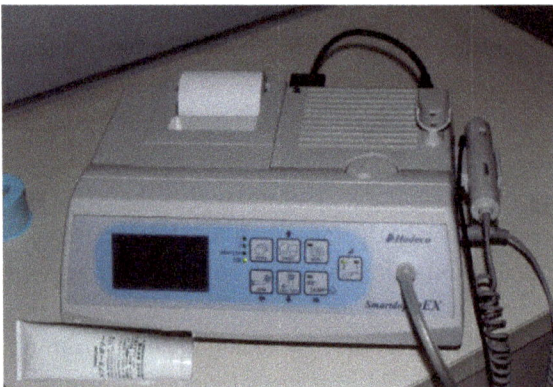

ABI machine with ultrasonic probe and Doppler jelly

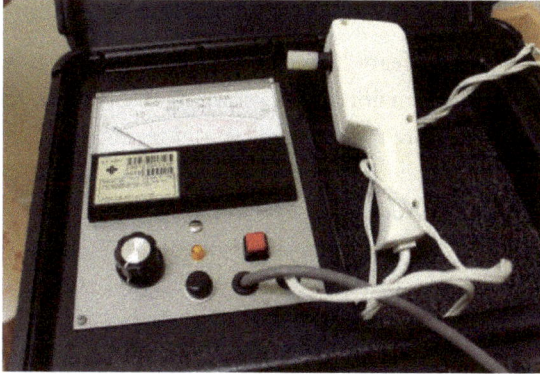

Biothesiometer

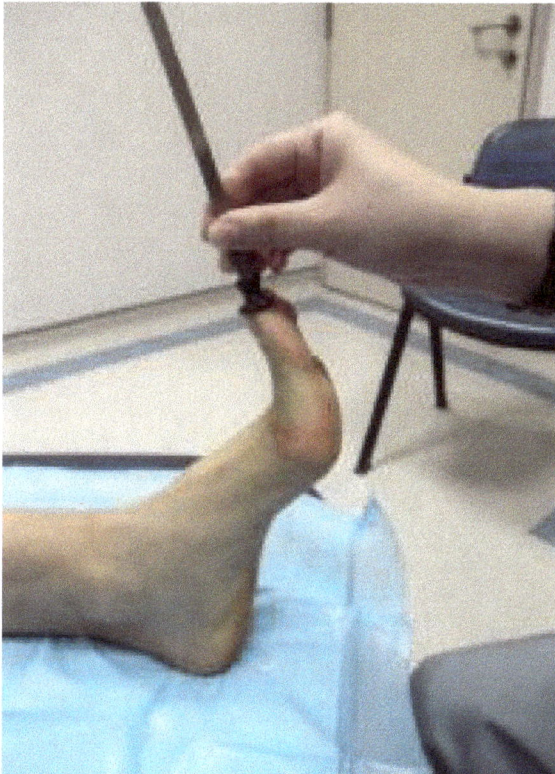

Tuning Fork Test

Conclusion

The NUH Diabetic Foot Team, together with the clinical pathway launched, successfully decreased the major amputation rate in NUH. It has encouraged other hospitals in Singapore to form similar foot teams. In addition, hospitals in neighbouring countries in the region (namely Malaysia, Indonesia and Hong Kong) are also setting up foot teams. In this way, the major amputation rate can also be reduced in our neighbouring countries.

NUH employs a two-pronged strategy. The first strategy is prevention by providing annual foot screening for all diabetics so that diabetic foot complications can be avoided. Secondly, when complications do arise, it is best treated by a team approach. This strategy can also be employed by other hospitals.

Appendix II

Publications by NUH Diabetic Foot Team

Books

1. A. Nather (ed.), *Diabetic Foot Problems* (World Scientific Publishing Co. Pte. Ltd. , Singapore, 2008). *Contributed 24 Chapters*
2. A. Nather and F. C. Han, The diabetic foot. In: S. Sivananthan, E. Sherry, *et al.* (eds.), *Mercer's Textbook of Orthopaedics and Trauma* (Hodder Education, 2011), Chapter 127.

Periodicals

1. A. Nather, S. B. Chionh, Y. H. Chan, J. L. L. Chew, C. B. Lin, S. H. Neo and E. Y. Sim, Epidemiology of diabetic foot problems and predictive factors for limb loss, *J. Diabetes Complications* **22**:77–82 (2008).
2. A. Nather, S. H. Neo, S. B. Chionh, S. C. F. Liew, E. Y. Sim and J. L. L. Chew, Assessment of sensory neuropathy in diabetic patients without diabetic foot problems, *J. Diabetes Complications* **22**:126–31 (2008).
3. A. Nather, S. B. Chionh, Y. Y. Han, P. L. Chan and A. Nambiar, Effectiveness of vacuum-assisted closure (VAC) therapy in the healing of chronic diabetic foot ulcers, *Ann. Acad. Med. Singapore* **39**(5):353–8 (2010).
4. A. Nather, S. B. Chionh, L. M. Tay, Z. Aziz, J. W. H. Teng, A. Nambiar, K. Rajeswari and A. Eramus, Foot screening for diabetics, *Ann. Acad. Med. Singapore* **39**(6):472–4 (2010).
5. A. Nather, S. B. Chionh, K. L. Wong, S. Q. O. Koh, Y. H. Chan, X. Y. Li and A. Nambiar, Socioeconomic profile of diabetic patients with and without foot problems, *Diabet. Foot Ankle* **1**:5523 (2010).

6. A. Nather, S. B. Chionh, K. L. Wong, X. B. Chan, L. Shen, P. A. Tambyah, A. Jorgensen and A. Nambiar, Value of team approach combined with clinical pathway for diabetic foot problems: a clinical evaluation, *Diabet. Foot Ankle* **1**:5731 (2010).

7. A. Nather, Y. H. Ng, K. L. Wong and J. A. Sakharam, Effectiveness of bridge VAC dressings in the treatment of diabetic foot ulcers, *Diabet. Foot Ankle* **2**:5893 (2011).

8. Z. Aziz, W. K. Lin, A. Nather and C. Y. Huak, Predictive factors for lower extremity amputations in diabetic foot infections, *Diabet. Foot Ankle* **2**:7463 (2011).

9. A. Nather, K. L. Wong, Z. Aziz, C. H. J. Ong, B. M. C. Feng and C. B. Lin, Assessment of sensory neuropathy in patients with diabetic foot problems, *Diabet. Foot Ankle* **2**:6367 (2011).

10. A. Nather, Short Commentary (Expert Opinion) for "Role of negative pressure wound therapy in healing of diabetic foot ulcers" by P. S. Nain, et al., *J. Surg. Tech. Case Rep.* **3**(1):10–11 (2011).

Appendix III

APADLP

During the First National and Regional Conference on Diabetic Foot Problems (DFPs) hosted in the National University of Singapore in November 2004, there were 220 participants from 4 countries — Malaysia, Indonesia, Hong Kong and Singapore. The stage was set to form a Regional Association with the 4 member countries. The Asia Pacific Association of Diabetic Foot Problems (APADFP) was set up with Dr. Aziz Nather as Founding President, Dr. R. Ramanathan from Malaysia as the President Elect, Dr. Mulyono Soedirman from Indonesia as the First Vice-President and Dr. Josephine Ip from Hong Kong as the Second Vice-President (Fig. 1).

The 1st regional conference on DFPs (Figs. 2 to 4) was an outstanding success with about 220 participants. The Guest-of-Honour was Dr. Balaji Sadasivan, Senior Minister of State for Health (Fig. 5).

The following year, a 2nd regional conference, known as the Asia Pacific Conference on Diabetic Foot Problems (APCDFP) was held in Putrajaya, Malaysia in 2005 (Fig. 6), with Dr. R. Ramanathan from Ipoh, Perak, Malaysia as the Chairperson in collaboration with Dr. Amara Naicker, Rehabilitation Physician of the Universiti Kebangsaan Malaysia (UKM) in Kuala Lumpur, Malaysia. This attracted about 200 participants.

At the business meeting, the Board Members decided to change the name of the association from APADFP to the Asia Pacific Association of Diabetic Limb Problems (APADLP). This was because diabetes involves upper limbs in 10% of cases.

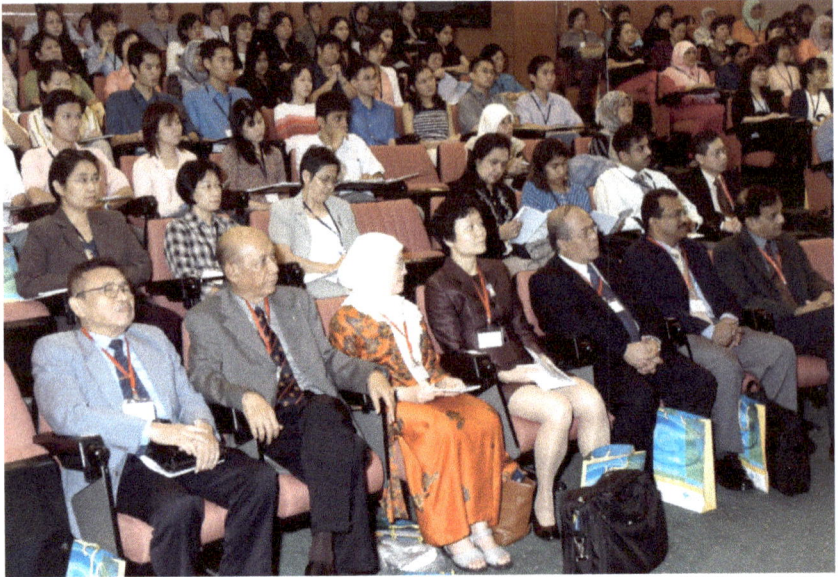

Figure 1.   Founding committee members of the APADFP

The 3rd Asia Pacific Conference on Diabetic Limb Problems (APCDLP) was held in Ancor, Jakarta, Indonesia in November 2006 (Fig. 7) with Dr. Mulyono Soedirman as the Organising Chairman (Fig. 8). It attracted about 200 participants.

With each year, the momentum of the Regional Association grew stronger. The 4th APCDLP was held in Hong Kong in November 2007 (Fig. 9), with Dr. Josephine Ip Wing-Yuk and Dr. Joseph Wong Wing Cheung as Co-Chairpersons from the University of Hong Kong and from Kwong Wah Hospital respectively. The National University Hospital (NUH) DFP Team ran in 2 out of the 3 Pre-conference Workshops during the Conference in Hong Kong. The Conference also attracted about 200 participants.

In 2008, the Conference returned to Singapore. The 5th APCDLP was held in NUH in October (Fig. 10). It was a great success with more than 250 participants.

The Guest-of-Honour for the 5th Conference was Professor K. Satku, Director of Medical Services in Singapore (Fig. 11). This was very appropriate as he was the man who had inspired us to set up a Diabetic Foot Team back in 2003. The team had actually spent 2 years writing a book on DFPs titled

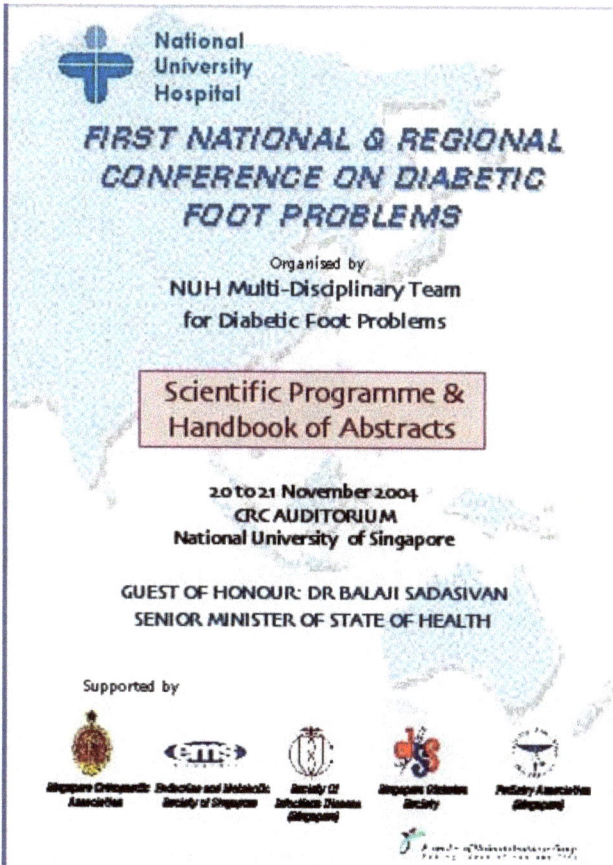

Figure 2. Poster for the 1st regional conference

"Diabetic Foot Problems" (Fig. 12) with our experience over the last 5 years of running the Diabetic Foot Service. This book was dedicated to Professor K. Satku.

This book was launched with great joy during the Opening Ceremony of the 5th APCDLP. The following year, this book became a best seller. It was the top, best selling medicine healthcare book for the month of May and June 2009, in the list of World Scientific. It was also one of the best sellers for podiatry and diabetic foot problems on Barnes and Nobles in 2009. The book was also in the best selling list on amazon.com in 2009, holding 2 positions — 42nd for the soft copy edition and 53rd for the hard copy.

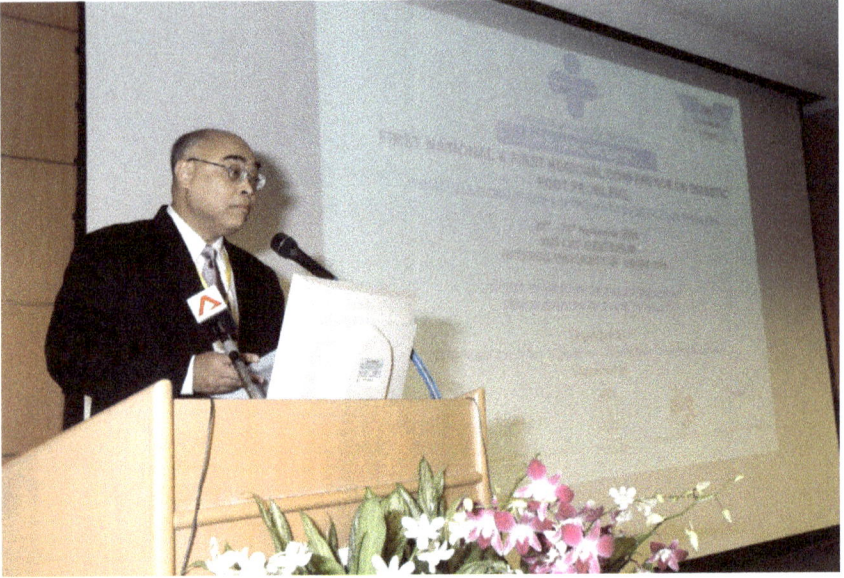

Figure 3. Dr. Aziz Nather giving his opening speech for the 1st regional conference

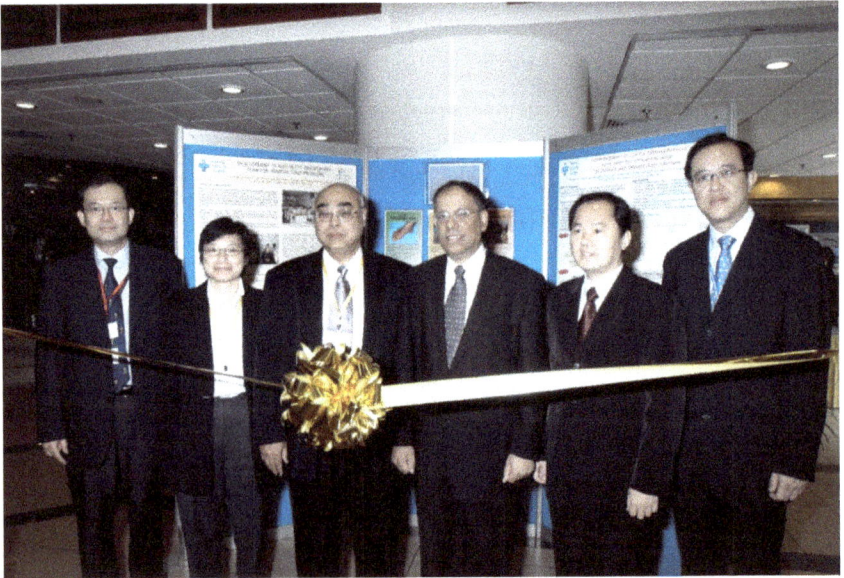

Figure 4. Opening ceremony of the 1st regional conference

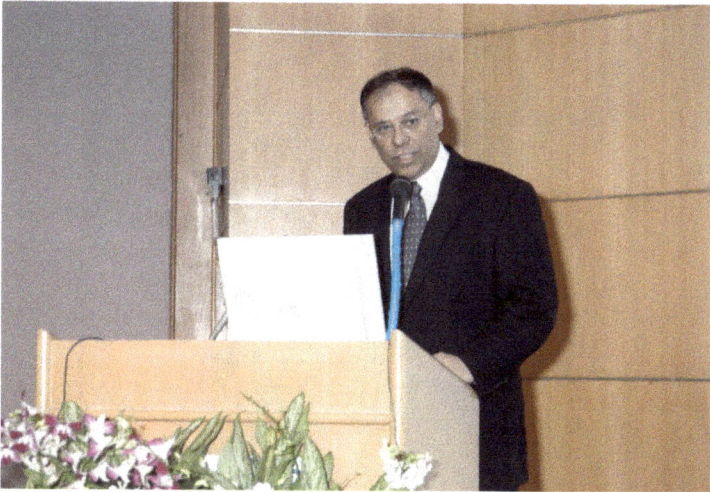

Figure 5. Dr. Balaji Sadasivan giving his opening speech for the 1st regional conference

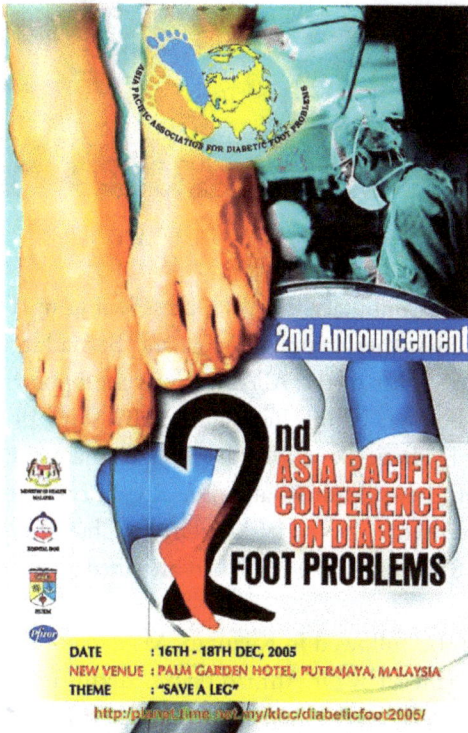

Figure 6. Poster for the 2nd APCDFP

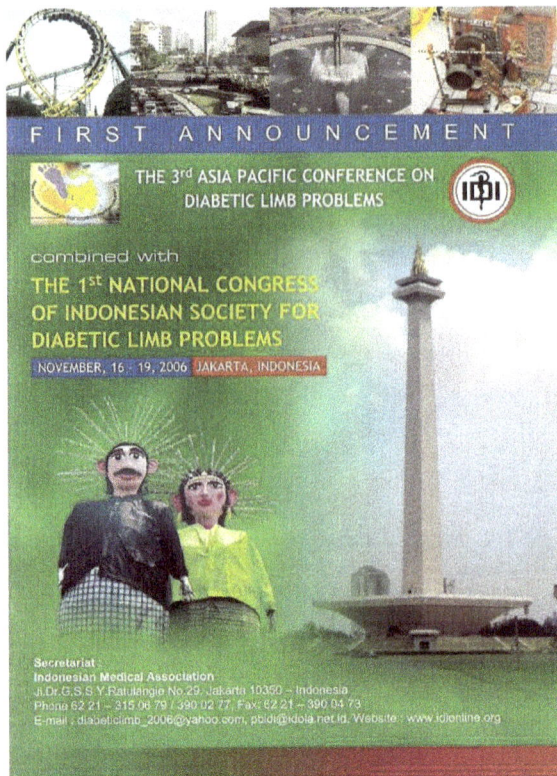

Figure 7.   Poster for the 3rd APCDLP

We received good publicity from the press including The Straits Times, TODAY English newspaper, radio 94.2 FM and Berita Harian (Fig. 13).

One of the highlights of the APADLP was the opportunity to hold the 6th APCDLP in Beijing, China in August 2009 (Fig. 14). There, we met the leaders of the Diabetic Foot World — Dr. Benjamin Lipsky, Dr. David Armstrong, Dr. Andrew Boulton and Dr. R.G. Frykberg (Fig. 15). They were Guest Speakers who were invited by Dr. Xu Zhangrong, the Organising Chairman (Fig. 16). This Conference also attracted more than 220 participants.

The 7th APCDLP followed in Kuantan, Malaysia in October 2010. This Conference was organised by Dr. Ahmad Hafiz Zulkifly from the International Islamic University Malaysia (IIUM). The NUH DFP Team ran one workshop at this Conference. There were 150 participants.

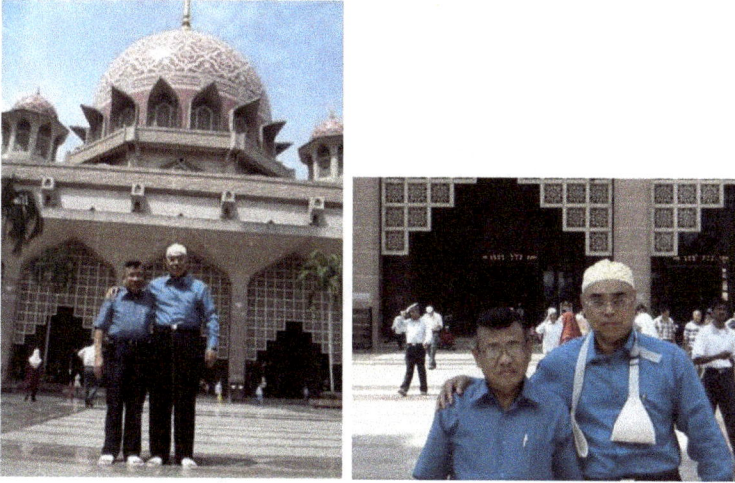

Figure 8. Dr. Aziz Nather with Dr. Mulyono Soedirman

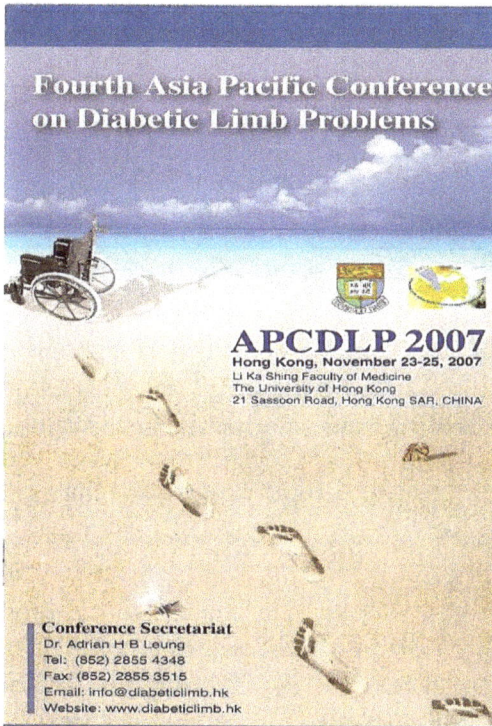

Figure 9. Poster for the 4th APCDLP

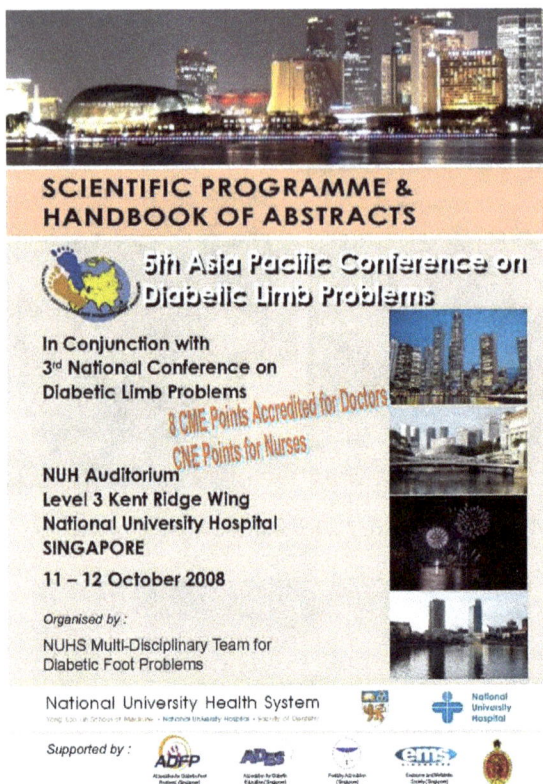

Figure 10.   Poster for the 5th APCDLP

Finally, the 8th APCDLP was recently held in Bandung, Indonesia in December 2011 (Fig. 17). The NUH DFP Team ran 2 workshops during this Conference. The Bandung Conference was also well-attended, with about 200 participants.

The future is bright for APADLP. The 9th APCDLP will be held in October 2012 in Hong Kong with Dr. Samson Chan as the Organising Chairman.

The 10th APCDLP will be held in Singapore in 10 November 2013. This will be a significant event in our association's history. Our 10th anniversary will be held in the very place that this association was founded!

For this meeting, a big conference is being organised, with 2 Pre-Conference Workshops. A new book titled "The Diabetic Foot" edited by

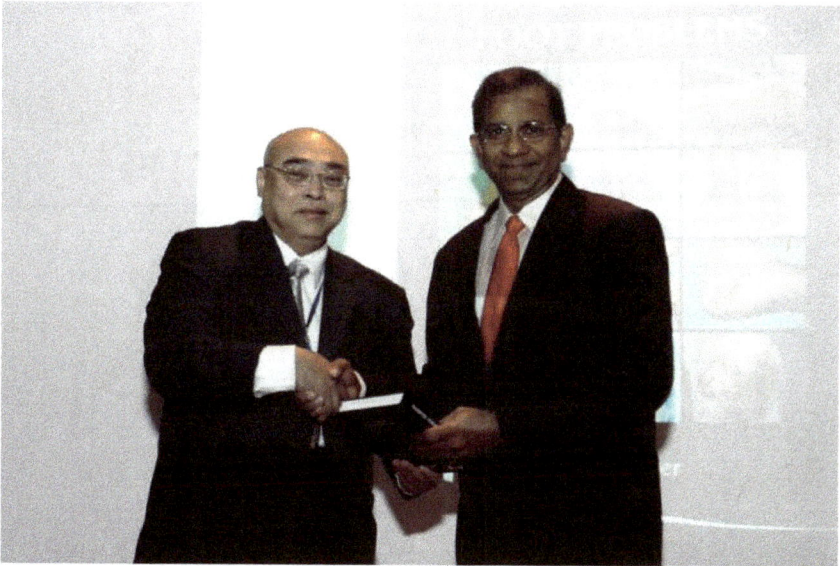

Figure 11. Dr. Aziz Nather presenting the book to Professor K. Satku

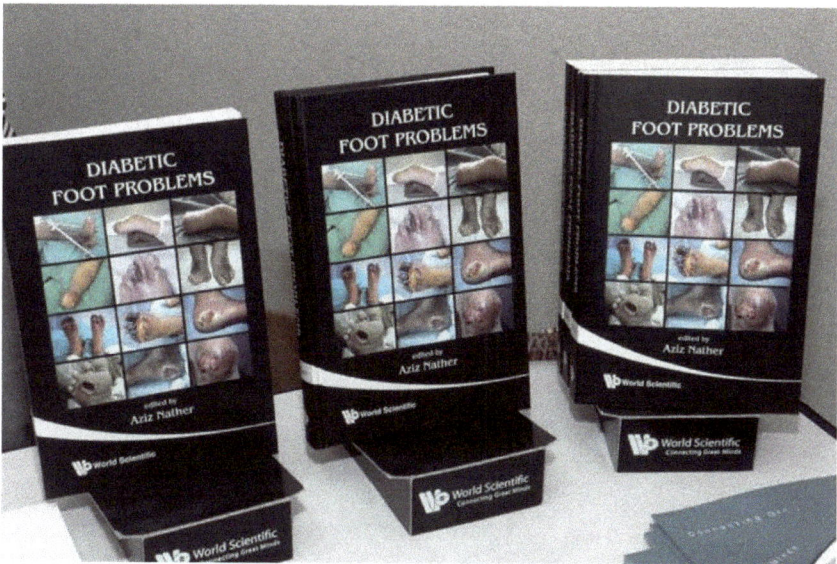

Figure 12. Launch of the book titled "Diabetic Foot Problems"

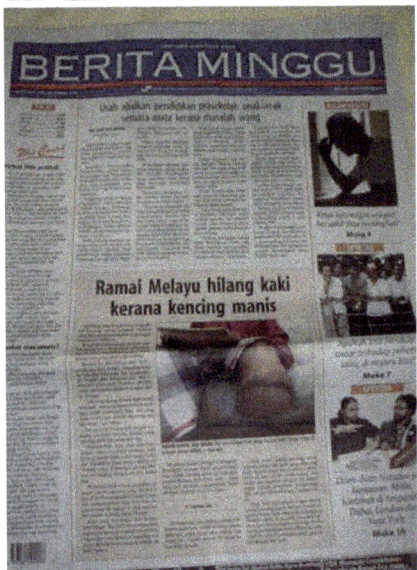

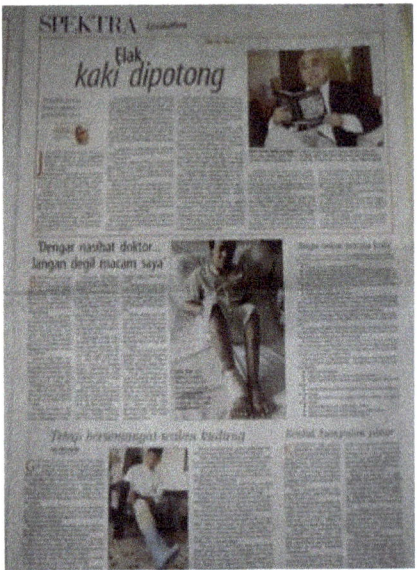

Figure 13. Newspaper articles: The Straits Times, TODAY and Berita Minggu

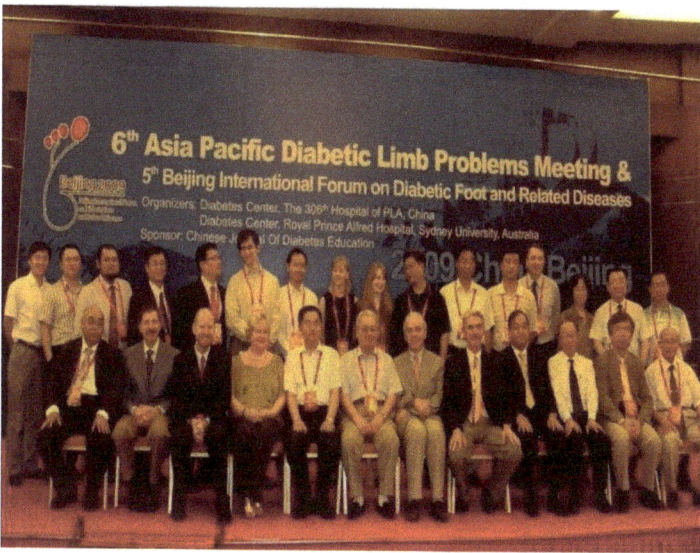

Figure 14. Organisers and Guest Speakers of the 6th APCDLP

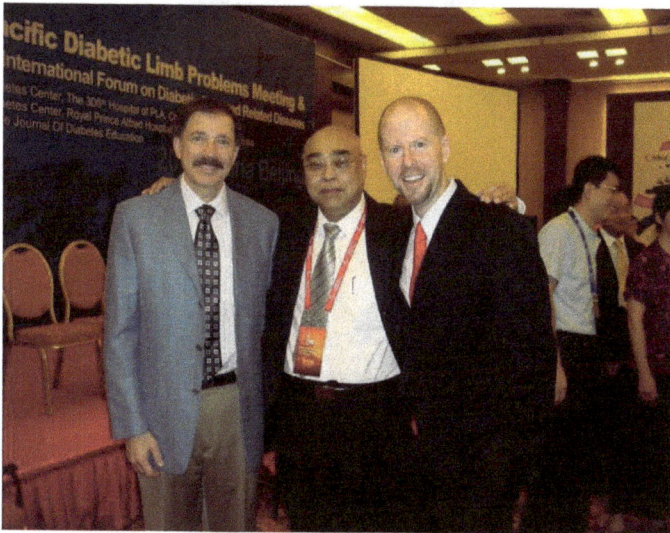

Figure 15. Dr. Benjamin Lipsky, Dr. Aziz Nather and Dr. David G. Armstrong

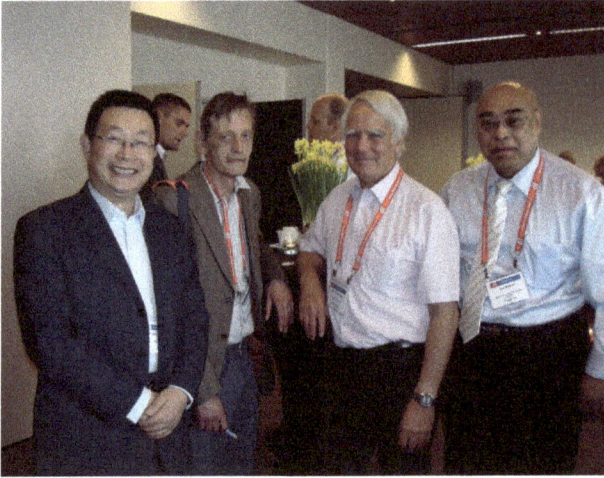

Figure 16. Dr. Xu Zhangrong (extreme left) at the 6th International Symposium on The Diabetic Foot

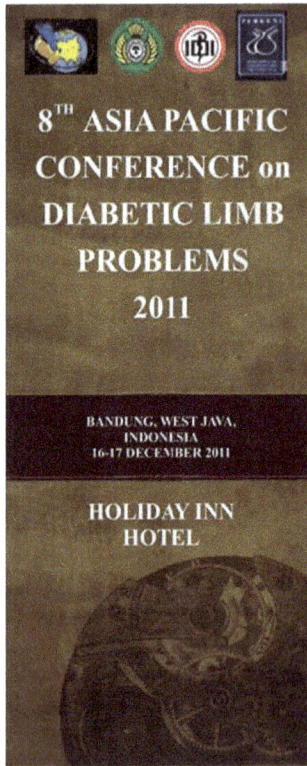

Figure 17. Poster for the 8th APCDLP

Dr. Nather, published by World Scientific in October 2012, will be launched during the Opening Ceremony of this Conference on 10 November 2013. It will be a great joy to see a second book launched on our 10th birthday and presented to the same man, Professor K. Satku, the man who inspired me to develop a diabetic foot service.

The development of the NUH DFP Team has catalysed the development of diabetic foot programmes throughout the country. It has also inspired the formation of Asia-Pacific Association for Diabetic Limb Problems. This led to the formation of DFP Teams in Malaysia (Terengganu, Kuala Lumpur, and Kelantan), Indonesia (Bandung and Makassar) and in Hong Kong.

ASEAN Plus Expert Group Forum on Management of Diabetic Foot Wounds

Formation

Formed in November 2012 with Associate Professor Aziz Nather, Singapore as Chairman of ASEAN Plus Expert Group Forum.

Mission

Our Mission is to provide patients with diabetic foot wounds with the best quality healthcare in ASEAN Plus countries.

Strategy

A two-prong strategy is adopted:

1) Forming an Expert Group Forum to discuss the management of diabetic foot wounds to produce clinical guidelines which we hope will eventually be adopted for use by all ASEAN Plus Countries.
2) Running a National Training Workshop on Management of Diabetic Foot Wounds to train Nurses and Allied Health Professionals to provide the best quality healthcare for such patients.

Objectives

Our objectives include:

- To discuss latest techniques used for management of diabetic foot wounds.
- To develop clinical guidelines for ASEAN Plus for the management of diabetic foot wounds.
- To organise National Training Workshop to train nurses and allied health professionals to provide the highest standard of quality care for patients with diabetic foot wounds.
- To publish a book "Best Practices in the Management of Diabetic Foot Wounds for ASEAN Plus" produced by ASEAN Plus Expert Group Forum, edited by A Nather, to be published by World Scientific Publishing Co. Pte Ltd at a later stage.

Composition of Expert Group Forum

Two members were invited from each ASEAN PLUS Country. Each member is an expert in the management of diabetic foot wounds. Member countries include Indonesia, Malaysia, Philippines, Singapore, Sri Lanka and Thailand.

Composition of ASEAN Plus Expert Group

INDONESIA

- Professor Sidartawan Soegondo
  Consultant/Endocrinologist/Diabetologist
  Cipto Mangunkusumo Hospital
  Jakarta, Indonesia

- Professor Mulyono Soedirman
  Orthopaedic Surgeon
  University Veteran Hospital
  Jakarta, Indonesia

MALAYSIA

- Dr Harikrishna K. R. Nair
  Wound Care Coordinator and Consultant
  Head, Diabetic Foot Care Unit

Kuala Lumpur Hospital
Kuala Lumpur, Malaysia
President, Malaysian Society of Wound Care Professionals

- Dr Anwar Hau Abdullah
  Consultant Orthopaedic Surgeon and Head
  Department of Orthopaedics
  Hospital Raja Perempuan Zainab 2
  Kota Bharu, Kelantan, Malaysia

PHILIPINES

- Dr Martin Anthony Villa
  Vascular Surgeon
  St Luke's Medical Centre
  Quezon City and Global City
  Dr James Dy Wound Healing Center
  (Chinese General Hospital)
  Manila, Philippines
  President, Philippines Wound Care Society

- Dr Luinio Tongson
  General Surgeon
  St Luke's Medical Centre
  Quezon City and Global City
  Dr James Dy Wound Healing Center
  (Chinese General Hospital)
  Manila, Philippines
  Vice — President, Philippines Wound Care Society

SINGAPORE

- Assoc Professor Aziz Nather
  Senior Consultant, Division of Foot & Ankle
  Chairman, NUH Diabetic Foot Team
  University Orthopaedics, Hand & Reconstructive Microsurgery Cluster
  National University Health System, Singapore
  Founding President and Current Honorary Secretary for Asia Pacific

Association of Diabetic Limb Problems
Corresponding Member of the International Working Group on the
Diabetic Foot (IWGDF), The Netherlands

- Dr Benjamin Chua
  General Surgeon
  Consultant and Director of Endovascular Surgery
  Department of General Surgery
  Singapore General Hospital

SRI LANKA

- Professor Mandika Wijayaratne
  Vascular Surgeon
  National Hospital of Sri Lanka
  Colombo, Sri Lanka
  President, Diabetic Association of Sri Lanka

- Dr Noel Somasundaram
  Endocrinologist
  National Hospital of Sri Lanka
  Colombo, Sri Lanka

THAILAND

- Professor Pramook Mutirangura
  Head, Department of Vascular Surgery
  Siriraj Hosptal
  Mahidol University
  Bangkok, Thailand

- Clinical Professor Apirag Chuangsuwanich
  Plastic Surgeon
  Siriraj Medical Hospital
  Bangkok, Thailand
  President of Society of Plastic and Reconstructive Surgeons of Thailand

Support

This forum is supported by Smith & Nephew Pte Ltd Singapore.

Inaugural ASEAN Plus Expert Group Forum

Is held in Hilton Hotel, Singapore on Saturday 10 November 2012 by Associate Professor Aziz Nather, Chairman of Forum in conjunction with the National Training Workshop for Nurses and Allied Health Professionals on the Management of Diabetic Foot Wounds held in National University Health System, Singapore on the same day.

The inaugural Forum and National Training Workshop is launched in Hilton Hotel by Professor K Satkunanantham, Director of Medical Services, Ministry of Health, Singapore.

Professor K Satku also launched this book: "The Diabetic Foot" edited by A Nather and published by World Scientific Publishing Co. Pte. Ltd.

10 November 2012

Associate Professor Aziz Nather
Chairman, ASEAN Plus Expert Group Forum
Chairman, NUH Diabetic Foot Team
Founding President and Current Honorary Secretary for Asia Pacific Association of Diabetic Limb Problems
Corresponding Member of the International Working Group on the Diabetic Foot (IWGDF), The Netherlands

www.ingramcontent.com/pod-product-compliance
Lightning Source LLC
Chambersburg PA
CBHW072255210326
41458CB00074B/1771